Aflatoxin
and
Food Safety

FOOD SCIENCE AND TECHNOLOGY

A Series of Monographs, Textbooks, and Reference Books

Editorial Advisory Board

Aflatoxin and Food Safety

Edited by
Hamed K. Abbas

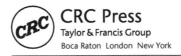

CRC Press
Taylor & Francis Group
Boca Raton London New York

CRC Press is an imprint of the
Taylor & Francis Group, an **informa** business

CRC Press
Taylor & Francis Group
6000 Broken Sound Parkway NW, Suite 300
Boca Raton, FL 33487-2742

First issued in paperback 2019

© 2005 by Taylor & Francis Group, LLC
CRC Press is an imprint of Taylor & Francis Group, an Informa business

No claim to original U.S. Government works

ISBN-13: 978 0 8247 2303 3 (hbk)
ISBN-13: 978-0-367-39192-8 (pbk)

Library of Congress Card Number 2005047024

Library of Congress Cataloging-in-Publication Data

Aflatoxin and food safety / Hamed K. Abbas, editor.
     p. cm. -- (Food science and technology series ; no. 149)
  Includes bibliographical references and index.
  ISBN 0-8247-2303-1 (alk. paper)
  1. Aflatoxins. 2. Food--Safety measures. I. Abbas, Hamed K. II. Title. III. Series: Food science and technology (CRC Press) ; 149.

RA1242.A344A35 2005
615.9'5295657--dc22   2005047024

Visit the Taylor & Francis Web site at
http://www.taylorandfrancis.com

and the CRC Press Web site at
http://www.crcpress.com

Dedicated to my family (Jean and my four children), whose patience, support, and inspiration are deeply appreciated. Also, to my late parents and my siblings in Iraq who put up with me during my formative years.

Preface

Aflatoxins are a class of toxins produced by *Aspergillus* species, including *A. flavus* Link, *A. parasiticus* Speare, and *A. nomius* Kurtzman, Horn & Hesseltine. These toxins are responsible for damage to 25% of the world's food crops. The fungi produce the contaminating toxins both pre- and postharvest. Aflatoxin is responsible for large economic losses to agriculture in the United States and other developed countries, but in developing countries, where the use of contaminated grain cannot always be avoided, aflatoxins also cause human and animal disease. Aflatoxin exposure contributes to the development of liver cancer in parts of the world where it is endemic, making it a significant contributor to a major public health problem. The presence of other mycotoxins, particularly fumonisins, along with aflatoxin in field samples brings additional concerns for the safety of food and feed supplies.

Until the 1980s, numerous reports and reviews were available on the impact of aflatoxins on livestock. From the 1990s to today, numerous works have appeared reporting studies on toxicological problems caused by aflatoxins, focusing mainly on the molecular biology of aflatoxin in both the fungus and host, aflatoxin management through conventional breeding, and genetic engineering to produce resistant lines of the susceptible crops and their release to general use. Biological control of aflatoxin using nontoxigenic strains of *Aspergillus flavus* in corn, peanut, and cotton made substantial progress during this period. Commercial use of this technology in the field is now showing promise for controlling aflatoxin contamination.

The goal of this book is to provide a comprehensive discussion regarding the progress made over the past 15 years in solving this problem by the world's finest aflatoxin scientists. The book began with the preparation of two special issues on the topic for the *Journal of Toxicology–Toxin Reviews*. Given the lack of books devoted to aflatoxin during the past decade and the low number devoted to other mycotoxins, a distinct need was identified for a book updating research progress in this area. Certainly, the field of aflatoxin research has continued to produce many important scientific publications that would benefit from being brought together in one resource. The general public's interest in aflatoxins has greatly increased in recent years due to publicity about biological terrorism, and scientists around the world share in this interest.

This volume should be of great interest to the scientific research community; to students in a wide range of biological, biomedical, and agricultural fields; to educators; to growers; and to government regulatory agencies in the United States and around the world. Every effort has been made to make this book a comprehensive resource on the subject for all interested persons.

The Editor

Hamed K. Abbas, Ph.D., is a lead scientist of the Mycotoxin Project and a Senior Research Plant Pathologist at the U.S. Department of Agriculture–Agricultural Research Service (USDA-ARS), Crop Genetics and Production Research Unit, Mid-South Area, Stoneville, Mississippi. Dr. Abbas completed his undergraduate and master's education at Baghdad University, Baghdad, Iraq, in 1977. He then immigrated to the United States, where he completed his doctorate in mycotoxin research at the Department of Plant Pathology, University of Minnesota, in 1987. Dr. Abbas has been involved in mycotoxin research throughout his career, initially working with biological control agents produced by fungi and bacteria. Over the last 3 years, Dr. Abbas has focused on aflatoxin and fumonisin contamination in cereal crops. Dr. Abbas has authored publications, including contributions to over 150 research journals, and is a sought-after speaker at scientific meetings. He has extensive experience with mycotoxins from the perspectives of both safety and biological control.

Acknowledgments

I am most grateful for the contributions of the authors as well as the support of many other individuals (especially Professor W. Thomas Shier, Bobbie J. Johnson, and Jennifer L. Tonos) who provided assistance during the preparation of this volume.

Contributors

Hamed K. Abbas
Crop Genetics and Production Research
  Unit
National Biological Control Laboratory
U.S. Department of Agriculture
Agricultural Research Service
Stoneville, Mississippi

Javier F. Betrán
Corn Breeding and Genetics
Department of Soil and Crop Sciences
Texas A&M University
College Station, Texas

Deepak Bhatnagar
Southern Regional Research Center
U.S. Department of Agriculture
Agricultural Research Service
New Orleans, Louisiana

Robert L. Brown
Southern Regional Research Center
U.S. Department of Agriculture
Agricultural Research Service
New Orleans, Louisiana

Paul M. Buckley
Corn Host Plant Resistance Research
  Unit
U.S. Department of Agriculture
Agricultural Research Service
Mississippi State, Mississippi

Bruce C. Campbell
Plant Mycotoxin Research Unit
Western Regional Research Center
U.S. Department of Agriculture
Agricultural Research Service
Albany, California

Kitty F. Cardwell
Cooperative State Research
Education and Extension Service
U.S. Department of Agriculture
Washington, D.C.

Jeffrey W. Cary
Southern Regional Research Center
U.S. Department of Agriculture
Agricultural Research Service
New Orleans, Louisana

Elizabeth A. Casman
Department of Engineering and Public
  Policy
Carnegie Mellon University
Pittsburgh, Pennsylvania

Perng-Kuang Chang
Southern Regional Research Center
U.S. Department of Agriculture
Agricultural Research Service
New Orleans, Louisiana

Zhi-Yuan Chen
Department of Plant Pathology and
  Crop Physiology
Louisiana State University Agricultural
  Center
Baton Rouge, Louisiana

Michael J. Clements
Corn Host Plant Resistance Research
  Unit
U.S. Department of Agriculture
Agricultural Research Service
Mississippi State, Mississippi

Thomas E. Cleveland
Southern Regional Research Center
U.S. Department of Agriculture
Agricultural Research Service
New Orleans, Louisiana

Anton E. Coy
Department of Crop and Soil Sciences
University of Georgia
Tifton, Georgia

Joe W. Dorner
National Peanut Research Laboratory
U.S. Department of Agriculture
Agricultural Research Service
Dawson, Georgia

Patrick F. Dowd
Crop Bioprotection Research Unit
National Center for Agricultural
  Utilization Research
U.S. Department of Agriculture
Agricultural Research Service
Peoria, Illinois

John Gilbert
Department for Environment, Food,
  and Rural Affairs
Central Science Laboratory
Sand Hutton, York, United Kingdom

Baozhu Z. Guo
Crop Protection and Management
  Research Unit
U.S. Department of Agriculture
Agricultural Research Service
Tifton, Georgia

Tom Hammond
Department of Plant Pathology
University of Wisconsin
Madison, Wisconsin

Leigh K. Hawkins
Corn Host Plant Resistance Research
  Unit
U.S. Department of Agriculture
Agricultural Research Service
Mississippi State, Mississippi

Sara H. Henry
The Center for Food Safety and Applied
  Nutrition
U.S. Food and Drug Administration
College Park, Maryland

C. Corley Holbrook
Crop Genetics and Breeding Research
  Unit
U.S. Department of Agriculture
Agricultural Research Service
Tifton, Georgia

James B. Holland
Department of Crop Science
North Carolina State University
U.S. Department of Agriculture
Agricultural Research Service
Raleigh, North Carolina

Bruce W. Horn
National Peanut Research Laboratory
U.S. Department of Agriculture
Agricultural Research Service
Dawson, Georgia

Tom Isakeit
Department of Plant Pathology
Texas A&M University
College Station, Texas

Eric T. Johnson
Crop Bioprotection Research Unit
National Center for Agricultural
  Utilization Research
U.S. Department of Agriculture
Agricultural Research Service
Peoria, Illinois

Marco A. Jonker
Laboratory for Food and Residue
  Analysis
National Institute for Public Health and
  the Environment
Bilthoven, The Netherlands

Nancy Keller
Department of Plant Pathology
University of Wisconsin
Madison, Wisconsin

Joan M. King
Department of Food Science
Louisiana State University Agricultural
  Center
Louisiana State University
Baton Rouge, Louisiana

Dewey R. Lee
Department of Crop and Soil Sciences
University of Georgia
Tifton, Georgia

Menghe H. Li
Thad Cochran National Warmwater
  Aquaculture Center
Mississippi State University
Stoneville, Mississippi

Robert E. Lynch
Crop Protection and Management
  Research Unit
U.S. Department of Agriculture
Agricultural Research Service
Tifton, Georgia

Bruce B. Manning
Thad Cochran National Warmwater
  Aquaculture Center
Mississippi State University
Stoneville, Mississippi

Chris M. Maragos
Mycotoxin Research Unit
U.S. Department of Agriculture
Agricultural Research Service
Peoria, Illinois

Kerry Mayfield
Soil and Crop Sciences
Texas A&M University
College Station, Texas

Tami McDonald
Department of Plant Pathology
University of Wisconsin
Madison, Wisconsin

J. David Miller
Department of Chemistry
Carleton University
Ottawa, Canada

Russell J. Molyneux
Plant Mycotoxin Research Unit
Western Regional Research Center
U.S. Department of Agriculture
Agricultural Research Service
Albany, California

Daan Noordermeer
Department of Plant Pathology
University of Wisconsin
Madison, Wisconsin

Gary Odvody
Agriculture Research and Extension
  Center
Texas A&M University
Corpus Christi, Texas

Gary A. Payne
Department of Plant Pathology
North Carolina State University
Raleigh, North Carolina

Javier Plasencia
Associate Professor
Departmento de Bioquímica
Facultad de Química
Universidad y Copilco, Mexico

Alfredo D. Prudente, Jr.
Department of Food Science
Louisiana State University Agricultural
  Center
Louisiana State University
Baton Rouge, Louisiana

Jane F. Robens
Food Safety and Health
U.S. Department of Agriculture
Agricultural Research Service
Beltsville, Maryland

Leilani A. Robertson
Department of Plant Pathology
North Carolina State University
Raleigh, North Carolina

Edwin H. Robinson
Thad Cochran National Warmwater
  Aquaculture Center
Mississippi State University
Stoneville, Mississippi

Thomas F. Schatzki
Plant Mycotoxin Research Unit
Western Regional Research Center
U.S. Department of Agriculture
Agricultural Research Service
Albany, California

Kimberly A. Scheidegger
Center for Integrated Pest Management
Raleigh, North Carolina

Vildes M. Scussel
Food Science and Technology
  Department
Center of Agricultural Sciences
Federal University of Santa Catarina
Florianopolis, Brazil

Gordon S. Shephard
PROMEC Unit
Medical Research Council
Tygerberg, South Africa

W. Thomas Shier
College of Pharmacy
University of Minneapolis
Minneapolis, Minnesota

Lili Tang
Department of Environmental
  Toxicology, and
The Institute of Environmental and
  Human Health
Texas Tech University
Lubbock, Texas

Hans P. van Egmond
Laboratory for Food and Residue
  Analysis
National Institute for Public Health and
  the Environment
Bilthoven, The Netherlands

Eugenia A. Vargas
RT LACQSA, CT LANAGRO MG
Belo Horizonte, Brazil

Jia-Sheng Wang
Department of Environmental
  Toxicology, and
The Institute of Environmental and
  Human Health
Texas Tech University
Lubbock, Texas

Mark A. Weaver
National Biological Control Laboratory
U.S. Department of Agriculture
Agricultural Research Service
Stoneville, Mississippi

Donald G. White
Department of Crop Sciences
University of Illinois
Urbana, Illinois

Neil W. Widstrom
Crop Genetics and Breeding Research
  Unit
U.S. Department of Agriculture
Agricultural Research Service
Tifton, Georgia

W. Paul Williams
Corn Host Plant Resistance Research
  Unit
U.S. Department of Agriculture
Agricultural Research Service
Mississippi State, Mississippi

David M. Wilson
Department of Plant Pathology
University of Georgia
U.S. Department of Agriculture
Agricultural Research Service
Tifton, Georgia

Gary L. Windham
Corn Host Plant Resistance Research
  Unit
U.S. Department of Agriculture
Agricultural Research Service
Mississippi State, Mississippi

Felicia Wu
Environmental and Occupational
  Health
University of Pittsburgh
Pittsburgh, Pennsylvania

Jiujiang Yu
U.S. Department of Agriculture
Agricultural Research Service
Southern Regional Research Center
New Orleans, Louisana

Yong-Qiang Zhang
Department of Plant Pathology
University of Wisconsin, Madison
Madison, Wisconsin

Table of Contents

1 The Costs of Mycotoxin Management in the United States

Jane Robens and Kitty F. Cardwell

CONTENTS

1.1 INTRODUCTION

Losses from mycotoxins in the United States are generally associated with regulatory losses, as opposed to lowered production, illness, or deaths from the effects of the toxins. This is particularly the case for human food, but increasingly it has become the case for animal feeds as strict feed quality control programs become the norm for large-scale animal production units. The Stoloff papers from the 1980s infer a lack of aflatoxin-related toxicity or carcinogenicity in humans in the United States.[6–8] Mycotoxin management costs are incurred by both producers and the federal and state governments to prevent mycotoxins from becoming a human and animal health threat. The Food and Drug Administration (FDA) has functioning mycotoxin regulatory programs for aflatoxin, fumonisins, and vomitoxin.[1,9,10,11]

Among all the mycotoxins, aflatoxin generates the greatest losses and the highest management costs due to its extremely high toxicity on a unit basis and its long history of stringent regulation. The peanut, corn, cottonseed, and tree nut industries all experience losses associated with meeting regulatory levels. The costs are inversely related to the regulatory level that must be met, and the necessity to meet lower concentration allowances increases the costs of crop management. In the United States, the FDA has used a 20-ppb tolerance almost since the initiation of their mycotoxin regulatory program, but industries that sell to European Union countries face regulatory allowances and buyer standards of much lower parts-per-billion concentrations.[3]

Few attempts have been made to estimate with accuracy the mycotoxin-related losses faced by various commodity groups in the United States. The Council on Agricultural Science and Technology (CAST) report, *Mycotoxins: Economics and Health Risks*, published in 1989, outlined the information regarding losses known at that time.[2] A chapter by the FDA's Peter Vardon in the CAST 2003 report on mycotoxins analyzes the potential current economic cost of mycotoxins in the United States.[13] Vardon estimated an annual range of losses from $0.5 million to over $1.5 billion from aflatoxin (corn and peanuts), fumonisin (corn), and deoxynivalenol (wheat). Uncertainties were built into the cost model based on commodity outputs, prices, and contamination levels based on surveillance samples and compliance with FDA regulatory limits. Vardon assumed that the livestock loss was directly proportional to the percentage of feed that was contaminated above FDA standards, and he calculated small livestock losses from aflatoxin and deoxynivalenol (DON). Not included were the costs of testing for the toxins, either to commodity producers or to the public through the FDA budget; the costs of growing less valuable alternative crops; or the costs of handling affected crops, among others.

In some cases it is very difficult to determine what is a mycotoxin loss and what is not, because the buyer may maintain that it is the threat of mycotoxins that necessitates paying a lower price, while in fact, the buyer may not want to deal with small quantities of corn or another commodity available from certain suppliers. A food safety issue can be used in domestic trade negotiations just as it can in international trade.

1.2 RESEARCH COSTS

The investment in research programs by the federal government, primarily to prevent mycotoxins in crops, can be considered a major cost of mycotoxin management. The Agricultural Research Service (ARS) of the U.S. Department of Agriculture (USDA) has a mycotoxin research program, for which the fiscal year 2000 budget was $17.7 million for approximately 60 scientists, that is primarily focused on prevention of the fungus and toxin production in the crop. This level of support was the total appropriated amount; it included the mycotoxin research share of administrative salaries, as well as the scientists and technicians and various support personnel, increasingly expensive energy costs, costs of services and building maintenance, etc. The USDA's Cooperative State Research Education and Extension Service (CSREES) reported a budget of $4.7 million for mycotoxin research, along with $5.1 million from states at their land grant institutions, and an additional $2.1 million from other federal agencies at these institutions (William Wagner, CSREES, June 2001, pers. comm.). The FDA also carries out research on mycotoxins at the

Center for Food Safety and Applied Nutrition, primarily on methodology development, effects of processing, and toxicology. This activity is assessed for 14 to 15 scientists at $1.5 million; however, the FDA calculation includes only the scientists' salaries and some immediate laboratory costs and does not include the agency administrative costs and infrastructure as does the ARS amount (John Newland, Center for Food Safety and Applied Nutrition, FDA, June 2001, pers. comm.).

1.3 TESTING AND INSURANCE

Analysis of product samples is needed to ensure that product offered to the market meets regulatory and market requirements. These considerable costs are incurred both by industry and by various government regulatory and action agencies. Industry costs, in particular, increase significantly during years when contamination of the crops is high. The average total value of commercial aflatoxin test kits on the market is approximately $10 million per year annually, or about 2 million tests for an average year. Sales increase rapidly in outbreak years (Robert Elder, USDA–ARS, May 2001, pers. comm.). In addition to the test kit costs, the range of charges for testing by official agencies and cooperative services is from $10 to $20 per sample, not including collection of the sample. For aflatoxin alone, testing can cost $30 to $50 million per year. For example, testing costs associated with corn production and marketing have been reported by the Grain Inspection Packers and Stockyards Administration (GIPSA), which conducts aflatoxin and DON testing for exported grains. For aflatoxin, GIPSA analyzes approximately 30,000 samples per year which generates approximately $290,000 in revenues. State and private laboratories with official sanction from the Federal Grain Inspection Service (FGIS) analyze approximately 27,000 samples per year which generates approximately $540,000 in revenues. For DON, the FGIS analyzes approximately 6000 samples per year which generates approximately $100,000 in revenues, while official agencies analyze an additional 18,000 samples to generate about $360,000 in revenues annually (John Giler, FGIS, May 2001, pers. comm.).

Grain sampling is part of the cost of testing commodities for mycotoxins. As part of the cost of testing corn for aflatoxin in southeast Texas, it is a considerable expense at $20 to $30 per test and one test per truckload of 30,000 to 60,000 pounds of commodity. This equates to a testing cost of $2 to $3 per acre (Jeff Nunley, South Texas Cotton and Grain Association, May 2001, pers. comm.). Also in southeast Texas, every 100 tons of cottonseed requires a test for aflatoxin, at a cost of about $125 (including sampling and transportation to the laboratory) per sample. Sample preparation for cottonseed costs more than for corn, which does not require dehulling or delinting, and the sample size differs (Peter Cotty, USDA–ARS, June 2001, pers. comm.).

The cost of litigation may also be significant for cottonseed producers. The identity of cottonseed is generally maintained through the market chain. If contamination above 0.5 ppb is detected in milk, the product may be traced to the dairies where the cattle are being fed contaminated cottonseed. The sellers, producers, and any other party who can be identified are likely to be sued. Feedlots for fattening beef cattle are wary of feeding cottonseed containing >20 ppb aflatoxin even though it may be legal up to 150 ppb (Jeff Nunley, South Texas Cotton and Grain Association, May 2001, pers. comm.). Insurance premiums and compliance with the recommendations of insurance companies are other major costs of managing mycotoxins. A private crop insurance company in Des Moines, IA, recommends that their insured producers sample a high percentage of their loads for the first 2 weeks of each season. Even if only a very small percentage of loads is found positive for the mycotoxin, they recommend that sampling continue on a random basis. This company states that testing costs for producers are $5 to $7 per test if carried out on a regular basis and $9 to $12 per test if done sporadically (David Frank, American Feed Industry Insurance Association, Des Moines, IA, June 2001, pers. comm.).

1.4 COMMODITY LOSS ESTIMATES FROM THE INDUSTRY

1.4.1 PEANUTS

Marshall Lamb at the ARS National Peanut Research Laboratory in Dawson, GA, has prepared a paper addressing losses from aflatoxin.[4] This paper surveys and analyzes actual losses in peanuts during the 1993 to 1996 crop years. Lamb estimated the net cost of aflatoxin to the farmer, the peanut buying point, and the sheller segments of the southeast peanut industry to be about $25 million per year. On a total segregation I farmer stock basis, aflatoxin cost the southeast peanut industry an average of $23.17 per ton, while the net cost of aflatoxin averaged $28.06 per acre. Peanuts are subject to a federal marketing order that proscribes very strict and complicated procedures for testing, segregating, and handling peanuts to prevent peanuts that do not meet FDA requirements for aflatoxin from becoming a part of the human food supply. The costs of aflatoxin result from both the decreased value of the crop as calculated from the quota support price and from expenses incurred in handling contaminated peanuts, including blanching, remilling, equipment, testing, and insurance. Lamb's calculation does not include the costs of production practices, particularly irrigation, that may be used to help prevent aflatoxin in the crop; however, the loan program for peanuts was changed by Congress after Lamb's study was completed, and the costs of aflatoxin contamination under the current commodity loan program would now be less because of a lower loan value for peanuts.

1.4.2 COTTON

Cottonseed is a byproduct of cotton fiber production; thus, cotton breeding and agronomic practices have not traditionally considered the need to prevent contamination of the seed. Aflatoxin contaminates cottonseed in Texas and in Arizona with sufficient frequency that it is a continuing concern of state regulatory officials in these states. The major market for cottonseed, either whole seed or meal, is feed for dairy cattle. In the late 1970s, aflatoxin from contaminated cottonseed fed to dairy cattle was detected in milk by state regulatory officials and the FDA. Dairy cattle excrete a much higher percentage of ingested aflatoxin in milk (metabolized to aflatoxin M_1) than is ever deposited in muscle meat of any species. In addition, the amounts of any residue allowed in milk are low, in this case <1 ppb. Cottonseed is still fed to dairy cattle, but tested and recognized contamination of milk is rare.[2]

Estimates for a single year do not provide a true picture of the extent of aflatoxin contamination because of its variability; thus, the Arizona Cotton Research and Protection Council combined their estimates from 1977 to 1999. During this 22-year period, Arizona had an average annual cottonseed production of 397,000 tons, with an average annual value of $42,205,000, for a total value of $928,510,000. Discounts on cottonseed with aflatoxin levels above 20 ppb vary from $20 to $50 per ton, with the majority falling in the $30 to $35 range. Based on these figures, the most conservative estimate of revenue losses due to aflatoxin contamination over the 22 year period is $96,074,000, or slightly over 10% (Table 1.1).

In addition to direct revenue losses due to aflatoxin discounts, regulatory restrictions prevent contaminated cottonseed from leaving the state (except under a restrictive permitting system), severely affecting marketing options for the Arizona growers. Costs of treatment to eliminate aflatoxin (ammoniation) plus interim shipping and storage fees would result in a cost benefit of $20 per ton or more if aflatoxin-free cottonseed could be shipped directly from gins to prime customers such as dairies.

In south Texas, Jeff Nunley estimated that testing costs alone could be as high as $150,000 for each of two major cottonseed processors that use cottonseed originating from south Texas. Cottonseed that contains high aflatoxin levels is segregated and processed separately, leading to additional costs at the processor level. These increased costs are ultimately reflected in lower values for cottonseed at the producer level. During the 1999 crop year, only about 30% of the cottonseed tested at the major cottonseed processing mills in south Texas had acceptable levels of aflatoxin (Table 1.1). While not all processors formally discounted their price for aflatoxin-contaminated cottonseed, discounts of $20 per ton for contaminated seed were common, with some discounts being larger. Based on an average $20 per ton discount, the loss of value to south Texas cotton producers for the 1999 crop from aflatoxin-contaminated seed would be slightly over $7,000,000. With a harvested acreage estimated at 960,000 acres, this loss equates to approximately $7.30 per harvested acre. In south Texas, contaminated cottonseed may be processed at an oil seed mill for crushing so some value is recouped for the contaminated crop; it may be sent to Indigo, CA, for ammoniation; or, finally, contaminated meal may be used for mushroom fertilizer.

1.4.3 CORN

Corn is contaminated with aflatoxin only sporadically, primarily when droughts occur, in the Corn Belt states, such as Iowa, Illinois, and Indiana. Severe losses from aflatoxin in Midwest corn did occur in 1983 and again in 1988. Corn is contaminated every year at one or more locations in the southern states of Georgia, Louisiana, Mississippi, Georgia, and North Carolina across to Texas. In 1998, corn losses in Mississippi, Louisiana, and Texas were extremely harsh and painful. Corn is grown to a very limited degree in Arizona but would be planted more frequently in many areas if it were not for aflatoxin contamination, which eliminates it as a potential rotation crop. Also in the south Texas Corpus Christi area, corn could be a valuable rotation crop for the primary cash crop of cotton, but, in order to avoid aflatoxin

TABLE 1.1
Reports of Direct Crop Revenue Losses Due to Mycotoxins

Crop	Location/Year(s)	Average Annual Production (Tons, 000)	Toxin	Average Contamination (%)	Estimated Annual Revenue Loss[a]	Source
Cotton	AZ/1977–1999	397	AF	55	4367 (at $20/ton)	Larry Antilla, Director of the Arizona Cotton Research and Protection Council, Phoenix AZ, April 2001
Cotton	Texas/1999	502	AF	70	7000 (at $20/ton)	Jeff Nunley, South Texas Cotton and Grain Association, May 2001
Peanut	Georgia		AF		25,000	Marshall Larr b[4]
Corn	Texas/1999 (4 districts in south Texas)	2100 (375 Bu)	AF	50	15,000 (at $0.4/Bu)	Jeff Nunley, South Texas Cotton and Grain Association, May 2001
Corn	Mississippi/1998	1400 (50 Bu)	AF	20 discounted, 4 abandoned	2000	Erick Larson, Mississippi Agricultural and Forestry Experiment Station, Mississippi State, MS, May 2001
Walnuts	California/2000	1236	AF	4	38,700	David Ramos. Davis California, March 2001
Almonds	California/1995–2001	366–830	AF		23,000–47,000	Merle Jacobs, Almond Board of California, Modesto, CA, March 2001
Barley	North Dakota, South Dakota, Minnesota/1993–1998		DON		406,000[a] (5 years)	John Mittleider, North Dakota Barley Council, Fargo, ND, June 2001
Wheat	North Dakota, South Dakota, Minnesota/1993–1998		DON		1,000,000[b]	Jim Baer, North American Millers, Washington, D.C., June 2001
Wheat	North Carolina/2003	60–80,000 Bu	DON		4000–8000	Paul Murphy, North Carolina State University, Raleigh, NC, February 2004

a Does not include abandoned acreage.
b Includes actual production losses.

contamination, 300,000 acres are planted to sorghum each year rather than to corn (Jeff Nunley, South Texas Cotton and Grain Association, May 2001, pers. comm.).

In Mississippi in 1998, a severe drought resulted in high aflatoxin contamination. These losses were in irrigated as well as dryland corn and were particularly onerous for farmers who had just planted corn for the first time. Of the 50-million-bushel crop, 20% had aflatoxin levels of 20 to 150 ppb and was sold at a discounted price, and another 4% was abandoned because it contained over 150 ppb; however, initially, approximately 50% of the crop was contaminated to the extent that many samples exceeded legal limits. Half of that amount was eventually sold for feed by farmers. Little of Mississippi corn is used directly for human consumption. Probe samples taken from truckloads for aflatoxin analysis of corn are generally smaller than optimal and more likely to be near 5 pounds than near 50 pounds. This is considered necessary to maintain the commercial flow of the commodity (Erick Larson, Mississippi Agricultural and Forestry Experiment Station, May 2001, pers. comm.).

The Georgia corn producers consider their markets to be limited by the perception, if not the reality, of contamination by aflatoxin. The acreage of corn in Georgia has been shrinking during the last 10 years as swine farms have left the state and been replaced by larger operations elsewhere. Swine producers are generally more content to use local Georgia corn than are poultry producers. This is probably due to the greater concern among poultry producers that aflatoxin may be harmful to broiler growth and even immune competency but also to the economics of corn transportation, handling, and distribution. Poultry operations are large and integrated with their own feed mills, and they do not want to handle local corn in truckload quantities but instead utilize trainloads of corn from the Midwest. They will use local corn shortly after it has been produced in the fall and when interruptions in the flow or arrival of trainloads of Midwest corn occur (Dewey Lee, University of Georgia, Albany, June 2001, pers. comm.).

1.4.4 TREE NUTS

Tree nuts such as almonds, walnuts, and pistachios may be contaminated with aflatoxin, though at lower levels than for cottonseed and corn; however. the problem is very significant to producers because: (1) the crop has a high unit value, and (2) much of the crop is sold to European markets that enforce limits significantly lower than those in the United States. For the 2000–2001 crop year, aflatoxin was found in 4% of the walnut samples tested by the industry. Because the crop size for the year 2000 was 236,000 tons, the walnut industry lost an estimated 18,880,000 pounds of walnut kernels to aflatoxin for the year's harvest. The 2000–2001 crop year experienced short tonnage (production) and higher market prices, and the cost of product lost has been estimated at $2.05 per pound of product; thus, the total direct dollar market value lost to the walnut industry was $38,704,000.

It is difficult to estimate the cost of aflatoxin to the almond industry; however, in almonds a strong correlation exists between aflatoxin and insect damage to kernels that places the nuts into an inedible category and thus can be used as an estimate of loss due to aflatoxin. Almond production utilizes several sophisticated techniques to sort the good from the inedible kernels, and handlers remove and dispose of their inedible almonds to non-human consumption channels. In California in the six crop years from 1995–1996 to 2000–2001, almond production ranged from 366,000,000 to 830,000,000 pounds, and exported almonds had a value of $623.8 million in 1999. If 3% of each year's production is considered inedible (aflatoxin contaminated), then the value of this 3% of the total crop was thus lost. That is, 10,980,000 to 24,900,000 pounds of almonds per year were considered inedible and their value was lost. Thus, based on a wholesale value of $1.50 to $3.00 per pound for uncontaminated, edible almonds, the market value lost by the producer for contaminated almonds ranged from $23,265,000 to $47,310,000 in this 6-year time period. The additional costs of transportation, sorting, and analytical tests for contaminated almonds are not included in the above loss figures.

1.4.5 BARLEY

Contamination with deoxynivalenol (DON), or vomitoxin produced by *Fusarium* head blight infection with *F. graminearum*, has caused serious losses to the barley producers in the affected area of Minnesota, North Dakota, and South Dakota. In barley, the loss is primarily due to vomitoxin (DON contamination), while that in wheat is due to both lowered grain production and toxin production. Wheat flowers outside of the boot and thus is inherently more susceptible to being infected with the fungal spores. Malters and brewers use a 0.5-ppm level of DON as a cutoff, but how it is used varies by company. DON-containing grain is discounted 5 to 10¢ per bushel for each 0.1 ppm that the grain exceeds 0.5 ppm. Anheuser–Busch is the most stringent, and anything in excess of 0.5 ppm vomitoxin in the barley grain or in malt that they may buy from other malters is unacceptable. Some malters, however, will accept grain with 2 to 3 ppm vomitoxin because in some cases the process of malting will lower the levels of vomitoxin; however, if the malting is carried out too long, the fungus will regrow and the levels will increase again.

Serious contamination with DON has occurred in Minnesota, North Dakota, and South Dakota each year since 1993. Prior to that, contamination was only sporadic. Barley growers believe that this was due to a change in long-term weather patterns, with the area now having higher rainfall and relative humidity. The acceptance rate for barley in the these states has not exceeded 35% since 1983. When barley is not acceptable for malting, it is used for animal feed, a use that brings a lesser rate of return. Growers need approximately $160 per acre to break even; malting barley usually yields about $160 per acre, but barley for animal feed yields only $100 per acre. The unavailability of barley as a reliable rotation crop is another loss to growers, with the preferred 3-year rotation in this area being first year, wheat; second year, feed grain; third year, oil seed; and back to wheat. Also included is the loss of the economic infrastructure that had grown up around handling and marketing the crop, particularly in eastern North Dakota. The barley producers in these three states have calculated a total loss of $406 million for the 6 years from 1993 through 1998. The total barley acreage has now declined over half from 1993 because the growers do not want to assume the high risk of growing malting barley. In 1993, 4,250,000 acres were planted with barley but in 2000 that number had declined to 1,950,000 acres (John Mittleider, North Dakota Barley Council, May 2001, pers. comm.).

1.4.6 WHEAT

Losses from *Fusarium* head blight (FHB; also known as scab) in wheat include both lowered grain yield and the presence of DON. In 1993, farm gate losses in the Red River Valley of North Dakota, South Dakota, and Minnesota were $200 to $400 million for this fungal infection and mycotoxin. In 1996, farmers suffered a $300 million loss raising soft wheat, and also in that year millers experienced significant replacement costs. Replacement costs include transportation of wheat from another area to meet contracted deliveries, as well as the higher price that must be paid for this wheat because of decreased availability. The industry estimates they have sustained total losses of $1 billion from wheat scab (Table 1.1) (Jim Baer, North American Millers Washington, D.C., June 2001, pers. comm.).

A North Dakota State University economist has estimated losses based on grain yields and prices (dollars per bushel) that might have been expected under normal conditions, in the absence of wheat head scab. Precipitation and temperature data were used to estimate "normal" production. The loss of production was calculated as the difference between actual and normal production, and then adjusted for acreage abandoned as a result of scab. Total direct and secondary economic losses from FHB in North Dakota for wheat and barley and in Minnesota for wheat were estimated at $545 million from 1998 to 2000. As significant as the direct loss is the finding of a significant secondary economic impact. For each dollar of lost net revenues for the producer, an additional $2.10, approximately, is lost in secondary economic activity by, for example, households, retail trade, finance, insurance and real estate, and personal business and professional services (William Nganji, North Dakota State University, Fargo, June 2001, pers. comm.).

By 2003, the weather patterns that had resulted in scab losses in the upper Midwest had changed, and the wheat growing areas in the Atlantic Seaboard states were now affected. In North Carolina, 50% of the winter wheat was estimated to be unsuitable for human consumption on the basis of the amounts of vomitoxin, although usually North Carolina's wheat is sold equally for human and animal consumption. Cleaning the wheat did not decrease the toxin levels as had previously been noted. A major cause of toxin contamination was the extremely high rain levels in all of 2003, including the time of head opening when the kernels are the most susceptible. This resulted in wheat being left in the field well beyond the usual harvest date because harvesting equipment could not be brought in. The total wheat production in North Carolina is usually 60 to 80 million bushels per year, but the loss in 2003 was estimated at $4 to $8 million (Paul Murphy, North Carolina State University, February 2004, pers. comm.).

Similar conditions were prevalent in Maryland, where winter wheat yields were almost halved. A poultry-producing major buyer did continue to buy this very reduced wheat crop at the usual unit price to continue their established harmonious relationships with the growers. The wheat producers in Maryland suffered most because of low crop yields, in contrast to North Carolina, where toxin contamination of relatively normal appearing wheat was often reported (J. Cofta, University of Maryland, February 2004, pers. comm.). These same weather conditions extended to the lower Midwest, and in Indiana FHB incidence in most fields ranged between 10% and 70%.

1.4.7 ANIMALS

Paul Sundberg of the National Pork Board (June 2001, pers. comm.) stated that swine producers do not recognize ongoing losses from aflatoxin, although they may occur in localized production areas in severely affected crop years. That only a very small number of cases of actual recognized toxicity in swine have been reported in the United States is the direct result of our food safety regulatory system. University scientists are apparently more concerned with the effects of aflatoxin in poultry feeds than are the poultry industries. Perhaps it is because they remember when a greater incidence of aflatoxin in corn at levels could decrease growth and increase disease susceptibility. To prevent contamination with aflatoxin above FDA guidelines, the poultry industry now relies on sampling of corn by the feed mills, which are often a part of the same integrated production and marketing operation. The sampling rate of the feed mills varies greatly depending on industry reports of the occurrence of aflatoxin in corn from specific localities in that year. When contamination is reported by the corn industry in specific states or when positives are found during routine sampling, the rate of sampling by the poultry industry is greatly increased.

A large integrated turkey producer reported conducting 2200 assays for aflatoxin, at a cost of approximately $2.67 per test for materials; they do not use the ELISA kits. They also reported conducting a total of 4200 tests for fumonisins, deoxynivalenol, and zearalenone in 2001 in their company laboratory, which serves their feed mill and production facilities. In the latter case, they used ELISA test kits costing approximately $7 apiece. These numbers of tests, which were skewed to test a greater proportion of the local southeast corn bought than of Corn Belt corn, were used to ensure the safety of approximately 400,000 T of corn (Neal Allen, Carolina Turkeys, Mt. Olive, NC, May 2002, pers. comm.).

1.5 DISCUSSION

In the United States, the FDA has established a tolerance of 20 ppb of aflatoxin for foods other than milk, but European markets are striving for a lower Codex importation standard of 2 ppb. Also in the United States, the production of susceptible crops is being reliably managed to meet the current FDA aflatoxin guidelines, with export crops for human use meeting the more stringent European guidelines; thus, the risk of exposure to aflatoxin and other mycotoxins under current regulations and handling practices is not considered to be a public health threat in the United States. Conservative calculations of estimated lost crop revenues and the cost of research and monitoring activities are between $500 million and $1.5 billion a year to manage mycotoxin-producing fungi to achieve this level of security, and this figure does not include secondary industry and international trade losses. Thus, the management of aflatoxins and other mycotoxins costs millions of dollars every year, and research into more definitive solutions must continue.

Suggested FDA advisory levels for *Fusarium* toxins range from 0 to 4 ppm and higher for some animal species. The FDA guidelines for these toxins are achievable without a major disruption of the corn production and marketing system; however, because fumonisins are found in maize and trichothecenes such as vomitoxin/DON are found in maize, wheat, and barley, the costs of *Fusarium* toxins to the United States could easily mount up as quickly as those of aflatoxin. Increased costs will be primarily related to fumonisin and vomitoxin testing at all levels of production and marketing and will of course vary greatly from year to year.

The most obvious cost of mycotoxins is their toxicity to humans and animals when they are present in food and feed in sufficient concentrations. Fortunately, this does not happen often in the United States, as possible toxic amounts are usually caught by one of the several levels of producer and government control. Where mycotoxins do not present a direct health threat to humans or animals, they can result in direct losses to producers when their crops exceed regulatory limits and the price is decreased, or the crop cannot be sold at all. Commodity handlers have the costs of testing and insurance and the occasional cost of moving or disposing of commodity for which the aflatoxin content was not initially recognized in time to prevent its acquisition. Society as a whole bears the costs of research to prevent mycotoxins as well as the costs of regulation at both federal and state levels. For example, corn producers could experience losses of revenue due to reduced prices for high-mycotoxin grain and increased costs for testing at grain elevators. For both aflatoxin and the *Fusarium* toxins the extent of losses to many producers depends in part on how willingly the elevator operators will accept high mycotoxin corn with the intent to handle it by commingling of loads, and this will vary with the overall level of contamination of the crop and the availability of clean corn. The existence of FDA guidelines has led to increased awareness of the possible presence of mycotoxins and greater care being taken by all producers and commodity handlers as well as livestock producers feeding their own animals on the farm.

Considering all the knowledge about the chemistry, modes of action, and toxic effects of mycotoxins on humans and animals and all the increased costs of production, solutions to the problems related to mycotoxins are still few and far between. Good agronomic practices may be helpful in marginal years but unless they include irrigation, they have little effect in years of even moderate drought. Reducing mycotoxin vulnerability of crops and competitively excluding toxic fungi are the most promising permanent solutions that have the potential to markedly reduce mycotoxin-related costs of production. Appropriate sampling and testing protocols that are also less expensive are also critical to reducing costs while ensuring that the FDA guidelines are being met.

REFERENCES

1. American Association of Veterinary Laboratory Diagnosticians (AAVLD), Recommendations concerning fumonisin B1 concentrations in feeds, *AAVLD Newslett.*, May 1993, pp. 25–26.
2. CAST, *Mycotoxins: Economic and Health Risks*, Task Force Report No. 116, Council for Agricultural Science and Technology, Ames, IA, 1989.
3. Hawk, A.L., Mycotoxins in grain marketing, in *Proc. 53rd Annual Corn and Sorghum Research Conf.*, Chicago, IL, 1998, pp. 299–303.
4. Lamb, M.C. and Sternitske, D.A., Cost of aflatoxin to the farmer, buying point, and sheller segments of the southeast U.S. peanut industries, *Peanut Sci.*, 28, 59–63, 2001.

5. Munkvold, G.P., *Potential Impact of FDA Guidelines for Fumonisins in Foods and Feeds*, APSnet Feature Article, American Phytopathological Society, St. Paul, MN, 2001.
6. Stoloff, L., Aflatoxin as a cause of primary liver-cell cancer in the United States, *Nutr. Cancer*, 5, 3–4, 1983.
7. Stoloff, L., A rationale for the control of aflatoxin in human foods, in *A Collection of Invited Papers Presented at the Sixth International IUPAC Symposium on Mycotoxins and Phycotoxins, Pretoria South Africa, July 22–25, 1985*, Elsevier Science, Amsterdam, 1986.
8. Stoloff, L., Aflatoxin is not a probable carcinogen: the published evidence is sufficient, *Reg. Toxicol. Pharmacol.*, 10, 272–283, 1989.
9. USFDA, Letter from Ronald Chesemore to State Agricultural Directors, State Feed Control Officials, and Food, Feed and Grain Trade Organizations on advisory levels for DON (vomitoxin) in food and feed, Public Health Service, U.S. Food and Drug Administration, U.S. Department of Health and Human Services, Rockville, MD, 1993.
10. USFDA, *Action Levels for Aflatoxins in Animal Feeds*, FDA Compliance Policy Guide, U.S. Food and Drug Administration, U.S. Department of Health and Human Services, Rockville, MD, 1994, pp. 384–385, Sec. 683.100.
11. USFDA, *Guidance for Industry: Fumonisin Levels in Human Foods and Animal Feeds*, Center for Food Safety and Applied Nutrition, Center for Veterinary Medicine, U.S. Food and Drug Administration, U.S. Department of Health and Human Services, Rockville, MD, 2000.
12. U.S. Wheat and Barley Scab Initiative, FHB plagues wheat in eastern U.S., *Fusarium Focus*, Fall 2003, pp 1–3.
13. Vardon, P.J., Potential economic costs of mycotoxins in the United States, in *Mycotoxins: Risks in Plant, Animal and Human Systems*, CAST Task Force Report No. 139, Council for Agricultural Science and Technology, Ames, IA, 2003, pp. 136–142.

2 Aflatoxin and Food Safety: Recent African Perspectives

Gordon S. Shephard

CONTENTS

2.1 INTRODUCTION

Food safety, with its emphasis on food quality, in the developing countries of Africa is an issue that frequently must be balanced by issues of food security with their emphasis on sufficiency of supply. Droughts during 2002 in a number of countries of southern Africa have made staple food supplies tenuous, while the reality for rural subsistence farmers is that, irrespective of food quality, the lack of economic alternatives frequently means that all food produced must be consumed by the local community. Even with adequate crops, poor traditional storage facilities can lead to fungal deterioration. Such a situation arose from excessive rains in Somalia over the period of late 1997 and early 1998.[1] Flood damage to grain (mainly sorghum) in underground storage areas resulted in visible fungal contamination of grain supplies for which no replacement food source was readily available. Given these harsh realities, it is not surprising that fungal contamination of staple foods in Africa is an area of major concern for food safety experts. Although only recognized during the previous century, human and animal mycotoxicoses resulting from fungal contamination have presumably existed for centuries in Africa. Indeed, a recent scientific reevaluation of the Biblical ten plagues of Egypt has postulated a mycotoxicological explanation for the tenth plague, namely that of the death of first-born sons.[2] In more recent times, outbreaks of gangrenous ergotism occurred in Ethiopia in 1978 after the consumption of grain contaminated with *Claviceps purpurea*,[3,4] and outbreaks of acute aflatoxicosis in Kenya in 1981 were attributed to the consumption of maize contaminated with aflatoxin.[5] Even more recently, the death of 12 people in the Meru North district of Kenya in 2001 was attributed to the consumption of maize contaminated with aflatoxin during storage in poorly ventilated facilities and plastic containers.[6] These fatal events highlight the problems of food safety, in general, and fungal contamination, in particular, in certain areas of Africa.1

Apart from outbreaks of acute aflatoxicosis, aflatoxin exposure contributes substantially to the disease burden of African communities. Studies on the correlation between the incidence of primary hepatocellular carcinoma and human exposure to aflatoxins in a number of African countries (Kenya, Mocambique, Swaziland) helped demonstrate the role of aflatoxin as a human carcinogen.[7] The relationship between aflatoxins and the childhood disease of kwashiorkor is not clear. Although kwashiorkor is widely thought to be a form of protein energy malnutrition, some characteristic features of the disease are known to be among the pathological effects caused by aflatoxins in animals. It has been suggested that either aflatoxins could play a causal role in the disease[8] or children suffering from the disease are at greater risk to the hazards of dietary aflatoxin.[9] Besides these direct effects of aflatoxin exposure, the extent to which the immunomodulatory effects of aflatoxins with depressed cell-mediated immunity[10] contribute to infectious disease burden is difficult to quantify but undoubtedly significant. A recent study in Gambian children ages 6 to 9 years has provided evidence for reduced immune function due to aflatoxin exposure.[11]

Aflatoxins are primarily produced by the fungi *Aspergillus flavus* Link and *A. parasiticus* Speare.[12,13] Optimal thermal conditions for fungal growth are 36 to 38°C, while maximum toxin production occurs at 25 to 27°C. Growth in storage facilities is favored by humidity above 85%. Because suitable conditions for its growth and toxin production occur in most areas of Africa, aflatoxin contamination of food is a universal problem across the continent. The frequent presence of aflatoxin contamination in

---

1 Further outbreaks of human aflatoxicosis, resulting in over 120 deaths, occurred in Kenya during 2004 (*CDC Morb. Mortal. Wkly Rep.*, 53, 790–793, 2004.).

staple food supplies in many communities has as a consequence the exposure of populations throughout their lives, including prenatal exposure of the fetus. Analysis of cord blood at birth in Ghana,[14] Kenya,[15] and Nigeria[14,16] has revealed that, although seasonal effects were present, around one third of assayed samples were positive for the presence of aflatoxins. Research in Gambia, in western Africa, not only has indicated that maternal exposure to aflatoxin can result in *in utero* exposure of the fetus but has also provided evidence to indicate that metabolic activation of aflatoxin B_1 (AFB$_1$) also occurs in the fetal liver.[17] Apart from prenatal exposure, infants in certain African regions are also further exposed to these carcinogens via their mothers' milk. Analysis of human breast milk from lactating mothers in Egypt,[18,19] Gambia,[20] Ghana,[14] Kenya,[8] Sierra Leone,[21] Sudan,[22] and Zimbabwe[23,24] has demonstrated post-natal consumption of various aflatoxins, including AFB$_1$, AFB$_2$, AFM$_1$, and AFM$_2$, by breastfed infants. Further studies have indicated that, after weaning, infants in Benin and Togo have enhanced aflatoxin exposure that is associated with impaired growth.[25,26]

Despite social and economic problems, some African states have addressed issues of food safety. The 1994/1995 survey of worldwide regulations for mycotoxins listed eight African countries that regulated maximum levels for either aflatoxin B_1 or aflatoxin M_1 or total aflatoxins in food.[27] These countries are Cote d'Ivoire, Egypt, Kenya, Malawi, Nigeria, Senegal, South Africa, and Zimbabwe. Subsequently, a further seven African countries (Algeria, Mauritius, Morocco, Mozambique, Sudan, Tanzania, and Tunisia) are known to have introduced specific mycotoxin regulations.[28] In addition, African researchers have maintained an interest in studies on the natural occurrence of mycotoxins, particularly aflatoxins. The purpose of this review is to summarize recent literature on the natural occurrence of aflatoxins in Africa published since 1990 as an indicator of the current research effort and the various areas of interest in the states across the continent. In order to maintain regional perspectives, the review has been subdivided into the geographical areas of southern, eastern, northern, and western Africa.

2.2 NATURAL OCCURRENCE IN COUNTRIES OF SOUTHERN AFRICA

2.2.1 Botswana

A survey in Botswana of the country's main dietary staples of maize and sorghum harvested during 1997 and 1998 showed an absence of aflatoxin contamination in maize and minor contamination in sorghum (3/19 positive; maximum 0.5 µg/kg total aflatoxin);[29] however, high levels of aflatoxins were determined in peanuts (15/29 positive; maximum 48 µg/kg total aflatoxin), peanut butter (15/21 positive; maximum 64 µg/kg), and phane (16/28 positive; maximum 10 µg/kg), which is an edible larval stage of the emperor moth. The high levels in peanuts indicate the need to introduce adequate control measures.

2.2.2 South Africa

South Africa has a well-developed commercial farming sector, and it is generally of importance in examining mycotoxin contamination of South African crops to distinguish between those produced under commercial farming conditions and those grown and stored by rural subsistence farmers. The main aflatoxin-producing fungi, *Aspergillus flavus* and *A. parasiticus*, only occur sporadically in both commercial and home-grown maize in South Africa and are not ear-rot pathogens under local conditions.[30] Extensive surveys of commercial maize crops have been performed since the first survey commissioned by the South African Maize Board in 1986, and they have consistently demonstrated a very low incidence of aflatoxin contamination in local maize. Analytical results reported by the Maize Board's laboratory showed an absence of aflatoxin (<2 μg/kg) in all of 456 and 496 samples of unprocessed commercial maize of the 1986 and 1987 crops, respectively.[31] Further analyses in 1988 (277 samples), 1989 (41 samples), 1990 (55 samples), and 1991 (166 samples) were also negative for aflatoxin.[31,32] In contrast, aflatoxin (maximum 20 μg/kg) was found in 5 of 118 samples from the 1992 crop, possibly due to extreme drought stress of the crop during the 1991/1992 growing season.[31] Low levels of aflatoxin were found in samples of the 1993 crop, with maximum levels of 2 and 5 μg/kg in white and yellow maize, respectively.[33] Analyses of 291 samples of white and yellow maize during the 1994/1995 marketing season showed mean levels at or below the detection limit of 1 μg/kg, with a maximum level of 6 μg/kg.[34] Analyses of maize products destined for both human (156 samples) and animal (62 samples) consumption during this period failed to detect (<1 μg/kg) any aflatoxin contamination. A study of mycotoxin contamination of maize (1989 crop) exported from South Africa to Taiwan also failed to detect aflatoxin (<0.5 μg/kg) in either preshipment or postshipment samples.[35] More recently, surveys of South African commercial maize have been performed by the Southern African Grain Laboratory. No aflatoxin was detected in the 90 samples from the 1999/2000 season,[36] and only one sample (22 μg/kg) was found contaminated in the 57 samples collected during the 2000/2001 season.[37] Studies of home-grown maize in the rural areas of eastern Transvaal (now Mpumalanga Province) and KwaZulu-Natal also showed only a sporadic incidence of aflatoxin in maize.[38] Although South African maize is virtually free of aflatoxin contamination, improper harvest and storage practices can give rise to fungal growth and consequently high levels of toxin. Individual samples of agricultural commodities specifically submitted over a 10-year period to a commercial testing service found aflatoxin contamination in 229 of the 1602 submitted samples, with levels in maize, other cereals, oil seeds, poultry feed, animal feed, forage, and soybean in the range of 1 to 500 μg/kg.[39]

Although the health implications of aflatoxin contamination of food have been known for a number of decades and maximum tolerated levels have been widely legislated by many countries, including South Africa, the need for reliable and regular monitoring of commodities is paramount. This has recently been demonstrated in South Africa by several reports, which first appeared in newspapers, that analysis of a sample of peanut butter being used in a national school feeding program showed contamination at a total aflatoxin level of 271 μg/kg.[40] In the absence of any official data being made available, it may be concluded that a lack of adequate control and testing of samples from certain peanut butter suppliers to this program has exposed significant numbers of young children to dietary aflatoxin. As part of an investigation into the adverse health effects of areca (betel) nut chewing, the possible aflatoxin contamination of raw, boiled, and baked nuts available from commercial suppliers was investigated.[41] Although the baked or boiled nuts infrequently contained low levels of aflatoxin (maximum 0.1 µg/kg AFB$_1$), ten samples of the raw nuts all contained aflatoxin in a range from 3.5 to 26.2 µg/kg (mean 8.9 µg/kg) total aflatoxin.

2.2.3 ZIMBABWE

Results of routine monitoring of groundnuts by the Zimbabwe Government Analyst Laboratory were reported at the 49th meeting of the Joint FAO/WHO Expert Committee on Food Additives (JECFA).[42] Seasonal variations were noted in that 46% of the samples analyzed during the 1995 season and 8% of the samples analyzed in the 1996 season were contaminated with aflatoxins at levels above 10 µg/kg. As noted in the introduction, previous studies in rural villages had indicated the presence of AFM$_1$ in human breast milk at levels up to 0.05 ng/mL, raising concerns regarding infant exposure.[23]

2.3 NATURAL OCCURRENCE IN COUNTRIES OF EAST AFRICA

2.3.1 ETHIOPIA

A survey in Addis Ababa of 60 ground red pepper samples and 60 samples of *Shiro*, a processed mixture of legumes (peas, chickpeas, and grass peas) and spices, demonstrated that, although moderate incidences of aflatoxin contamination occur (13.33% and 8.33%, respectively), the levels of contamination can be very high (range 250 to 525 µg/kg and 100 to 500 µg/kg, respectively).[43] Only AFB$_1$ was detected in this survey.

2.3.2 KENYA

Despite reports of human aflatoxicoses in Kenya[5,6] and reports of its presence in umbilical cord blood[15] and human breast milk,[8] little published information is available on the levels of aflatoxins in human foods in Kenya. Maize represents a major dietary cereal, and it is estimated that maize meal is consumed in Kenya at a rate of about 0.4 kg/person/day.[44] A survey of maize meal from various commercial sources in Nairobi revealed the presence of aflatoxins in maize at levels between 0.4 and 20 µg/kg.[44] In rural areas, the retention of traditional food processing and storage practices can lead to mycotoxin contamination of food. In ethnic communities in eastern and central Kenya, maize is pounded in water and then dried prior to storage; however, insufficient drying can lead to fungal deterioration, and foods collected from these regions can have aflatoxin levels as high as 2000 µg/kg.[45]

2.3.3 TANZANIA

Local foods and beverages have been investigated as possible sources of aflatoxin exposure. In a study on local traditionally cured fish (salted, sun dried, or smoke dried) purchased in the Morogoro municipality, 3 fish varieties (10 samples each) were free of aflatoxin, while in 3 other varieties, one sample from each variety contained aflatoxin at levels between 6.7 and 18.5 µg/kg.[46] Due to the large quantities of beer that are consumed in various communities, this beverage is an important source of mycotoxin exposure in many countries around the world. In a study of 15 brewed alcoholic beverages purchased from local brewers in Dar es Salaam, 9 contained AFB_1 at levels between 10 and 50 µg/L.[47] Of the 9 contaminated samples, 8 were prepared from maize, millet, sorghum, or mixtures thereof, while the last brew had reported ingredients of sugarcane and honey. The remaining brews that were analyzed and found negative for aflatoxin were prepared from mixtures of sugarcane, palm juice, honey, yeast, and tea leaves. The effects of beer contamination can be serious, as these locally brewed beverages generally contain low levels of alcohol and some local inhabitants can consume up to 5 to 6 L/day.

2.4 NATURAL OCCURRENCE IN COUNTRIES OF NORTH AFRICA

2.4.1 EGYPT

Compared to many other African countries, an extensive literature on aflatoxin contamination of a wide range of foods in Egypt has appeared over the previous decade. Egyptian researchers have investigated the natural occurrence of aflatoxins in a range of human foods including milk,[18,48] cheeses,[18] dried fruits,[49] spices,[50–52] peanuts,[48,53] cottonseeds,[54] processed meat,[51,55] maize,[56] coconut,[57] hazelnuts,[58] walnuts,[58] corn flakes,[59] soybean,[56,60] fruit drinks,[61] wheat,[48] rice,[48] barley,[48] herbs,[52] medicinal plants,[52] dried vegetables,[52] lentils, and various other legumes.[48]

A recent survey of dairy products in Egypt showed AFM_1 in 3 of 15 cows' milk samples (mean 6.3 µg/kg) and in 1 of 10 dried milk samples (5 µg/kg), as well as AFB_1, AFM_1, and AFG_1 in various cheese types, with individual levels as high as 10 µg/kg.[18] A previous survey reported an AFM_1 level of 15 µg/kg in 1 of 15 milk powders analyzed.[48] AFM_1 levels of this magnitude would imply very high levels of AFB_1 in animal feed. A survey of a range of Egyptian animal feeds conducted some years before the milk analysis revealed that, apart from peanut shells contaminated at 400 µg/kg AFB_1, mixed feed used for milk production was the next most highly contaminated feed and contained up to 50 µg/kg each of AFB_1 and AFG_1.[62] Furthermore, cottonseed cake used for animal feed in Egypt can have aflatoxin levels as high as 200 µg/kg.[54]

As part of a project to assess aflatoxin exposure in the Egyptian population, common Egyptian foods, such as nuts, spices, herbs, medicinal plants, dried vegetables, and cereal grains susceptible to aflatoxin contamination, were sampled in Cairo.[52] The incidence of aflatoxin contamination ranged from 21.4% in cereal grains with AFB_1 levels of 6 to 92 µg/kg (mean, 36 µg/kg) to nuts and seeds with a contamination rate of 82.4% and a range of AFB_1 levels of 4 to 74 µg/kg (mean, 24 µg/kg). An extensive survey of cereal grains collected from four Egyptian governorates during 1996/1997 showed that maize (57 samples) was the most contaminated commodity with rates of 86.7 to 100% in the 4 governorates and levels as high as 200 µg/kg (individual means in the 4 governorates ranged from 63.6 to 107.7

μg/kg).[56] Contamination levels in yellow corn and gluten were lower, while soybean meal was the least contaminated (0 to 5.8% of samples; maximum, 25 μg/kg). A previous study on soybean seeds had found 35 out of 100 samples positive at levels up to 35 μg/kg.[60]

As in other countries, locally purchased nuts can show considerable contamination, and studies conducted by various researchers have shown levels in hazelnuts up to 175 μg/kg[58] and local peanuts up to 1056 μg/kg.[48] An extensive survey of 215 samples of fresh and processed meat products, including beefburger, hot dogs, sausages, and luncheon meat, and 130 samples of spices used in the meat industry showed an absence of aflatoxins in fresh meat, canned meat, salami, beefsteak, and minced meat.[51] The presence of aflatoxins in other processed meat products correlated positively with the addition of spices to the product. An independent survey of spices found 16 samples of the 120 analyzed to be contaminated at levels up to 35 μg/kg.[50]

2.4.2 LIBYA

In the first report on the natural occurrence of aflatoxins in Libya, 20 of 25 sheep, cattle, and camel feedstuffs were found to be contaminated with various mixtures of AFB_1, AFB_2, AFG_1, and AFG_2 as detected and confirmed by thin-layer chromatography;[63] however, exact levels of contamination were not reported.

2.4.3 MOROCCO

During the period from September 1989 to June 1991, a survey on the occurrence of AFB_1 in Moroccan poultry feeds and their ingredients was conducted; it involved 315 samples from 30 farms and 4 feed mills.[64] Whereas only 4% of mixed feed samples from feed mills contained AFB_1, 17% of samples from the poultry farms showed contamination, indicating the need for improved agricultural hygiene practices to prevent fungal growth in feeding troughs. The maximum AFB_1 level found in mixed feed from the mills was 110 μg/kg, whereas the maximum level in farm samples was 200 μg/kg, apart from one farm suffering an outbreak of aflatoxicosis where levels between 2000 and 5625 μg/kg were determined.

2.4.4 SUDAN

The natural occurrence of aflatoxins in peanuts,[65,66] peanut butter,[66] cereal grains,[67] and legume seeds[67,68] has been investigated. Groundnuts are an important crop and a major export product in Sudan. The two main peanut producing regions are the irrigated central region and the rain-fed western region. Each region is subdivided into 4 districts. A survey of aflatoxin contamination in each district was conducted in which 5 samples were collected at harvest from each of 5 areas in each district (25 samples per district).[65] In the irrigated central region, no aflatoxin was detected in any samples, whereas in the rain-fed western region contaminated samples were found in all districts ranging from a 10% contamination rate with a mean of 0.19 ± 0.08 μg/kg in Casgeal to 100% contamination with a mean of 8.37 ± 0.61 μg/kg in El Hamdi. The difference in the results from the two regions is partly related to the insect damage that was noted in crops in the western region that was absent in peanuts harvested in the central region. In the three towns of the capital, Khartoum, 81 samples of peanut paste and roasted peanuts were collected. The maximum levels of aflatoxin were in red roasted groundnuts from Khartoum North (14.3 µg/kg). A more recent survey of peanuts and peanut products collected from local markets in the same two growing regions concluded that, in addition to harvest differences, local storage conditions led to elevated levels of aflatoxin contamination in locally available products.[66] Of the samples collected in the central region, mean AFB_1 levels were 8.5 ± 6.8 µg/kg, whereas in the humid western region, mean levels were 87.4 ± 197.3 µg/kg. In Sudan, the western region is also a region of high risk for hepatocellular carcinoma relative to the central region.

Surveys of cereal and legume seeds collected in two cities of Sudan showed aflatoxin contamination in dukhun (millet), dura (sorghum), sesame, wheat, and maize, with the last cereal being the most contaminated with levels between 10 and 15 µg/kg.[67] The legumes in these studies (haricot beans, broad beans, chickpeas, lupins, groundnuts, cowpeas, and lentils) also showed various levels of contamination below 15 µg/kg, except for cowpeas, in which no aflatoxins were detected.[67,68]

2.5 NATURAL OCCURRENCE IN COUNTRIES OF WEST AFRICA

2.5.1 BENIN

Extensive surveys of maize, the most important cereal grown and consumed in Benin, were conducted between 1993 and 1995 in randomly selected villages across the country's four agroecological zones, ranging from coastal savannah in the south to southern Guinea savannah, northern Guinea savannah, and Sudan savannah in the north.[69-71] In a survey of preharvest maize, the southern and northern Guinea savannas had the highest total (AFB_1 plus AFB_2) aflatoxin levels with mean values in contaminated samples of 241.2 and 109.5 µg/kg in 1994 and 262.9 and 80.6 µg/kg in 1995, respectively.[71] Most of the maize sampled from farmers' stores in the 4 zones contained less than 5 µg/kg aflatoxin, although between 2.2 and 5.8% of samples from the 4 zones contained levels above 100 µg/kg at harvest.[69] During 6 months' storage, increases in toxin levels in samples from 2 of the 4 zones were observed, with the greatest increase being in the dry most northern zone (Sudan savannah) in which percentage contamination below 5 µg/kg dropped from 90.1% to 67.8%, the percentage contamination below 20 µg/kg increased from 8.8% to 25.8%, and the percentage of samples above 100 µg/kg increased from 2.2 to 24.2%. Apart from storage, other factors related to higher aflatoxin levels were insect damage, the use of local plants as storage protectants, and the use of certain storage structures or storage practices such as on or under the house roof.

2.5.2 CAMEROON

As in Benin, maize is an important cereal crop in Cameroon. During 1996 and 1997, two surveys of maize were performed in the Humid Forest and Western Highlands agroecological zones of Cameroon in which low incidence rates of both *Aspergillus flavus* infection and aflatoxin contamination were found, indicating that aflatoxin is not a problem in Cameroon-grown maize.[72]

2.5.3 GHANA

Aflatoxin contamination in two of the primary agricultural products of Ghana (namely, groundnuts and maize) has been investigated. Stored (6 to 8 months) groundnut samples were obtained from 12 of the major markets in all 10 regions of Ghana.[73] Samples randomly selected from sellers were bulked and visually sorted into damaged and undamaged kernels. The degree of damage ranged from 1.5 to 9.25%. Relatively low levels of total aflatoxin (50% contamination rate; 0.1 to 12.2 µg/kg) were detected in the undamaged kernels, while levels from 5.7 to 22,168 µg/kg were found in the damaged kernels. These results would suggest that a partial solution to the groundnut contamination problem in Ghana could be found by implementing sorting procedures.

In Ghana, maize is a dietary staple, especially among people in the coastal communities, where it is consumed as a fermented maize product (kenkey) among the Ga and Fanti tribes. Kenkey is a fermented maize dumpling produced at a household level and sold in urban areas as a ready-to-eat staple food. The traditional process for kenkey production involves steeping of maize kernels for 1 to 2 days, milling, and then mixing of the dough, which is left to undergo spontaneous fermentation for 2 to 3 days.[74] A portion of fermented dough is cooked and mixed with raw fermented dough to form a ball, which is then finally boiled for 3 hours in maize husks or banana leaves. Samples of fresh and fermented dough and kenkey balls collected at various sites in Accra revealed considerable aflatoxin contamination, with levels of total aflatoxin in the dough between 100.2 and 183.7 µg/kg, while 15 of 16 kenkey samples were contaminated between 6.15 and 196.1 µg/kg (mean, 50.55 µg/kg).[75] A study of aflatoxin contamination of 15 maize samples collected from processing sites in Accra revealed that 8 samples contained total aflatoxin ranging from 2 µg/kg to as high as 662 µg/kg.[76] Studies on the kenkey-making process reveal a potential for increasing contamination levels during the initial stages of fermentation, while the final cooking step can lead to reductions in AFB_1 of between 38 and 80%.[74] Hence, it has been suggested that in a Hazard Analysis Critical Control Point (HACCP) system for kenkey production, two critical control points (raw maize ingredients and final cooking) are possible at which reduction in aflatoxin can be exercised.[77]

2.5.4 GAMBIA

In order to assess total aflatoxin intakes of individuals in Gambia, a range of cooked foodstuffs was collected from a rural village and analyzed for aflatoxins.[78] The highest contamination levels were in groundnut sauce in which 18 of 20 samples were contaminated (19 to 944 µg/kg; mean, 162 µg/kg); however, significant contamination was found in other foods, such as maize (9/10 positive; range, 2 to 35 µg/kg; mean, 9.7 µg/kg), millet (9/9 positive; range, 1 to 27 µg/kg; mean, 9.8 µg/kg), sorghum (2/8 positive; levels of 2 and 16 µg/kg), rice (14/20 positive; range, 2 to 19 µg/kg; mean, 7.9 µg/kg), and leaf sauces (3/3 positive; levels of 21, 26, and 34 µg/kg). It is clear that in Gambia, aflatoxin contamination appears widespread in different foodstuffs.

2.5.5 NIGERIA

The tropical environment of parts of Nigeria provides optimal conditions for fungal growth and mycotoxin production. The natural occurrence of aflatoxins in a wide range of food commodities in Nigeria has been investigated: maize,[79,80] maize-based snacks,[80] maize-based weaning food,[81] garri, beans, yam flour, cassava flour,[82] melon seeds,[83] and groundnuts.[84] Low levels of aflatoxin have been detected in many of these commodities. Recent studies on groundnuts have reported total aflatoxin levels as high as 64 mg/kg in raw nuts.[84] Besides groundnuts, a major concern is aflatoxin contamination of maize that is processed into traditional foods such as corn cakes and corn rolls for which children are major consumers.[80] A study of maize, corn cakes, and corn rolls sampled from farms and producers in southwestern Nigeria showed that 45, 80, and 12% of samples were contaminated with mean total aflatoxin of 200, 233, and 55 µg/kg in the positive samples, respectively.[80] Levels as high as 1070 µg/kg were found in corn cake. Of particular concern is neonatal exposure to aflatoxins. The presence of aflatoxins in umbilical cord blood at birth has been reported in Nigeria,[14] while in a study of hospital meals or of patients' mothers' food, 12 of 48 maize-based gruels used as weaning food for children were found to be contaminated at levels as high as 19.7 µg/kg.[81] A range of animal feedstuffs, including groundnut cake, poultry mash, and cow feed, has been shown to be contaminated, with the former being the worst affected commodity (87% of 23 samples; mean aflatoxin level, 382 µg/kg; maximum level, 1862 µg/kg).[79]

2.5.6 SENEGAL

Groundnuts are an important crop in west Africa, and the problem of aflatoxin contamination is a significant constraint on their production. The extent of this problem is illustrated by field trials of various cultivars conducted in Senegal, Niger, and Burkina Faso in which mean contamination over a range of cultivars ranged from 1 to 450 µg/kg with a mean of 143 µg/kg.[85] Aflatoxin levels in peanut oil and food prepared by local small-scale production plants are also high.[86] Samples taken from two regions over 2 consecutive years were determined to have mean levels of total aflatoxin ranging between 57 and 82 µg/kg.

2.5.7 SIERRA LEONE

In Sierra Leone, fish is an important source of dietary protein and is generally smoke-dried for storage. Examination of 20 samples of dried fish from homes and markets revealed the presence of *Aspergillus flavus* in 14 samples, as well as the presence of aflatoxin.[87] No quantification of toxin was recorded. The presence of mycotoxigenic fungi on foods such as sesame seeds has been investigated,[88] while the analysis of urine samples collected from 1993 to 1994 from 434 children ages 5 to 14 years revealed widespread exposure to both aflatoxins and ochratoxin A in Sierra Leone.[89]

2.6 CONCLUSION

It is clear from this review that aflatoxin contamination in agricultural crops is widespread in Africa and that an awareness of this situation exists across the continent; however, in many areas, the insufficiency of food supplies is a major impediment to improvements in food safety. Increased pressure on limited food resources and the attendant malnutrition exacerbates the mycotoxin problem by increasing the likelihood of human consumption of contaminated foodstuffs and by rendering the population more susceptible to the consequent adverse health effects. In addition to the research on the natural occurrence of aflatoxins addressed in this review, a number of scientists have investigated the use of indigenous African plants as possible natural protectants against insect and fungal damage during storage;[73,90–92] nevertheless, such use must be carefully evaluated, as these practices may exacerbate the aflatoxin contamination problem.[69] The effects of rural village food processing techniques as possible means of decontamination have also been investigated in Zambia,[93] Nigeria,[94] and Ghana[4] and must be considered more widely. The concerns of African agricultural and biomedical scientists over mycotoxin exposure in African populations and the need for appropriate government measures were expressed in a resolution adopted at the International Coordination Workshop on Mycotoxins in Foods in Africa, held in Cotonou, Benin, in November 1995.[95] This resolution aimed to promote an awareness of the need for concerted action to address these issues on the African continent. As Africa enters the 21st century, it is to be hoped that questions of food safety will receive increased attention.

REFERENCES

1. Golden, M.H.N., Personal communication, 2002 (http://www.sare.org/htdocs/hypermail/html-home/27–html/0162.htm).
2. Marr, J.S. and Malloy, C.D., An epidemiologic analysis of the ten plagues of Egypt, *Caduceus*, 12, 7–24, 1996.
3. King, B., Outbreak of ergotism in Wollo, Ethiopia, *Lancet*, 1(8131), 1411, 1979.
4. Demeke, T., Kidane, Y., and Wuhib, E., Ergotism: a report on an epidemic, 1977–78, *Ethiopian Med. J.*, 17, 107–113, 1979.
5. Ngindu, A., Johnson, B.K., Kenya, P.R., Ngira, J.A., Ocheng, D.M., Nandwa, H., Omondi, T.N., Jansen, A.J., Ngare, W., Kaviti, J.N., Gatei, D., and Siongok, T.A., Outbreak of acute hepatitis caused by aflatoxin poisoning in Kenya, *Lancet*, 1(8285), 1346–1348, 1982.
6. Anon., *The Nation*, Nairobi, October 3, 2001 (archive no. 20011007.2427 at http://www.promedmail.org/).
7. Van Rensberg, S.J., Role of epidemiology in the evaluation of mycotoxin health risks, in *Mycotoxins in Human and Animal Health*, Rodricks, J.V., Hesseltine, C.W., and Mehlman, M.A., Eds., Pathotox Publishers, Park Forest South, IL, 1977, pp. 699–711.

8. Hendrickse, R.G., Clinical implications of food contaminated by aflatoxins, *Ann. Acad. Med.*, 20, 84–90, 1991.
9. Adhikari, M., Ramjee, G., and Berjak, P., Aflatoxin, kwashiorkor, and morbidity, *Nat. Toxins*, 2, 1–3, 1994.
10. Pestka, J.J. and Bondy, G.S., Immunotoxic effects of mycotoxins, in *Mycotoxins in Grain*, Miller, J.D. and Trenholm, H.L., Eds., Eagan Press, St. Paul, MN, 1994, pp. 339–358.
11. Turner, P.C., Moore, S.E., Hall, A.J., Prentice, A.M., and Wild C.P., Modification of immune function through exposure to dietary aflatoxin in Gambian children, *Environ. Health Perspect.*, 111, 217–220, 2003.
12. Marasas, W.F.O. and Nelson, P.E., Aflatoxicosis, in *Mycotoxicology*, Marasas, W.F.O. and Nelson, P.E., Eds., Pennsylvania State University Press, University Park, PA, 1987, pp. 25–31.
13. Tuite, J., The genus *Aspergillus*, in *Mycotoxic Fungi, Mycotoxins, Mycotoxicoses: An Encyclopedic Handbook*, Wyllie, T.D. and Morehouse, L.G., Eds., Marcel Dekker, New York, 1977, pp. 21–39.
14. Lamplugh, S.M., Hendrickse, R.G., Apeagyei, F., and Mwanmut, D.D., Aflatoxins in breast milk, neonatal cord blood, and serum of pregnant women, *Br. Med. J.*, 296, 968, 1988.
15. De Vries, H.R., Maxwell, S.M., and Hendrickse, R.G., Foetal and neonatal exposure to aflatoxins, *Acta Paediatr. Scand.*, 78, 373–378, 1989.
16. Abula, E.O., Uriah, N., Aigbefo, H.S., Oboh, P.A., and Agbonlahor, D.E., Preliminary investigation on the aflatoxin in cord blood of jaundiced neonates, *West Afr. J. Med.*, 17, 184–187, 1998.
17. Wild, C.P., Rasheed, F.N., Jawla, M.F.B., Hall, A.J., Jansen, L.A.M., Montesano, R., *In utero* exposure to aflatoxin in West Africa, *Lancet*, 337(8757), 1602, 1991.
18. El-Sayed, A.M.A.A., Neamat-Allah, A.A., and Soher, E.A., Situation of mycotoxins in milk, dairy products and human milk in Egypt, *Mycotoxin Res.*, 16, 91–100, 2000.
19. El-Sayed, A.M.A.A., Soher, E.A., and Neamat-Allah, A.A., Human exposure to mycotoxins in Egypt, *Mycotoxin Res.*, 18, 23–30, 2002.
20. Zarba, A., Wild, C.P., Hall, A.J., Montesano, R., Hudson, G.J., and Groopman, J.D., Aflatoxin M$_1$ in human breast milk from The Gambia, West Africa, quantified by combined monoclonal antibody immunoaffinity chromatography and HPLC, *Carcinogenesis*, 13, 891–894, 1992.
21. Jonsyn, F.E., Maxwell, S.M., and Hendrickse, R.G., Ochratoxin A and aflatoxins in breast milk samples from Sierra Leone, *Mycopathologia*, 131, 121–126, 1995.
22. Coulter, J.B.S., Lamplugh, S.M., Suliman, G.I., Omer, M.I.A., and Hendrickse, R.G., Aflatoxins in human breast milk, *Ann. Trop. Paediatr.*, 4, 61–66, 1984.
23. Wild, C.P., Pionneau, F.A., Montesano,R., Mutiro, C.F., and Chetsanga, C.J., Aflatoxin detected in human breast milk by immunoassay, *Int. J. Cancer*, 40, 328–333, 1987.
24. Nyathi, C.B., Mutiro, C.F., Hasler, J.A., and Chetsanga, C.J., Human exposure to aflatoxins in Zimbabwe, *Central Afr. J. Med.*, 35, 542–545, 1989.
25. Gong, Y.Y., Egal, S., Hounsa, A., Turner, P.C., Hall, A.J., Cardwell, K.F., and Wild, C.P., Determinants of aflatoxin exposure in young children from Benin and Togo, West Africa: the critical role of weaning, *Int. J. Epidemiol.*, 32, 556–562, 2003.
26. Gong, Y.Y., Cardwell, K.F., Hounsa, A., Egal, S., Turner, P.C., Hall, A.J., and Wild, C.P., Dietary aflatoxin exposure and impaired growth in young children from Benin and Togo: cross-sectional study, *Br. Med. J.*, 325, 20–21, 2002.

27. FAO, *Worldwide Regulations for Mycotoxins 1995: A Compendium*, Food and Nutrition Paper 64, Food and Agriculture Organization, Rome, Italy, 1997.
28. Van Egmond, H.P. and Jonker, M.A., Worldwide regulations on aflatoxins, *Aflatoxin and Food Safety*, Abbas, H.K., Ed., Marcel Dekker, Boca Raton, FL, 2006, pp. 77–93.
29. Siame, B.A., Mpuchane, S.F., Gashe, B.A., Allotey, J., and Teffera, G., Occurrence of aflatoxins, fumonisin B_1, and zearalenone in foods and feeds in Botswana, *J. Food Protect.*, 61, 1670–1673, 1998.
30. Marasas, W.F.O., Medical relevance of mycotoxins in southern Africa, *Microbiol. Ailments Nutr.*, 6, 1–5, 1988.
31. Viljoen, J.H., Marasas, W.F.O., and Thiel, P.G., Fungal infection and contamination of commercial maize, in *Cereal Science and Technology: Impact on a Changing Africa*, Taylor, J.R.N., Randall, P.G., and Viljoen, J.H., Eds., CSIR, Pretoria, South Africa, 1993, pp. 837–853.
32. Rheeder, J.P., Sydenham, E.W., Marasas, W.F.O., Thiel, P.G., Shephard, G.S., Schlechter, M., Stockenström, S., Cronje, D.W., and Viljoen, J.H., Fungal infestation and mycotoxin contamination of South African commercial maize harvested in 1989 and 1990, *S. Afr. J. Sci.*, 91, 127–131, 1995.
33. Rava, E., Viljoen, J.H., Kallmeyer, H., and De Jager, A., Fungi and mycotoxins in South African maize of the 1993 crop, *Mycotoxin Res.*, 12, 15–24, 1996.
34. Rava, E., Mycotoxins in maize products of the 1994/1995 marketing season, *Mycotoxin Res.*, 12, 25–30, 1996.
35. Rheeder, J.P., Sydenham, E.W., Marasas, W.F.O., Thiel, P.G., Shephard, G.S., Schlechter, M., Stockenström, S., Cronje, D.W., and Viljoen, J.H., Ear-rot fungi and mycotoxins in South African corn of the 1989 crop exported to Taiwan, *Mycopathologia*, 127, 35–41, 1994.
36. Anon., *Grain Quality of the 1999/2000 South African Maize Crop*, Southern African Grain Laboratory, Pretoria, South Africa, 2001, pp. 1–50.
37. Anon., *Grain Quality of the 2000/2001 South African Maize Crop*, Southern African Grain Laboratory, Pretoria, South Africa, 2002, pp. 1–50.
38. Dutton, M.F., Robertson, E.J., Mathews, C., and Beck, B.D.A., Occurrence of mycotoxins in maize in a rural area in South Africa and methods of prevention of contamination and elimination, in *Cereal Science and Technology: Impact on a Changing Africa*, Taylor, J.R.N., Randall, P.G., and Viljoen, J.H., Eds., CSIR, Pretoria, South Africa, 1993, pp. 823–835.
39. Dutton, M.F. and Kinsey, A., A note on the occurrence of mycotoxins in cereals and animal feedstuffs in Kwazulu Natal, South Africa 1984–1993, *S. Afr. J. Anim. Sci.*, 26, 41–57, 1996.
40. PROMEC Unit, *Aflatoxin in Peanut Butter*, MRC Policy Brief No. 3, Medical Research Council, Tygerberg, South Africa, 2001.
41. Van der Bijl, P., Stockenström, S., Vismer, H.F., and Van Wyk, C.W., Incidence of fungi and aflatoxins in imported areca nut samples, *S. Afr. J. Sci.*, 92, 154–156, 1996.
42. Henry, S., Bosch, F.X., Bowers, J.C., Portier, C.J., Petersen, B.J., and Barraj, L., Aflatoxins, in *Safety Evaluation of Certain Food Additives and Contaminants*, prepared for the 49th Meeting of the Joint FAO/WHO Expert Committee on Food Additives, WHO, Geneva, Switzerland, 1998, pp. 359–468,
43. Fufa, H. and Urga, K., Screening of aflatoxins in *Shiro* and ground red pepper in Addis Ababa, *Ethiop. Med. J.*, 34, 243–249, 1996.

44. Muriuki, G.K. and Siboe, G.M., Maize flour contaminated with toxigenic fungi and mycotoxins in Kenya, *Afr. J. Health Sci.*, 2, 236–241, 1995.

45. Mwangi, C.M., *Human Exposure to Mycotoxins in Relation to Feeding Habits in Certain Districts in Kenya* [abstract P1.17], Pan-African Environmental Mutagen Society, Cape Town, South Africa, 1996, p. 68.

46. Mugula, J.K. and Lyimo, M.H., Microbiological quality of traditional market cured fish in Tanzania, *J. Food Safety*, 13, 33–41, 1992.

47. Nikander, P., Seppälä, T., Kilonzo, G.P., Huttunen, P., Saarinen, L., Kilima, E., and Pitkänen, T., Ingredients and contaminants of traditional alcoholic beverages in Tanzania, *Trans. Roy. Soc. Trop. Med. Hyg.*, 85, 133–135, 1991.

48. El-Gohary, A.H., Aflatoxin in some foodstuffs with special reference to public health hazard in Egypt, *Indian J. Animal Sci.*, 66, 468–473, 1996.

49. Zohri, A.A. and Abdel-Gawad, K.M., Survey of mycoflora and mycotoxins of some dried fruits in Egypt, *J. Basic Microbiol.*, 4, 279–288, 1993.

50. El-Kady, I.A., El-Maraghy, S.S.M., and Mostafa, M.E., Natural occurrence of mycotoxins in different spices in Egypt, *Folia Microbiol.*, 40, 297–300, 1995.

51. Aziz, N.H. and Youssef, Y.A., Occurrence of aflatoxins and aflatoxin-producing moulds in fresh and processed meat in Egypt, *Food Addit. Contamin.*, 8, 321–331, 1991.

52. Selim, M.I., Popendorf, W., Ibrahim, M.S., Sharkawy, S.E., and El Kashory, E.S., Aflatoxin B_1 in common Egyptian foods, *J. AOAC Int.*, 79, 1124–1129, 1996.

53. El-Maghraby, O.M.O. and El-Maraghy, S.S.M., Mycoflora and mycotoxins of peanut (*Arachis hypogaea* L.) seeds in Egypt. 1. Sugar fungi and natural occurrence of mycotoxins, *Mycopathologia*, 98, 165–170, 1987.

54. Mazen, M.B., El-Kady, I.A., and Saber, S.M., Survey of mycoflora and mycotoxins of cotton seeds and cotton seed products in Egypt, *Mycopathologia*, 110, 133–138, 1990.

55. Ismail, M.A. and Zaky, Z.M., Evaluation of the mycological status of luncheon meat with special reference to aflatoxigenic moulds and aflatoxin residues, *Mycopathologia*, 146, 147–154, 1999.

56. El-Tahan, F.H., El-Tahan, M.H., and Shebl, M.A., Occurrence of aflatoxins in cereal grains from four Egyptian governorates, *Nahrung*, 44, 279–280, 2000.

57. Zohri, A.A. and Saber, S.M., Filamentous fungi and mycotoxin detected in coconut, *Zentralbl. Mikrobiol.*, 148, 325–332, 1993.

58. Abdel-Hafez, A.I.I., and Saber, S.M., Mycoflora and mycotoxin of hazelnut (*Corylus avellana* L.) and walnut (*Juglans regia* L.) seeds in Egypt, *Zentralbl. Mikrobiol.*, 148, 137–147, 1993.

59. El-Sayed, A.M.A.A., Soher, E.A., and Sahab, A.F., Occurrence of certain mycotoxins in corn and corn-based products and thermostability of fumonisin B_1 during processing, *Nahrung*, 47, 222–225, 2003.

60. El-Kady, I.A. and Youssef, M.S., Survey of mycoflora and mycotoxins in Egyptian soybean seeds, *J. Basic Microbiol.*, 33, 371–378, 1993.

61. Abdel-Sater, M.A., Zohri, A.A., and Ismail, M.A., Natural contamination of some Egyptian fruit juices and beverages by mycoflora and mycotoxins, *J. Food Sci. Technol. Mysore*, 38, 407–411, 2001.

62. Abdelhamid, A.M., Occurrence of some mycotoxins (aflatoxin, ochratoxin A, citrinin, zearalenone and vomitoxin) in various Egyptian feeds, *Arch. Anim. Nutr. Berlin*, 40, 647–664, 1990.

63. El-Maraghy, S.S.M., Fungal flora and aflatoxin contamination of feedstuff samples in Beida Governorate, Libya, *Folia Microbiol.*, 41, 53–60, 1996.

64. Kichou, F. and Walser, M.M., The natural occurrence of aflatoxin B_1 in Moroccan poultry feeds, *Vet. Hum. Toxicol.*, 35, 105–108, 1993.

65. Elamin, N.H.H., Abdel-Rahim, A.M., and Khalid, A.E., Aflatoxin contamination of groundnuts in Sudan, *Mycopathologia*, 104, 25–31, 1988.
66. Omer, R.E., Bakker, M.I., Van't Veer, P., Hoogenboom, R.L.A.P., Polman, T.H.G., Alink, G.M., Idris, M.O., Kadaru, A.M.Y., and Kok, F.J., Aflatoxin and liver cancer in Sudan, *Nutr. Cancer*, 32, 174–180, 1998.
67. Abdel-Rahim, A.M., Osman, N.A., and Idris, M.O., Survey of some cereal grains and legume seeds for aflatoxin contamination in the Sudan, *Zentralbl. Mikrobiol.*, 144, 115–121, 1989.
68. El-Nagerabi, S.A.F. and Elshafie, A.E., Incidence of seed-borne fungi and aflatoxins in Sudanese lentil seeds, *Mycopathologia*, 149, 151–156, 2000.
69. Hell, K., Cardwell, K.F., Setamou, M., and Poehling, M.-H., The influence of storage practices on aflatoxin contamination in maize in four agroecological zones of Benin, west Africa, *J. Stored Prod. Res.*, 36, 365–382, 2000.
70. Hell, K., Cardwell, K.F., Setamou, M., and Schulthess, F., Influence of insect infestation on aflatoxin contamination of stored maize in four agroecological regions in Benin, *Afr. Entomol.*, 8, 169–177, 2000.
71. Setamou, M., Cardwell, K.F., Schulthess, F., and Hell, K., *Aspergillus flavus* infection and aflatoxin contamination of preharvest maize in Benin, *Plant Dis.*, 81, 1323–1327, 1997.
72. Ngoko, Z., Marasas, W.F.O., Rheeder, J.P., Shephard, G.S., Wingfield, M.J., and Cardwell, K.F., Fungal infection and mycotoxin contamination of maize in the Humid Forest and the Western Highlands of Cameroon, *Phytoparasitica*, 29, 352–360, 2001.
73. Awuah, R.T. and Kpodo, K.A., High incidence of *Aspergillus flavus* and aflatoxins in stored groundnut in Ghana and the use of microbial assay to assess the inhibitory effects of plant extracts on aflatoxin synthesis, *Mycopathologia*, 134, 109–114, 1996.
74. Kpodo, K., Sorensen, A.K., and Jakobsen, M., The occurrence of mycotoxins in fermented maize products, *Food Chem.*, 56, 147–153, 1996.
75. Jespersen, L., Halm, M., Kpodo, K., and Jakobsen, M., Significance of yeasts and moulds occurring in maize dough fermentation for "kenkey" production, *Int. J. Food Microbiol.*, 24, 239–248, 1994.
76. Kpodo, K., Thrane, U., and Hald, B., *Fusaria* and fumonisins in maize from Ghana and their co-occurrence with aflatoxins, *Int. J. Food Microbiol.*, 61, 147–157, 2000.
77. Nickelsen, L. and Jakobsen, M., Quantitative risk analysis of aflatoxin toxicity for the consumers of "kenkey," a fermented maize product, *Food Control*, 8, 149–159, 1997.
78. Hudson, G.J., Wild, C.P., Zarba, A., and Groopman, J.D., Aflatoxins isolated by immunoaffinity chromatography from foods consumed in The Gambia, West Africa, *Nat. Toxins*, 1, 100–105, 1992.
79. Atawodi, S.E., Atiku, A.A., and Lamorde, A.G., Aflatoxin contamination of Nigerian foods and feedingstuffs, *Food Chem. Toxicol.*, 32, 61–63, 1994.
80. Adebajo, L.O., Idowu, A.A., and Adesanya, O.O., Mycoflora, and mycotoxins production in Nigerian corn and corn-based snacks, *Mycopathologia*, 126, 183–192, 1994.
81. Oyelami, O.A., Maxwell, S.M., and Adeoba, E., Aflatoxins and ochratoxin A in the weaning food of Nigerian children, *Ann. Trop. Paediatr.*, 16, 137–140, 1996.
82. Ibeh, I.N., Uraih, N., and Ogonor, J.I., Dietary exposure to aflatoxin in Benin City, Nigeria: a possible public health concern, *Int. J. Food Microbiol.*, 14, 171–174, 1991.
83. Ekundayo, C.A. and Idzi, E., Mycoflora and nutritional value of shelled melon seeds (*Citrulus vulgaris* Schrad.) in Nigeria, *Plant Foods Hum. Nutr.*, 40, 215–222, 1990.
84. Thomas, A.E., Coker, H.A.B., Odukoya, O.A., Isamah, G.K., and Adepoju-Bello, A., Aflatoxin contamination of *Arachis hypogaea* (groundnuts) in Lagos area of Nigeria, *Bull. Environ. Contam. Toxicol.*, 71, 42–45, 2003.

85. Waliyar, F., Ba, A., Hassan, H., Bonkoungou, S., and Bosc, J.P., Sources of resistance to *Aspergillus flavus* and aflatoxin contamination in groundnut genotypes in West Africa, *Plant Dis.*, 78, 704–708, 1994.

86. Diop, Y., Ndiaye, B., Diouf, A., Fall, M., Thiaw, C., Thiam, A., Barry, O., Ciss, M., and Ba, D., Artisanal peanut oil contamination by aflatoxins in Senegal, *Ann. Pharm. Fr.*, 58, 470-474, 2000.

87. Jonsyn, F.E. and Lahai, G.P., Mycotoxic flora and mycotoxins in smoke-dried fish from Sierra Leone, *Nahrung*, 5, 485–489, 1992.

88. Jonsyn, F.E., Seedborne fungi of sesame (*Sesamum indicum* L.) in Sierra Leone and their potential aflatoxin/mycotoxin production, *Mycopathologia*, 104, 123–127, 1988.

89. Jonsyn-Ellis, F.E., Seasonal variation in exposure frequency and concentration levels of aflatoxins and ochratoxins in urine samples of boys and girls, *Mycopathologia*, 152, 35–40, 2000.

90. Udoh, J.M., Cardwell, K.F., and Ikotun, T., Storage structures and aflatoxin content of maize in five agroecological zones of Nigeria, *J. Stored Prod. Res.*, 36, 187–201, 2000.

91. Tantaoui-Elaraki, A. and Beraoud, L., Inhibition of growth and aflatoxin production in *Aspergillus parasiticus* by essential oils of selected plant materials, *J. Environ. Pathol. Toxicol. Oncol.*, 13, 67–72, 1994.

92. Mahmoud, A.L., Inhibition of growth and aflatoxin biosynthesis of *Aspergillus flavus* by extracts of some Egyptian plants, *Lett. Appl. Microbiol.*, 29, 334–336, 1999.

93. Njapau, H., Muzungaile, E.M., and Changa, R.C., The effect of village processing techniques on content of aflatoxins in corn and peanuts in Zambia, *J. Sci. Food Agric.*, 76, 450-456, 1998.

94. Adegoke, G.O., Otumu, E.J., and Akanni, A.O., Influence of grain quality, heat, and processing time on the reduction of aflatoxin B_1 levels in "tuwo" and "ogi": two cereal-based products, *Plant Foods Hum. Nutr.*, 45, 113–117, 1994.

95. Cardwell, K. and Miller, J.D., Mycotoxins in foods in Africa, *Nat. Toxins*, 4, 103–107, 1996.

3 Aflatoxin and Food Safety: Recent South American Perspectives

Vildes M. Scussel

CONTENTS

3.1 INTRODUCTION

Food safety in the South American continent and its relation to mycotoxins is a quite broad and diversified subject. This continent varies widely in geographical location, climate, soil, types of agricultural commodities, and cultural habits, to name a few. Differences in economics have led to diverse tolerance levels and differences in the way that individual countries may regulate foods contaminated with mycotoxins. Several of the countries lack regulations or even minimal monitoring programs. Governments and scientists of major grain-producing countries in South America — Brazil, Argentina, Colombia, are Venezuela — are well aware of the problems associated with some mycotoxins and have the most data published in the literature. Less developed South American countries such as Bolivia, French Guyana, Guyana, Paraguay, Peru, and Suriname lack resources and funding to monitor levels of mycotoxins in foods. What has convinced South American countries to take mycotoxins seriously is the export of commodities and the use of grains by the meat industries to feed their animals. The reason why South America refuses batches of imported grains is not always due to levels of mycotoxin contamination but often is due to the price of the commodity; therefore, food consumed by the South American populace is not always the safest and could have adverse health effects. Most of the published data report aflatoxin (AFL; AFB_1, AFB_2, AFG_1, and AFG_2) contamination in peanuts and corn and their products, but some staple foods, such as black beans and rice, also are monitored in some of the countries, in addition to wheat, coffee, Brazil nuts, and the presence of aflatoxin M_1 (AFM_1) in milk. Animals exposed to AFL-contaminated feed are another important consideration, as some South American countries have high levels of AFL residues in meat liver and milk products. It is important to emphasize that, due to their high grain production and export, some South American countries have implemented control measures to reduce the levels of AFLs. By implementing training programs, good harvesting practices, and grain-drying procedures, as well as emphasizing the adverse effects on public health, levels of AFLs and toxigenic fungi have decreased quite considerably in recent years.

3.1.1 GRAIN PRODUCTION

South America has a high grain production sector. Brazil, Venezuela, and Argentina are the main general exporting countries with exports of 57.8, 29.5, and 26.7 billion free on board (f.o.b.), respectively, followed by Chile, Colombia, Peru, Ecuador, and Uruguay (18.5, 12.3, 7.3, 4.8, and 2.24 billion f.o.b., respectively).[49] The primary grains are corn, coffee, soybean, and rice, mainly produced in Brazil, Argentina, Colombia, and Venezuela. Peanuts are produced in Argentina, Brazil, Suriname, Chile, Paraguay, Venezuela, and Uruguay.

3.1.2 PATTERNS OF DIET AND AFL-RELATED FOOD

Central and South America are the seventh largest consumers of cereal products internationally and the sixth largest consumer of milk internationally (Table 3.1). Most South American countries have middle-income economies.[83] The continent has three dominant food cultures: (1) Indo-America, along the mountains (Colombia, Ecuador, Peru, and Bolivia), where the traditional staple foods are maize, beans, and potatoes; (b) Tropi-America (Venezuela and north of Brazil), where the traditional diets contain a large proportion of starchy roots and tubers (cassava, yam) in addition to beans and rice; and (3) the temperate prairies, where the diets are high in animal foods but are otherwise Mediterranean in nature and include cereals. Table 3.2 shows

TABLE 3.1
Consumption of Some Major Food Groups Worldwide as Percentage of Total Energy

Country	Cereals (%)	Other Starchy Food (%)	Vegetables and Fruits (%)	Meat (%)	Milk and Dairy Products (%)
Australia and New Zealand	26.2	6.5	8.6	34.5	15.1
Caribbean	37.3	15.1	11.5	10.8	8.6
Central and South America	43.1	12.9	5.0	13.6	9.4
China	73.3	10.8	5.0	15.1	1.4
Eastern Europe	38.2	7.9	7.9	20.1	12.9
India	67.1	5.8	5.0	1.43	8.6
Asia (low income)	75.6	7.2	4.3	2.9	5.0
Asia (middle income)	58.2	7.9	8.6	9.4	2.9
North Africa	62.7	5.8	8.6	5.0	5.8
Northern and Central Europe	22.7	11.5	9.35	25.9	15.8
Oceania	27.6	51.1	17.9	10.8	0.7
Southern Europe	28.0	7.9	11.5	28.1	15.1
Sub-Saharan Africa	48.4	45.3	2.9	5.8	5.0
United States and Canada	24.4	6.5	10.1	26.6	15.8

Source: Data from World Cancer Research Fund and American Institute for Cancer Research.[83]

that the diets of most countries in South America are based on cereals and other starchy foods.[83] In Brazil and Paraguay, rice and beans are relatively important and stable parts of the diet, while in Uruguay and Argentina, rice, beans, and wheat are significant. Clearly, the diets of these South American countries include cereals that can be contaminated by AFLs when exposed to factors that allow the growth of fungi. Starchy roots are often a source of fungal growth in Paraguay, Bolivia, and Colombia. Foods that can be indirectly contaminated with AFLs when they are obtained from animals given AFB_1-contaminated feed include beef, pork, chicken, liver, eggs, and milk. Thus, AFLs may be found in the starchy foods (cereal, pulses, roots), high-protein foods (beef, chicken, liver), and alcoholic beverages of a typical South American diet.

3.1.3 REGULATION

Due to social and economic concerns, some South American countries have addressed food safety issues and established maximum residue levels (MRLs) for AFLs and other mycotoxins. Table 3.3 shows the MRL for AFLs established by

TABLE 3.2
Consumption of Some Major Food Groups in South America as Percentage of Total Energy

South American Regions	Country	Cereals (%)	Other Starchy Food (%)	Vegetables and Fruits (%)	Meat (%)	Milk and Dairy Products (%)
Eastern	Brazil	34.9	19.8	6.9	17.6	13.5
Northern	Colombia	33.1	32.3	5.8	17.6	12.3
	Ecuador	35.9	21.3	4.8	12.7	15.2
	French Guyana	31.5	13.5	13.8	43.6	16.4
	Guyana	49.0	15.1	4.8	13.3	15.8
	Suriname	50.8	7.8	6.4	17.0	11.1
	Venezuela	51.8	14.1	3.7	13.9	11.7
Southern	Argentina	31.5	12.0	9.0	44.9	18.1
	Chile	46.5	9.4	10.1	20.0	12.9
	Uruguay	34.6	9.4	7.4	38.2	35.7
Western	Bolivia	42.8	32.3	7.4	24,9	4.7
	Paraguay	31.0	41.2	11.1	31.5	7.0
	Peru	46.4	21.4	6.9	15.2	10.5

Source: Data from World Cancer Research Fund and American Institute for Cancer Research.[83]

Mercosul countries (southern area of South American trade comprised of Argentina, Brazil, Paraguay, and Uruguay), as well as for Suriname, Venezuela, Peru, and Colombia. The Mercosul countries have established a MRL for total AFLs (AFB_1 + AFB_2 + AFG_1 + AFG_2) of 20 μg/kg for all food products that contain either peanuts or corn. Furthermore, the Mercosul countries have established MRLs on milk products of 0.5 μg/kg (natural) and 5.0 μg/kg (powdered). Each country that belongs to Mercosul also has its own regulations. For example, Argentina allows only 5 μg/kg of AFB_1 in peanuts, corn, and related products.[3,20] Zero tolerance for AFB_1 is mandated for all baby food products. It appears as though Colombia, Suriname Venezuela, and Uruguay should modify their MRLs for AFLs, as they remain high (30 μg/kg) for cereal, peanuts, and related food products.

3.1.4 AFLATOXIN EXPOSURE IN THE SOUTH AMERICAN POPULATION

Without governmental policies and thresholds to regulate AFL levels in food supplies, the human population in South America is continuously exposed to these mycotoxins. Although some data suggest that exposure to food contaminated with AFLs can lead to hepatocellular carcinoma (HCC), published data on acute and chronic human aflatoxicosis outbreaks in South American communities are lacking. Although the data are scarce or nonexistent, AFL exposure remains an important issue with regard to food safety and public health. Safety assessments must be undertaken by South American countries, as data suggest that long-term exposure might lead to HCC development or other diseases.[79] An Argentina study performed by Lopes et al.[39] showed 0.47 ng/mL AFB_1 in one of 13 blood samples from donors with hepatic diseases.

Evaluation of AFL exposure by measuring toxin levels in contaminated foods can be difficult to interpret due to the heterogeneous distribution of AFLs. Additionally, the dietary intake of a given food can be highly variable and unreliably reported. Genetic variability in AFB_1 metabolism may also influence the level of exposure at the individual level; therefore, an alternative for evaluating AFL exposure is to estimate levels using specific biological markers (biomarkers) based on an understanding of the metabolism of the compound. For AFB_1, these include aflatoxin–N7–guanine (AFB_1–N7-gua) in the urine, or aflatoxin–albumin (AFB_1–alb) in the blood. Using the AFB_1–alb biomarker assay approach, a study was carried out by Haas et al.[34] to assess the level of exposure to AFB_1 in a Brazilian population. A blood sample was taken from urban residents ($n = 50$; ages 18 to 52) in 1999 at the Blood Center of Antonio Carlos de Camargo Hospital, São Paulo. Serum albumin was extracted and digested and AFB_1–alb adduct levels were determined by enzyme-linked immunosorbent assay (ELISA). AFB_1–alb adducts were detected in 31/50 (62%) samples (range, 0 to 57.3 pg AFB_1–lys adducts per mg of blood albumin [pg/mg]). The mean level for those individuals who tested positive was 14.9 pg/mg. Males had the two highest levels, measured at 57.1 and 57.3 pg/mg. The levels in this study were similar to those observed in the Philippines.[78] This was the first study from South America that determined human AFB_1 exposure using the biomarker approach. These data warrant further investigation of both the sources and consequences of exposure to this potent toxin in Brazil and other South American countries.

The purpose of this review is to summarize recent literature published since 1993 that addresses the natural occurrence of AFLs in South America. This information serves as an indicator of the current research effort and the various areas of interest in the countries across the continent. Due to the small quantity of South American data published in English-language journals, data reported in Spanish- or Portuguese-language journals, good-quality data published in Latin American Mycotoxicology conference proceedings, and official data obtained from South American private and governmental accredited laboratories of mycotoxin analysis are presented here. In order to maintain regional perspectives, the review has been subdivided into the geographical areas of Northern (Ecuador, Colombia, French Guyana, Guyana, Suriname, Venezuela), Southern (Argentina, Chile, Uruguay), Eastern (Brazil, a major region by itself), and Western (Bolivia, Peru, Paraguay) South America. Most of the AFL data are from the Eastern region.

3.2 CLIMATE

Aflatoxins are produced by *Aspergillus flavus* Link and *A. parasiticus* Speare. The optimal thermal conditions for growth of these fungi are from 36 to 38°C, while maximum toxin production occurs between 25 and 27°C. Fungal growth in storage facilities is favored by relative humidity above 85%. Because suitable conditions for their growth and toxin production occur in most areas of South America, AFL

TABLE 3.3

Aflatoxin Regulation for Foods Consumed by Humans in Countries of South America

Country	Food Raw	Food Products	Aflatoxin Type	MRL (μg/kg)[a]
Argentina	—	Baby food	AFB_1	0
	Peanuts	Peanut products (AFB_1, 5 μg/kg)	$AFB_1 + AFB_2 + AFG_1 + AFG_2$	20
	Corn	Corn products (AFB_1, 5 μg/kg)	$AFB_1 + AFB_2 + AFG_1 + AFG_2$	20
	—	Soy meal	AFB_1	30
	Milk	Milk powder	AFM_1	0.05
	—	Milk products	AFM_1	0.5
Brazil[3,5]	Peanuts (with/without hull-peel)	Peanut (toasted, roasted)	$AFB_1 + AFB_2 + AFG_1 + AFG_2$	20
		Peanut butter	$AFB_1 + AFB_2 + AFG_1 + AFG_2$	20
	Corn (whole, broken, smashed)	Corn flours (whole with no germ)	$AFB_1 + AFB_2 + AFG_1 + AFG_2$	20
	Milk	—	AFM_1	0.5
	Milk	Milk powder	AFM_1	5.0
Colombia	Foods	Foods	$AFB_1 + AFB_2 + AFG_1 + AFG_2$	20
	Cereal (sorghum, millet)	—	$AFB_1 + AFB_2 + AFG_1 + AFG_2$	30
	Oilseeds	—	$AFB_1 + AFB_2 + AFG_1 + AFG_2$	10
	Sesame seeds	—	$AFB_1 + AFB_2 + AFG_1 + AFG_2$	20

Country				
Mercosul[20]	Peanuts (with/without hull-peel)	Peanuts (toasted, roasted), peanut butter	$AFB_1 + AFB_2 + AFG_1 + AFG_2$	20
	Corn	Corn flour (whole/no germ)	$AFB_1 + AFB_2 + AFG_1 + AFG_2$	20
	—	Corn meal	$AFB_1 + AFB_2 + AFG_1 + AFG_2$	20
	Milk	—	AFM_1	0.5
	—	Milk powder	AFM_1	5.0
Peru	All foods	All foods	$AFB_1 + AFB_2 + AFG_1 + AFG_2$	10
Suriname	Peanuts	Peanut products	AFB_1	5
	Pulses	—	AFB_1	5
	Corn	—	$AFB_1 + AFB_2 + AFG_1 + AFG_2$	30
Uruguay	Peanuts	Peanut products	$AFB_1 + AFB_2 + AFG_1 + AFG_2$	30
	Food and spices	—	$AFB_1 + AFB_2 + AFG_1 + AFG_2$	20
	—	Soy products	$AFB_1 + AFB_2 + AFG_1 + AFG_2$	30
	—	Dried fruits	$AFB_1 + AFB_2 + AFG_1 + AFG_2$	30
	Cocoa	—	$AFB_1 + AFB_2 + AFG_1 + AFG_2$	10
	—	Baby food	$AFB_1 + AFB_2 + AFG_1 + AFG_2$	3
	Milk	Milk products	AFM_1	0.5
Venezuela	—	Rice flour	$AFB_1 + AFB_2 + AFG_1 + AFG_2$	5

[a] Maximum residue level.

contamination of food is problematic in most parts of the continent. Variable climate conditions and the specific type of commodity can also lead to differences in the prevalence of fungal species in the regions and therefore the toxins produced.[69] The climate in South America is quite diversified, with equatorial and tropical climates in the northern and western regions and subtropical and temperate climates in the central and southern portions of the continent. South America contains areas of dense forests, deserts, and prairies, which make parts of it excellent for growing crops, as well as fungi. Depending on the variations in temperature and relative humidity, AFLs as well as other mycotoxins, such as deoxynivalenol (DON), T-2 toxin, fumonisins (FBs), and zearalenone (ZEA) produced by *Fusarium* spp., occur in the Southern region of South America, including southeastern and southern Brazil. An exception would be the dry climate (semiarid in the north and arid in the south) of Argentina, northern Chile, and the sea coast of Peru.

3.2.1 DROUGHTS AND FOOD SUPPLY

Maintaining food safety and food quality must be balanced by food security and sufficiency of supply. In some areas, food shortages are caused by recurrent climate variations such as drought or too much rain, which lead to crop spoilage by fungi or AFL contamination (fungus stress). Many subsistence farming communities in South America depend on consumption of homegrown crops, regardless of their quality. This is especially true in countries such as Peru, Bolivia, Suriname, or Paraguay, which have lower incomes (resulting in a lack of information, regulations, laboratories for mycotoxin analysis, and monitoring programs). Droughts during the winter of 2003 in a number of countries of southern South America reduced the supply of staple foods. The reality for rural subsistence farmers, throughout all South American countries, is that, regardless of food quality, a lack of economic alternatives frequently means that all food produced must be consumed by the local community. This leads to a AFB_1 exposure. In addition, even with adequate crops, poor traditional storage facilities can lead to fungal deterioration of crops. Considering the above, it is not surprising that fungal contamination of South American staple foods is an area of major concern for food safety experts.

3.3 NATURAL OCCURRENCE OF AFLATOXINS IN SOUTH AMERICAN COUNTRIES

3.3.1 EASTERN SOUTH AMERICA: BRAZIL

3.3.1.1 Brazil Agriculture and Mycotoxins

Brazil is the fifth largest country in the world, with an area of $8,551,996$ km^2; it is the largest country in South America. It has one third of the world's total tropical rain forests, and the four main climate zones of the world (equatorial, tropical, subtropical, and temperate) are represented within. This climate diversity offers optimal conditions of temperature and moisture for the growth of various species of fungi and production of mycotoxins. Moreover, Brazil's soil is very rich in organic matter, allowing significant production of grain and other food commodities. In fact, Brazil has the greatest economic potential of South America and is the main exporter of agricultural products, including soybean, coffee, corn, sugar, and cocoa.

Brazil is divided into five regions (North, Northeast, Central-West, South, and Southeast). The North and Northeast regions have average temperatures of 26°C and rainfall greater than 2500 mm/year. The Central-West and Southeast regions have dry winters, wet summers, and rainfall from 1000 to 1500 mm/year. The South region has milder temperatures with rains of 1500 to 2000 mm/year. It has four very well-defined seasons and balanced amounts of rainfall throughout the year. In fact, it has a climate similar to that of Argentina and Uruguay (in the southern region of South American).

Brazil's well-developed commercial farming sector is located mainly in the South and Central-West regions, where most grain (corn and soy) production is produced for export. Agricultural cooperatives that are spread throughout those regions have high-quality grain and farming equipment and storage facilities that are shared by the members, and they practice excellent grain handling and storage procedures. Prevention and control procedures to reduce mycotoxin formation in crops are very well established by the cooperatives. Nevertheless, mycotoxin-contaminated foods are still present, especially during drought or other stress conditions such as flood or high insect proliferation in the field. The major concern in Brazil is still AFLs. Peanuts are the main crop affected. The prevalence of AFL contamination in corn is lower. Other mycotoxins such as ochratoxin A (OTA), ZEA, DON, and FBs are known to contaminate corn, beans, and wheat in Brazil; however, depending on the Brazilian region, their occurrence varies. Some regions must monitor AFLs and OTA contamination in crops, as well as some *Fusarium* toxins. Conversely, in the southern region of Brazil, *Fusarium* toxins (FBs, trichothecenes, and ZEA) are the biggest concern, but the presence of AFL contamination is constantly being monitored in the South.

With regard to Brazilian laboratory accreditation and monitoring programs, the Brazilian Agriculture Ministry (MA) has established laboratory accreditation for AFL analysis. The MA's reference laboratory is located in the state of Minas Gerais (MG). For a laboratory to be accredited, it must meet several criteria set by the reference laboratory. This includes practices and procedures related to methodology, safety, reference standard handling, sampling procedures, and staff training. Monitoring programs have been carried out throughout the country by the MA[4] and the Ministry of Health (MH) through the Sanitary Vigilance Agency.

3.3.1.2 Aflatoxins in the Brazilian Diet

In Brazil, a large amount of research has been conducted on AFLs and other mycotoxin food contamination as it relates to human health. Studies include the identification of various toxigenic fungi genera and species, mapping of different crop regions, method development, and agronomic and storage practices to reduce AFL contamination. AFLs are currently being monitored in several different foods (in addition to peanuts and corn), as well as AFM_1 in milk. Most data reported on mycotoxins are focused in the Southeast and South regions of Brazil. These data are primarily on processed peanuts and corn but also include beans, rice, wheat, Brazil nuts, dried fruits, and other commodities; however, the data have primarily been obtained for peanuts, corn, and milk due to Brazilian regulatory policies on those foods:

- *Peanuts* — Most of Brazil's peanut production comes from the state of São Paulo.[21] Table 3.4 shows data obtained for AFL contamination from the South and Southeast regions of Brazil for commercialized raw and processed peanuts. The percentage of positive samples varied from about 8 to 80% of total samples, regardless of the harvesting year. Levels ranged from 2 to 16,862 µg/kg. The high level detected in peanut commercialized in Rio Grande do Sul corresponded to a single sample.[44] These data show that AFL contamination in peanuts and peanut products in Brazil is still a serious problem. Occasionally, disturbingly high levels of AFL have been identified in peanuts from São Paulo and Rio Grande do Sul. High AFL levels in peanuts suggest that more adequate control measures should be introduced. São Paulo has improved its agricultural practices for harvesting, storing, and processing peanuts in order to reduce contamination. It is important to emphasize that most of the peanut products in South region came from São Paulo, but these same products were packed and commercialized in the southern states of Rio Grande do Sul, Santa Catarian, or Parana. The most recent data collected for quantifying levels of AFLs were obtained from official and private laboratories that monitor commercialized foods in Brazil.
- *Brazilian staple foods* — The country's main dietary staples include rice and black beans (*Phaseolus vulgaris* L.) but also processed wheat and corn. Although some AFLs have been detected in all of these commodities, the occurrence is not as frequent as for peanuts, and levels of contamination are lower (Table 3.5). In fact, the most prevalent mycotoxin in black beans is OTA.[14] Brazilian corn also has less AFL contamination compared to peanuts. Most reports suggest levels ranging from 2 to 256.4 µg/kg. Only one sample out of 30 from São Paulo was contaminated with 500 µg/kg of AFLs.[58] In a recent survey, 84 corn samples were collected from supermarkets in Santa Catarina for AFL analysis. Only 7 were contaminated with AFLs, with a maximum of 256.4 µg/kg and a mean of 38.6 µg/kg.[37] Wheat contamination has always been reported to be lower than that of peanuts. The detected reported levels were shown to be 38 µg/kg in both 1990 and 2003.[2,72]
- *Milk and dairy products* — When corn and other AFL-contaminated crops are used for feeding dairy cattle, AFB_1 will be metabolized to AFM_1. Levels of AFM_1 have been identified in cows' milk ranging from 0.073 to 2.920 µg/kg (MRL_{Brazil}, 0.5 µg/kg); therefore, AFLs and AFM_1 are currently being monitored in cow silage and feeds and in milk to ensure milk quality for the Brazilian population. As shown in Table 3.6, the state of Minas Gerais reported that cheese from the city of Belo Horizonte had maximum AFM_1 levels of 6.920 µg/kg.[59] In contrast, milk analyzed in

Santa Catarina in 2001 and 2003 did not contain AFM_1 up to the limit of quantification (0.005 µg/kg). These data suggest that high-quality silage and feed are being used to feed milking cows in this region of Brazil.

- *Brazil nuts* — Brazil nuts are an important product for the northern economy of Brazil (especially for the states of Acre, Amazon, Para, and Macapa); however, some constraints are placed on their export due to AFL contamination when sold in shells. Studies have been carried out to evaluate AFL contamination and to assess the risk points prior to harvesting or processing of Brazil nuts. Cartaxo et al.[7] studied the occurrence of filamentous fungi and AFL contamination of Brazil nuts in the shell. Nuts were collected from dense rain forest in the state of Acre after pods fell naturally from trees, and they were analyzed for fungi and AFLs. *Aspergillus flavus* and *A. niger* were the predominant species throughout the harvesting period (90 days). Although fungus was detected, no AFL contamination was observed, suggesting that environmental conditions in the forest are not suitable for toxin production. However, the presence of fungi indicates the need for rigorous quality control of temperature and humidity, especially during transport and storage of in-shell Brazil nuts. When Brazil nuts are shelled, AFLs are seldom detected, as shown in Table 3.7.[67]

3.3.1.3 Population Exposure vs. Staple Foods

Cancer is the second leading cause of death in Brazil. HCC is the eighth most common cancer in the world, and it is the cause of approximately 4% of deaths in Brazil;[22] however, the lack of a proper registry for cases of cancer in several regions of Brazil suggests that the real situation could be worse. In a study carried out by the Brazilian Institute of Cancer, out of a total 2066 HCC cases registered from 1981 to 1985, 166, 110, and 45 cases were from Paraná, Rio Grande do Sul, and Santa Catarina states, respectively (southern region of Brazil). On the other hand, 608 registered cases were from the state of São Paulo (Southeast region).[35,36] Very few Brazilian data have been reported internationally, but they include data from the three Brazilian states of Para, Goias, and Rio Grande do Sul. These states have reported female/male HCC cases of 7/6, 42/34, and 117/83 out of a total of 2093/2794, 3095/3702, and 5436/5865 cases of cancer registered in their respective capital cities (Belem, Goiania, and Porto Alegre).[55]

Brazil has an internationally recognized reputation for AFL contamination in foods, especially peanuts and to a lesser extent their products; however, only one report in the literature has been cited concerning the levels of Brazilian population exposure to AFB_1 and its relations to HCC. Haas et al.[34] reported a mean level of 14.9 pg of AFB_1–lys per mg using blood samples collected from individuals during the *Fiestas juninas* (winter parties where the main foods consumed are made with peanuts and corn). These observations in Brazil were similar to those in the Philippines using the AFB_1 biomarker (AFB_1–alb adducts) detection method.

A relationship between AFB_1 and hepatitis virus (HBV) in the etiology of HCC has been reported.[84,85] Major risk factors for HCC in high-risk areas are chronic infection with HBV and dietary exposure to AFLs. HBV infection can alter hepatic

TABLE 3.4
Aflatoxin Contamination in Raw and Processed Peanuts Commercialized in Different Brazilian Regions

Brazilian Region	State	Year	Aflatoxins	Positive/Total Sample	Positive Sample (µg/kg)		Detection	Ref.
					Range	Mean		
Southeast	SP	1994	$AFB_1 + AFG_1$[a]	32/66	28–997 (B_1) 14–149 (G_1)	NA	TLC	Brigido et al.[6]
	SP	1990–1996	$AFB_1 + AFG_1$	279/1115	63–948	NA	TLC	Fonseca et al.[21]
	SP	1995–1996	$AFB_1 + AFG_1$	41/80	1099 (max.)	266	TLC	Freitas and Brigido[25]
	SP	1990–1991	$AFB_1 + AFG_1$	205/316	4–195	NA	TLC	Freitas and Baldolato[24]
	SP	NA	$AFB_1 + AFG_1$	3/25	2–1000	NA	TLC	Miranda[47]
	SP	1996–1997	AFLs	53/108	29–1178	NA	TLC	Oliveira et al.[54]
	SP	1994	$AFB_1 + AFG_1$	142/321	5–2440	305	TLC	Sabino et al.[62]
	SP	1995–1997	AFB1 + AFG1	62/137	5–536	NA	TLC	Sabino et al.[63]
	SP	NA	AFLs	9.6/10	0.2–44.7	NA	TLC	Stefanovitz et al.[74]
	SP	NA	$AFB_1 + AFG_1$	51/99	8–2152	NA	HPLC	Sylos et al.[75]
	SP	NA	AFLs	8/30	5–233	NA	TLC	Sylos et al.[75]
	SP	NA	AFLs	209/272	222	NA	TLC	Vieira et al.[82]

Southern	RS	NA	AFLs	36/59	805 (max)	NA	TLC	Baldissera et al.[1]
	RS	1997	AFLs	36/213	3.2–25.6	NA	TLC	Pitch et al.[57]
	RS	1986–2000	AFLs	43/524	584–16,862	NA	HPLC	Mallmann[42]
	RS	1998–1999	AFLs	63/210	5–2227	NA	TLC	Nordin[52]
	RS	1997–2000	AFLs	157/544	3–6018	NA	TLC	Nordin[52]
	SC	1997	AFLs	5/72	2[b]–53	NA	TLC	Costa and Scussel[15]
	SC	1997–1998	AFLs	12/131	57–127	NA	TLC	Costa and Scussel[16]
	SC	1998–2000	AFLs	72/246	2[b]–74	NA	TLC	Costa and Scussel[16]
	SC	2000–2002	AFLs	17/147	2[b]–120	NA	TLC	Costa et al.[17]
	SC	1998–1999	AFLs	16/106	33.4–127.3	NA	TLC	Scussel et al.[66]
	SC	2001–2003	$AFB_1 + AFG_1$	19/214	2[b]–641	221.2	TLC	Scussel et al.[67]
Others	FD	1985–1995	$AFB_1 + AFG_1$	89/450	<10–600	NA	TLC	Silva et al.[70]
	PE	1989–1991	$AFB_1 + AFG_1$	21/43	25–518	NA	TLC	Colaço et al.[11]

[a] Brazilian regulation up to 1996 = $AFB_1 + AFG_1$ (30 µg/kg).

[b] LDQ: 2 µg/kg (limit of quantification).

Note: AFLs: aflatoxins (AFB_1, AFB_2, AFG_1, AFG_2); AM, Amazonas; BA, Bahia; FD, Federal District; GO, Goiás; HPLC, high-performance liquid chromatography; MG, Minas Gerais; MG/S, Mato Grosso do Sul; NA, data not available; PE, Pernambuco; PR, Paraná; RJ, Rio de Janeiro; RS, Rio Grande do Sul; SC, Santa Catarina; SP, São Paulo; TLC, thin-layer chromatography.

TABLE 3.5
Aflatoxin Contamination in Raw and Processed Food Commercialized in Different Brazilian Regions

| Brazilian | | | | | Positive/Total | Positive Sample (μg/kg) | | | |
Region	State	Commodity	Year(s)	Aflatoxins	Sample	Range	Mean	Detection	Ref.
Southeastern	MG	Corn	1992–1993	AFLs	0/40	NA	NA	TLC	Nicacio et al.[50]
	SP	Corn	1991	AFLs	1/30	500	NA	TLC	Pozzi et al.[58]
	SP	Organic and morning cereals	1991	AFLs	0/103	NA	NA	TLC	Soares and Furlanni[71]
	SP	Wheat	1990	AFLs	0/20	NA	NA	TLC	Furlong et al.[26]
	SP	Wheat, products	1991	AFLs	0/38	NA	NA	TLC	Soares and Furlanni[72]
Southern	SC	Beans	1997–1998	AFB$_1$	4/72	2[b]	2	TLC	Costa[14]
	SC	Corn	2001–2002	AFLs	1/30	18	NA	TLC	Costa et al.[17]
	SC	Corn	2001–2003	AFLs	7/84	2–256.4	38.6		Laboratório de Micotoxicologia (Labmico)[37]
	RS	Corn	1986–1997	AFLs	1273/2460	NA	36.2	TLC	Santurio, et al.[64]
	SC	Dried fruits	2003	AFLs	3/90	2–6	3.3	TLC	Robert et al.[61]
	RS	Beans	1997–2000	AFLs	2/100	21–38	29.5	TLC	Nordin[52]
	RS	Corn products	1997–2000	AFLs	59/296	3.18–67	NA	TLC	Nordin[52]
	RG	Corn for feed	1993–1994	AFB$_1$	1/115	10	10	TLC	Nordin and Luchese[51]
	RG	Sorghum	1993–2003	AFLs	NA/804	60–146	0–96	TLC	Laboratório de Micotoxicologia (Labmico)[38]
	PR	Wheat and wheat flour	2003	AFBs	0/38	ND	NA	TLC	Birck et al.[2]

Others								
RS	Wheat	1988–1990	AFLs	0/16	NA	NA	TLC	Furlong et al.[27]
Several states[a]	Beans	1996–1997	AFLs	92/481	53.4/160.3	NA	TLC	Scussel et al.[65]
FD	Beans/rice/corn/wheat/feed	1985–1995	AFB$_1$ + AFG$_1$	0/114	NA	NA	TLC	Silva et al.[70]
SP, PR, MGS, MG, GO	Corn	1993–1994	AFB$_1$	97/292	2–89	NA	TLC	Gloria et al.[29]
	Corn	1993–1994	AFB$_2$	33/292	1–17	NA	TLC	Gloria et al.[29]
	Corn	1993–1994	AFG$_1$	13/292	2–85	NA	TLC	Gloria et al.[29]
	Corn	1993–1994	AFG$_2$	7/292	1–6	NA	TCL	Gloria et al.[29]
AM	Feed	1995	AFLs	0/60	NA	NA	TLC	Oliveira et al.[54]
FD	Nuts	1985–1995	AFB$_1$ + AFG$_1$	1/117 +	1200	1200	TLC	Silva et al.[70]

[a] Bahia, Ceara, Goiás, Minas Gerais, Mato Grosso do Sul, Paraná, Rio Grande do Sul, Santa Catarina, and São Paulo.

[b] LDQ: 2 µg/kg (limit of quantification).

Note: AC, Acre; AFLs, aflatoxins (AFB$_1$, AFB$_2$, AFG$_1$, AFG$_2$).; AM, Amazonas; BA, Bahia; FD, Federal District; GO, Goiás; HPLC, high-performance liquid chromatography; MG, Minas Gerais; MGS, Mato Grosso do Sul; NA, data not available; PE, Pernambuco; PR, Paraná; RJ, Rio de Janeiro; RS, Rio Grande do Sul; SC, Santa Catarina; SP, São Paulo; TLC, thin-layer chromatography.

TABLE 3.6
Aflatoxin Contamination in Milk, Milk Products, and Eggs Commercialized In Different Brazilian States

Brazilian Region	State	Commodity	Year(s)	Aflatoxins	Positive/Total Sample	Positive Sample (μg/kg) Range	Positive Sample (μg/kg) Mean	Detection	Ref.
Southeast	MG	Cheese	2000	AFM_1	56/75	0.020–6.920	0.62	HPLC	Prado et al.[59]
	SP	Cheese, yogurt	1990	AFM_1	0/66	ND	ND	HPLC	Sylos and Rodríguez–Amaya[76]
	RJ	Egg	NA	AFB_1	2/120	2–5	3	TLC	Fraga et al.[23]
	RJ	Egg	NA	AFM_1	0/120	ND	ND	TLC	Fraga et al.[23]
	SP	Milk (pasteurized)	1992	AFM_1	4/52	0.073–0.370	0.156	HPLC	Sylos and Rodríguez–Amaya[76]
	SP	Milk *in natura*	1992–1993	AFM_1	0/144	ND	ND	TLC	Correa et al.[13]
	SP	Milk powder (dissolved)	1992–1993	AFM_1	33/300	0.100–1.000	0.270	ELISA	Oliveira et al.[54]
South	RS	Milk *in natura*	1995–1996	AFM_1	11/240	0.198–2.920	NA	HPLC	Mallman et al.[43]
	RS	Milk *in natura* (Tetra Pak)	1995–1996	AFM_1	3/35	0.197–0.418	NA	HPLC	Mallman et al.[43]
	SC	Milk *in natura*[a]	2001	AFM_1	0[a]/20	ND	ND	HPLC	Labmico[37]
	SC	Milk *in natura* (Tetra Pak)	2003	AFM_1	0[b]/25	ND	ND	HPLC	Seo et al.[68]

[a] Tetra Pak carton and polyethylene bags: LDQ, 2 μg/kg (limit of quantification).
[b] LDQ, 0.5 ppb.

Note: ELISA, enzyme-linked immunosorbent assay; HPLC, high-performance liquid chromatography; MG, Minas Gerais; NA, data not available; ND, not detected; RJ, Rio de Janeiro; RS, Rio Grande do Sul; SC, Santa Catarina; SP, São Paulo; TLC, thin-layer chromatography.

metabolism of AFL, leading to increased DNA damage for a given level of exposure. The potency of AFB_1 as a hepatocarcinogenic agent increases some 30-fold in the presence of HBV. A survey on the type and incidence of hepatic diseases (cirrhosis, hepatitis, and HCC) in children and adults (based on registrations at the cancer reference hospital Joana de Gusmao, located in Santa Catarina) was carried out by Hass and Scussel.[33] The incidence of cirrhosis and hepatitis was 46% and 40% of the cases, respectively, while the number of reported HCC cases was 14%. Sixty-four percent of the hepatitis cases were caused by virus infection, and 22% were autoimmune. Hepatitis A and B (HAV and HBV) was found in 7.1% and 21.4%, respectively, of the total virus cases. Although the HCC incidence in Santa Catarina has been low in relation to other hepatic disease studies between 1980 and 1997, the authors emphasize that the hepatitis virus was well represented, especially HBV. In adults, the incidence of hepatitis and HCC were lower (14.3% and 11.7% of the cases, respectively). Apart from HBV that could lead to HCC in the Santa Catarina populace, one should take into account diet and the possibility of AFB_1 contamination. The populace of the southeast and southern regions of Brazil consumes large quantities of peanut snacks and a hard peanut paste (*pacoquinha*) that is preferred by children, who are most sensitive to the toxic effects of AFB_1.

3.3.2 COUNTRIES OF SOUTHERN SOUTH AMERICA: ARGENTINA, CHILE, AND URUGUAY

The countries of South America's southern region are also referred to as the countries of the Southern Cone and are the major exporters of beef and grain. Their terrains consist of desert, grasslands, temperate forests, and glaciers. Argentina and Uruguay have mild winters and regular rainfall throughout the year. Several studies have been published on mycotoxins in Argentina and Uruguay, but data are lacking with regard to the actual AFL exposure of the populace in the southern regions of those countries. The contamination of agricultural crops, such as wheat, corn, sunflower seeds, and soybean, by *Fusarium* toxins is a major concern in these two countries. Peanuts grown for export that are contaminated with AFLs are also an issue, especially in Argentina. Although Uruguay is smaller compared to other South American agricultural countries, it has been investigating mycotoxins in a temperate climate environment. These include esporodesmins, cyclopiazonic acid, and ergot toxins. Uruguay also monitors AFLs throughout the country. Table 3.8 shows data from the southern region for several commodities. Data reported by Resnick et al.[60] showed that AFL contamination in the corn crop was greatest in Argentina from 1990 to 1992, reaching a maximum of 200 µg/kg in 1991. Conversely, for the 1994 and 1995 planting seasons in Argentina, no AFL contamination was observed in 30 samples of corn.[31] During the 1993 to 1995 planting seasons in Uruguay, 71 corn samples were analyzed for the presence of AFL, and contamination reached levels as high as 20 µg/kg. A greater number of samples were analyzed for crops such as wheat, barley, soybean, dried fruits, and vegetables than for corn, and they presented AFL contamination up to the MRL allowed by the Mercosul (20 µg/kg). In Chile, AFL contamination in foodstuffs and feeds has not yet been defined. Research

TABLE 3.7
Aflatoxin Contamination in Tree Nuts Commercialized in Different Brazilian States with Respective LOD[c] and LOQ[d]

Tree Nuts[a]	Sample			Positive Samples (μg/kg)				Detection (μg/kg)				Ref.
	State	Total	Year(s)	Range	Mean	>LOQ[a]	<LOQ	TLC		HPLC		
								LOD	LOQ	LOD	LOQ	
Brazil nuts, in shell	MA	120	2002[b]	8.0/686	171.4	30	ND	2.0	2.0	—	—	Nutricon[53 d]
Brazil nuts, shelled	SP	164	2001–2003	1.0/1.076	179	148	16	<1	≥1	—	—	Esalq[19 c]
	RS	14	2000–2003	ND	ND	ND	ND	5	5	—	—	Cientec[10 c]
	SC	63	2003	ND	ND	ND	ND	2	2	—	—	Laboratório de Micotoxicologia (Lamic)[37 c]
Almonds	SP	09	2001–2003	27.5/27.5	27.5	1	8	<1	≥1	—	—	Esalq[19 c]
Hazelnuts	RS	04	2001–2002	ND	ND	ND	ND	5	5	—	—	Laboratório de Micotoxinas (Lamic)[38 c]
Cashew nuts	SP	23	2002–2003	2.0/8.0	4.4	11	12	<1	≥1	—	—	Esalq[19 d]
Walnuts	RS	14	1993–1903	3.0	0.8	2	12	—	—	—	1	Laboratório de Micotoxinas (Lamic)[38 c]
Pecans	RS	13	2000	ND	ND	ND	ND	5	5	—	—	Cientec[10 c]

[a] Brazil nut samples (in-shell) from Amazon were collected in the Amazon forest and analyzed prior to processing (vapor shelling) for export; those from other states (without shell and peeled) were collected from supermarkets and commercialized in Brazil (packed in plastic containers); other tree nuts (with shell and peel except for cashew nuts) were collected from supermarkets and commercialized in Brazil (packed in plastic bags).

[b] Accredited laboratory data.

[c] Randomly sampled from supermarkets.

[d] Sampling performed by the Ministry of Agriculture, Brazil.

Note: AFLs, aflatoxins (AFB$_1$ + AFB^2 + AFG$_1$ + AFG$_2$); LOD, limit of detection; LOQ, limit of quantification; MA, Amazon; ND, not detected; RS, Rio Grande do Sul; SC, Santa Catarian; SP, São Paulo.

TABLE 3.8

Aflatoxin Contamination in Raw and Processed Food from Southern Region of the South American Continent

Country	Commodity	Crop Year	Aflatoxin	Positive/Total Sample	Range	Mean	Detection	Ref.
					Positive Sample (µg/kg)			
Argentina	Corn[a]	1988, 1993, 1994	AFB$_1$	0/682	ND	ND	TLC	Resnick et al.[60]
Argentina		1990	AFB$_1$	123/491	160 (max)	8	—	Resnick et al.[60]
Argentina		1991	AFB$_1$	90/288	200 (max)	9	—	Resnick et al.[60]
Argentina		1992	AFB$_1$	94/349	30 (max.)	4	—	Resnick et al.[60]
Argentina	Corn[a]	1994–1995	AFLs	0/30	ND	ND	TLC	Gonzáles et al.[31]
Argentina	Polenta[b]	1996	AFB$_1$	65/135	tr–24	NA	TLC	Garbini et al.[28]
Argentina	Cornmeal, flakes[a]	1997	AFLs	0/38	ND	NA	TLC	Solovey et al.[73]
Chile	Several food	1997–2000	AFLs	46/201	0.2–268	NA	HPTLC	Vega et al.[81]
Chile	Peanuts	2001–2003	AFLs	2/466	1.3–17	NA	HPTLC	Vega et al.[80]
Uruguay[c]	Wheat	1993–1995	AFLs	29/123	2–20	NA	TLC	Piñeiro et al.[56]
	Barley, malt	1993–1995	AFLs	12/137	2–20	NA	TLC	Piñeiro et al.[56]
	Rice, soybean, meat products	1993–95	AFLs	0/140	ND	NA	TLC	Piñeiro et al.[56]
	Corn	1993–1995	AFLs	1/71	<20	NA	TLC	Piñeiro et al.[56]
	Oilseeds	1993–1995	AFLs	9/80	2–20	NA	TLC	Piñeiro et al.[56]
	Dried fruits	1993–1995	AFLs	6/157	2–20	NA	TLC	Piñeiro et al.[56]
	Dried vegetables	1993–1995	AFLs	2/100	2–20	NA	TLC	Piñeiro et al.[56]
	Cocoa beans	1993–1995	AFLs	3/91	2–20	NA	TLC	Piñeiro et al.[56]
	Milk	1993–1995	AFM$_1$	7/22	2–20	NA	TLC	Piñeiro et al.[56]
	Butter	1993–1995	AFM$_1$	0/14	ND	ND	TLC	Piñeiro et al.[56]

[a] Buenos Aires, Cordoba, Santa Fe. [b] Hard porridge made with corn flour and hot water. [c] Various regions of the country.

Note: AFLs, aflatoxins (AFB$_1$, AFB$_2$, AFG$_1$, AFG$_2$); HPTLC: high-performance thin-layer chromatography; NA, data not available; ND, rot detected; TLC, thin-layer chromatography; tr, trace (no LDC reported).

projects investigating AFL-producing fungi and their toxigenicity, as well as environment stress to Chilean crops, would provide insight as to whether AFL contamination of foodstuffs is an issue in this country.

3.3.3 COUNTRIES OF NORTHERN SOUTH AMERICA: COLOMBIA, ECUADOR, FRENCH GUYANA, GUYANA, SURINAME, AND VENEZUELA

Countries in the northern region of South America are located near the Ecuador. This implies a region of high humidity with constant rainfalls and hot temperatures throughout the year. The main crops produced in those countries are rice, corn, and coffee. Although rice is produced in all the countries, corn is grown mainly in Colombia, Venezuela, Guyana, and French Guyana. Coffee is the main crop of Colombia and Venezuela. The northern region has countries of Creole culture such as Colombia and Venezuela, thus beans and rice are the primary source of energy. In contrast, in countries of indigenous Inca cultures such as Ecuador, corn is the staple food. Data on mycotoxins in this area have been published only from Colombia and Venezuela. Venezuela carried out work on AFL decontamination with ammonia,[44] and both countries have set standards for AFL contamination in foodstuffs. The Colombian government allows a MRL for AFL of 30 µg/kg in cereals, 20 µg/kg in sesame seeds, 10 µg/kg in oil seeds, and 20 µg/kg in all other foodstuffs. Venezuela regulates for AFLs in rice, with a MRL of 5 µg/kg. Table 3.9 shows levels of AFL contamination in foods as reported by Colombian and Venezuelan officials. Three hundred corn samples were analyzed in Colombia but only 38 were contaminated with AFLs. Diaz et al.[18] reported a maximum level of 103 µg/kg in 2003. Colombia also grows peanuts, which can contain AFLs; however, this issue seems to be more prevalent in animal feedstuffs. Interestingly, feed and feedstuffs produced in 1995 and 1996 had relatively low levels of AFL contamination (mean, 11 and 8 µg/kg; maximum, 66 and 10 µg/kg for AFB_1 and AFB_2, respectively).[9] AFLs were detected in 16.7% of the samples in Venezuela when various peanut-related products (toasted in shell, packed in bags or canned, prepared with sugar and ground as peanut butter) were analyzed. Peanut butter reportedly had the highest levels of AFLs, at 91 µg/kg.[8] Venezuela analyzed corn grown in the crop year 1995/1996 for mycoflora and AFLs. Although the authors[45] of the report did not provide information with regard to the total number of samples contaminated, AFL levels for each region surveyed were as follows: Region I reported trace levels up to 931.7 µg/kg, and region II reported between 508 and 931.7 µg/kg, which are very high AFL contamination levels.

In Ecuador, French Guiana, Guiana, and Suriname, agricultural commodities include rice, corn, cocoa, coffee, and manioc. While AFL or other mycotoxin are probably contaminating their crops, data are very difficult to obtain. A study performed in Ecuador reported AFL contamination in 63% of the samples that were used to feed milking cows.[41] The maximum level of AFL reported was 320 µg/kg. The authors expressed concerns regarding the possibility that AFM_1 transferred via contaminated milk could expose the public, especially children, and cause health-related problems in the future.

TABLE 3.9

Aflatoxin Contamination in Raw and Processed Food from Northern Region of South America

Country	Commodity	Crop Year	Aflatoxin	Positive/Total Sample	Positive Sample (µg/kg) Range	Positive Sample (µg/kg) Mean	Detection	Ref.
Colombia	Feedstuffs	1995–1996	AFB$_1$	39/154	1–66	11	HPLC	Céspedes and Diaz[9]
	Feedstuffs	1995–1996	AFB$_2$	13/154	1–10	8	HPLC	Céspedes and Diaz[9]
Colombia	Feed	1995–1996	AFB$_1$	19/46	2–23	7	HPLC	Céspedes and Diaz[9]
	Feed	1995–1996	AFB$_2$	2/46	1–2	2	HPLC	Céspedes and Diaz[9]
Colombia	Corn	2002	AFB$_1$	38/300	103 (max.)	NA	HPLC	Diaz et al.[18]
Ecuador	Feed (milking cows)	2000	AFLs	25/39	21–320	NA	NA	Lucio et al.[41]
Venezuela	Peanuts:	1997	AFLs	9/54:	NA	–	TLC	Carrara et al.[8]
	Canned			2/16		9		
	Toasted in shell			2/16		28.5		
	In bags			3/15		23		
	Toasted with sugar			2/7		4		
	Peanuts, buttered	1997	AFLs	11/15	tr–91	NA	TLC	Carrara et al.[8]
	Sorghum	NA	AFB$_1$, AFB$_2$, AFG$_1$	31/47	0.375–2.5	NA	TLC	Melendez and Martinez[46]
	Corn	1996	AFB$_1$	2/20	NA	NA	TLC	Loreto and Martinez[40]
	Rice	1996	AFLs	0/20	ND	NA	TLC	Loreto and Martinez[40]
	Corn	1995–1996[a]	AFLs	NA	0–931.7	NA	ELISA	Mazzani et al.[45]
	Corn	1995–1996[b]	AFL	NA	508–908	NA	ELISA	Mazzani et al.[45]

[a]Sabana Larga. [b]Sabana Para.

Note: AFLs, aflatoxins (AFB$_1$, AFB$_2$, AFG$_1$, AFG$_2$); ELISA, enzyme-linked immunosorbent assay; HPLC, high-performance liquid chromatography; NA, data not available; ND, not detected; TLC, thin-layer chromatography; tr, trace (no LDC reported).

3.3.4 COUNTRIES OF WESTERN SOUTH AMERICA: BOLIVIA, PARAGUAY, AND PERU

The indigenous culture (Inca) of Bolivia, Paraguay, and Peru relies on corn and potato as their staple foods. Paraguay produces peanuts, corn, soybean, and wheat. The most prevalent crops in Peru and Bolivia include coffee, rice, corn, and cocoa. Those commodities are considered good substrates for aflatoxigenic fungi growth. They are located in a region where the climate is suitable for fungal growth, but published data are nonexistent or difficult to gather. Bolivia has reported some data on AFL contamination in Brazil nuts and milk (Table 3.10). Although the number of nut samples was not representative of the Bolivian production, a low contamination was detected.[48] No AFM_1 was contaminating the 40 milk samples surveyed by Gonzales and Morales.[32] These countries are the most impoverished in South America, and minimal regulations, monitoring programs, and data are available to evaluate public exposure levels of AFLs.

3.4 ORGANIZATION OF THE SOUTH AMERICAN MYCOTOXICOLOGY RESEARCH COMMUNITY

It is important to mention that Latin American scientists working in mycotoxin research organized the Latin American Society of Mycotoxicology (LASM) in 1996. The society brings together scientists from Mexico, Central America, and South America and provides a forum for mycotoxin discussion, organizes conferences, promotes mycotoxin training courses, and promotes harmonization of methodology and sampling plans. These efforts have led to more reliable data from Latin America. The LASM produces official documents to inform governmental and community sectors on the risks of mycotoxins for human and animal health. Also, it maintains an online database at the LA Mycotoxicology Network site (http://www.ufrrj.br/slam/), where members and nonmembers can share information on current Latin American publications.

3.5 CONCLUSIONS

This review article suggests that some countries of South America (Brazil, Argentina, Uruguay, Venezuela, and Colombia) are addressing the needs of the region by monitoring levels of AFLs in spite of constraints in human and material resources; however, these research activities must be extended to other South American countries, as well. Data on AFL exposure using biomarkers has been carried out only in Brazil. Contamination of raw and processed food consumed by the population of South America is a reality; therefore, the South American scientific community should consider evaluating levels of human exposure to AFB_1 by means of biomarkers. This technique seems to provide improved reliability compared to evaluating exposures through AFL detection in food.[79] It is necessary to set regulations and control measurements for AFL for all South American countries in order to protect the population's health and to promote fair trade at the international level.

TABLE 3.10
Aflatoxin Contamination in Raw and Processed Food from Western Region of South America

Country	Commodity	Crop Year	Aflatoxin	Positive/Total Sample	Positive Sample (µg/kg)		Detection	Ref.
					Range	Mean		
Bolivia	Brazil nuts, raw	NA	AFLs	NA/49	2.4–8.8	NA	TLC	Morales and Flores[48]
	Brazil nuts, processed	NA	AFLs	0/71	ND	ND	TLC	Morales and Flores[48]
Bolivia	Milk	NA	AFM$_1$	5/40	NA	NA	HPLC	Gonzales and Morales[32]

Note: AFLs, aflatoxins (AFB$_1$, AFB$_2$, AFG$_1$, AFG$_2$); NA, data not available; ND, not detected; HPLC, high-performance liquid chromatography; TLC, thin-layer chromatography.

REFERENCES

1. Baldissera, M.A., Ahmad, S.H.E., Pranke, P.H.L., Heinrichs, C.M., Zanadrea, S., and Santurio, J.M., Incidência de aflatoxinas em amendoim farinha de milho, in *VII Encontro de Micotoxinas*, São Paulo, Brazil, May, 4–7, 1992, p. 12.
2. Birck, N.M.M., Lorini, I., and Scussel, V.M., Sanitary conditions and mycotoxins in wheat grains (*Triticum aestivum*) and flour (common and special) through milling process, in *IV Congresso Latinoamericano de Micotoxicologia*, Havana, Cuba, September 24–26, 2003 (disc).
3. Brazil Ministry of Agriculture, MAARA/Ordinance No. 183, March, 21, 1996, published in *Brazilian Official Journal*, March 25, 1996.
4. Brazil Ministry of Agriculture, MAARA/Ministry Directive No. 230, June 10, 1997, published in *Brazilian Official Journal*, June 11, 1997.
5. Brazil Ministry of Agriculture, MAARA/Ministry Directive No. 9, March 24, 2000, published in *Brazilian Official Journal*, March 30, 2000.
6. Brigido, B.M., Badolato, M.I.C., and Freitas, V.P.S., Contaminação de amendoim e seus produtos comercializados na região de Campinas SP por aflatoxinas durante o ano de 1994, *Rev. Inst. Adolfo Lutz*, 55, 85–90, 1995.
7. Cartaxo, C., Souza, J., Correa, T., Costa, P., and Freitas-Costa, O., Occurence of aflatoxins and filamentous fungi contamiantion in Brazil nuts left inside the forest, in *IV Congresso Latinoamericano de Micotoxicologia*, Havana, Cuba, September 24–26, 2003 (disc).
8. Carrara, E., Maritnez, A.J., and Diaz, G., Incidência de aflatoxinas em mani, productos de mani y semillas comestibles, in *II Congresso Latinoamericano de Micotoxicologia*, Maracay, Venezuela, July, 14–18, 1997, p. 82.
9. Cespedes, A.E. and Diaz, CI.J., Analysis of aflatoxins in poultry and pig feeds and feedstuffs used in Colombia, *J. AOAC Int.*, 80, 1215–1219, 1997.
10. Cientec Laboratório de Micotoxinas–RS, *Fundação de Ciência e Tecnologia Registry*, Nordin, N.S.D., Coordinator, Porto Alegre, Rio Grande do Sul, Brazil, 2003.
11. Colaço, W., Feraz, U., and Albuquerque, L.R., Incidência de aflatoxinas em amendoim e produtos derivados consumidos na cidade de Recife, no período de 1999 e 1991, *Rev. Inst. Adolfo Lutz*, 54(1), 1–4, 1994.
12. Companhia Nacional de Abastecimento (Conab), 2003 (http://www.conab.gov.br/).
13. Correa, B. et al., Distribution of molds and aflatoxins in dairy cattle feeds and raw milk, *Rev. Microbiol.*, 28, 279–283, 1997.
14. Costa, L.L.F., Fungos toxigenicos e micotoxinas em feijão (*Phaseolus vulgaris* L.) cultivado no Estado de Santa Catarina, Masters thesis, Florianópolis, SC, Brazil, 2000, 89 pp.
15. Costa, L.L.F. and Scussel, V.M., Ocorrência de micotoxinas em produtos alimentícios comercializados em Florianópolis: Estado de Santa Catarina, in *IX Encontro Nacional de Micotoxinas*, Florianópolis, Brazil, May 18–21, 1998, p. 130.
16. Costa, L.L.F. and Scussel, V.M., Fungi and aflatoxin production in peanuts from southern region of Brazil, in *IXth Internacional Congress of Bacteriology and Applied Microbiology*, Sydney, Australia, August, 16–20, 1999, p. 265.
17. Costa, L.L.F., Scussel, V.M., and Lang, R.M., Aflatoxinas em grãos destinados ao consumo humano comercializados no Estado de Santa Catarina, in *XXIVth Congresso Nacional de Milho e Sorgo, Florianópolis*, Brazil, September 5–10, 2002, p. 116.
18. Diaz, G., Ocorrência natural de aflatoxinas, ocratoxina A, zearalenona e fumonisinas em alimentos de consumo humano y animal em Colômbia, in *IV Congresso Latinoamericano de Micotoxicologia*, Havana, Cuba, September 24–26, 2003 (disc).

19. Esalq–Laboratório de Micotoxicologia, *Escola Superior de Agricultura Luiz de Queiros Registry*, Fonseca, H. and Gloria, E.M, Coordinators, Piracicaba, São Paulo, Brazil, 2003.

20. Fonseca, H., Micotoxinas website, 2003 (http://www.micotoxinas.com.br).

21. Fonseca, H., Calori-Domingues, M.A., Gloria, E.M. Zambello, I.V., and Segatti-Piedade, F., Ocorrência de aflatoxinas em amendoim no Estado de São Paulo nos anos 1990 e 1996, in *IX Encontro Nacional de Micotoxinas*, Florianópolis, Brazil, May, 18–21, 1998, p. 118.

22. Fundação Oncocentro de São Paulo (FOSP), http://www.eu.ansp.br.

23. Fraga, M.E., Direito, G.M., Santana, D.M.N., Barros, G.C., and Rosa, C.A.R., Determinação por cromatografia por camada delgada de aflatoxinas (B1 e M1) e aflaxicol em ovos destinados ao comércio, *Rev. Bras. Med. Vet.*, 18, 172–175, 1996.

24. Freitas, V.P.S. and Baldolato, M.I.C., Incidência de aflatoxinas em paçoca de amendoim consumidas na cidade de Campinas, Estado de São Paulo, *Rev. Inst. Adolfo Lutz*, 52(112), 83–97, 1992.

25. Freitas, V.P.S. and Brigido, B.M., Occurrence of aflatoxins B_1, B_2, G_1 and G_2 in peanuts and their products marketed in the region of Campinas, Brazil, in 1995 and 1996, *Food Addit. Contam.*, 15, 807–811, 1998.

26. Furlong, E.B., Soares, L.M.V., Lasca, C.C., and Kohara, E.Y., Mycotoxins and fungi in wheat during 1990 in test plots in the state of São Paulo, Brazil, *Mycopathology*, 131, 185–119, 1995.

27. Furlong, E.B., Soares, L.M.V., Lasca, C.C., and Kohara, E.Y., Mycotoxins and fungi in wheat stored in elevators in the state of Rio Grande do Sul, Brazil, *Food Addit. Contam.*, 12, 683–688, 1995.

28. Garbini, S., Galli, S., Tomchinsky, E., Delli Santi, V., Gandia, S., Rizzo, I., Varsavsky, E., and Frade, H., Aflatoxinas: control en alimentos a base de harina de maiz, in *II Congresso Latinoamericano de Micotoxicologia*, Maracay, Venezuela July 14–18, 1997, p. 82.

29. Gloria, E.M., Fonseca, H., and Souza, I.M., Occurrence of mycotoxins in maize delivered to the food industry in Brazil, *Tropical Sci.*, 37, 107–110, 1997.

30. Gonzales, H.H.L., Resnik, St., Boca, R.T., and Marasas, W.F.O., Mycoflora of Argentinian corn harvested in the main production area in 1990, *Mycopathology*, 130, 29–36, 1995.

31. Gonzalez, H.H.L., Martinez, E.J., Pacin, A.M., Resnik, S.L., and Sydenharn, E.W., Natural co-occurrence of fumonisins, deoxynivalenol, zearalenone and aflatoxins in field trial corn in Argentina, *Food Addit. Contam.*, 16, 565–570, 1999.

32. Gonzales, S. and Morales, D., Determinación de la concentracion de aflatoxina M1 presente em la leche cruda de vaca proveniente del altiplano Boliviano, in *III Congresso Latinoamericano de Micotoxicologia*, Cordoba, Argentina, November 6–10, 2000, p. 75.

33. Haas, P. and Scussel, V.M., Hepatocellularcercinoma and hepatic diseases in patients from Santa Catarina State, Brazil, in mycotoxin contamination: health risk and prevention, in *Proc. Int. Symp. of Mycotoxicology*, Mycotoxin Supplement, Chiba, Japan, 1999, pp. 231–236.

34. Hass, P., Gong, Y.Y., Turner, P.C., Wild, C.P., and Scussel, V.M., Study of aflatoxin exposure in Brazilian population using the AFB_1–albumin biomarker, in *IV Congresso Latinoamericano de Micotoxicologia*, Havana, Cuba, September 24–26, 2003 (disc).

35. Instituto Nacional do Câncer (INCA), Ministério da Saúde, *Registro Nacional de Patologia Tumoral: Diagnósticos de Câncer Brasil, 1981/1985*, Ministério da Saúde, Rio de Janeiro, 1991, p. 143.

36. Instituto Nacional de Câncer (INCA), Ministério da Saúde, http://www.inca.org.br.

37. Laboratório de Micotoxicologia (Labmico), *Labmico Registry*, Scussel, V.M., Coordinator, Universidade Federal de Santa Catarina, Florianópolis, SC, Brazil, 2003.
38. Laboratório de Micotoxinas (Lamic), *Labmico Registry*, Mallman, C.A., Coordinator, Universidade Federal de Santa Maria, Santa Maria, Rio Grande do Sul, Brazil, 2003.
39. Lopes, C., Ramos, L., Garcia, C., Giolito, I., Yujnovsky, F., and Rodríguez, F., Determinación de aflatoxina B_1 em suero humano por HPLC, in *III Congreso Latinoamericano de Micotoxicologia*, Cordoba, Argentina, November 6–10, 2000, p. 50.
40. Loreto, I.R. and Martinez, A., Utilización de uma técnica de screening para la determinación de micotoxinas em arroz y maiz, in *II Congreso Latinoamericano de Micotoxicologia*, Maracay, Venezuela, July 14–18, 1997, p. 89.
41. Lucio, C., Dolores, E., Fierro, V., and German, A., Evaluación del contenido de micotoxinas em balanceados que utilizan los proveedores de pasteurizadora Quito, S.A., in *II Congreso Latinoamericano de Micotoxicologia*, Maracay, Venezuela, July 14–18, 1997, p. 115.
42. Mallman, C.A., Universidade Federal de Santa Maria, Brazil (http://www.ufsm.br/mycotoxins).
43. Mallman, C.A., Santurio, J.M., Schneider, L.G., Almeida, C.A.A., Fontana, F.Z., and Pozzobon, M.C., Prevalência e sazonalidade da aflatoxina M1 no leite produzido e comercializado no município de Santa Maria, in *II Congreso Latinoamericano de Micotoxicologia*, Maracay, Venezuela, July 14–18, 1997, p. 91.
44. Martinez, A.J., Metodo de amoniacion para raciones contaminadas por aflatoxinas y fumonisinas, in *Atualidades em Micotoxinas e Armazenagem de Grãos*, Scussel, V.M., Ed., Florianópolis, SC, Brazil, 2000, pp. 203–207.
45. Mazzani, C., Borges, O., Luzon, O., Barrientos, V., and Quijada, P., *Aspergillus flavus* e aflatoxinas em granso de cultivares de maislanco em fincas del estado Yaracuy (Venezuela), in *II Congreso Latinoamericano de Micotoxicologia*, Maracay, Venezuela, July 14–18, 1997, p. 96.
46. Meléndez, B. and Martinez, A., Niveles de aflatoxinas em sorgo (sorghum bicolor L. Moench) y su relacion com el contenido de taninos, in *Micotoxinas: Perspectiva Latinoamericana,* Cruz, L.C.H., Ed., Editora Universidade Rurale, Rio de Janeiro, 1996, pp. 157–160.
47. Miranda, M.S., Diagnostico de contaminação por micotoxinas no estado da Bahia 1992/1997, in *Proc. Int. IUPAC Symp. on Mycotoxins and Phycotoxins*, Rome, May 10–14, 1996, p. 95.
48. Morales, D. and Flores, S., Deteccion de la contaminacion com aflatoxina B_1 y G_1 em las diferentes etapas de prodution de la castana (*Bertholleta excelcia*), in *II Congreso Latinoamerciano de Micotoxicologia*, Maracay, Venezuela, July 14–18, 1997, p. 98.
49. Nationmaster, www.nationmaster.com.
50. Nicacio, M.A.S., Prado, G., and Linardi, V.R., Determinação de aflatoxina e identificação da microbiota fungica em milho pos-colheita, *Arq. Biol. Tecnol.*, 38, 851–857, 1995.
51. Nordin, N. and Luchese, R.L.H., Detecção de aflatoxina e zearalenona emmeliho destinado a alimentação animal, *Bol. Soc. Bras. Ciên. Tecnol. Ali.*, 32, 35–39, 1998.
52. Nordin, N.S.D., *Mycotoxin Analysis for Federative Republic of Brazil*, Japan International Agency Country Report, 2000, pp. 41–59.
53. Nutricon Laboratory of Physical, Chemical, and Mycotoxins, *Nutrition Food Analysis Registry*, Pacheco, A.M., Coordinator, Manaus, Amazonas, Brazil, 2003.
54. Oliveira, C.A.F., Germano, P.M.L., Bird, C., and Pinto, C.A., Immunochemical assessment of alfatoxin M_1 in milk powder consumed by infants in São Paulo, Brazil, *Food Addit. Contam.*, 14, 7–10, 1997.

55. Parkin, S.L.W., Ferlay, J., Raymond, L., and Young, J., Cancer incidence in five continents, *IARC Sci. Publ.*, 7, 143, 1997.

56. Pineiro, M., Dawson, R., and Costarrica, M.L., Monitoring program for mycotoxin contamination in Uruguayan food and feeds, *Nat. Toxins*, 4, 242–245, 1996.

57. Pitch, P.H., Nordin, N.S.D., and Noll, I.B., Detecção de aflatoxinas em produtos derivados de milho comercializados na região de Porto Alegre, in *IX Encontro Nacional de Micotoxinas*, Florianópolis, Brazil, May 18–21, 1998, p. 120.

58. Pozzi, C.R., Correa, B., Gambale, W., Paula, C.L., Chacon-Reche, N.O., and Meirelles, M.C.A., Postharvest and stored corn in Brazil: mycoflora interactionm abiotic fictors and mycotoxin ocurrence, *Food Addit. Contam.*, 12, 313–319, 1995.

59. Prado, G., Oliveira, M.S., Pereira, M.L., Abrantes, F.M., Santos, L.G., and Veloso, T., Ocorrência de aflatoxina M1 em amostras de queijo minas comercializado na cidade de Belo Horizonte–Minas Gerais, in *III Congresso Latinoamericano de Micotoxicologia*, Cordoba, Argentina, November 6–10, 2000, p. 103.

60. Resnik, S., Neira, S., Pacin, A., Martinez, E., Apro, N., and Latreite, R., A survey of the natural occurrence of aflatoxins and zearalenone in Argentine field maize: 1983–1994, *Food Addit. Contam.*, 13, 115–120, 1996.

61. Robert, F., Souza, M., Hass, P., Peres, M., Costa, L.L.F., and Scussel, V.M., Mycotoxin evaluation on raisins and other dried fruits, in *IV Congresso Latinoamericano de Micotoxicologia*, Havana, Cuba, September 24–26, 2003 (disc).

62. Sabino, M., Inomata, E.I., Lanusdo, L.C.A., Milanez, T.V., Navas, S.A., and Zorzetto, M.A.P., A survey of the occurrence of aflatoxins in groundnuts (peanuts) and groundnut products in São Paulo, Brazil, in 1994, *Rev. Inst. Adolfo Lutz*, 58, 53–57, 1999.

63. Sabino, M., Milanez, T.V., Lamardo, LC.A., Inomata, E.I., Zorzetto, M.A.P., Navas, S.A., and Stofer, M., Occurrence of aflatoxins in peanuts and peaunt products consumed in the state of São Paulo, Brazil, from 1995 to 1997, *Rev. Microbiol.*, 30, 85–88, 1999.

64. Santurio, J.M., Mallman, C.A., Baldissera, M.A., Maixner, A.E., Montagner, S.T., Goulart K., and Sano, R., Prevalência e sazonalidade de micotoxinas em comodidades e rações no sul do Brasil, in *II Congresso Latinoamericano de Micotoxinas*, Maracay, Venezuela, July 14–18, 1997, p. 77.

65. Scussel, V.M., Costa, L.L.F., Souza, G., Gasparin, J.D., Ribeiro, D., Silva, E.L., and Baldi, F., Estudo da relação entre bolores e ocorrência de micotoxinas em feijão (*Phaseolus vulgaris* L.) classes preto, cores e branco, reavaliação da Portaria 161/87 sub-item 4.5.1.1.1.do MA/SNA, Research Report, Brazilian Beans, Universidade Federal de Santa Catarina, Florianópolis, SC, 1997, 86 pp.

66. Scussel, V.M., Costa, L.L.F., and Souza, G.D., Afaltoxin in raw and processed peanuts commercialized in Santa Catarina State, Brazil, in *Proc. Int. Symp. of Mycotoxicology*, Mycotoxin Supplement, Chiba, Japan, 1999, pp. 220–225.

67. Scussel, V.M., Robert, F., Souza, M., Gonzaga, L., and Haas, P., Quality and mycotoxin evaluation of shelled and in-shell Brazil nuts (*Bertholletia exclesia*), in *Proc. Int. IUPAC Symp. on Mycotoxins and Phycotoxins*, 2004.

68. Seo, S.T., Selaro, M., Gonzaga, L., and Scussel, V.M., Physical chemical chracteristics and aflatoxin M_1 evaluation in milk long life type commercialized in Florianópolis, Southern Brazil, in *IV Congresso Latinoamericano de Micotoxicologia*, Havana, Cuba, September 24–26, 2003 (disc).

69. Shephard, S.S., Aflatoxin and food safety: recent African perspectives, *Toxin Rev. J. Toxicol.*, 22(2), 271–290, 2003.

70. Silva, S.C., Oliveira, J.N., and Caldas, E.D., Aflatoxinas em alimentos comercializados no Distrito Federal de 1985 a 1995, *Rev. Inst. Adolfo Lutz*, 56, 49–52, 1996.

71. Soares, L.M.V. and Furlanni, R.P.Z., Survey of mycotoxins in wheat and wheat products sold in health food stores of the city of Campinas, State of São Paulo, *Rev. Microbiol.*, 27, 41–45, 1996.

72. Soares, L.M.V. and Furlanni, R.P.Z., Survey of aflatoxins, ochratoxin A, zearalenone and esterimatocistine in health foods and breakfast cereals commercialized in the city of Campinas, São Paulo, *Ciên. Tecnol. Ali.*, 16, 126–129, 1996.

73. Solovey, M.M.S., Somosa, C., Cano, G., Pacin, A., and Resnick, S., A survey on fumonisins, deoxynivalenol, zearalenone, and aflatoxin contamination in corn-based food products in Argentina, *Food Addit. Contam.*, 16, 325–329, 1999.

74. Stefanovitz, A.H.O., Fonseca, H., Domingues, M.A.C., and Gloria, E.M., Aflatoxin contamination in different types of peanut kernels by Brazilian official classification, in *Proc. Int. IUPAC Symp. Mycotoxins and Phycotoxins*, Rome, May 27–31, 1996, p. 40.

75. Sylos, C.M., Ocorrência de aflatoxinas, ácido ciclopiazonico e ocratoxina A em alguns alimentos, in *III Congresso Latinoamericano de Micotoxicologia*, Cordoba, Argentina, November 6–10, 2000, p. 122.

76. Sylos, C.M. and Rodriguez-Amaya, D.B., Ocurrence of aflatoxin M_1 in milk and dairy products commercialized in Campinas, Brazil, *Food Addit. Contam.*, 13, 169–172, 1996.

77. Sylos, C.M., Rodriguez-Amaya, D.B., Santurio, J.M., and Baldissera, M.A., Occurrence of aflatoxins and cyclopiazonic acid in Brazilian peanut and corn, in *III Congresso Latinoamericano de Micotoxicologia*, Cordoba, Argentina, November 6–10, 2000, p. 132.

78. Tan, C.K., Lo, D.S.T., Law, N.M. et al., Blood aflatoxin levels in patients with hepatocellular carcinoma in Singapore, *Singapore Med. J.*, 36, 612–614, 1995.

79. Van Rensberg, S.J., Role of epidemiology in the evaluation of mycotoxin health risks in mycotoxins in human and animal health, *Mycotoxins in Human and Animal Health*, Rodricks, J.V. et al., Eds., Pathotox Publishers, Park Forest South, IL, 1977, pp. 699–711.

80. Vega, H.M.R., Saelzer, G., Rios, E., Herlitz, C., Bastias, M., and Veja, M., Contaminación por micotoxinas de alimentos y piensos em Chile: resultados del trienio 1997–2000, in *III Congresso Latinoamericano de Micotoxicologia*, Cordoba, Argentina, November 6–10, 2000, p. 123.

81. Vega, M. Chile, micotoxinas, globalizacion. Las micotoxinas son um problema?, in *IV Congresso Latinoamericano de Micotoxicologia*, Havana, Cuba, September 24–26, 2003 (disc).

82. Vieira, A.P., Pinho, B., and Badiale-Fulong, E., Avaliação da qualidade e ocorrência de micotoxinas em farinhas, pães, pizzas comercializadas na zona sul do Rio Grande do Sul, in *Proc. IX Int. IUPAC Symp. on Mycotoxins and Phycotoxins*, Rome, May, 12–16, 1996, p. 112.

83. World Cancer Research Fund and AICR, Patterns of diet, in *Food, Nutrition and the Prevention of Cancer: A Global Perspective*, Potter, J.D., Ed., American Institute for Cancer Research, Washington, D.C., 1997, 670 pp.

84. Wild, C.P., Fortuin, M., Donato, F., Whittle, H.C., Hall, A.J., Wolf, C.R., and Montesano, R., Aflatoxin, liver enzymes, and hepatitis B virus infection in Gambia children, *Cancer Epidemiol. Biomarkers Prev.*, 2(6), 555–561, 1993.

85. Wild, C.P., Hasegawa, R., Barraud, L., Chutimatawin, S., Chapot, B., Ito, N.E., and Montesano, R., Aflatoxin–albumin adducts: a basis for comparative carcinogenesis between animals and humans, *Cancer Epidemiol. Biomarkers Prev.*, 5, 179–189, 1995.

4 Aflatoxins in Maize: A Mexican Perspective

Javier Plasencia

CONTENTS

4.1 INTRODUCTION

Aflatoxins are secondary metabolites produced by *Aspergillus flavus* and *A. parasiticus* that occur in nuts and cereal crops. These compounds have a high acute toxicity, as well as immunosuppressive, mutagenic, teratogenic, and carcinogenic activities and are classified as group 1 carcinogens by the International Agency for Research on Cancer (IARC).[1] Aflatoxin contamination of maize (*Zea mays* L.) is a problem almost everywhere this crop is grown; however, distinct environmental and cultural conditions determine the severity of the problem in each region. Mexico is the center of origin for maize, and its agricultural production is characterized by a wide diversity of genotypes grown under distinct environmental conditions. Most of the maize produced in Mexico is grown under nonirrigated conditions, mainly in subsistence agriculture by peasants for their own consumption or for selling at a local market. Most of the corn varieties produced under these conditions are open-pollinated landraces, which are locally adapted genotypes of corn selected empirically for many years and the seeds of which are saved and planted next season. Maize consumption in Mexico is high in comparison with other countries and most of it is consumed in the form of alkaline-cooked products such as tortillas. The

TABLE 4.1

Production Statistics of Maize in Distinct Geographical Areas in Mexico in Irrigated and Nonirrigated Surfaces

Producing Region	Irrigated			Nonirrigated		
	Harvested Area (ha)	Production (ton)	Yield (ton/ha)	Harvested Area (ha)	Production (ton)	Yield (ton/ha)
Northwest	317,372	2,685,712	8.46	71,215	80,234	1.12
Northeast	120,105	636,593	5.30	446,462	422,637	0.94
North-Central	5281	18,151	3.43	1604	917	0.57
Southeast	101,407	304,189	2.99	2,981,047	5,057,125	1.69
Central	237,694	1,109,276	4.66	1,362,064	3,353,222	2.46
West	283,933	1,529,351	5.38	1,889,636	4,955,961	2.62
Total	1,065,792	6,283,272	—	6,752,028	13,870,096	—

Note: Data correspond to the spring/summer and fall/winter cycles in 2001.

Source: Ministry of Agriculture, Mexico (SAGARPA), www.sagarpa.gob.mx.

average consumption of tortillas in Mexico is estimated to be as high as 325 g per day per person. In this chapter, aflatoxin contamination is examined in terms of the particular conditions of maize production, and consumption in Mexico and significant efforts directed toward reducing mycotoxin incidence in the field and in storage and decreasing exposure in foods are reviewed.

4.2 MAIZE PRODUCTION IN MEXICO

Maize production systems in most regions in Mexico differ from those in the rest of North America. In most parts of the country, especially in the south, maize production is characterized by small-scale, labor-intensive agriculture. Plow agriculture relies on improved seeds and fertilizers provided by federal and state agencies. Also, a very traditional maize-growing system known as slash-and-burn agriculture is practiced on the hillsides and is characterized by intercropping with beans, squash, or peppers.[2,3] Maize is grown in all 32 states in Mexico; these states are divided into six geographical regions with quite distinct environmental and production conditions (Table 4.1). Approximately 86% of the corn production area is nonirrigated, has low fertilizer and pesticide input, and employs open-pollinated genotypes adapted to the region. Such practices result in low yields that vary from 0.6 to 2.6 ton/ha, and the production in these regions accounts for 69% of the national production. In contrast, irrigated surfaces account for only 14% of the total maize production area in the country but contribute 31% of the total grain production. This agricultural system is especially productive in northwest Mexico, in the states of Sonora and Sinaloa, and it more resembles production systems in the United States, as hybrid seed is employed with high fertilizer and pesticide input. Also, higher yields are obtained (8.5 ton/ha) which are also comparable to those obtained in the United States.[4]

In Mexico, 7.9 million ha are planted annually with maize distributed throughout several different types of environments. According to the international center for maize and wheat breeding (CIMMYT), in Mexico approximately 39.5% of the maize is grown in lowland tropical environment, mainly in southeastern and western Mexico. Approximately 40% of the maize is grown on highlands, distributed throughout southeastern and central Mexico, and the remaining 20.5% corresponds to subtropical production with practically no production in temperate zones. A distinct feature of maize cultivation is the wide diversity of genotypes grown.[4] Only 21% of the maize planted in Mexico utilizes improved seeds and commercial hybrids, and the remaining 79% of the area devoted to maize is planted with farm-saved seed from open-pollinated genotypes called *landraces*.[5] A landrace is comprised of a population of individuals with similar genotypes that possess distinguishable characteristics from other populations. Some modern races of maize, derived from the natural outcrossing of older races, are widely grown in Mexico. Landrace *Vandeño* is grown in the southern Pacific coast (west), *Tuxpeño* in the lowlands of the Gulf of Mexico (southeast), *Chalqueño* and *Celaya* in the center of the country, and *Tabloncillo* on the west coast. Most of these landraces perform well and have been employed as progenitors in crosses to develop inbreds and varieties adapted to certain growing regions.[6] In contrast to hybrid corn production, most peasant farmers save seed from these open-pollinated varieties from one harvest to plant again next season. Such practice facilitates cross-pollination among races, resulting in the high genetic diversity of maize genotypes.

4.3 AFLATOXIN INCIDENCE IN MAIZE AND MAIZE-DERIVED PRODUCTS

Aflatoxin incidence has been documented in Mexico by surveys in different regions of maize and maize-derived products. Probably one of the most significant episodes of aflatoxin contamination of maize occurred at Tamaulipas in northeastern Mexico where aflatoxin levels above 100 µg/kg were reported in practically all corn harvested in 1989. The government response was to implement a supervising program to analyze the crop for the following years, resulting in 87% of the crop being quarantined due to high aflatoxin levels.[7] About 60,000 tons of contaminated maize (295 µg/kg average total aflatoxins) were stored in a warehouse, and various approaches were considered to reduce aflatoxin levels and utilize the grain. Sieving the whole kernel achieved only a discrete reduction to 66 µg/kg; ammonium decontamination was considered, but it was not economically viable. Finally, the contaminated corn was sold to a company devoted to alcohol production.[8]

A contrasting case is that in the state of Sonora in northwest Mexico, where a survey to determine aflatoxin incidence was conducted using 133 corn samples harvested in 1996, 1997, and 1998. Only 33% of the samples contained aflatoxins at levels of 1 to 18 µg/kg, and the higher aflatoxin content determined in this survey was still below the 20-µg/kg imposed by sanitary regulations.[9]

TABLE 4.2
Action Levels of Aflatoxin in Maize Intended
for Various Uses in Animal Feeding,
According to Regulation NOM-188 of the
Mexican Ministry of Health

Species/ Production Stage	Maximum Level Allowed (μg/kg)
Poultry (egg production)	100
Swine (25–45 kg)	100
Swine (above 45 kg)	200
Mature swine for breeding	100
Ruminants	100
Finishing beef cattle	300

Studies on aflatoxin occurrence in foods intended for human consumption have also been conducted, mainly in urban areas. Maize grain and tortillas sampled from 50 nixtamal mills and tortilla stores, respectively, were analyzed for aflatoxin content, and the authors reported 45 to 272 fluorescent particles in a 4.54-kg sample, indicating aflatoxin levels well above 20 μg/kg.[10] Chemical analyses by thin-layer chromatography (TLC) detected aflatoxin B_1 in 72% of the maize or tortilla samples tested, whereas aflatoxins B_2, G_1, and G_2 were not found. Aflatoxin B_1 content varied from 5 to 500 μg/kg, although most of the positive samples contained 40 μg/kg.[10]

In a more recent survey conducted in the city of Monterrey in northern Mexico, aflatoxin content was analyzed in kernelled corn employed for tortilla making. The authors employed high-performance liquid chromatography (HPLC) separation with fluorescent detection and found aflatoxins B_1 and G_1 in 36 out of the 41 samples tested. Aflatoxin B_1 concentrations ranged from 5 to 465 μg/kg and aflatoxin G_1 from 1.6 to 57 μg/kg. Most of the samples tested (58%) contained aflatoxin levels above the permitted 20-μg/kg regulatory level.[11]

4.4 AFLATOXIN REGULATIONS IN MEXICO

Regulations for aflatoxin levels in cereals are imposed by two sets of guidelines published by the Ministry of Health. Regulation NOM-188-SSA1-2002 establishes the maximum level of aflatoxins allowed in cereals intended for human and animal consumption, as well as the sanitary requirements for the transport and storage of products.[12] Action levels are set at 20 μg/kg (ppb) total aflatoxins, and when this concentration is exceeded the cereal can only be used for animal consumption (see Table 4.2). This regulation is also applied for imported cereals and establishes guidelines for sampling, subsampling, and analyses of total aflatoxins in cereals by the HPLC method with fluorescence detection. The resolution to establish such regulatory levels was made by officials from various government agencies, such as Ministry of Health, Ministry of Agriculture, and Ministry of Commerce, who are

TABLE 4.3

Maximum Allowable Levels of Aflatoxin in Nixtamalized Products for Human Consumption, According to Regulations NOM-187 and NOM-188 of the Mexican Ministry of Health

Product	Maximum Level (µg/kg)
Masa	12
Nixtamalized maize tortillas	
Nixtamalized maize tostadas	
Nixtamalized flour for the preparation of tortillas and tostadas	
Wheat tortillas	20
Whole-grain tortillas	
Flour for the preparation of wheat tortillas	
Whole grain for tortilla preparation	

supported by researchers from academic institutions and representatives from the grain-handling industry. These action levels are comparable to those established by the U.S. Food and Drug Administration (FDA) for food and feed[13] and are consistent with the regulatory levels in many countries.[14] In addition, guideline NOM-187-SSA1/SCFI-2002 sets the sanitary specifications that businesses devoted to producing *masa*, tortillas, and tostadas must meet.[15] Maximum aflatoxin levels permitted are set at 12 µg/kg for *masa*, tortillas, and other related products (see Table 4.3). No regulations have been established for aflatoxin M levels in milk.

4.5 BREEDING FOR RESISTANCE TO AFLATOXIN CONTAMINATION

Because maize is a cross-pollinated crop, high heterozygosity and genetic variability are maintained. The development of inbred lines by controlled self-pollination through several generations has achieved some homozygosity. By crossing two unrelated inbred lines, the vigor lost during inbreeding is recovered to produce hybrid corn. The development of hybrid corn has led to remarkable improvements in lodging resistance, disease resistance, cold tolerance, drought tolerance, insect resistance, and seed quality. As with most plant diseases, genetic resistance is the most effective and economical means to reduce *Aspergillus flavus* infection and aflatoxin contamination; however, the identification of maize genotypes with significant resistance to *A. flavus* has not been an easy task due to the multiple interactions among host, pathogen, and environment.

Four major genetically controlled components for which variability exists appear to be involved in determining the fate of *A. flavus*–maize interactions: (1) resistance to the infection process, (2) resistance to toxin production, (3) plant resistance to insect damage, and (4) tolerance to environmental stress.[16] The latter two components have an indirect influence because their effects only reduce aflatoxin contamination and do not prevent it. Although differences among genotypes have been found, heritability of the trait appears to be low, and the genotype/environment interactions may often mask true differences among genotypes.

One of the main challenges to identifying resistance is that the inoculation technique should achieve functional levels of inoculum while still resembling a natural infection process.[17] *Aspergillus flavus* is a weak pathogen that was first thought to infect kernels exclusively through wounds produced by insects. Although insect injury is not an essential prerequisite for kernel infection, it is difficult to achieve high levels of infection without first causing mechanical damage to the kernel; however, injury-type inoculation (e.g., pinboard method) overcomes any physical barrier of the pericarp or other structural portion of the kernel intended to prevent fungal invasion, and any morphological type of resistance would be missed in the evaluation.[18] The use of silk inoculation represents a more natural infection process. When resistance selection studies have relied on natural infection, the distinction of genotypes is complicated, although gross distinctions can be made.[19]

Isolates of *Aspergillus flavus* show a wide diversity in aflatoxin production, and no conclusive evidence supports the supposition that aflatoxin biosynthesis facilitates kernel infection. The qualitative and quantitative variations in aflatoxin production by different isolates of *A. flavus* have not been addressed in studies designed to differentiate genotypes for resistance to aflatoxin contamination, as many studies have employed one isolate, NRRL 3357, primarily because of its stability in producing aflatoxin B_1.[20–23] By using a single isolate that is not representative of the entire population, sources of resistance could be missed in the selection process.

Distribution of *Aspergillus flavus* within a single ear usually follows an aggregated pattern, further complicating the selection of resistant genotypes, as differentiation is usually based on aflatoxin levels. Ear-to-ear variation in aflatoxin content is evident from a study in which *A. flavus*-infected ears were analyzed, and it was found that all of them contained detectable levels of aflatoxin ranging from 1 to 1560 ng/g. Such variability is also observed within an ear; when individual kernels were analyzed, most of them (72%) did not contain aflatoxins, but other kernels contained levels ranging from 400 to 80,000 ng/g.[24] Clustering of aflatoxin in the ears requires large, representative samples of ears, and this is often difficult because typically little material is available in any breeding program. Although controlling the production of aflatoxin is the ultimate desired trait, the percentage of kernels infected with *A. flavus* is a suitable alternative to test as well.[25]

In contrast to the United States, where practically 100% of the total acreage is grown with maize hybrids, in Mexico the open-pollinated varieties prevail. A 2-year study to compare resistance to aflatoxin contamination among four maize hybrids and eight open-pollinated varieties (OPVs) was conducted in the United States at eight locations relying on natural infection. Aflatoxin levels for the 12 entries ranged from a low of 37 ppb for "Yellow Creole" (OPV) to a high of 772 ppb for "Huffman" (OPV). This latter variety yielded a level well above the rest of the entries. The mean aflatoxin level for the eight open-pollinated varieties was 214 ppb (range, 37 to 772 ppb), which was significantly higher than the mean of 63 ppb (range, 42 to 81) for the four hybrids. The hybrids as a group generally appeared to be less prone to aflatoxin contamination than the open-pollinated varieties; however, aflatoxin levels for two of the OPV were in the range of the hybrids.[19]

Because drought stress is frequently associated with higher aflatoxin levels and given the difficulties in selecting *Aspergillus flavus-* or aflatoxin-resistant hybrids, a complementary approach to this problem is the breeding of drought-tolerant varieties. CIMMYT has succeed in developing drought-tolerant cultivars, either by avoiding stress through early flowering or truly performing well in terms of yield under drought conditions;[4,26] however, some maize genotypes, such as "Huffman," are drought tolerant but yield higher aflatoxin levels in the field under appropriate conditions.[19,25]

Although selecting maize genotypes with high resistance levels to *Aspergillus flavus* infection has been a very difficult task due to multiple environmental interactions and low heritability, some genotypes highly resistant to *A. flavus* infection and aflatoxin contamination have been characterized. Germplasm GT-MAS:gk, released in 1992 and registered as a source of resistance,[27] is a maize population originating from an open-pollinated ear that shows high heterogeneity in resistance to *A. flavus* and maturity.[28] A more refined analysis of the genetic variation of this population was performed with randomly amplified polymorphic DNA (RAPD), and its association with resistance to *A. flavus* and aflatoxin production established three distinct groups. Group I contained the most resistant individuals, group II had the least resistance, and group III was intermediate.[29] Biochemical and molecular analyses within this population have identified differences in wax and cutin layers content of the kernel pericarp[30] and the expression of antifungal proteins in the maize kernels[31] as being responsible for this enhanced resistance to *A. flavus*.

The resistant genotypes within GT-MAS:gk germplasm are an interesting case of a heterogeneous population derived from open-pollinated varieties. Mexican maize landraces constitute, as well, broad heterogeneous populations that might serve as source of resistance to *Aspergillus flavus*. Recently, plant breeders of maize landraces, or *criollos*, are recognizing them as valuable sources of good agronomic qualities such as yield, ear length and diameter, flowering time, and plant height,[32] but no assessment of resistance to *A. flavus* has been performed yet. Despite the multiple environmental interactions and low heritability, it has been demonstrated that genetic resistance to aflatoxin contamination can be identified within maize populations, thus it is worthwhile to take advantage of the wide genetic diversity in maize landraces to pursue the incorporation of this trait into Mexican varieties. The CIMMYT maize germplasm bank is an excellent and reliable source, as are the collections obtained by plant breeders in different states.

Alternative sources of resistance are the wild relatives of maize. In Mexico, the center of origin of *Zea mays*, other species have been identified. One of them, *Z. diploperennis*, was recognized in Jalisco, Mexico, as a diploid and perennial species that readily crosses with *Z. mays* to produce fertile plants.[33] Crosses between inbred Mo20W × teosinte yielded hybrids that consistently show significantly lower concentrations of aflatoxin B_1 than other hybrids tested. Plants were subjected to naturally occurring infection in three different locations, and it was demonstrated that the resistance observed was inherited and not due to environmental variation.[34]

4.6 TRANSGENIC MAIZE AND AFLATOXIN CONTROL IN MEXICO

Although the role of insects in fostering *Aspergillus* colonization of maize kernels is well documented, little evidence suggests that transgenic corn expressing insecticidal proteins has a significant effect on reducing aflatoxin contamination.[35] In contrast, several studies have reported a protective effect of Cry-type proteins in maize against *Fusarium* kernel rot and fumonisin accumulation.[35] Cry-type proteins constitute a family of insecticidal proteins from *Bacillus thuringiensis*, the genes of which have been incorporated into several crops to confer protection against insect pests. In corn, several hybrids expressing distinct Cry-type proteins have been developed and widely used in the United States, Canada, Argentina, and other maize-producing countries.

In experiments set up at two locations, 11 transgenic corn hybrids expressing CryIA protein and their corresponding nontransgenic counterparts were evaluated for *Aspergillus* ear rot and aflatoxin levels. No significant differences were found between these groups, but a possible resistance mechanism could have been missed because *Aspergillus* was inoculated with a pinboard, thus overcoming one physical barrier against insects.[36]

A different hybrid, Mon840, expresses Cry2Ab protein and apparently provides more protection against lepidopteran pests. This hybrid was analyzed to determine whether it is more resistant to aflatoxin contamination than other transgenic hybrids as well as nontransgenic hybrids. This study relied on natural insect infestation of corn earworm and fall armyworm, and *Aspergillus flavus* was silk-inoculated in drought-stressed plants. The results of the 2-year study showed that aflatoxin content in the Mon840 hybrid was significantly lower than nontransgenic Bt and Cry1Ab hybrids during the first year and significantly lower than nontransgenic Bt hybrids in the second year.[37]

Although the use of transgenic hybrids combined with crop management shows some promise in controlling fungal kernel rot and aflatoxin contamination in maize, this technology has not been implemented in Mexico due to a moratorium imposed by the Mexican government on planting transgenic maize. The government's precautionary approach is based on the Cartagena Protocol on Biosafety.[38] Because Mexico is the center of origin of maize, efforts have been made to prevent gene flow from transgenic hybrids to maize landraces and to other *Zea* species. A stringent regulation has been imposed that bans planting transgenic maize seed until scientific and technical data determine the importance of gene flux in areas with high biodiversity in maize landraces and wild relatives to assess the potential consequences. Despite this moratorium, controversial evidence of the presence of transgenes in Mexican open-pollinated varieties has been found,[39] and discussions are now taking place regarding what detrimental effects, if any, these transgenes could have.

4.7 *ASPERGILLUS* MANAGEMENT IN THE FIELD

Preharvest *Aspergillus flavus* colonization of maize and aflatoxin contamination also occur, and several environmental factors have been associated with fungal infection. In maize grown at 32 to 38°C, approximately 73% kernel infection was observed, whereas only 7.5% infection was observed in maize grown at 21 to 26°C.[40] Relative humidity above 86% also favors colonization and aflatoxin production in the field. Drought-stressed plants also have a higher incidence of infection by *A. flavus*.[41] Another significant field study was conducted in northeastern Mexico to evaluate the consequences of certain crop management practices on aflatoxin contamination levels in maize. When a well-adapted hybrid (H-422) was planted early, before mid-February, at a density of 55,000 plants per ha with adequate irrigation and insect control, very low aflatoxin levels (0 to 6 μg/kg) were recorded in the 3-year study. In contrast, late planting of hybrid G-2340 at a high density (75,000 plants per ha) with neither irrigation nor insect control yielded significantly increased aflatoxin levels (63 to 167 μg/kg). Among the variables tested, the two main factors closely associated with aflatoxin contamination were late planting and ear insect damage.[42] Most of the insect specimens collected at harvest time were sap beetles, representing a five-species complex. The findings obtained from this study were implemented as part of a mandatory corn management system in the northeastern region to increase yields and reduce aflatoxin contamination levels.

Insects have long been recognized as playing a role in aflatoxin contamination of maize, although initial attempts to identify species that might vector *Aspergillus flavus* were inconclusive. Moths of the corn earworm, *Helicoverpa zea*, and European corn borer, *Ostrinia nubilalis*, have been implicated as vectors of this fungus.[43] A 5-year study carried out in northeastern Mexico identified three predominant micro-leopterans species in maize: *Carpophilus freemani*, a sap beetle; *Sitophilus zeamais*, a maize weevil; and *Cathartus quadricollis*, a squarenecked grain beetle. *C. freemani* constitutes nearly 90% of all collected species, and its incidence increased up to 28-fold in damaged ears. Crop phenology studies demonstrated that the sap beetle remains abundant during all maize grain developmental stages, and its presence shows a strong association with *Aspergillus flavus* infection and aflatoxin contamination.[44] Insecticide application is a significant factor of *A. flavus* management in Mexico.

4.8 *ASPERGILLUS* MANAGEMENT DURING STORAGE

Initially, *Aspergillus flavus* and other *Aspergillus* spp. were considered exclusively storage fungi, and aflatoxin contamination was believed to be primarily a storage problem that is very severe in many rural areas that lack the infrastructure for drying and other appropriate storage conditions. Usually, corncobs are harvested at moisture contents that vary between 25 and 30% and are dried under the sunlight to reach a moisture content of 12 to 14%. Research has been conducted to determine the optimum temperature and moisture content of grains during storage to prevent *Aspergillus* spp. growth and aflatoxin production. In maize inoculated with *A. flavus* and stored at 27°C for 30 days with varying moisture contents, an association between moisture content and aflatoxin levels was established. At 16% moisture, aflatoxin levels reached 116 μg/kg, while at 22% moisture aflatoxin levels of 2166 μg/kg were obtained.[45] In this same study, the authors tested the protective effects of propionic acid salts (6.5 to 12.5 L/ton) on fungal growth and aflatoxin production. All grains treated with ammonium, calcium, or sodium propionates yielded very low *Aspergillus flavus* growth and aflatoxin levels (2 to 5.6 μg/kg) at all moisture contents; however, when grain viability was tested in all treatments, low germination rates were observed, suggesting the need to reduce the fungistatic dose.[45]

Insect damage is invariably associated with *Aspergillus flavus* infection during storage, and a stronger correlation is observed at high insect infestation, particularly by the maize weevil (*Sitophilus zeamais*), a primary pest of stored grain; thus, control of the insect populations with insecticides can reduce *A. flavus* infection in stored maize, but these options are expensive for small farmers in countries such as Mexico. Moreover, several insect pests have developed resistance to various pesticides, and the strict environmental regulations for the use of some products have limited the available options for insect control. A genetic approach to identifying maize geno-types with increased resistance to insect infestation and eventually to *Aspergillus* infection has been taken on by CIMMYT researchers, who tested 21 maize varieties against 5 insect pests, including coleopteran and lepidopteran species, during storage at 26.5°C and 75% relative humidity. Some maize varieties showed a range of resistance to coleopteran pests but not to lepidopteran species, indicating different resistance mechanisms. Most of the varieties tested were landraces obtained in Mexico, from the highlands, mid-altitude environments, or tropics.[46] Although the authors did not test the resistance to *A. flavus* infection and aflatoxin production, this landrace collection provides a starting point for research on the advantages of the wide genetic diversity present in Mexican maize landraces. Ideally, management of stored grain to prevent aflatoxin contamination must include utilizing resistance to insects and fungi, as well as controlled environmental conditions.

4.9 GRAIN TREATMENTS TO REDUCE AFLATOXIN LEVELS

The most practical and economical action to reduce aflatoxin levels is to prevent *A. flavus* colonization and aflatoxin production in the field; however, when the grains have been contaminated, several approaches might reduce aflatoxin levels in corn. A government program implemented by the national agricultural research institute (INIFAP) to reduce mycotoxin levels in corn-based feeds tested Mexican alumino-silicates characterized as Atapulgita and Fuller earth. The protective effect was evaluated by mixing the aluminosilicates at 0.05% and 1% with chicken feed that contained over 100 µg/kg aflatoxin during a 3-week feeding assay. The performance of these materials was comparable to that of novasil, a commercial aluminosilicate, based on the chickens' weight gain and feed efficiency.[47] When higher doses of aflatoxins occur in feeds, the protective effect of aluminosilicates is not as notable. Lara et al.[48] tested organoaluminosilicates (0.3%) in a long-term feeding study of hens fed a diet containing 4000 µg/kg aflatoxin, and they evaluated egg yield. In hens fed with the aflatoxin, diet egg production was reduced 20%, while for hens fed a contaminated diet amended with the organoaluminosilicate, egg production decreased by only 10%. Thus, the binding material provided a 50% protection.

Chemical inactivation of aflatoxins in corn has been achieved with high efficiency by ammoniation, by utilizing either the high-pressure/high-temperature format or the atmospheric pressure/ambient temperature format. The former is employed primarily for feedmill operations, and the latter is employed for on-farm use.[49] Inactivation efficiency has been evaluated by analyzing the micronucleus and sister chromatid exchange rate in peripheral blood cells of mice fed with contaminated maize. Animals fed with aflatoxin contaminated/inactivated corn had 45% lower levels of induced cytogenetic damage than those animals fed with the contaminated maize.[50,51] Although efficient, ammoniation is expensive and unaffordable for most farmers in Mexico, especially those involved in subsistence agriculture.

The use of binding agents to reduce aflatoxin levels in feeds is a common practice in large poultry farms in Mexico that perform tests to determine aflatoxin levels in feeds. Further research would be helpful to develop and test binding materials in Mexico in order to reduce costs and avoid importing foreign technology.

4.10 FATE OF AFLATOXINS IN PROCESSED MAIZE PRODUCTS

Maize use and consumption in Mexico are different than in the United States, as approximately 60% of the total maize used (imports and production) is intended for human consumption, in contrast to 4% in the United States. Maize is a staple in Mexico, and most of it is consumed as nixtamalized products such as tortillas. Per capita consumption of this type of food is estimated at 120 kg per year. In rural zones, maize accounts for 70% of the total calories and 50% of the protein intake. Nixtamalization is a pre-Columbian process that consists of cooking maize grains in a lime (CaO) solution for up to an hour and then steeping it overnight. The steeping liquor is discarded, and the cooked maize or nixtamal is rinsed to remove the excess calcium hydroxide and pericarp. The softened maize grains are ground to produce *masa*, from which tortillas are made. These flat, round cakes are later baked on a hot plate. This alkaline cooking procedure improves flavor, starch gelatinization, water uptake, and niacin availability because the bound forms of niacinogen and niacytin are released during hydrolysis. Studies on protein content and availability report contrasting results; although a higher protein efficiency ratio has been found in tortillas in comparison to raw corn, other authors have suggested that cross-linking, racemization, degradation, and formation of Maillard browning complexes with sugars lead to reduced protein digestibility and nitrogen retention in lime-cooked products. These contradictory results are primarily due to such distinct variables as corn genotype, lime concentration, and cooking/steeping time.[52]

The effect of nixtamalization on aflatoxin levels has been studied as well, also with contrasting results. Researchers have employed both naturally contaminated corn and aflatoxin-amended corn for these experiments. Abbas et al.[53] employed naturally contaminated corn to prepare nixtamal by boiling the kernels in 2% lime and baking at 110°C. Through TLC analyses, the authors found the average concentrations of aflatoxins B_1 and B_2 in the tortillas were only 40% and 28% lower, respectively, than those in the corn kernels. The thermal and alkaline treatment to which the corn is subjected during nixtamalization hydrolyzes the lactone ring of the aflatoxin molecule, generating a salt that might be solubilized and further decarboxylated;[54] however, acidification of the final product causes reformation of the aflatoxin molecules that were not degraded. This recyclization could be of toxicological significance, as the acid environment in the stomach would contribute to it. In another study, Price and Jorgensen[55] studied the effects of nixtamalization on naturally contaminated corn that was cooked in various lime concentrations with different cooking times. When the nixtamal was prepared by boiling the kernels for 1 hour in 0.25% limewater, aflatoxin levels were reduced from 142 to 38 μg/kg, representing a 73% reduction; however, upon acidification, the aflatoxin levels in the tortilla increased to 110 μg/kg due to reformation of the lactone ring. Most of the studies on the effect of nixtamalization on reducing aflatoxin levels report that pH values increase up to 13 in the steeping liquor. Nevertheless, the pH of the final product only increases less than 1 pH unit, from 5.83 in the corn kernel to 6.73 in the tortilla, due to the potent buffer capacity of the endosperm contents.[54] The preparation of tortilla chips, for example, involves a deep-frying step, which further reduces aflatoxin levels as higher temperatures are employed. During tortilla chip preparation, frying at 190°C reduced the aflatoxin content 75% in naturally contaminated maize containing 43 μg/kg total aflatoxins.[54]

Apparently significant differences exist in the chemical stability of the B- and G-aflatoxin series. When tortillas prepared from corn contaminated with the four most abundant aflatoxins (B_1, B_2, G_1, G_2) were analyzed, a 100% reduction was observed in aflatoxins G_1 and G_2, which are more susceptible to alkaline hydrolysis than the B-series aflatoxins.[56]

Extrusion is a food-preparation technology in which mixing, shearing, cooking, puffing, and drying take place in a single continuous process. This method has been adapted to prepare *masa* for tortillas as it offers several advantages, such as lower energy consumption and less liquid waste. In addition, the tortillas have superior nutritional properties, including higher levels of amino acids, vitamins, fiber, and protein than the traditional tortillas prepared by nixtamalization.[57] Studies comparing traditional nixtamalization and extrusion processes for reducing aflatoxin content showed that the traditional nixtamalization reduces levels of aflatoxin B_1 by 94%, whereas the extrusion process decreases them by 46%. In an attempt to achieve a 100% reduction with the extrusion process, 0.3% lime and 1.5% hydrogen peroxide were added, but at these concentrations the taste and aroma of the tortillas were negatively affected.[58] In a similar study, the authors employed *Aspergillus*-inoculated samples of corn (29 and 93 μg/kg) to test the traditional nixtamalization and the extrusion processes. Reductions of 90% and 70% were achieved with the traditional and the extrusion processes, respectively.[59]

The levels of aflatoxins and byproducts obtained after the nixtamalization process and the effects due to high consumption of tortillas and related products are not fully resolved. Serious epidemiological and toxicological research must be done in this area to determine the extent to which this is a public health issue in Mexico.

4.11 CONCLUSIONS

Although significant research on *Aspergillus flavus* infection and aflatoxin contamination in Mexico has been conducted, more information is necessary to determine the incidence of this toxin and other mycotoxins in maize. In most parts of Mexico, maize is grown under nonirrigation conditions, predisposing plants to drought stress and *A. flavus* infection; however, no studies have directly compared aflatoxin contamination levels in distinct agricultural systems. Management of *A. flavus* infection and aflatoxin contamination should rely on agronomic strategies such as early planting to avoid drought stress, complemented with insect control and adequate storage conditions. Unfortunately, most of these practices are not economically feasible for small subsistence peasants in southeast and central Mexico. The wide diversity of maize genotypes represented in landraces offers the opportunity to encourage resistance to kernel rot and aflatoxin contamination, and further research is required to identify such sources of resistance and compare them to other characterized germplasms, such as the GT-MAS:gk population. The unique conditions of maize production and consumption in Mexico warrant the development of an integrated research program to characterize the aflatoxin production potential of *Aspergillus* spp. in distinct growing regions in Mexico, as well as the characterization of maize genotypes, including locally adapted landraces, open-pollinated varieties, and hybrids in terms of aflatoxin resistance. An assessment of the aflatoxin production potential of *A. flavus* isolates from maize in distinct geographical regions in Mexico would contribute to selecting and characterizing strains to be employed in breeding programs and to obtain epidemiological data on the incidence of this toxigenic pathogen. Finally, risk assessment of aflatoxin consumption in Mexico due to maize-derived products contamination must be conducted with respect to total aflatoxin ingestion via nixtamalized products. Analytical techniques and validation methods for aflatoxin analysis in this type of foods must be developed by Mexican laboratories in order to determine the degree of exposure of Mexican population to aflatoxins. Such studies should be considered to determine action level limits for regulatory purposes.

REFERENCES

1. Peraica, M., Radic, B., Lucic, A., and Pavlovic, M., Toxic effects of mycotoxins in humans, *Bull. World Health Org.*, 77(9), 754–766, 1999.
2. Brush, S.B., *In situ* conservation of landraces in centers of crop diversity, *Crop Sci.*, 35(2), 346–354, 1995.
3. Brush, S.B., Bio-cooperation and the benefits of crop genetic resources: the case of Mexican maize, *World Dev.*, 26(5), 755–766, 1998.
4. Pingali, P. L. and Pandey, S., Meeting world maize needs: technological opportunities and priorities for the public sector, in *CIMMYT 1999–2000 World Maize Facts and Trends — Meeting World Maize Needs: Technological Opportunities and Priorities for the Public Sector,* Pingali, P.L., Ed., CIMMYT, Mexico, 2001, pp. 1–20.
5. Perales, R.H., Brush, S.B., and Qualset, C.O., Landraces of maize in Central Mexico: an altitudinal transect, *Econ. Bot.*, 57(1), 7–20, 2003.
6. Reyes-Castaneda, P., *El maiz y su cultivo*, AGT Editor, Mexico, 1990, 460 pp.
7. Lopez, M.J., Carvajal, M., and Ituarte, B., Supervising programme of aflatoxins in Mexican corn, *Food Addit. Contam.*, 12(3), 297–312, 1995.
8. Carvajal, M. and Arroyo, G., Management of aflatoxin contaminated maize in Tamaulipas, Mexico, *J. Agric. Food Chem.*, 45(4), 1301–1305, 1997.

9. Garcia-Aguirre, G., Martinez-Flores, R., and Melgarejo-Hernandez, J., Inspeccion para aflatoxinas en el maiz almacenado o transportado en el estado de Sonora, 1998, *Ann. Inst. Biol. Mexico*, 72(2), 187–193, 2001.

10. Torreblanca, R.A., Bourges, R.H., and Morales J., Aflatoxin in maize and tortillas in Mexico: mycotoxin carryover from grain to tortillas in Mexico, in *Aflatoxin in Maize: Proceedings of the Workshop*, Zuber, M.S., Lillehoj, E.B., and Renfro, B.L., Eds., CIMMYT, Mexico, 1987, pp. 310–317.

11. Torres-Espinosa, E., Acuna-Askar, K., Naccha-Torres, L.R., Montoya-Olvera, R., and Castrellon-Santa Anna, J.P., Quantification of aflatoxins in corn distributed in the city of Monterrey, Mexico, *Food Addit. Contam.*, 12(3), 383–386, 1995.

12. Secretaria de Salud, *Norma Oficial Mexicana NOM-188-SSA1-2002: Productos y servicios — Control de aflatoxinas en cereales para consumo humano y animal, Especificaciones sanitarias*, Diario Oficial de la Federacion, Mexico, 2002, pp. 23–42.

13. Wood G.E. and Trucksess M. W., Regulatory control programs for mycotoxin-contaminated food, in *Mycotoxins in Agriculture and Food Safety*, Sinha, K.K. and Bhatnagar, D., Eds., Marcel Dekker, New York, 1998, pp. 459–481.

14. FAO, *Worldwide Regulations for Mycotoxins 1995: A Compendium*, Food and Nutrition Paper 64, Food and Agriculture Organization, United Nations, Rome, Italy, 1997, pp. 1–41.

15. Secretaria de Salud, *Norma Oficial Mexicana, NOM-187-SSA1/SCFI-2002: Productos y Servicios — Masa, tortillas, tostadas y harinas preparadas para su elaboración y establecimientos donde se procesan, Especificaciones sanitarias*, Información comercial, Métodos de prueba, Diario Oficial de la Federación, Mexico, 2003, pp. 9–37.

16. Widstrom, N.W., Breeding strategies to control aflatoxin contamination of maize through host plant resistance, in *Aflatoxin in Maize: Proceedings of the Workshop*, Zuber, M.S., Lillehoj, E.B., and Renfro, B.L., Eds., CIMMYT, Mexico, 1987, pp. 212–220.

17. Windham, G.L., Williams, W.P., Buckley, P.M., and Abbas, H.K., Inoculation techniques used to quantify aflatoxin resistance in corn, *J. Toxicol. Toxin Rev.*, 22(2–3), 317–329, 2003.

18. Scott, G.E. and Zummo, N., Host-plant resistance: screening techniques, in *Aflatoxin in Maize: Proceedings of the Workshop*, Zuber, M.S., Lillehoj, E.B., and Renfro, B.L., Eds., CIMMYT, Mexico, 1987, pp. 221–235.

19. Zuber, M.S., Darrah, L.L., Lillehoj, E.B., Josephson, L.M., Manwiller, A., Scott, G.E., Gudauskas, R.T., Horner, E.S., Widstrom, N.W., Thompson, D.L., Bockholt, A.J., and Brewbaker J.L., Comparison of open-pollinated maize varieties and hybrids for preharvest aflatoxin contamination in the southern United States, *Plant Dis.*, 67(2), 185–187, 1983.

20. LaPrade, J.C. and Manwiller, A., Aflatoxin production and fungal growth on single cross corn hybrids inoculated with *Aspergillus flavus*, *Phytopathology*, 66(5), 675–677, 1976.

21. Zuber, M.S., Calvert, O.H., Kwolek, W.F., Lillehoj, E.B., and Kang, M.S., Aflatoxin B_1 production in an eight-line diallel of *Zea mays* infected with *Aspergillus flavus*, *Phytopathology*, 68(9), 1346–1349, 1978.

22. Scott, G.E. and Zummo, N., Sources of resistance in maize to kernel infection by *Aspergillus flavus* in the field, *Crop Sci.*, 28(3), 504–507, 1988.

23. Scott, G.E., Zummo, N., Lillehoj, E.B., Widstrom, N.W., Kang, M.S., West, D.R., Payne, G.A., Cleveland, T.E., Calvert, O.H., and Fortnum, B.A., Aflatoxin in corn hybrids field inoculated with *Aspergillus flavus*, *Agron. J.*, 83(3), 595–598, 1991.

24. Lillehoj, E.B. and Zuber, M.S., Variability in corn hybrid resistance to preharvest aflatoxin contamination, *J. AOCS*, 12, 970–973, 1981.

25. Tubajika K.M. and Damann K.E., Sources of resistance to aflatoxin production in maize, *J. Agric Food Chem.*, 49(5), 2652–2656, 2001.

26. Meng, E. and Ekboir, J., Current and future trends in maize production and trade, in *CIMMYT 1999–2000 World Maize Facts and Trends: Meeting World Maize Needs — Technological Opportunities and Priorities for the Public Sector*, Pingali, P.L., Ed., CIMMYT, Mexico, 2001, pp. 35–44.

27. McMillan, W.W., Widstrom, N.W., and Wilson, D.M., Registration of GT-MAS:gk maize germplasm, *Crop Sci.*, 33, 882, 1993.

28. Guo, B.Z., Butron, A., Li, H., Widstrom, N.W., and Lynch, R.E., Restriction fragment length polymorphism assessment of the heterogeneous nature of maize population GT-MAS:gk and field evaluation of resistance to aflatoxin production by *Aspergillus flavus*, *J. Food Prot.*, 65(1), 167–171, 2002.

29. Guo, B.Z., Li, R.G., Widstrom, N.W., Lynch, R.E., and Cleveland, T.E., Genetic variation within maize population GT-MAS:gk and the relationship with resistance to *Aspergillus flavus* and aflatoxin production, *Theor. Appl. Genet.*, 103(4), 533–539, 2001.

30. Guo, B.Z., Russin, J.S., Cleveland, T.E., Brown, R.L., and Widstrom, N.W., Wax and cutin layers in maize kernels associated with resistance to aflatoxin production by *Aspergillus flavus*, *J. Food Prot.*, 58, 296–300, 1995.

31. Guo, B.Z., Chen, Z.Y., Brown, R.L., Lax, A.R., Cleveland, T.E., Russin, J.S., Mehta, A.D., Selitennikoff, C.P., and Widstrom, N.W., Germination induces accumulation of specific proteins and antifungal activities in corn kernels, *Phytopathology*, 87, 1174–1178, 1997.

32. Carballoso-Torrecilla, V., Mejia-Contreras, A., Balderrama-Castro, S., Carballo-Carballo, A., and Gonzalez-Cossio, F.V., Divergence in native maize populations in high valleys of Mexico, *Agrociencia*, 34(2), 167–174, 2000.

33. Iltis, H.H., Doebley, J.F., Guzman-M.R., and Pazy, B., *Zea diploperennis* (Gramineae): a new teosinte from Mexico, *Science*, 203, 186–187, 1979.

34. Wallin, J.R., Widstrom, N.W., and Fortnum, B.A., Maize populations with resistance to field contamination by aflatoxin B_1, *J. Sci. Food Agric.*, 54, 235–238, 1991.

35. Dowd, P.F., Insect management to facilitate preharvest mycotoxin management, *J. Toxicol. Toxin Rev.*, 22(2–3), 327–350, 2003.

36. Maupin, L.M., Clements, M.J., Walker, S.L., and White, D.G., Effect of CryIA(b) on *Aspergillus* ear rot and aflatoxin production in commercial corn hybrids, *Mycopathologia*, 155(1), 106, 2002.

37. Odvody, G.N. and Chilcutt, C.F., Aflatoxin and insect response in south Texas of near-isogenic corn hybrids with Cry1Ab and Cry2Ab events, *Mycopathologia*, 155(1), 107, 2002.

38. Galvez, A., Mexico, in *The Cartagena Protocol on Biosafety: Reconciling Trade in Biotechnology with Environment and Development*, Bail, C., Falkner, R., and Marquard, H., Eds., Earthscan Publications and the Royal Institute of International Affairs, London, 2002, pp. 207–211.

39. Quist, D. and Chapela, I.H., Transgenic DNA introgressed into traditional maize landraces in Oaxaca, Mexico, *Nature*, 414, 541–543, 2001.

40. Jones, R.K., Duncan, H.E., Payne, G.A., and Leonard, K.J., Factors influencing infection by *Aspergillus flavus* in silk-inoculated corn, *Plant Dis.*, 64(9), 859–863, 1980.

41. Jones, R.K. and Duncan, H.E., Effect of nitrogen fertilizer, planting date, and harvest date on aflatoxin production in corn inoculated with *Aspergillus flavus*, *Plant Dis.*, 65, 741–744, 1981.

42. Rodriguez-del-Bosque, L.A., Impact of agronomic factors on aflatoxin contamination in preharvest field corn in northeastern Mexico, *Plant Dis.*, 8(9), 988–993, 1996.

43. Wicklow, D.T., Epidemiology of *Aspergillus flavus* in corn, in *Aflatoxin in Corn: New Perspectives*, Shotwell, O.D. and Hurburgh, C.R., Eds., Iowa State University, Ames, 1991, pp. 315–328.

44. Rodríguez-del-Bosque, L.A., Leos-Martínez, J., and Dowd, P.F., Effect of ear wounding and cultural practices on abundance of *Carpohilus freemani* (Coleoptera: Nitidulidae) and other microlepidopterans in maize in northeastern Mexico, *J. Econ. Entomol.*, 91(4), 796–801, 1998.

45. Moreno-Martínez, E., Vázquez-Badillo, M., and Facio-Parra, F., Use of propionic acid salts to inhibit aflatoxin production in stored grains of maize, *Agrociencia*, 34(2), 477–484, 2000.

46. Savidan, A., Tritrophic Interactions in Maize Storage Systems, Ph.D. dissertation, University of Neuchatel, 2002, 224 pp.

47. Marquez-Marquez, R., Tejada-de-Hernandez, L., and Madrigal-Bujaidar, E., Genotoxicity of aflatoxin B_1 and its ammonium derivatives, *Food Addit. Contam.*, 12(3), 425–429, 1995.

48. Lara, J., Medina, J.C., Aviles, J.L., Fierro, J.A., Garcia, I., and Munoz, J., Use of an organoaluminosilicate to reduce the toxic effect of a mixture of aflatoxin and zearalenone on the egg production of laying hens, in *Proc. Second World Mycotoxin Forum*, The Netherlands, February, 2003.

49. Lopez-Garcia, R. and Park, D.L., Effectiveness of post-harvest procedures in management of mycotoxin hazards, in *Mycotoxins in Agriculture and Food Safety*, Sinha, K.K. and Bhatnagar, D., Eds., Marcel Dekker, New York, 1998, pp. 407–433.

50. Marquez-Marquez, R., Madrigal-Bujaidar, E., and Tejada-de-Hernandez, L., Genotoxic evaluation of ammonium inactivated aflatoxin B_1 in mice fed with contaminated corn, *Mutat. Res.*, 299(1), 1–8, 1993.

51. Marquez-Marquez, R.N. and Tejada-de-Hernandez, L., Aflatoxin adsorbent capacity of two Mexican aluminosilicates in experimentally contaminated chicken diets, *Food Addit. Contam.*, 12(3), 431–433, 1995.

52. Rooney, L.W. and Serna-Saldivar, S.O., Food uses of whole corn and dry-milled fractions, in *Corn Chemistry and Technology*, White, P.J. and Johnson, L.A., Eds., American Association of Cereal Chemists, St. Paul, MN, 2003, pp. 399–429.

53. Abbas, H.K., Mirocha, C.J., Rosiles, R., and Carvajal, M., Effect of tortilla preparation process on aflatoxins B_1 and B_2 in corn, *Mycotoxin Res.*, 4, 33–36, 1988.

54. Torres, P., Guzmán-Ortiz, M., and Ramírez-Wong, B., Revising the role of pH and thermal treatments in aflatoxin content reduction during the tortilla and deep frying processes, *J. Agric. Food Chem.*, 49(6), 2825–2829, 2001.

55. Price, R.L. and Jorgensen, K.V., Effects of processing on aflatoxin levels and on mutagenic potential of tortillas made from naturally contaminated corn, *J. Food Sci.*, 50(2), 347–357, 1985.

56. Arriola, M.C., Porres, E., Cabrera, S., Zepeda, M., and Rolz, C., Aflatoxin fate during alkaline cooking of corn for tortilla preparation, *J. Agric. Food Chem.*, 36(3), 530–533, 1988.

57. Gomez-Aldapa, C.A., Martinez-Bustos, F., Figueroa-Cardenas, J.D., Ordorica-Falomir, C.A., and Gonzalez-Hernandez, J., Chemical and nutritional changes during preparation of whole corn tortillas prepared with instant flour obtained by extrusion process, *Arch. Latinoam. Nutr.*, 46, 315–319, 1996.

58. Elias-Orozco, R., Castellanos-Nava, A., Gaytan-Martínez, M., Figueroa-Cardenas, J.D., and Loarca-Piña, G., Comparison of nixtamalization and extrusion processes for a reduction in aflatoxin content, *Food Addit. Contam.*, 19(9), 878–885, 2002.
59. Mendez-Albores, J.A., Arambula-Villa, G., Loarca-Piña, M.G., Gonzalez-Hernandez, J., Castano-Tostado, E., and Moreno-Martinez, E., Aflatoxins' fate during the nixtamalization of contaminated maize by two tortilla-making processes, *J. Stored Prod. Res.*, 40(1), 87–94, 2004.

5 Worldwide Regulations on Aflatoxins*

Hans P. van Egmond and Marco A. Jonker

CONTENTS

5.1 INTRODUCTION

Food legislation and inspection already existed in ancient times.[1] A need has always been felt for some control on the quality of foodstuffs. Such control is intended to protect the health of the consumer and to prevent misrepresentation with respect to the composition of food. In the days of early food legislation, the protection of food was mostly local, and municipal ordinances were promulgated for that purpose. Later, when auxiliary sciences such as bacteriology, chemistry, and microbiology developed, statutory regulations were initiated in many countries, leading, at the beginning of the twentieth century, to the adoption of official food legislation and regulations.

---

* The opinions expressed are those of the authors and do not necessarily represent the decisions or the stated policy of the National Institute for Public Health and the Environment.

Currently, food regulations not only prohibit the introduction, delivery for introduction, or receipt in commerce of adulterated or misbranded food, but they also often include specific regulations that impose limits or tolerances on the concentration of particular contaminants in foods. Such contaminants may be of industrial or natural origin. Among the natural contaminants (mycotoxins, phycotoxins, bacterial toxins), the most detailed and extensive regulations exist for the mycotoxins, and now approximately 100 countries in the world have established regulations for mycotoxins. These regulations always include the aflatoxins. Currently, virtually all countries with fully developed market economies have established specific limits and regulations for aflatoxins in food and feed. This is not always the case in the developing countries. The fact that countries do not have specific regulations for mycotoxins in food and feed does not mean that mycotoxin problems do not exist or that they are ignored. Often, countries can fall back on general food legislation to protect their citizens and livestock from the harmful effects of these compounds.

Of the mycotoxins, the aflatoxins were the first to be regulated, a process beginning in the late 1960s. For many years, regulations for other mycotoxins remained scarce. This situation is changing now, and mycotoxins for which currently proposed or active limits and regulations exist include the naturally occurring aflatoxins, aflatoxin M_1, agaric acid, deoxynivalenol, diacetoxyscirpenol, ergot alkaloids, fumonisins (B_1, B_2, and B_3), HT-2 toxin, ochratoxin A, patulin, phomopsins, sterigmatocystin, T-2 toxin, and zearalenone. In this article, however, the focus is on the aflatoxins. Those interested in learning about the specific regulations established or in development for the other mycotoxins are referred to the full FAO document.[2]

5.2 MAIN FACTORS INFLUENCING MYCOTOXIN REGULATIONS

Several factors, of both a scientific and socioeconomic nature, may influence the establishment of mycotoxin limits and regulations. These include:

- Availability of toxicological data
- Availability of data on the occurrence of mycotoxins in various commodities
- Knowledge of the distribution of mycotoxin concentrations in lots
- Availability of analytical methods
- Legislation in other countries with which trade contracts exist
- Need for sufficient food supply

5.2.1 HAZARD IDENTIFICATION AND HAZARD CHARACTERIZATION

Regulations are primarily made on the basis of known toxic effects. With regard to the mycotoxins currently considered most significant (aflatoxins, ochratoxin A, patulin, fumonisins, zearalenone, and some trichothecenes, including deoxynivalenol), the Joint Expert Committee on Food Additives (JECFA), a scientific advisory body of the World Health Organization (WHO) and the Food and Agriculture Organization (FAO), has recently reevaluated the hazards these mycotoxins present.[3]

JECFA provides a mechanism for assessing the toxicity of additives, veterinary drug residues, and contaminants. Safety evaluations of contaminants incorporate various steps in a formal health risk assessment approach.

The qualitative indication that a contaminant can cause adverse effects on health (hazard identification) is usually included in the information presented to JECFA for evaluation. Similarly, qualitative and quantitative evaluations of the nature of the adverse effects (hazard characterization) are embodied in the datasets that are present. The evaluation of toxicological data carried out by JECFA normally results in the estimation of a provisional tolerable weekly intake (PTWI) or a provisional tolerable daily intake (PTDI). The use of the term "provisional" reflects the tentative nature of the evaluation, in view of the paucity of reliable data on the consequences of human exposure at levels approaching those with which JECFA is concerned. In principle, the evaluation is based on the determination of a no-observed-adverse-effect level (NOAEL) in toxicological studies and the application of an uncertainty factor. The uncertainty factor means that the lowest NOAEL in animal studies is divided by 100 (10 for extrapolation from animals to humans, and 10 for variation between individuals) to arrive at a tolerable intake level. In cases where the data are inadequate, JECFA uses a higher safety factor.

This hazard assessment approach does not apply for toxins where carcinogenicity is the basis for concern, as is the case with the aflatoxins. Assuming that a no-effect concentration limit cannot be established for genotoxic compounds such as the aflatoxins, any small dose will have a proportionally small effect. Not allowing any amount of aflatoxins would then be appropriate, if these were not natural contaminants that can never completely be eliminated without outlawing the contaminated food or feed. In these cases, JECFA does not allocate a PTWI or PTDI; instead, it recommends that the level of the contaminant in food should be reduced so as to be as low as reasonably achievable (ALARA). The ALARA level, which may be viewed as the irreducible level for a contaminant, is defined as the concentration of a substance that cannot be eliminated from a food without involving the discard of that food altogether or without severely compromising the availability of major food supplies. This covers the case of the JECFA evaluations of aflatoxins made in 1998.

At their 1998 meeting, JECFA considered estimates of the carcinogenic potency of aflatoxins and the potential risks associated with their intake. At that meeting, JECFA reviewed a wide range of studies, conducted in both animals and humans, that provided qualitative and quantitative information about the hepatocarcinogenicity of aflatoxins.[4] The Committee evaluated the potency of these contaminants, linked those potencies to intake estimates, and discussed the potential impact of hypothetical standards for aflatoxin B_1 (10 and 20 µg/kg, which are often occurring limits for aflatoxin B_1; see section on general observations) on the overall risk for certain populations. The conclusion was made that reducing the standard from 20 µg/kg to 10 µg/kg would not result in any observable difference in the rates of liver cancer.

In February 2001, a special JECFA session was devoted to mycotoxins.[3] The mycotoxins evaluated or reevaluated at this 56th JECFA meeting included fumonisins B_1, B_2, B_3, and B_4; ochratoxin A; deoxynivalenol; T-2 and HT-2 toxins; and aflatoxin M_1. The evaluation of aflatoxin M_1 was the most interesting, as JECFA responded to a request by the Codex Committee on Food Additive and Contaminants at its Thirty-Second Session[5] to "examine exposure to aflatoxin M_1 and to conduct a quantitative risk assessment" to compare the application of two standards for contamination of milk (0.05 µg/kg and 0.5 µg/kg, limits currently applied in the European Union and the United States, respectively). The calculations showed that, with worst-case assumptions, the projected risks for liver cancer attributable to the use of the proposed maximum aflatoxin M_1 levels of 0.05 µg/kg and 0.5 µg/kg are very small, and no significant health benefit would be gained if the 0.5-µg/kg limit were reduced to 0.05 µg/kg. In the further development of tolerable daily intake (TDI) levels to maximum tolerated levels for aflatoxins in food and feed for national or international (Codex Alimentarius) purposes, factors other than hazard assessment play a role; these will be discussed below.

5.2.2 Exposure Assessment

In addition to information about toxicity, exposure assessment is another ingredient of risk assessment. Reliable data on the occurrence of mycotoxins in various commodities and food intake data are needed to prepare exposure assessments. The quantitative evaluation of the likely intake of mycotoxins is quite difficult. At its 56th Meeting, JECFA stressed the importance of the use of validated analytical methods and the application of analytical quality assurance (see also Section 5.2.4) to ensure that the results of surveys provide a reliable assessment of intake.[3] In most of the JECFA reviews of mycotoxins, the analytical data on the levels of contamination were often inadequate from developed countries and nonexistent for developing countries. Because most mycotoxin contamination is heterogeneous (including the naturally occurring aflatoxins), sampling is an important consideration in the development of information on the levels of contamination (see also Section 5.2.3).[6]

In the European Union, efforts to assess exposure are undertaken within SCOOP (Scientific Cooperation on Questions Relating to Food) projects, funded by the European Commission. The SCOOP projects are targeted to make the best estimates of intake of several mycotoxins by European Union inhabitants. In the 1990s, these activities resulted in a report on the exposure assessment of aflatoxins,[7] and later SCOOP reports for several other mycotoxins followed. The SCOOP data are being used by the European Commission's European Food Safety Authority (EFSA) for its evaluation and advisory work on the risks to public health arising from dietary exposure to certain mycotoxins.

5.2.3 Sampling Procedures

The distribution of the concentration of mycotoxins in products is an important factor to be considered in establishing regulatory sampling criteria. The distribution can be very heterogeneous, as is the case with aflatoxins in peanuts. The number of contaminated peanut kernels in a lot is usually very low, but the contamination level within a kernel can be very high. If care is not taken for representative sampling, the aflatoxin concentration in an inspected lot may be wrongly estimated. Theoretically, consumption of peanuts could lead to an accidental high single dose of aflatoxins, rather than a chronic intake at a relatively low level. A similar situation could occur with pistachio nuts and figs. The risk to both consumer and producer must be considered when establishing sampling criteria for products in which mycotoxins are heterogeneously distributed. The design of sampling procedures has been an international concern for a long time; for example, Codex Alimentarius[5] and FAO[8] have been active in this area. Discussions in working groups of these international organizations are continuously carried out to find a harmonized international approach. Examples of official sampling plans for aflatoxins are those for peanuts and corn practiced in the United States and for peanuts in the European Union. The U.S. Department of Agriculture (USDA) requires three 22-kg laboratory samples to average less than 15 ng total aflatoxins per g for acceptance. In the European Union, one 30-kg laboratory sample is required to test less than 15 ng total aflatoxins per g for raw peanuts destined for further processing, and three 10-kg laboratory samples must all test less than 4 ng total aflatoxins per g (and 2 ng aflatoxin B_1 per g) for finished peanuts sold for direct human consumption. Although the approaches are different, the U.S. peanut industry in cooperation with USDA has recently developed an origin certification program (OCP) with several key European Union countries that import U.S. peanuts into Europe. These key markets, in a memorandum of understanding, have agreed to recognize the sampling and testing of U.S. peanuts for aflatoxin before their export to these markets.[9] Documents showing positive lot identification and aflatoxin test results can be used to certify that the peanuts meet European Union aflatoxin regulations. For the OCP, the U.S. exporter uses a first 22-kg sample test result for screening lots. A second USDA 22-kg sample is tested according to European Union protocol for lot certification. The OCP will reduce lots rejected at the port of entry, reduce the disruption in supply for the importer, reduce economic losses for the exporter and the importer, and maintain European Union standards for consumer safety. The origin certification program is an example of an agreement between two countries that is mutually beneficial to both while maintaining high standards for consumer safety.[10]

5.2.4 METHODS OF ANALYSIS

Legislation calls for methods of control. Reliable analytical methods will have to be available to make enforcement of the regulations possible. Tolerance levels that do not have a reasonable expectation of being met are wasteful in the resources that they utilize and may well condemn products that are perfectly fit for consumption.[11] In addition to reliability, simplicity is desired, as it will influence the amount of data that will be generated and the practicality of the ultimate measures taken. The reliability of analysis data can be improved through the use of methods that fulfill certain performance criteria (as can be demonstrated in interlaboratory studies). AOAC International and CEN (the European Standardization Committee, equivalent to the International Standards Organization [ISO]) have a number of standardized methods of analysis for mycotoxins available that have been validated in formal interlaboratory studies, and this number is gradually growing. The latest edition of the *Official Methods of Analysis* of AOAC International[12] contains approximately 40 validated methods for mycotoxin determination, including many aflatoxin detection methods. CEN has produced a document that provides criteria for mycotoxin methods.[13] This document gives information concerning the method performance that can be expected from experienced analytical laboratories. The CEN criteria are reflected as method performance requirements in official European Union legislation on aflatoxins.[14]

In addition, the application of analytical quality assurance (AQA) procedures is recommended, including the use of (certified) reference materials, especially when a high degree of comparison and accuracy is required. Further developments in AQA and the use of reference materials are likely to emerge in the future for the control of mycotoxins in foods and feeds. Several (certified) reference materials for mycotoxins have been developed or are currently being redeveloped in projects funded by the European Commission's Standards, Measurements, and Testing Programme (previously named Bureau Communautaire de Référence [BCR]). BCR reference materials for aflatoxins include various milk powders with aflatoxin M_1; a chloroform calibrant solution with aflatoxin M_1; peanut butter with aflatoxins B_1, B_2, G_1, and G_2; peanut meal with aflatoxin B_1; and animal feedstuff with aflatoxin B_1. They are currently available worldwide. Certified reference materials are relatively expensive and supplies are limited; therefore laboratories are advised to develop their own reference materials for routine use, the toxin content of which should be established on the basis of the certified materials.

Besides the application of (certified) reference materials, regular participation in interlaboratory comparisons (e.g., proficiency testing schemes) is becoming increasingly important as part of AQA measures that a laboratory must undertake to demonstrate acceptable performance. A number of proficiency testing schemes for aflatoxins exist at the international level, including those organized by FAPAS® (Food Analysis Performance Assessment Scheme),[15] operated from Europe by the Central Science Laboratory in the United Kingdom, and those organized by the American Oil Chemists' Society (AOCS) in the United States.

Good analytical methodology and AQA are prerequisites for adequate food law enforcement. Also important, especially in free-trade areas, is how enforcement bodies handle such issues as measurement uncertainty. Within the European Union and the European Free Trade Area, approaches are not yet harmonized, which may lead to different action levels for, for example, aflatoxins. Therefore, the Food Law Enforcement Practitioners (FLEP) mycotoxins working party has recommended a uniform approach.[16]

5.2.5 TRADE CONTRACTS

Preferably, regulations should be brought into harmony with those in force in other countries with which trade contracts exist. In fact, this approach has been applied in the European Union, Mercosur, and Australia/New Zealand, where harmonized regulations for aflatoxins now exist. Strict regulative actions may lead importing countries to ban or limit the importing of commodities such as certain food grains and animal feedstuffs, which can make it difficult for exporting countries to find or maintain markets for their products. For example, the stringent regulations for aflatoxin B_1 in animal feedstuffs in the European Union[17] led European animal feed manufacturers to switch from groundnut meal to other protein sources to include in feeds; this had an impact on the export of groundnut meal of some developing countries.[18] The distortion of the market caused by regulations in importing countries may lead to the export of less contaminated foods and feeds, leaving inferior foods and feeds for the local market. Some countries apply different limits for aflatoxins in certain products depending on the destination.

The World Bank issued a report in 2001 describing a study on the impact of adopting international food safety standards and harmonization of standards on global food trade patterns.[19] Several scenarios led to estimates of the effects of aflatoxin regulatory standards in 15 importing (4 developing) countries on exports from 31 (21 developing) countries. In one of the scenarios, the authors examined trade flow if all countries adopted an international standard for aflatoxin B_1 in food of 9 μg/kg (which would be equivalent to the Codex guidelines of 15 μg/kg for total aflatoxins), in contrast to all importing countries remaining at the (generally lower) limits of 1998. Doing so would lead to an increase in cereal and nut trade among these countries by US$ 6.1 billion (or 51%).

5.2.6 FOOD SUPPLY

The regulatory philosophy should not jeopardize the availability of basic commodities at reasonable prices. Especially in developing countries, where food supplies are already limited, drastic legal measures may lead to a lack of food and excessive prices. People living in these countries cannot exercise the option of starving to death today in order to live a better life tomorrow. At the time of writing, for example, the dramatic food security situation in parts of Africa is leading to measures that prioritize food sufficiency above food safety. Mycotoxins are an important problem as evidenced by occasional outbreaks of human mycotoxicoses and the role of aflatoxins in liver cancer in west Africa and fumonisins in esophageal cancer in South Africa.[20]

5.2.7 SYNOPSIS

Weighing the various factors that play a role in the decision-making process of establishing mycotoxin tolerances is not trivial. Common sense is a major factor for reaching a decision. Public health officials are confronted with a complex problem: Mycotoxins, and particularly aflatoxins, should be excluded from food and feed as much as possible. Because the substances are present in foods as natural contaminants, however, human exposure cannot be completely prevented, and exposure of the population to some level of mycotoxins has to be tolerated. Despite the dilemmas, mycotoxin regulations, and particular those for aflatoxins, have been established in the past decades in many countries, and newer regulations are still being drafted.

5.3 AFLATOXIN REGULATIONS AND DEVELOPMENTS

Numerous articles about limits and regulations for mycotoxins and their rationales have been published.[1,21-30] The most recent comprehensive survey was undertaken in 2002/2003 and was published as an FAO Food and Nutrition Paper in 2004.[2]

5.3.1 The International FAO Inquiry 2002/2003

In 2002/2003, an international inquiry was held among the Agricultural Services of the Dutch Embassies around the world, with the request to gather up-to-date information from local authorities on the situation regarding mycotoxin regulations in as many countries of the world as possible. When this procedure did not lead to the desired information, personal contacts were used. The questions in the inquiry concerned:

- Existence of mycotoxin regulations
- Types of mycotoxins and products for which regulations are in force or proposed, together with maximum permissible levels
- Authorities responsible for control of mycotoxins
- Use of official and published methods of sampling and analysis

By the end of 2003, data were received from 94 countries. Together with information gathered in previous inquiries, detailed information is now available about the existence or absence of specific mycotoxin limits and regulations in food and feed in 122 countries. Some conclusions with respect to current limits and regulations for aflatoxins can be made from a review of these data.

5.3.2 Observations

Figure 5.1 shows countries with and without regulations for mycotoxins. On a worldwide basis, approximately 100 countries had mycotoxin regulations for foods or feeds in 2003, an increase of approximately 30% compared to 1995. The total population in these countries represents approximately 87% of the world's inhabitants. In fact, all countries with mycotoxin regulations at least have regulatory limits for aflatoxin B_1 or the sum of aflatoxins B_1, B_2, G_1, and G_2 in foods or feeds, a situation that was also observed in 1995. The number of countries regulating aflatoxins has significantly increased over the years. The aflatoxin regulations are often detailed and specific for various foodstuffs, dairy products, and feedstuffs.

In Table 5.1, an attempt has been made to compare medians, ranges, and numbers for countries that had legally established limits for aflatoxins in foodstuffs and in animal feedstuffs intended to be used for dairy cattle in the years 1995[30] and 2003[2] so trends are visible. Such a comparison is not easy to make and is subject to future adjustments because not all data used may be fully correct. Another limitation is that some countries have many regulations specifying different tolerated levels for individual foods and feeds, while others have set only one tolerated level (e.g., for "all foods" or for "all feeds"); therefore, simplifications were made. For food, selections were made of limits established for aflatoxin B_1 and total aflatoxins for the category "all foods," or, if this category was not mentioned in the regulations, for those foodstuffs considered closest to this category. Similarly, for the comparison of aflatoxin M_1 limits, a selection was made of regulatory levels set for milk (whereas many countries also had specific limits for milk products as milk powder, cheese, and infant foods). Finally, for aflatoxins in animal feedstuffs, some countries have

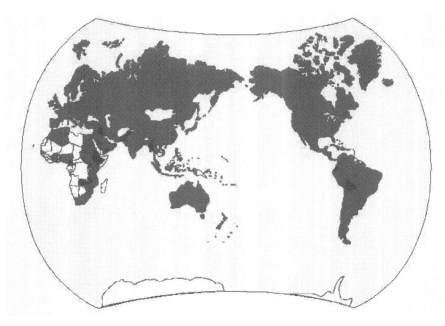

FIGURE 5.1 Countries with and without regulations for aflatoxins. Light gray, known to have regulations; dark gray, known to have no specific regulations; white, unknown.

many limits, often dictated by the destination of the feedstuff. To compare the limits between countries for aflatoxin B_1 and total aflatoxins in animal feedstuffs, those were selected that were known or assumed to be relevant for feedstuffs for dairy cattle. These are often the most stringent from the human health point of view, because of the carryover of aflatoxin B_1 into aflatoxin M_1 in milk and dairy products. For all five categories for which some characteristics are summarized in Table 5.1, frequency distributions of the 2003 situation were prepared and are shown in Figures 5.2 to 5.6. Table 5.1 and these figures lead to the following comments.

Compared to the situation in 1995, the maximum tolerated levels for aflatoxin B_1 in food did not change dramatically in 2003, although the range of limits narrowed slightly (1 to 20 µg/kg), and 2 µg/kg is now a limit in force in 29 countries (see Figure 5.2). Most of these countries belong to the European Union (where, since 1998, harmonized limits for aflatoxin B_1 and the sum of the aflatoxins B_1, B_2, G_1, and G_2 are in force) or the European Free Trade Association (EFTA) or are candidate European Union countries, many of which have brought their national regulations already into harmony with the European Union in anticipation of their future membership. Another major limit is visible at 5 µg/kg, which is followed by 21 countries, spread over Africa, Asia/Oceania, Latin America, and Europe. The United States and Canada do not have a single limit for aflatoxin B_1.

As in 1995, also in 2003 many countries regulated the aflatoxins with limits for the sum of the aflatoxins B_1, B_2, G_1, and G_2, sometimes in combination with a specific limit for aflatoxin B_1. The range of limits (1 to 35 µg/kg) narrowed slightly as compared to 1995, whereas the median limit (10 µg/kg) was slightly higher. The

TABLE 5.1

Maximum Tolerated Levels for Aflatoxins in 1995 and 2003 and Number of Countries Having Relevant Regulations

Aflatoxin/Matrix Combination	1995			2003		
	Median (μg/kg)	Range (μg/kg)	Countries (No.)	Median (μg/kg)	Range (μg/kg)	Countries (No.)
Aflatoxin B_1 in foodstuffs	4	0–30	33	2	1–20	61
Aflatoxins $B_1 + B_2 + G_1 + G_2$ in foodstuffs	8	0–50	48	10	1–35	76
Aflatoxin M_1 in milk	0.05	0–1	17	0.05	0.05–15	60
Aflatoxin B_1 in feedstuffs	5	5–50	25	5	5–50	39
Aflatoxin $B_1 + B_2 + G_1 + G_2$ in feedstuffs	20	0–1000	17	20	0–50	21

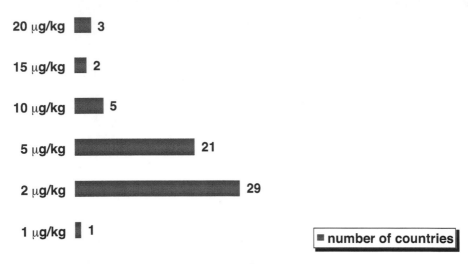

FIGURE 5.2 Occurrence of specific limits for aflatoxin B$_1$ in food.

most frequently occurring limit (see Figure 5.3) is at 4 µg/kg (applied by 29 countries), again a limit found back in the harmonized regulations in the European Union, EFTA, and candidate European Union countries, where dual limits both for aflatoxin B$_1$ and for total aflatoxins are enforced. Another major peak occurs at 20 µg/kg, applied by 17 countries, half of them in Latin America (where it is also a Mercosur harmonized limit) and several in Africa. Also, the United States, one of the first countries to establish an aflatoxin action limit, follows the 20-µg/kg limit. Over the years, the desire to limit total aflatoxins in foodstuffs has remained, resulting in 76

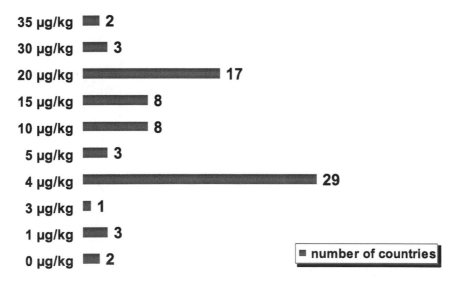

FIGURE 5.3 Occurrence of specific limits for the sum of aflatoxins in food.

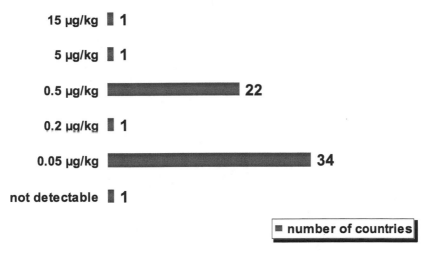

FIGURE 5.4 Occurrence of specific limits for aflatoxin M_1 in milk.

countries in 2003 applying such regulatory levels (as compared to 61 countries with a specific limit for aflatoxin B_1). Whether a regulatory level for the sum of the aflatoxins, which requires more analytical work than for aflatoxin B_1 alone, contributes significantly to better protection of public health than a regulatory level for aflatoxin B_1 alone is debatable. Aflatoxin B_1 is the most important of the aflatoxins, considered from the viewpoints of both toxicology and occurrence. It is unlikely that commodities will contain aflatoxins B_2, G_1, and G_2 and not aflatoxin B_1, and the concentration of the sum of the aflatoxins B_2, G_1, and G_2 is generally less than the concentration of aflatoxin B_1 alone. Typical occurrence ratios for aflatoxins B_1 and B_2 (mainly produced by *Aspergillus flavus*) average approximately 4:1. Typical occurrence ratios for aflatoxin B_1 and the sum of the aflatoxins B_2, G_1, and G_2 (the G toxins are mainly produced by *A. parasiticus*) average approximately 1:0.8, although variations do occur for both ratios. Regulatory authorities in those countries that apply a regulatory level for the sum of the aflatoxins should critically inspect the analytical data of monitoring agencies to see how frequently the availability of data on the sum of the aflatoxins (beyond that on aflatoxin B_1) has been indispensable to adequately protect the consumer. Analysis of one target component (aflatoxin B_1) could be sufficient and more practical.

Regulations for aflatoxin M_1 are now seen in 60 countries, a more than threefold increase as compared to 1995. It is again the European Union, EFTA, and candidate European Union countries that contribute in major part to the largest peak seen in Figure 5.4 at 0.05 µg/kg, but some other countries in Africa, Asia, and Latin America also apply this limit. The other peaking limit is at 0.5 µg/kg. This higher regulatory level is applied in the United States and several Asian and European countries, and it occurs most frequently in Latin America, where it is established as a harmonized Mercosur limit. The tenfold difference between the two most prevailing limits for aflatoxin M_1, which have existed for many years, has given rise to debates within

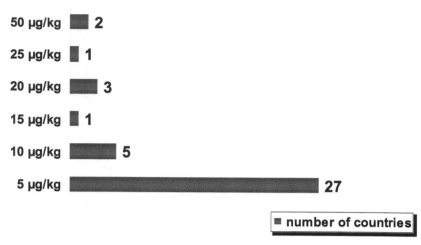

FIGURE 5.5 Occurrence of specific limits for aflatoxin B_1 in feed for dairy cattle.

Codex Alimentarius that have led to their request to JECFA to reevaluate the human health risk of aflatoxin M_1. Apart from these sub-µg/kg regulatory levels, a few countries indicated in the 2003 inquiry that they regulate aflatoxin M_1 in milk at levels of 5 and 15 µg/kg. These levels are not realistic, and probably these are mistakes that will need to be adjusted during the correction stages of the document currently drafted for the coming FAO document.

For feedstuffs many aflatoxin regulations exist. Those that are applied for feed for dairy cattle are summarized in Figure 5.5. Whereas many more countries now regulate aflatoxin B_1 in feedstuffs for dairy cattle than in 1995 (39 in 2003 vs. 25 in 1995), this increase is only slightly visible for the countries that regulate the sum of the naturally occurring aflatoxins (21 in 2003 vs. 17 in 1995). This is understandable and logical from the point of view that it is aflatoxin M_1, the metabolite of aflatoxin B_1, that causes health concerns. Consequently, limiting aflatoxin B_1 in animal feeds is the most effective means of controlling aflatoxin M_1 in milk. Figure 5.5 shows that a limit of 5 µg/kg dominates the distribution pattern of aflatoxin B_1 regulations. This limit is applied in the European Union and EFTA countries, is followed in many of the candidate European Union countries, and is only sporadically seen outside Europe. Strict application will normally be effective to ensure that aflatoxin M_1 levels in milk remain below 0.05 µg/kg (where these countries have set their corresponding limit for aflatoxin M_1 in milk).

The number of regulations for the sum of the aflatoxins in feedstuffs is considerably less than those existing for aflatoxin B_1 only. The limits may vary, depending on the destination of the feedstuff. Figure 5.6 depicts the distribution of the limits for total aflatoxins in animal feeds that are given to dairy cattle. A relatively flat distribution is apparent, with the most frequently occurring limit being 20 µg/kg. A further analysis reveals that regulatory levels for the sum of the aflatoxins B_1, B_2, G_1, and G_2 occur in the feed regulations of all the world's continents, but in particular in the Americas.

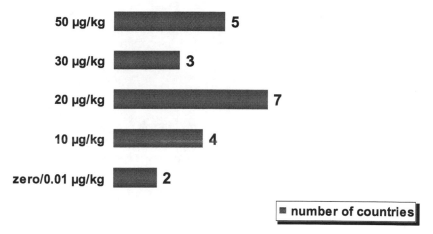

FIGURE 5.6 Occurrence of specific limits for the sum of aflatoxins in feed for dairy cattle.

5.4 CONCLUDING REMARKS

Comparing the situations in 1995 and 2003, in 2003 more countries were known to have regulations for aflatoxins in more commodities and products, and tolerance limits generally showed a slight tendency to decrease. Regulations have become more diverse and detailed and establish newer requirements regarding official procedures for sampling and analytical methodology, reflecting the general concerns that governments have regarding the potential effects of aflatoxins on the health of humans and animals. At the same time, harmonization of tolerance levels is taking place in some free-trade zones (European Union, EFTA, Mercosur, Australia/New Zealand), and harmonization has taken place for goods involved in international commerce.[31]

Harmonization is a slow process because of the different views and interests of those involved in the process. Whereas harmonized tolerance levels would be beneficial from the point of view of trade, one might argue this would not necessarily be the case from the point of view of (equal) human health protection around the world. Risk assessment is the product of hazard assessment and exposure assessment. The hazard of aflatoxins to individuals is probably more or less the same all over the world (although other factors sometimes play a role as well, such as hepatitis B virus infection in relation to the aflatoxin hazards). Exposure is not the same around the world because of differences in levels of contamination and dietary habits.

National governments or regional communities should encourage and fund activities that contribute to reliable exposure assessment of aflatoxins in their regions. Examples of such activities are the SCOOP tasks, undertaken in the European Union in support of risk evaluations on some mycotoxins. The availability of inexpensive, validated, and easily performed analytical methodology and the application of analytical quality assurance are basic ingredients that can result in obtaining meaningful data on the occurrence of aflatoxins.

The regulations enacted for aflatoxins in foods and feeds and those under development should be the result of sound cooperation between interested parties, drawn from science, consumers, industry, and policymakers. Only then can realistic protection be achieved.

ACKNOWLEDGMENTS

The authors wish to thank the Food and Agriculture Organization of the United Nations for permission to make use of material collected during the international inquiry on worldwide limits and regulations for mycotoxins carried out by the National Institute for Public Health and the Environment in 2002/2003 under contract with FAO, as well as material published in 1997 in FAO Food and Nutrition Paper 81, *Worldwide Regulations for Mycotoxins 1995: A Compendium*. The detailed results of the 2002/2003 inquiry have been published by the FAO.[2]

REFERENCES

1. van Egmond, H.P., Current situation on regulations for mycotoxins: overview of tolerances and status of standard methods of sampling and analysis, *Food Addit. Contam.*, 6, 139–188, 1989.
2. FAO, *Worldwide Regulations for Mycotoxins 2003: A Compendium*, Food and Nutrition Paper 81, Food and Agriculture Organization, United Nations, Rome, Italy, 2004.
3. FAO, *Safety Evaluation of Certain Mycotoxins in Food*, FAO Food and Nutrition Paper 74, prepared for the 56th Meeting of the Joint FAO/WHO Expert Committee on Food Additives (JECFA), Food and Agriculture Organization, United Nations, Rome, 2001, p. 701.
4. WHO, *Safety Evaluation of Certain Food Additives and Contaminants*, Food Additives Series 40, prepared for the 49th Meeting of the Joint FAO/WHO Expert Committee on Food Additives (JECFA), WHO International Programme on Chemical Safety, World Health Organization, Geneva, 1998, 87 pp.
5. Codex Alimentarius Commission, Joint FAO/WHO Food Standards Programme, Report of the 32nd Session of the Codex Committee of Food Additives and Contaminants, Beijing, People's Republic of China, March 20–24, 2000.
6. Page, S.W., Risk assessment for mycotoxins 2003 [abstract], in *Final Programme: Abstracts of Lectures and Posters*, Vol. 31, The Second World Mycotoxin Forum, Noordwijk aan Zee, The Netherlands, February 17–18, 2003.
7. European Commission, *Reports on Tasks for Scientific Cooperation*, report of experts participating in Task 3.2.1: Risk Assessment of Aflatoxins, Report EUR 17526 EN, Directorate-General for Industry, Office for Official Publications of the European Communities, Luxembourg, 1997, 157 pp.
8. FAO, *Sampling Plans for Aflatoxin Analysis in Peanuts and Corn*, Food and Nutrition Paper 55, Food and Agriculture Organization, United Nations, Rome, Italy, 1993, 76 pp.
9. Trucksess, M.W., Whitaker, T.B., van Egmond, H.P., Wilson, D.M., Solfrizzo, M., Abramson, D., Dorner, J.,Ware, G.M., Maragos, C., Hald, B., Sabino, M., Eppley, R.M., and Hagler, W.M., General referee report committee on natural toxins and food allergens–mycotoxins, *J. AOAC Int.*, 86, 1–10, 2003,

10. Adams, J. and Whitaker, T.B., Peanuts, aflatoxin and the Origin Certification Program, in *Meeting the Mycotoxin Menace*, Barug, D., van Egmond, H.P., López Garciá, R., Van Osenbruggen, W.A., and Visconti, A., Eds., Wageningen Academic Publishers, The Netherlands, 2004, pp. 183–196.

11. Smith, J.W., Lewis, C.W., Anderson, J.G., and Solomons, G.L., *Mycotoxins in Human and Animal Health*, technical report, European Commission, Directorate XII, Science, Research and Development, Agro-Industrial Research Division, EUR 16048 EN, Brussels, Belgium, 1994, 300 pp.

12. Horwitz, W., Natural toxins, in *Official Methods of Analysis of AOAC International*, 17th ed., AOAC International, Gaithersburg, MD, 2000.

13. CEN, *Food Analysis, Biotoxins, and Criteria for Analytical Methods of Mycotoxins*, Report No. CR 13505, Comité Européen de Normalisation, Brussels, Belgium, 1999, 8 pp.

14. European Commission, Commission Directive 98/53/EC of 16 July 1998, laying down the sampling methods and the methods for analysis for the official control of the levels for certain contaminants in foodstuffs, *Off. J. Eur. Commun.*, L201, 93–101, 1998.

15. Richard, J.L., Payne, G.A., Desjardins, A.E., Maragos, C., Norred, W.P., Pestka, J.J., Phillips, T.D., van Egmond, H.P., Vandon, P.J., Whitaker, T.B., and Wood, G., *Mycotoxins: Risks in Plant, Animal and Human Systems*, CAST Task Force Report 139, Council for Agricultural Science and Technology, Ames, IA, 2003, pp. 101–103.

16. Jeuring, H.J., The implementation of EU controls on imported food, in *Meeting the Mycotoxin Menace*, Barug, D., van Egmond, H.P., López Garciá, R., Van Osenbruggen, W.A., and Visconti, A., Eds., Wageningen Academic Publishers, The Netherlands, 2004, pp. 155–163.

17. Commission of the European Communities, Commission Directive of 13 February 1991 amending the Annexes to Council Directive 74/63 EEC on undesirable substances and products in animal nutrition (91/126/EEC), *Off. J. Eur. Commun.*, L60, 16–17, 1991.

18. Bhat, R., *Mycotoxin Contamination of Foods and Feeds*, working document, Third Joint FAO/WHO/UNEP International Conference on Mycotoxins, MYC-CONF/99/4a, Tunis, Tunisia, March 3–6, 1999.

19. Wilson, J.S. and Otsuki, T., *Global Trade and Food Safety: Winners and Losers in a Fragmented System*, Report of Development Research Group (DECRG), The World Bank, Washington, D.C., 2001, 34 pp.

20. Shepherd, G.S., Mycotoxins worldwide: current issues in Africa, in *Meeting the Mycotoxin Menace*, Barug, D., van Egmond, H.P., López Garciá, R., Van Osenbruggen, W.A., and Visconti, A., Eds., Wageningen Academic Publishers, The Netherlands, 2004, pp. 81–88.

21. Krogh, P., Mycotoxin tolerances in foodstuffs, *Pure Appl. Chem.*, 49, 1719–1721, 1977.

22. Schuller, P.L., van Egmond, H.P., and Stoloff, L., Limits and regulations on mycotoxins, in *Proc. Int. Symp. on Mycotoxins*, Naguib, K., Naguib, M.M., Park D.L., and Pohland, A.E., Eds., Cairo, Egypt, September 6–8, 1983, pp. 111–129.

23. Stoloff, L., van Egmond, H.P., and Park, D.L., Rationales for the establishment of limits and regulations for mycotoxins, *Food Addit. Contam.*, 8, 213–222, 1991.

24. Gilbert, J., Regulatory aspects of mycotoxins in the European Community and USA, in *Fungi and Mycotoxins in Stored Products*, Champ, B.R., Highley, E., Hocking A.D., and Pitt, J.J., Eds., proceedings of an international conference, Bangkok, Thailand, April 23–26, 1991 (*ACIAR Proc.*, 36, 194–197, 1991).

25. van Egmond, H.P., Regulatory aspects of mycotoxins in Asia and Africa, in *Fungi and Mycotoxins in Stored Products*, Champ, B.R., Highley, E., Hocking A.D., and Pitt, J.J., Eds., proceedings of an international conference, Bangkok, Thailand, April 23–26, 1991 (*ACIAR Proc.*, 36, 198–204, 1991).

26. van Egmond, H.P. and Dekker, W.H., Worldwide regulations for mycotoxins in 1994, *Nat. Toxins*, 3, 332–336, 1995.

27. Boutrif, E. and Canet, C., Mycotoxin prevention and control: FAO programmes, *Revue de Médicine Vétérinaire*, 149, 681–694, 1998.

28. Rosner, H., Mycotoxin regulations: an update, *Revue de Médicine Vétérinaire*, 149, 679–680, 1998.

29. van Egmond, H.P., *Worldwide Regulations for Mycotoxins*, working document, Third Joint FAO/WHO/UNEP International Conference on Mycotoxins, MYC-CONF/99/8a, Tunis, Tunisia, March 3–6, 1999.

30. FAO, *Worldwide Regulations for Mycotoxins 1995: A Compendium*, Food and Nutrition Paper 64, Food and Agriculture Organization, United Nations, Rome, Italy, 1997, 43 pp.

31. Kloet, D.G., Harmonization of standards for mycotoxins in the Codex Alimentarius, in *Food Safety of Cereals: A Chain-Wide Approach to Reduce Fusarium Mycotoxins*, Scholten, O.E., Ruckenbauer, P., Visconti, A., Van Osenbruggen, W.A., and den Nijs, A.P.M., Eds., European Commission, Brussels, 2002, pp. 62–63.

6 Ecology and Population Biology of Aflatoxigenic Fungi in Soil

Bruce W. Horn

CONTENTS

6.1 INTRODUCTION

Species belonging to *Aspergillus* section *Flavi* are among the most intensively studied of all fungi, due largely to their formation of carcinogenic aflatoxins in agricultural commodities that impact animal and human health.[1,2] Apart from the health concerns of aflatoxins, the economic cost of these mycotoxins is enormous, amounting to approximately $25 million annually to the peanut industry in the southeastern United States alone.[3] Aflatoxigenic fungi are common components of soil mycobiota and are actively involved in decomposition and nutrient cycling.[4,5] Members of section *Flavi* utilize a wide range of carbon and nitrogen sources[6,7] and produce a diversity of enzymes for degrading plant components such as cellulose, pectin, lignin, and lipids.[8–11] These fungi also invade developing seeds of crops, and the primary inoculum for infection originates from soil; therefore, an understanding of the activities and population structure of aflatoxigenic fungi in soil is a prerequisite for developing effective measures to control aflatoxin contamination.

6.2 AFLATOXIGENIC SPECIES

Relatively few fungi are capable of synthesizing aflatoxins, but two species, *Aspergillus flavus* and *A. parasiticus*, are widespread and important colonists of agricultural commodities. *A. flavus* commonly contaminates corn, peanuts, cottonseed, and tree nuts with aflatoxins before harvest and during storage.[12–16] The species typically produces aflatoxins B_1 and B_2 and cyclopiazonic acid[17] and is extremely variable in mycotoxin production, with strains ranging in toxigenicity from nonproducers to potent producers of aflatoxins.[18] In contrast, *A. parasiticus* is most prevalent in peanuts and synthesizes aflatoxins G_1 and G_2 in addition to the B aflatoxins but not cyclopiazonic acid.[17,19] *A. parasiticus* generally produces high levels of aflatoxins, and nonaflatoxigenic strains are rare.[17,20]

Aspergillus flavus as a species is genetically complex and has been subdivided into several groups based on morphology, mycotoxin profile, and molecular characters. Morphologically, *A. flavus* isolates can be categorized either as the typical L strain with sclerotia >400 μm in diameter or as the S strain, which is dominated by abundant small sclerotia <400 μm in diameter.[21] For the purposes of this review, mention of *A. flavus* will imply the L strain unless otherwise specified. The S strain was first recognized as an undescribed taxon by Hesseltine et al.[22] and was formally described as variety *parvisclerotigenus* by Saito and Tsuruta.[23] The type culture of *A. flavus* var. *parvisclerotigenus* produces only B aflatoxins, but other S-strain isolates produce both B and G aflatoxins.[22–27] Only S-strain isolates that produce B aflatoxins have been identified in the United States; both types of the S strain occur in Argentina, West Africa, Southeast Asia, and Australia.

Based on randomly amplified polymorphic DNA (RAPD) analyses and sequencing of gene regions, *Aspergillus flavus* is nonmonophyletic and is separable into two genetic groups that cannot be readily distinguished morphologically.[25,28] Group I consists of both L and S strains that produce only B aflatoxins, and group II is comprised of S strains that produce B or B + G aflatoxins. *A. parasiticus* as currently defined may similarly be comprised of several distinctive genetic groups.[20,29] Research on the population biology of aflatoxigenic fungi is dependent on the accuracy of species identifications and recognition of important intraspecific genetic groups. The current taxonomic uncertainty may to some degree compromise population studies and is reminiscent of earlier studies in which *A. flavus*, *A. parasiticus*, and perhaps other species in section *Flavi* were lumped together as the "*A. flavus* group" and, as a consequence, much valuable information was lost.

Sterigmatocystin, an intermediate in the aflatoxin pathway, is synthesized as an endpoint metabolite by several *Aspergillus* species (including *A. nidulans*) and even by representatives of other fungal genera.[30,31] Because this initial portion of the aflatoxin pathway is fairly widespread, it is not surprising that other aflatoxigenic species have been discovered in recent years. *A. nomius* is very similar to *A. flavus* morphologically but produces both B and G aflatoxins and is quite distinct in molecular characters from other members of section *Flavi*.[32,33] This species parasitizes insects and also has been isolated from soil. Another species, *A. bombycis*, has been isolated (along with *A. nomius*) from insect frass in silkworm-rearing houses in Japan and Indonesia.[33] *A. pseudotamarii* was described from two isolates from

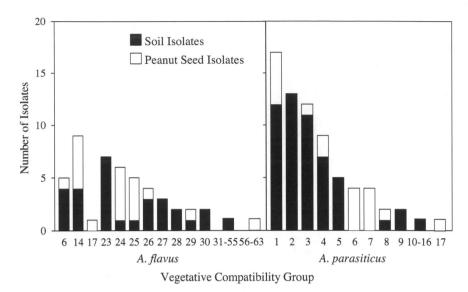

FIGURE 6.1 Diversity of *Aspergillus flavus* and *A. parasiticus* VCGs from a single peanut field in Georgia. (From Horn, B.W. and Greene, R.L., *Mycologia*, 87, 324–332, 1995. With permission.)

Japan and Brazil,[34,35] and *A. ochraceoroseus*, the only species outside of section *Flavi* reported to produce aflatoxins, has been isolated only from African forest soils.[36,37] Unlike *A. flavus* and *A. parasiticus*, these aflatoxigenic species, although interesting, do not have a major impact on agriculture.

6.3 GENETIC DIVERSITY OF SOIL POPULATIONS

The high diversity within *Aspergillus flavus* populations as revealed by colony morphology in the laboratory has long been recognized. Isolates differ in phenotype according to sclerotium production (nonsclerotial to predominantly sclerotial), conidial head formation (densely sporulating to mostly mycelial), and conidial color (bright yellow green to dark green).[17,38,39] The wide range in the production of aflatoxins and cyclopiazonic acid by *A. flavus* isolates is equally reflective of this variability.[15,18,40]

Vegetative compatibility reactions within a population are another measure of diversity in aflatoxigenic fungi. In *Aspergillus* species, hyphal anastomosis between two individuals is genetically controlled by a series of *het* loci in which the occurrence of different alleles at one or more loci results in incompatibility.[41] Vegetatively compatible individuals within a population together form subpopulations called vegetative compatibility groups (VCGs). Papa[42] first examined the diversity of *A. flavus* VCGs in corn kernels from 15 counties in the state of Georgia. Subsequent studies involved VCG analyses of soil populations of *A. flavus* in a cotton field in Arizona[43] and in a peanut field in Georgia[44] (Figure 6.1). In *A. flavus* isolates from the latter study, DNA fingerprints were unique for each VCG and were generally

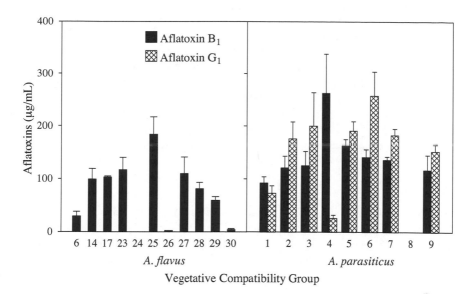

FIGURE 6.2 Production of aflatoxins B_1 and G_1 within VCGs of *Aspergillus flavus* and *A. parasiticus*. Standard deviations are indicated. *A. parasiticus* VCG 8 produces 226 ± 23.6 μg/mL *O*-methylsterigmatocystin (intermediate in the aflatoxin pathway). (From Horn, B.W. et al., *Mycologia*, 88, 574–587, 1996. With permission.)

identical for isolates within a VCG, providing an independent confirmation of the use of VCGs as a measure of genetic variability within populations.[45] Genetic diversity in *A. flavus* soil populations is very high, even within a small soil sample, and VCG or genotype diversity values (number of VCGs or genotypes divided by total number of isolates) range from 0.49 to 0.84.[42–44,46] DNA-fingerprint, RAPD, and VCG analyses of *A. parasiticus* soil populations from Australia and the United States indicate that this species also is highly diverse genetically (Figure 6.1).[44,47,48]

Most of the phenotypic diversity in populations of *Aspergillus flavus* and *A. parasiticus* can be attributed to differences among VCGs. Morphological characters (sclerotium number, size, and shape; conidial color) and mycotoxin production (aflatoxin B_1; cyclopiazonic acid) are more similar within a VCG than between VCGs (Figure 6.2).[17,26,49] Aflatoxigenic and nonaflatoxigenic strains of both species are segregated into separate VCGs and are rarely found together in the same VCG.[17,49]

The VCGs of *Aspergillus flavus* and *A. parasiticus* appear to be widely distributed. *A. parasiticus* VCG 1 and several nontoxigenic *A. flavus* VCGs have been isolated from agricultural soils from across a large section of the United States.[18,50] These distributions may reflect long-range dispersal or may be due to introductions from planting infected seed. It is not known to what degree VCGs are comprised of individuals that are clonal and genetically identical. In several instances, vegetatively compatible isolates of *A. flavus* have been shown to differ genetically.[45,49]

The origins of genetic diversity in soil populations of aflatoxigenic fungi and the selective forces that maintain this diversity are not understood. *Aspergillus flavus* and *A. parasiticus* have no known sexual stage. The high VCG diversity in soil suggests that heterokaryosis, which occurs only between vegetatively compatible individuals, is not common. The parasexual cycle has been reported for *A. flavus* and *A. parasiticus*[51,52] and could result in mitotic recombination, but this cycle requires heterokaryosis as a precondition and has not been demonstrated in *Aspergillus* species outside of the laboratory. Geiser et al.[28] have proposed that *A. flavus* has a population structure indicative of recombination based on a lack of congruence of five gene trees. Similar evidence for recombination has been reported for *A. nomius*.[33] Data suggesting cryptic recombination do not explain the method of recombination, how often recombination occurs, or when recombination occurred in the history of species.

6.4 GEOGRAPHIC DISTRIBUTION

Patterns in the distribution of *Aspergillus flavus* and *A. parasiticus* in soil have been observed at spatial scales ranging from single fields to large geographic regions and have even been examined, to a limited extent, on a worldwide basis. These distribution patterns reflect differences in propagule density, species incidence, and degree of toxigenicity.

6.4.1 REGIONAL SURVEYS

Extensive sampling of single fields has shown that *Aspergillus flavus* and *A. parasiticus* are not randomly distributed in soil but rather show an aggregated form of distribution based on propagule density[53,54] and VCG incidence.[44] Localized colonization of soil substrates by aflatoxigenic fungi may create patches of higher propagule density, particularly if accompanied by extensive sporulation. Similarly, colonization by a single fungal individual would result in clonal aggregations of an identical VCG.

Orum et al.[55,56] examined soil populations of *Aspergillus flavus* S strain in cotton fields within a relatively small geographic area in Yuma County in Arizona. Variances in S-strain incidence and density at different spatial scales of sampling (20 to 100 km; 10 to 15 km; 1 to 5 km; 150 to 300 m) were compared and found to be highest among fields (scale of 1 to 5 km).[55] Subsequent sampling of fields adjacent to the original fields and with different crop histories revealed similar S-strain incidences, suggesting that patches extended beyond field boundaries and that factors other than crop composition and agricultural practices were responsible for the distribution patterns.[56] Analyses of soil populations in Arizona were further complicated by the rapid changes in S-strain incidence from one year to the next, particularly within a 30-km^2 area of the study in which populations may have been influenced by weather-related factors. Bayman and Cotty[43] similarly showed that the profile of *A. flavus* VCGs in soil from a cotton field shifted dramatically during consecutive years, and the dominant VCG during one year was not detected in the following year. Current knowledge of the population dynamics of aflatoxigenic fungi cannot definitively explain these fluxes in genotype composition. Rapid population changes may be due to large-scale dispersal of a genotype into an area or to selection of a particular genotype under specific crop conditions, or the apparent changes may simply reflect nonrepresentative sampling of the population.

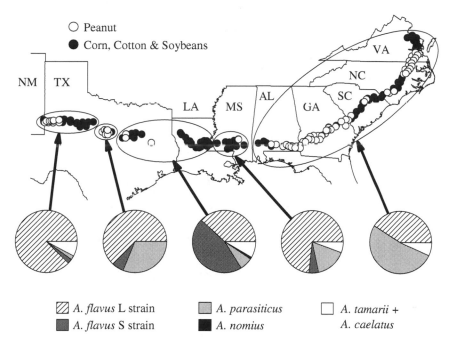

FIGURE 6.3 Incidences of species (as percentages of *Aspergillus* section *Flavi*) in soil along a transect in the United States. *A. tamarii* and *A. caelatus* are nonaflatoxigenic species. State abbreviations: NM, New Mexico; TX, Texas; LA, Louisiana; MS, Mississippi; AL, Alabama; GA, Georgia; SC, South Carolina; NC, North Carolina; VA, Virginia. (From Horn, B.W. and Dorner, J.W., *Mycologia*, 90, 767–776, 1998. With permission.)

Aflatoxigenic fungi show vertical patterns of distribution in agricultural soils, the details of which are largely uncharacterized. Conidia of *Aspergillus flavus* and *A. parasiticus* are extremely hydrophobic and when applied to the soil surface do not readily move downward beyond the upper 6 cm of soil despite repeated rainfall events.[57] Nevertheless, sizable populations of species from section *Flavi* are present in cultivated fields up to 30 cm in depth,[57,58] possibly due to the mixing of soil during plowing or to colonization of organic matter at such depths.

6.4.2 CONTINENTAL SURVEYS

Few single research projects have attempted large-scale comparisons of soil populations of aflatoxigenic fungi over geographic areas that encompass differences in climate, soil type, and cropping systems. The most studied area, the southern United States, is characterized by high temperatures and periodic droughts during the growing season and, therefore, has a high incidence of aflatoxin contamination in susceptible crops. Horn and Dorner[50] established a 3300-km transect from eastern New Mexico to northern Virginia in the southern United States and examined soil populations in peanut fields from four major peanut-growing regions as well as fields with other crops in regions where peanuts are not cultivated (Figure 6.3). *Aspergillus flavus* was the dominant aflatoxigenic fungus across the transect; the L strain was present in all regions whereas the S strain was more restricted in distribution and was most prevalent in the cotton-growing regions of Louisiana and the eastern half of Texas. Fields from peanut-growing regions had significantly higher densities and incidences of *A. parasiticus* than fields from regions where other crops are traditionally grown, not an unexpected finding because *A. parasiticus* infects peanuts more than aerial crops such as corn and cotton.[13,59] *A. nomius* was detected at low incidences only in the Mississippi Delta region of Louisiana and Mississippi. Positive correlations in soil density between species from section *Flavi* as well as between those species and total filamentous fungi suggest that environmental factors were affecting fungal populations as a whole and that regional differences could not be easily explained by climate alone. In another study, soil populations were characterized from three cotton-growing regions of southeastern (Louisiana, Mississippi, Alabama) and southwestern (Arizona) United States.[60] The incidence of *A. flavus* S strain was high in the Mississippi Delta region, as reported in the previously described transect, and in Arizona.

Supplementing these surveys of the southern United States with other more limited studies from the literature to cover additional regions of the country may broaden our understanding of distribution patterns, although doing so introduces inaccuracies arising from differences in sampling techniques, medium composition, incubation conditions, and taxonomic interpretations; nevertheless, trends in fungal distribution can be discerned, particularly for *Aspergillus parasiticus*. Soil populations of *A. parasiticus* are associated with peanut cultivation in the southeastern United States,[50] but such an association is not apparent in other areas of the country. Horn and Dorner[50] reported sizable *A. parasiticus* populations in Virginia north of the peanut-growing region, and the species also has been reported from soils in pistachio and fig orchards from California[61,62] and in corn fields from the Midwest.[46,48,63,64] *A. parasiticus* has not been detected in cotton fields and uncultivated land from the desert regions of southern Arizona,[60,65] and the species does not survive beyond one year when added to soil in that region.[66] Therefore, crop composition appears to greatly influence *A. parasiticus* populations in the southern United States, but climate may be a more important determinant in other regions.

Several studies outside of the United States have shown geographic patterns in the distribution of aflatoxigenic fungi. A survey of soil populations from northern Japan southward into Indonesia indicated that *Aspergillus flavus* and *A. parasiticus* are more prevalent in the southern regions.[67,68] In the Republic of Bénin, West Africa, average yearly rainfall decreases with increasing latitude.[69] In association with this moisture gradient, *A. flavus* L-strain densities in soil from cornfields were significantly higher in the southern, wetter regions, whereas densities of the S strain were higher in the northern, drier regions next to the Sahara Desert.

The aflatoxin-producing potential of *Aspergillus flavus* populations appears to be correlated with latitude. Soil populations of *Aspergillus flavus* are predominantly aflatoxigenic in the southern United States, with >95% of isolates producing aflatoxins in the peanut-growing region of southern Alabama and Georgia (Figure 6.4).[18] In contrast, aflatoxin-producing isolates of *A. flavus* often comprise <50% of soil

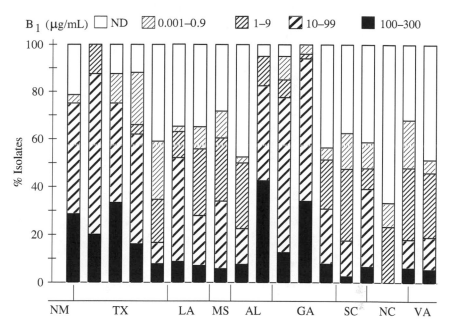

FIGURE 6.4 Production of aflatoxin B_1 by L-strain isolates of *Aspergillus flavus* from agricultural soils along a transect extending from New Mexico to Virginia. See Figure 6.3 for a map of the transect and abbreviations of states. ND, not detected. (From Horn, B.W. and Dorner, J.W., *Appl. Environ. Microbiol.*, 65, 1444–1449, 1999. With permission.)

isolates at the higher latitudes of the midwestern corn belt.[46,64,70] The least aflatoxigenic populations among four major peanut-growing regions in the United States were in the northernmost area of North Carolina and Virginia.[18] Cotty[60] also reported that *A. flavus* toxigenicity is negatively correlated with latitude. A similar pattern in distribution has been shown for Japan, where increasing latitude is associated with lower aflatoxigenicity of *A. flavus* populations.[67] Decreasing temperature with increasing latitude may be the common environmental variable associated with these observations.

6.4.3 WORLDWIDE SURVEYS

Many *Aspergillus* species from section *Flavi* are distributed worldwide and have been found wherever soil fungi have been examined. *Aspergillus* species in general appear to be most abundant in subtropical and warm temperate regions, particularly in agricultural soils, and decrease in density and species diversity with increasing latitude.[4,71] Klich[72] compiled data from over 100 studies and examined the global distribution of species within section *Flavi*. *A. flavus* occurred at greater than expected frequencies at 26 to 35° latitude (subtropical to warm temperate), and *A. parasiticus* occurred at slightly greater than expected frequencies in the tropics (0 to 15°). Because *A. flavus* was present at expected frequencies in all biomes (forest, grassland, wetland, desert, and cultivated), it was suggested that temperatures optimal for growth (25 to

TABLE 6.1

Soil Populations of *Aspergillus flavus* and *A. parasiticus* from Cultivated Fields and Neighboring Forests in Southwestern Georgia

Habitat	*Aspergillus flavus* Density (CFU/g)[a]	*Aspergillus flavus* Relative Density (%)[b]	*Aspergillus parasiticus* Density (CFU/g)	*Aspergillus parasiticus* Relative Density (%)
Cultivated fields:				
Peanut	1286	0.88	909	0.62
Peanut	432	0.51	358	0.42
Peanut	194	0.20	427	0.43
Corn	782	0.25	1112	0.36
Corn	152	0.20	90	0.12
Corn	84	0.08	161	0.15
Neighboring forests:				
Oak	ND[c]	—	32	0.007
Oak/sweetgum	32	0.006	ND	—
Oak/hickory	16	0.004	16	0.004
Pine	16	0.015	16	0.015
Pine	ND	—	ND	—
Pine	ND	—	ND	—

[a] Colony-forming units per gram of soil (dry weight).
[b] Relative density = percentage of total filamentous fungi.
[c] ND, not detected.

40°C) instead of habitat might account for the high frequency of this species at subtropical to warm-temperate latitudes.[72] However, the data were based entirely on the occurrence of species (rare and abundant species were given equal weights) in published studies. A compilation that incorporates the absolute and relative densities of species may greatly modify these conclusions. Certainly *A. flavus* densities are much higher in cultivated fields than in natural habitats such as forests (Table 6.1) and prairies,[63] and desert ecosystems are known to harbor high populations of *A. flavus*.[65]

6.5 ADAPTATIONS FOR SURVIVAL IN SOIL

Aspergillus flavus and *A. parasiticus* are well adapted for survival in soil and may exist as conidia, sclerotia, or hyphae. Identification of hyphae and conidia in soil, either by direct observation or indirectly through dilution plating, presents many difficulties.[4] Aspergilli sporulate profusely in nature, and colonies resulting from dilution plating, a widely used technique for assessing soil populations, likely arise from quiescent conidia; therefore, population data obtained through dilution plating suggest the potential of these fungi for colonization of plants and other substrates but say little about their current activity in soil.

Conidia of aflatoxigenic fungi when added to soil slowly lose their viability.[73,74] Wicklow et al.[75] examined differences in conidium viability of *Aspergillus flavus* and *A. parasiticus* for 3 years between northern (Illinois) and southern (Georgia) regions of the United States. *A. flavus* conidia were not detected in soil from either location by the end of the experiment; surprisingly, *A. parasiticus* conidia remained largely viable in Illinois but not in Georgia. The high soil densities of aflatoxigenic fungi in Georgia despite the increased conidium mortality may be due to the addition of large quantities of inoculum from crops contaminated with aflatoxins, the result of high temperatures and frequent droughts in the southern United States.[75] Thus, population fluxes in soil reflect conidium mortality that is countered by the influx of inocula from infected crops and/or colonization of organic matter.[76]

Sclerotia are commonly produced by strains of *Aspergillus flavus* and *A. parasiticus* in culture[17,21,46,48,64] and likely serve as resistant structures for surviving adverse environmental conditions.[77] Although the sclerotia are morphologically similar to stromata of *Petromyces alliaceus* (anamorph = *A. alliaceus*), a species in section *Flavi* that sporadically produces ascospores within stromata,[78] a sexual stage has never been linked to *A. flavus* and *A. parasiticus* sclerotia. Wicklow et al.[75] demonstrated that the majority of sclerotia survived burial in Illinois and Georgia for 3 years; survivability was less on the soil surface.[79] Sclerotia of *A. flavus* have been reported from nature on preharvest corn kernels[80] and in the pith of corncobs that had overwintered on the soil surface.[81] In addition, *A. parasiticus* sclerotia have been detected on insect-damaged peanut seeds,[74] and large numbers of the small sclerotia of *A. flavus* S strain can form in developing cotton bolls.[82]

The mode of infection by sclerotia of aflatoxigenic fungi and the importance of sclerotia in agricultural ecosystems are poorly understood. Sporogenic germination in which conidial heads form on the sclerotium surface has been demonstrated under laboratory conditions and on the soil surface of a cornfield.[83,84] Soil densities of *Aspergillus flavus* and *A. parasiticus* greatly increase in the vicinity of buried sclerotia, presumably due to conidia produced by sporogenic germination.[75] Sclerotia of both species also may germinate in soil by producing mycelium and thereby directly invade the substrate. Stack and Pettit[85] reported colonization of organic matter through myceliogenic germination of *A. flavus* sclerotia. Similarly, peanuts became highly infected with *A. parasiticus* when soil in experimental control plots was inoculated with sclerotia.[74] Without any evidence of sporogenic germination, it was surmised that infection likely occurred through invasion by mycelium from germinating sclerotia.

Wicklow et al.[80] documented the dispersal of sclerotia onto soil during combine harvesting of five cornfields in the southern United States. Small numbers of *A. flavus* sclerotia were recovered from insect-damaged kernels before harvest and from chaff and debris exiting the combine exhaust. Extensive sampling of soil following harvest resulted in the recovery of only two sclerotia from the most heavily infected field. Because soil from those same fields contained high densities of *A. flavus* propagules (700 to 7400 CFU/g) that presumably represent conidia and hyphae, the importance of sclerotia may be minimal. Sclerotia may instead be of greater importance in natural habitats or fallow fields where soil populations of aflatoxigenic fungi are very low and where preferred substrates such as seeds are either rare or not immediately available.

6.6 SOIL AS A SOURCE OF PRIMARY INOCULUM

Soil serves as a reservoir for primary inoculum that is responsible for the infection of crops susceptible to aflatoxin contamination. The aerial fruiting of crops such as corn, cotton, and tree nuts dictates important differences in the manner of infection compared to the subterranean fruiting of peanuts.[14] Aerial crops become infected by *Aspergillus flavus* conidia that are dispersed by wind and vectored by insects, though it is often difficult to determine whether the conidia originated as primary inoculum from soil or as secondary inoculum from currently infected crops. Sporulation on crop debris deposited on the soil surface is clearly one source of inoculum. This has been demonstrated experimentally through biological control in which nontoxigenic strains of *A. flavus* and *A. parasiticus* sporulate profusely on inoculated grain that has been distributed onto the soil surface. Corn and cottonseed become infected with nontoxigenic strains, which reduce aflatoxin contamination by competing with native aflatoxigenic strains.[86,87] Olanya et al.[88] showed that *A. flavus* sporulates on waste corn deposited on the soil surface, creating a linear dispersal gradient of airborne conidia away from the corn deposits. Second, windborne dust containing *A. flavus* conidia may directly infect crops. Cotton bolls in Arizona became contaminated with aflatoxins when soil was artificially blown over the crop,[89] and dust associated with disking has been implicated in infection of pistachio nuts.[61] Finally, insects disperse conidia of aflatoxigenic fungi directly from soil to the crop. Soil insects in cornfields harbor *A. flavus* and *A. parasiticus* both externally and internally.[90] Lussenhop and Wicklow[91] showed that nitidulid beetles are involved in infection of corn ears in the southern United States. Buried ears that had overwintered supported visible *A. flavus* sporulation and were associated with nitidulid beetles, 68% of which were contaminated with *A. flavus* at the time of corn silking. The beetles were attracted to developing ears wounded by other insects such as the corn earworm, and ears became infected with a phenotypically distinct strain of *A. flavus* transmitted from the buried ears.

In contrast to aerial crops, peanuts are infected through direct contact with soil. Seeds from visibly undamaged pods become infected through a little-understood route of invasion involving hyphal penetration of the pod pericarp.[92–94] In the more frequent mode of infection, pods and seeds are damaged by various arthropods and become highly susceptible to invasion by aflatoxigenic fungi. Larvae of the lesser cornstalk borer (*Elasmopalpus lignosellus*) are responsible for the scarification and penetration of pods in the southeastern United States,[95,96] whereas in tropical regions of the world white grubs (scarab beetle larvae), termites, and millipedes may cause considerable damage.[97–99] These arthropods are most damaging to peanut pods in dry soil at elevated temperatures, conditions that are also conducive to drought stress in peanut plants. Drought-stressed peanuts have a lowered resistance to invasion by aflatoxigenic fungi due in part to cessation of phytoalexin production.[100]

The strong correlation between insect damage and aflatoxin contamination in peanuts is well established, but the sources of inoculum and their relative importance require further study. Direct exposure of the freshly created wound site to surrounding soil would allow for invasion by *Aspergillus flavus* and *A. parasiticus*. Conidia of these fungi are normally quiescent in soil, even within the geocarposphere of developing peanut pods.[73,101] Injury to the pod stimulates the germination of *A. flavus* conidia in soil adjacent to the wound[101] due to release of sugars and amino-N compounds.[102] Wound sites on peanut seeds also may become infected from inoculum transmitted by arthropods. Lesser cornstalk borer larvae and fungus-feeding mites harbor *A. flavus* conidia both externally and internally and vector them to peanuts.[95,103] Dispersal by these arthropods in peanuts is likely for only limited distances in the soil environment compared to the potentially long distances by flying insects in aerial crops. Lesser cornstalk borer larvae migrate for short distances and have been captured in pitfall traps between peanut rows;[104,105] however, the internal incidences of *A. flavus* in surface-sterilized larvae are often low (<10%),[95] suggesting that *A. flavus* is incidental from the soil environment and does not comprise secondary inoculum from neighboring infected pods. Detailed monitoring of the movement of individual larvae in soil during feeding is needed to clarify the association between larval damage and colonization by aflatoxigenic fungi.

Demonstration of the effect of soil population density on crop infection by aflatoxigenic fungi under field conditions has proven difficult, particularly with aerial crops where primary inoculum cannot be easily identified. Peanuts appear to be relatively insensitive to propagule density. Griffin and Garren[106] estimated that pod infection is possible with as few as 2.0 propagules of *Aspergillus flavus* in a 0.5-mm layer of the geocarposphere. Furthermore, an increase in soil density of *A. parasiticus* conidia from 100 to 10^5 CFU/g resulted in an increase of only 5% in the incidence of seed infection in drought-stressed peanuts.[74] Drought and elevated soil temperatures responsible for increased peanut susceptibility to invasion by *A. flavus* and *A. parasiticus* may be more important than soil propagule density in determining the severity of peanut seed infection.

6.7 SOIL POPULATION DYNAMICS IN RELATION TO CROPS

Soils from mesic habitats such as forests and prairies harbor very low populations of aflatoxigenic fungi compared to cultivated fields from the same areas, indicating that agricultural practices greatly increase soil populations (Table 6.1).[63] Pettit et al.[58] reported that when peanuts were grown continuously on previously nonagricultural land, *Aspergillus flavus* was detected in soil by the latter part of the second year. Agricultural soils planted in annual crops are characterized by considerable exposure to sunlight, resulting in increased evaporation and mean maximum temperatures, both of which are conducive to drought stress in plants and invasion by aflatoxigenic fungi.[107–109] High population densities of *A. flavus* (both L and S strains) occur in nonagricultural soils of the hot, arid Sonoran Desert of the southwestern United States where the seeds and pericarps of native leguminous trees are extensively invaded and contaminated with aflatoxins.[65] Desert environments may represent the preferred native habitat of *A. flavus*, and agricultural practices in nonarid regions may to some degree create localized desert-like conditions favorable for aflatoxigenic fungi.

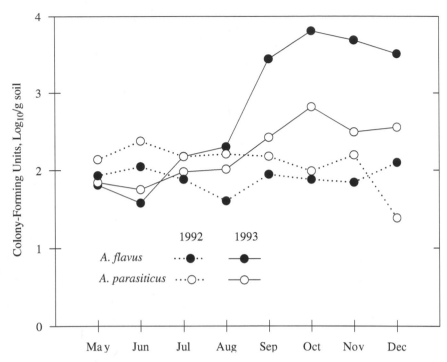

FIGURE 6.5 Soil populations of *A. flavus* and *A. parasiticus* from two cornfields in southwestern Georgia. Corn was combine-harvested in August following nondrought (1992) and drought (1993) conditions. (From Horn, B.W. et al., *Appl. Environ. Microbiol.*, 61, 2472–2475, 1995. With permission.)

Numerous studies have failed to demonstrate any short-term effect of crop rotation on soil populations of aflatoxigenic fungi.[53,55,63,64,69,70,106] Soil populations may instead depend upon the long-term effects of periodic droughts on susceptible crops. Horn and Dorner[50] speculated that differences in the soil density of *Aspergillus flavus* among four major peanut-growing regions in the United States could be explained by climatic differences in the frequency of drought.

During drought years that are associated with extensive aflatoxin contamination, combine harvesting of corn releases prodigious numbers of conidia into the air and scatters *Aspergillus flavus*-infected debris onto the soil surfaces.[80,108,110] Soil population densities of *A. flavus* may increase many-fold immediately following harvest.[80] Horn et al.[76] examined the effects of corn and peanut cultivation on soil populations of *A. flavus* and *A. parasiticus* in three fields in the southeastern United States. Population densities of both species remained fairly stable, with the exception of a corn field that was exposed to drought (Figure 6.5). In that instance, soil densities of *A. flavus* increased from 200 to 6400 CFU/g following harvest. Infected drought-stressed plants, therefore, periodically replenish soil populations of aflatoxigenic fungi. This population fluctuation was observed in 40 Iowa corn fields where soil populations during the drought year 1988 averaged 1200 CFU/g following harvest and subsequently dropped to 700 and 396 CFU/g by 1989 and 1990, respectively.[64] Those same fields were not exposed to further drought and, consequently, densities continued to decline to 14 CFU/g in 1991 and 0.3 CFU/g by 1993.[70] Infrequent droughts also may account for the changes in the genetic composition of *A. flavus* populations in soil as reported by Bayman and Cotty.[43] The decrease in soil populations between droughts may result in a low population base in which the genetic composition has changed over time; therefore, drought-induced *A. flavus* outbreaks in a single field are, to some degree, independent of one another due to their origins from different soil populations that serve as a source of primary inoculum.

In addition to the direct dispersal of conidia to soil during harvest, debris from crops such as corn, peanuts, and tree nuts can support colonization and sporulation by aflatoxigenic fungi once deposited onto soil.[61,64,70,80,81,91,111] Angle et al.[63] reported that 40 and 85% of soil populations of *Aspergillus flavus* and *A. parasiticus*, respectively, were associated with corn residues in Missouri; however, it was not known whether those residues arose from crops infected before harvest or from noninfected debris that was subsequently invaded by soil inhabitants. Aspergilli are important decomposers of organic matter in soil,[4] and several studies suggest that the invasion of crop debris directly from soil contributes to soil populations. Griffin and Garren[111] showed that rye, which is often planted as a winter crop before peanuts, led to an increase in *A. flavus* populations when deep-plowed into soil during the following spring. Similarly, root segments of peanut, cotton, soybean, snapbean, and sorghum became colonized by *A. flavus* when buried in soil.[112]

Because *Aspergillus parasiticus* primarily invades subterranean peanuts and rarely infects aerial crops, the relationship between crop infection and soil populations differs from that of *A. flavus* in several important respects. *A. parasiticus* appears to be more adapted to the soil environment than *A. flavus*[13,76] and as a consequence exhibits less dependence on crop infection for maintaining soil populations. Soil populations of *A. parasiticus* can be relatively high in areas where peanuts are not cultivated and where the low infection rate of aerial crops cannot account for the population levels.[46,50,63] Even in peanut fields where infection with *A. parasiticus* contributes to soil populations, other environmental parameters often appear to predominate. Carter et al.[47] reported that in the peanut-growing region of southeastern Australia, the proportion of *A. parasiticus* to *A. flavus* in soil has increased over a 20-year period from 1:1 to 10:1. The high genetic diversity of *A. parasiticus* strains from this entire period suggests that the increase was due to a build-up of native strains rather than the preponderance of an aggressive, newly introduced strain. Because peanuts had been grown in the region for more that 70 years, it was further hypothesized that the population increase was the result of changing environmental conditions or cultivation practices rather than due solely to the presence of peanuts. The peanut-growing region studied had suffered from protracted drought conditions during the 1990s that may have favored *A. parasiticus*, and the introduction of winter crops may have lowered soil levels of *A. flavus* relative to *A. parasiticus*, whose populations are better adapted to survival in soil. Horn et al.[74] reported that the proportion of *A. parasiticus* to *A. flavus* in soil inexplicably increased from 3:7 at planting to 1:1 upon instigation of drought despite a low incidence of seed infection by *A. parasiticus*. Populations of aflatoxigenic fungi in the geocarposphere have been reported to remain unchanged[101,113] or increase[114,115] during pod development. Those studies showing population increases have not distinguished between the direct effect of pods on the geocarposphere and the effect of established pod infections that secondarily produce conidia.

6.8 SELECTIVE EFFECTS OF CROPS

Aflatoxigenic fungi in agricultural ecosystems have two components to their life cycle, one as colonizers of organic matter in soil and the other as facultative parasites of crops. A comparison of the population structure of *Aspergillus flavus* and *A. parasiticus* with other fungal species may provide insight into the selective forces influencing the different life-cycle stages. Soil populations of *A. flavus* and *A. parasiticus* and soil populations of nonpathogenic *Fusarium oxysporum* demonstrate extremely high VCG diversities.[44,116] In contrast, *F. oxysporum* isolates pathogenic to crops have a low VCG diversity due to strong selection for pathogenicity in strains.[117,118] This suggests that *A. flavus* and *A. parasiticus* have population characteristics consistent with a saprobic existence, with diversity perhaps being maintained in the soil environment, and that genetic diversity in aflatoxigenic fungi is not diminished through infection of crops.[17] Bayman and Cotty[43] and Horn and Greene[44] reported considerable overlap between the *A. flavus* and *A. parasiticus* VCGs present in soil and those infecting crops (Figure 6.1).

Although genetic diversity within a species is often similar between soil and crop populations, diversity among species between the two populations can be quite different. The most striking example is the preferential infection of corn by *Aspergillus flavus*.[59,90] Horn et al.[76] reported that despite an equal proportion of *A. flavus* and *A. parasiticus* in soil, corn ears were infected only with *A. flavus*, which resulted in a large increase in soil populations of *A flavus* relative to *A. parasiticus* following harvest (Figure 6.5). Because *A. flavus* and *A. parasiticus* are both carried to corn by soil insects,[90] selection for *A. flavus* likely occurs in the crop. This is supported by research showing that *A. parasiticus* readily infects corn when artificially inoculated alone[81,119] but is out-competed by *A. flavus* when the two species are coinoculated.[120] Even in peanuts, a crop that is commonly infected with *A. parasiticus*, *A. flavus* appears to be the more aggressive species.[59,74]

A continuing question concerning the population structure of aflatoxigenic fungi in agricultural ecosystems is do certain crops select for aflatoxigenicity? Schroeder and Boller[15] examined *Aspergillus flavus* populations from different crops in Texas and reported that 96% of isolates from peanuts produced aflatoxins as opposed to 79, 49, and 35% in cottonseed, sorghum, and rice, respectively. Vaamonde et al.[27] similarly found a high incidence of aflatoxigenic *A. flavus* in peanuts (73%) relative to wheat (13%) and soybeans (5%). The aflatoxin-producing ability of soil isolates from those same fields in both studies was not examined but would indicate whether certain strains were preferentially selected from the soil population. Horn and Dorner[18] postulated that the high density of *A. flavus* in soil from the peanut-growing region of southern Alabama and Georgia is due to seed infection resulting from frequent droughts and that the high percentage of aflatoxigenic isolates (Figure 6.4) is the result of selective forces imposed by peanuts. Nevertheless, most crops are colonized by a mixture of aflatoxigenic and nonaflatoxigenic strains of *A. flavus*,[15,46] and nontoxigenic strains applied to soil for biological control readily compete with native aflatoxigenic strains for available infection sites.[86,87,121] Further research is necessary to resolve any possible crop effects on the aflatoxin-producing potential of *A. flavus* populations.

6.9 CONCLUSIONS

Any explanation for the role of aflatoxins in the life cycle of *Aspergillus flavus* must address the apparent lack of a selective advantage in crops for strains that produce aflatoxins.[122] Aflatoxin production instead may be of importance in soil habitats where ecological niches are more diverse than in crops and where strains may be partitioned in some manner according to their aflatoxin-producing ability. Adverse environmental conditions likely associated with the soil environment, including elevated temperature, low pH, and nutrient deprivation, help maintain the aflatoxin-producing ability in *A. flavus* over successive generations.[123] Insight into not only the role of aflatoxins in the fungal life cycle but also, ultimately, effective ways to control aflatoxin contamination of crops may rest with soil.

REFERENCES

1. Hussein, H.S. and Brasel, J.M., Toxicity, metabolism, and impact of mycotoxins on humans and animals, *Toxicology*, 167, 101–134, 2001.
2. Peraica, M., Radić, B., Lucić, A, and Pavlović, M., Toxic effects of mycotoxins in humans, *Bull. World Health Org.*, 77, 754–766, 1999.
3. Lamb, M.C. and Sternitzke, D.A., Cost of aflatoxin to the farmer, buying point, and sheller segments of the southeast United States peanut industry, *Peanut Sci.*, 28, 59–63, 2001.
4. Klich, M.A., Tiffany, L.H., and Knaphus, G., Ecology of the aspergilli of soils and litter, in Aspergillus: *Biology and Industrial Applications*, Bennett, J.W. and Klich, M.A., Eds., Butterworth-Heinemann, Boston, 1992, pp. 329–353.
5. White, J.P. and Johnson, G.T., Aflatoxin production correlated with nitrification in *Aspergillus flavus* group species, *Mycologia*, 74, 718–723, 1982.
6. Davis, N.D., Diener, U.L., and Agnihotri, V.P., Production of aflatoxins B_1 and G_1 in chemically defined medium, *Mycopathol. Mycol. Appl.*, 31, 251–256, 1967.
7. Hesseltine, C.W., Sorenson, W.G., and Smith, M., Taxonomic studies of the aflatoxin-producing strains in the *Aspergillus flavus* group, *Mycologia*, 62, 123–132, 1970.
8. Betts, W.B. and Dart, R.K., Initial reactions in degradation of tri- and tetrameric lignin-related compounds by *Aspergillus flavus*, *Mycol. Res.*, 92, 177–181, 1989.
9. Cotty, P.J., Cleveland, T.E., Brown, R.L., and Mellon, J.E., Variation in polygalacturonase production among *Aspergillus flavus* isolates, *Appl. Environ. Microbiol.*, 56, 3885–3887, 1990.
10. Long, K., Ghazali, H.M., Ariff, A., Man, Y.C., and Bucke, C., Substrate preference of mycelium-bound lipase from a strain of *Aspergillus flavus* Link, *Biotechnol. Lett.*, 20, 369–372, 1998.
11. Olutiola, P.O., Cellulase enzymes in culture filtrates of *Aspergillus flavus*, *Trans. Br. Mycol. Soc.*, 67, 265–268, 1976.

12. Diener, U.L., Pettit, R.E., and Cole, R.J., Aflatoxins and other mycotoxins in peanuts, in *Peanut Science and Technology*, Pattee, H.E. and Young, C.T., Eds., American Peanut Research and Education Society, Yoakum, TX, 1982, pp. 486–519.

13. Diener, U.L., Cole, R.J., Sanders, T.H., Payne, G.A., Lee, L.S., and Klich, M.A., Epidemiology of aflatoxin formation by *Aspergillus flavus*, *Ann. Rev. Phytopathol.*, 25, 249–270, 1987.

14. Payne, G.A., Process of contamination by aflatoxin-producing fungi and their impact on crops, in *Mycotoxins in Agriculture and Food Safety*, Sinha, K.K. and Bhatnagar, D., Eds., Marcel Dekker, New York, 1998, pp. 279–306.

15. Schroeder, H.W. and Boller, R.A., Aflatoxin production of species and strains of *Aspergillus flavus* group isolated from field crops, *Appl. Microbiol.*, 25, 885–889, 1973.

16. Siriacha, P., Kawashima, K., Kawasugi, S., Saito, M., and Tonboon-Ek, P., Postharvest contamination of Thai corn with *Aspergillus flavus*, *Cereal Chem.*, 66, 445–448, 1989.

17. Horn, B.W., Greene, R.L., Sobolev, V.S., Dorner, J.W., Powell, J.H., and Layton, R.C., Association of morphology and mycotoxin production with vegetative compatibility groups in *Aspergillus flavus*, *A. parasiticus*, and *A. tamarii*, *Mycologia*, 88, 574–587, 1996.

18. Horn, B.W. and Dorner, J.W., Regional differences in production of aflatoxin B_1 and cyclopiazonic acid by soil isolates of *Aspergillus flavus* along a transect within the United States, *Appl. Environ. Microbiol.*, 65, 1444–1449, 1999.

19. Dorner, J.W., Cole, R.J., and Diener, U.L., The relationship of *Aspergillus flavus* and *Aspergillus parasiticus* with reference to production of aflatoxins and cyclopiazonic acid, *Mycopathologia*, 87, 13–15, 1984.

20. Tran-Dinh, N., Pitt, J.I., and Carter, D.A., Molecular genotype analysis of natural toxigenic and nontoxigenic isolates of *Aspergillus flavus* and *A. parasiticus*, *Mycol. Res.*, 103, 1485–1490, 1999.

21. Cotty, P.J., Virulence and cultural characteristics of two *Aspergillus flavus* strains pathogenic on cotton, *Phytopathology*, 79, 808–814, 1989.

22. Hesseltine, C.W., Shotwell, O.L., Smith, M., Ellis, J.J., Vandegraft, E., and Shannon, G., Production of various aflatoxins by strains of the *Aspergillus flavus* series, in *Toxic Micro-Organisms*, Herzberg, M., Ed., U.S. Government Printing Office, Washington, D.C., 1970, pp. 202–210.

23. Saito, M. and Tsuruta, O., A new variety of *Aspergillus flavus* from tropical soil in Thailand and its aflatoxin productivity, *Proc. Jpn. Assoc. Mycotoxicol.*, 37, 31–36, 1993.

24. Cotty, P.J. and Cardwell, K.F., Divergence of West African and North American communities of *Aspergillus* section *Flavi*, *Appl. Environ. Microbiol.*, 65, 2264–2266, 1999.

25. Geiser, D.M., Dorner, J.W., Horn, B.W., and Taylor, J.W., The phylogenetics of mycotoxin and sclerotium production in *Aspergillus flavus* and *Aspergillus oryzae*, *Fungal Genet. Biol.*, 31, 169–179, 2000.

26. Novas, M.V. and Cabral, D., Association of mycotoxin and sclerotia production with compatibility groups in *Aspergillus flavus* from peanut in Argentina, *Plant Dis.*, 86, 215–219, 2002.

27. Vaamonde, G., Patriarca, A., Fernández Pinto, V., Comerio, R., and Degrossi, C., Variability of aflatoxin and cyclopiazonic acid production by *Aspergillus* section *Flavi* from different substrates in Argentina, *Int. J. Food Microbiol.*, 88, 79–84, 2003.

28. Geiser, D.M., Pitt, J.I., and Taylor, J.W., Cryptic speciation and recombination in the aflatoxin-producing fungus *Aspergillus flavus*, *Proc. Natl. Acad. Sci. USA*, 95, 388–393, 1998.

29. Kumeda, Y., Asao, T., Takahashi, H., and Ichinoe, M., High prevalence of B and G aflatoxin-producing fungi in sugarcane field soil in Japan: heteroduplex panel analysis identifies a new genotype within *Aspergillus* section *Flavi* and *Aspergillus nomius*, *FEMS Microbiol. Ecol.*, 45, 229–238, 2003.

30. Barnes, S.E., Dola, T.P., Bennett, J.W., and Bhatnagar, D., Synthesis of sterigmatocystin on a chemically defined medium by species of *Aspergillus* and *Chaetomium*, *Mycopathologia*, 125, 173–178, 1994.

31. Cole, R.J. and Schweikert, M.A., *Handbook of Secondary Fungal Metabolites*, Vol. 1, Academic Press, New York, 2003, 1006 pp.

32. Kurtzman, C.P., Horn, B.W., and Hesseltine, C.W., *Aspergillus nomius*, a new aflatoxin-producing species related to *Aspergillus flavus* and *Aspergillus tamarii*, *Antonie van Leeuwenhoek*, 53, 147–158, 1987.

33. Peterson, S.W., Ito, Y., Horn, B.W., and Goto, T., *Aspergillus bombycis*, a new aflatoxigenic species and genetic variation in its sibling species, *A. nomius*, *Mycologia*, 93, 689–703, 2001.

34. Goto, T., Ito, Y., Peterson, S.W., and Wicklow, D.T., Mycotoxin producing ability of *Aspergillus tamarii*, *Mycotoxins*, 44, 17–20, 1997.

35. Ito, Y., Peterson, S.W., Wicklow, D.T., and Goto, T., *Aspergillus pseudotamarii*, a new aflatoxin producing species in *Aspergillus* section *Flavi*, *Mycol. Res.*, 105, 233–239, 2001.

36. Klich, M.A., Mullaney, E.J., Daly, C.B., and Cary, J.W., Molecular and physiological aspects of aflatoxin and sterigmatocystin biosynthesis by *Aspergillus tamarii* and *A. ochraceoroseus*, *Appl. Microbiol. Biotechnol.*, 53, 605–609, 2000.

37. Maggi, O. and Persiani, A.M., Mycological studies of the soil, in *Comparative Studies on Microfungi in Tropical Ecosystems: Mycological Studies in South Western Ivory Coast Forest*, Rambelli, A., Persiani, A.M., Maggi, O., Lunghini, D., Onofri, S., Riess, S., Dowgiallo, G., and Puppi, G., Eds., MAB, UNESCO, Rome, 1983, pp. 69–94.

38. Klich, M.A. and Pitt, J.I., Differentiation of *Aspergillus flavus* from *A. parasiticus* and other closely related species, *Trans. Br. Mycol. Soc.*, 91, 99–108, 1988.

39. Raper, K.B. and Fennell, D.I., *The Genus* Aspergillus, Williams & Wilkins, Baltimore, MD, 1965, 686 pp.

40. Joffe, A.Z., Aflatoxin produced by 1626 isolates of *Aspergillus flavus* from groundnut kernels and soils in Israel, *Nature*, 221, 492, 1969.

41. Leslie, J.F., Fungal vegetative compatibility, *Annu. Rev. Phytopathol.*, 31, 127–150, 1993.

42. Papa, K.E., Heterokaryon incompatibility in *Aspergillus flavus*, *Mycologia*, 78, 98–101, 1986.

43. Bayman, P. and Cotty, P.J., Vegetative compatibility and genetic diversity in the *Aspergillus flavus* population of a single field, *Can. J. Bot.*, 69, 1707–1711, 1991.

44. Horn, B.W. and Greene, R.L., Vegetative compatibility within populations of *Aspergillus flavus*, *A. parasiticus*, and *A. tamarii* from a peanut field, *Mycologia*, 87, 324–332, 1995.

45. McAlpin, C.E., Wicklow, D.T., and Horn, B.W., DNA fingerprinting analysis of vegetative compatibility groups in *Aspergillus flavus* from a peanut field in Georgia, *Plant Dis.*, 86, 254–258, 2002.

46. Wicklow, D.T., McAlpin, C.E., and Platis, C.E., Characterization of the *Aspergillus flavus* population within an Illinois corn field, *Mycol. Res.*, 102, 263–268, 1998.

47. Carter, D., Bui, T., Walsh, S., and Tran-Dinh, N., RAPD analysis of *Aspergillus parasiticus* isolates from peanut growing soils in Queensland, Australia, *J. Food Mycol.*, 1, 31–39, 1998.

48. McAlpin, C.E., Wicklow, D.T., and Platis, C.E., Genotypic diversity of *Aspergillus parasiticus* in an Illinois corn field, *Plant Dis.*, 82, 1132–1136, 1998.

49. Bayman, P. and Cotty, P.J., Genetic diversity in *Aspergillus flavus*: association with aflatoxin production and morphology, *Can. J. Bot.*, 71, 23–31, 1993.

50. Horn, B.W. and Dorner, J.W., Soil populations of *Aspergillus* species from section *Flavi* along a transect through peanut-growing regions of the United States, *Mycologia*, 90, 767–776, 1998.

51. Papa, K.E., The parasexual cycle in *Aspergillus flavus*, *Mycologia*, 65, 1201–1205, 1973.

52. Papa, K.E., The parasexual cycle in *Aspergillus parasiticus*, *Mycologia*, 70, 766–773, 1978.

53. Griffin, G.J., Garren, K.H., and Taylor, J.D., Influence of crop rotation and minimum tillage on the population of *Aspergillus flavus* group in peanut field soil, *Plant Dis.*, 65, 898–900, 1981.

54. Griffin, G.J., Smith, E.P., and Robinson, T.J., Population patterns of *Aspergillus flavus* group and *A. niger* group in field soils, *Soil Biol. Biochem.*, 33, 253–257, 2001.

55. Orum, T.V., Bigelow, D.M., Nelson, M.R., Howell, D.R., and Cotty, P.J., Spatial and temporal patterns of *Aspergillus flavus* strain composition and propagule density in Yuma County, Arizona, soils, *Plant Dis.*, 81, 911–916, 1997.

56. Orum, T.V., Bigelow, D.M., Cotty, P.J., and Nelson, M.R., Using predictions based on geostatistics to monitor trends in *Aspergillus flavus* strain composition, *Phytopathology*, 89, 761–769, 1999.

57. Horn, B.W., Greene, R.L., Sorensen, R.B., Blankenship, P.D., and Dorner, J.W., Conidial movement of nontoxigenic *Aspergillus flavus* and *A. parasiticus* in peanut fields following application to soil, *Mycopathologia*, 151, 81–92, 2001.

58. Pettit, R.E., Taber, R.A., and Schroeder, H.W., Prevalence of *Aspergillus flavus* in peanut soils, *J. Am. Peanut Res. Assoc.*, 5, 195, 1973.

59. Hill, R.A., Wilson, D.M., McMillian, W.W., Widstrom, N.W., Cole, R.J., Sanders, T.H., and Blankenship, P.D., Ecology of the *Aspergillus flavus* group and aflatoxin formation in maize and groundnut, in *Trichothecenes and Other Mycotoxins*, Lacey, J., Ed., John Wiley & Sons, Chichester, 1985, pp. 79–95.

60. Cotty, P.J., Aflatoxin-producing potential of communities of *Aspergillus* section *Flavi* from cotton producing areas in the United States, *Mycol. Res.*, 101, 698–704, 1997.

61. Doster, M.A. and Michailides, T.J., Development of *Aspergillus* molds in litter from pistachio trees, *Plant Dis.*, 78, 393–397, 1994.

62. Doster, M.A., Michailides, T.J., and Morgan, D.P., *Aspergillus* species and mycotoxins in figs from California orchards, *Plant Dis.*, 80, 484–489, 1996.

63. Angle, J.S., Dunn, K.A., and Wagner, G.H., Effect of cultural practices on the soil population of *Aspergillus flavus* and *Aspergillus parasiticus*, *Soil Sci. Soc. Am. J.*, 46, 301–304, 1982.

64. Shearer, J.F., Sweets, L.E., Baker, N.K., and Tiffany, L.H., A study of *Aspergillus flavus/parasiticus* in Iowa crop fields: 1988–1990, *Plant Dis.*, 76, 19–22, 1992.

65. Boyd, M.L. and Cotty, P.J., *Aspergillus flavus* and aflatoxin contamination of leguminous trees of the Sonoran Desert in Arizona, *Phytopathology*, 91, 913–919, 2001.

66. Wilson, D.M., Holbrook, C.C., and Matheron, M.E., *Aspergillus flavus* and *A. parasiticus* used as peanut plot inoculum to study preharvest aflatoxin contamination, *Proc. Am. Peanut Res. Educ. Soc.*, 28, 30, 1996.

67. Manabe, M., Tsuruta, O., Tanaka, K., and Matsuura, S., Distribution of aflatoxin-producing fungi in soil in Japan, *Trans. Mycol. Soc. Jpn.*, 17, 436–444, 1976.

68. Manabe, M. and Tsuruta, O., Geographical distribution of aflatoxin-producing fungi inhabiting in Southeast Asia, *Jpn. Agric. Res. Q.*, 12, 224–227, 1978.

69. Cardwell, K.F. and Cotty, P.J., Distribution of *Aspergillus* section *Flavi* among field soils from the four agroecological zones of the Republic of Bénin, West Africa, *Plant Dis.*, 86, 434–439, 2002.

70. McGee, D.C., Olanya, O.M., Hoyos, G.M, and Tiffany, L.H., Populations of *Aspergillus flavus* in the Iowa cornfield ecosystem in years not favorable for aflatoxin contamination of corn grain, *Plant Dis.*, 80, 742–746, 1996.

71. Christensen, M. and Tuthill, D.E., *Aspergillus*: an overview, in *Advances in* Penicillium *and* Aspergillus *Systematics*, Samson, R.A. and Pitt, J.I., Eds., Plenum Press, New York, 1985, pp. 195–209.

72. Klich, M.A., Biogeography of *Aspergillus* species in soil and litter, *Mycologia*, 94, 21–27, 2002.

73. Griffin, G.J., *Fusarium oxysporum* and *Aspergillus flavus* spore germination in the rhizosphere of peanut, *Phytopathology*, 59, 1214–1218, 1969.

74. Horn, B.W., Dorner, J.W., Greene, R.L., Blankenship, P.D., and Cole, R.J., Effect of *Aspergillus parasiticus* soil inoculum on invasion of peanut seeds, *Mycopathologia*, 125, 179–191, 1994.

75. Wicklow, D.T., Wilson, D.M., and Nelsen, T.C., Survival of *Aspergillus flavus* sclerotia and conidia buried in soil in Illinois or Georgia, *Phytopathology*, 83, 1141–1147, 1993.

76. Horn, B.W., Greene, R.L., and Dorner, J.W., Effect of corn and peanut cultivation on soil populations of *Aspergillus flavus* and *A. parasiticus* in southwestern Georgia, *Appl. Environ. Microbiol.*, 61, 2472–2475, 1995.

77. Coley-Smith, J.R. and Cooke, R.C., Survival and germination of fungal sclerotia, *Ann. Rev. Phytopathol.*, 9, 65–92, 1971.

78. Klich, M.A., *Identification of Common* Aspergillus *Species*, Centraalbureau voor Schimmelcultures, Utrecht, The Netherlands, 2002, 116 pp.

79. Wicklow, D.T., Survival of *Aspergillus flavus* sclerotia in soil, *Trans. Br. Mycol. Soc.*, 89, 131–134, 1987.

80. Wicklow, D.T., Horn, B.W., Burg, W.R., and Cole, R.J., Sclerotium dispersal of *Aspergillus flavus* and *Eupenicillium ochrosalmoneum* from maize during harvest, *Trans. Br. Mycol. Soc.*, 83, 299–303, 1984.

81. Zummo, N. and Scott, G.E., Relative aggressiveness of *Aspergillus flavus* and *A. parasiticus* on maize in Mississippi, *Plant Dis.*, 74, 978–981, 1990.

82. Garber, R.K. and Cotty, P.J., Formation of sclerotia and aflatoxins in developing cotton bolls infected by the S strain of *Aspergillus flavus* and potential for biocontrol with an atoxigenic strain, *Phytopathology*, 87, 940–945, 1997.

83. Wicklow, D.T. and Donahue, J.E., Sporogenic germination of sclerotia in *Aspergillus flavus* and *A. parasiticus*, *Trans. Br. Mycol. Soc.*, 82, 621–624, 1984.

84. Wicklow, D.T. and Wilson, D.M., Germination of *Aspergillus flavus* sclerotia in a Georgia maize field, *Trans. Br. Mycol. Soc.*, 87, 651–653, 1986.

85. Stack, J.P. and Pettit, P.E., Germination of *Aspergillus flavus* sclerotia in soil, *Phytopathology*, 74, 799, 1984.

86. Cotty, P.J., Influence of field application of an atoxigenic strain of *Aspergillus flavus* on the populations of *A. flavus* infecting cotton bolls and on the aflatoxin content of cottonseed, *Phytopathology*, 84, 1270–1277, 1994.

87. Dorner, J.W., Cole, R.J., and Wicklow, D.T., Aflatoxin reduction in corn through field application of competitive fungi, *J. Food Prot.*, 62, 650–656, 1999.

88. Olanya, O.M., Hoyos, G.M., Tiffany, L.H., and McGee, D.C., Waste corn as point source of inoculum for *Aspergillus flavus* in the corn agroecosystem, *Plant Dis.*, 81, 576–581, 1997.

89. Lee, L.S., Lee, Jr., L.V., and Russell, T.E., Aflatoxin in Arizona cottonseed: field inoculation of bolls by *Aspergillus flavus* spores in wind-driven soil, *J. AOCS*, 63, 530–532, 1986.

90. Lillehoj, E.B., McMillian, W.W., Guthrie, W.D., and Barry, D., Aflatoxin-producing fungi in preharvest corn: inoculum source in insects and soils, *J. Environ. Qual.*, 9, 691–694, 1980.

91. Lussenhop, J. and Wicklow, D.T., Nitidulid beetles (Nitidulidae: Coleoptera) as vectors of *Aspergillus flavus* in pre-harvest maize, *Trans. Mycol. Soc. Jpn.*, 31, 63–74, 1990.

92. Cole, R.J., Hill, R.A., Blankenship, P.D., and Sanders, T.H., Color mutants of *Aspergillus flavus* and *Aspergillus parasiticus* in a study of preharvest invasion of peanuts, *Appl. Environ. Microbiol.*, 52, 1128–1131, 1986.

93. Frank, Z.R., Smulevitch, Y., and Lisker, N., Preharvest kernel invasion in groundnut genotypes by *Aspergillus flavus* and its relation to the pod surface area, *Euphytica*, 75, 207–213, 1994.

94. Xu, H., Annis, S., Linz, J., and Trail, F., Infection and colonization of peanut pods by *Aspergillus parasiticus* and the expression of the aflatoxin biosynthetic gene, *nor-1*, in infection hyphae, *Physiol. Molec. Plant Pathol.*, 56, 185–196, 2000.

95. Bowen, K.L. and Mack, T.P., Relationship of damage from the lesser cornstalk borer to *Aspergillus flavus* contamination in peanuts, *J. Entomol. Sci.*, 28, 29–42, 1993.

96. Lynch, R.E. and Wilson, D.M., Enhanced infection of peanut, *Arachis hypogaea* L., seeds with *Aspergillus flavus* group fungi due to scarification of peanut pods by the lesser cornstalk borer, *Elasmopalpus lignosellus* (Zeller), *Peanut Sci.*, 18, 110–116, 1991.

97. Lynch, R.E., Wightman, J.A., and Ranga Rao, G.V., Insects and arthropods, in *Compendium of Peanut Diseases*, 2nd ed., Kokalis-Burelle, N., Porter, D.M., Rodríguez-Kábana, R., Smith, D.H., and Subrahmanyam, P., Eds., APS Press, St. Paul, MN, 1997, pp. 65–69.

98. Lynch, R.E., Ouedraogo, A.P., and Dicko, I., Insect damage to groundnut in semi-arid tropical Africa, in *Agrometeorology of Groundnut, Proceedings of an International Symposium*, ICRISAT, Andhra Pradesh, India, 1986, pp. 175–183.

99. Umeh, V.C., Waliyar, F., and Traoré, A., *Aspergillus* species colonization of termite-damaged peanuts in parts of West Africa and its control prospects, *Peanut Sci.*, 27, 1–6, 2000.

100. Dorner, J.W., Cole, R.J., Sanders, T.H., and Blankenship, P.D., Interrelationship of kernel water activity, soil temperature, maturity, and phytoalexin production in preharvest aflatoxin contamination of drought-stressed peanuts, *Mycopathologia*, 105, 117–128, 1989.

101. Griffin, G.J., Conidial germination and population of *Aspergillus flavus* in the geocarposphere of peanut, *Phytopathology*, 62, 1387–1391, 1972.

102. Hale, M.G. and Griffin, G.J., The effect of mechanical injury on exudation from immature and mature peanut fruits under axenic conditions, *Soil Biol. Biochem.*, 8, 225–227, 1976.

103. Aucamp, J.L., The role of mite vectors in the development of aflatoxin in groundnuts, *J. Stored Prod. Res.*, 5, 245–249, 1969.

104. Johnson, S.J. and Smith, J.W., Ecology of *Elasmopalpus lignosellus* parasite complex on peanuts in Texas, *Ann. Entomol. Soc. Am.*, 74, 467–471, 1981.

105. Jones, D. and Bass, M.H., Evaluation of pitfall traps for sampling lesser cornstalk borer larvae in peanuts, *J. Econ. Entomol.*, 72, 289–290, 1979.

106. Griffin, G.J. and Garren, K.H., Population levels of *Aspergillus flavus* and the *A. niger* group in Virginia peanut field soils, *Phytopathology*, 64, 322–325, 1974.

107. Hill, R.A., Blankenship, P.D., Cole, R.J., and Sanders, T.H., Effects of soil moisture and temperature on preharvest invasion of peanuts by the *Aspergillus flavus* group and subsequent aflatoxin development, *Appl. Environ. Microbiol.*, 45, 628–633, 1983.

108. Jones, R.K., Duncan, H.E., and Hamilton, P.B., Planting date, harvest date, and irrigation effects on infection and aflatoxin production by *Aspergillus flavus* in field corn, *Phytopathology*, 71, 810–816, 1981.

109. Klich, M.A., Relation of plant water potential at flowering to subsequent cottonseed infection by *Aspergillus flavus*, *Phytopathology*, 77, 739–741, 1987.

110. Hill, R.A., Wilson, D.M., Burg, W.R., and Shotwell, O.L., Viable fungi in corn dust, *Appl. Environ. Microbiol.*, 47, 84–87, 1984.

111. Griffin, G.J. and Garren, K.H., Colonization of rye green manure and peanut fruit debris by *Aspergillus flavus* and *Aspergillus niger* group in field soils, *Appl. Environ. Microbiol.*, 32, 28–32, 1976.

112. Stack, J.P. and Pettit, P.E., Colonization of organic matter substrates in soil by *Aspergillus flavus*, *Proc. Am. Peanut Res. Educ. Soc.*, 16, 45, 1984.

113. Kloepper, J.W. and Bowen, K.L., Quantification of the geocarposphere and rhizosphere effect of peanut (*Arachis hypogaea* L.), *Plant Soil*, 136, 103–109, 1991.

114. McDonald, D., The influence of the developing groundnut fruit on soil mycoflora, *Trans. Br. Mycol. Soc.*, 53, 393–406, 1969.

115. Subrahmanyam, P. and Rao, A.S., Rhizosphere and geocarposphere mycoflora of groundnut (*Arachis hypogaea* Linn.), *Proc. Indian Acad. Sci.*, 85B, 420–431, 1977.

116. Gordon, T.R. and Okamoto, D., Vegetative compatibility groupings in a local population of *Fusarium oxysporum*, *Can. J. Bot.*, 69, 168–172, 1991.

117. Bosland, P.W. and Williams, P.H., An evaluation of *Fusarium oxysporum* from crucifers based on pathogenicity, isozyme polymorphism, vegetative compatibility, and geographic origin, *Can. J. Bot.*, 65, 2067–2073, 1987.

118. Larkin, R.P., Hopkins, D.L., and Martin, F.N., Vegetative compatibility within *Fusarium oxysporum* f.sp. *niveum* and its relationship to virulence, aggressiveness, and race, *Can. J. Microbiol.*, 36, 352–358, 1990.

119. Wilson, D.M., McMillian, W.W., and Widstrom, N., Use of *Aspergillus flavus* and *A. parasiticus* color mutants to study aflatoxin contamination of corn, in *Biodeterioration*, Vol. 6, Barry, S., Houghton, D.R., Llewellyn, G.C., and O'Rear, C.E., Eds., CAB International, Slough, U.K., 1986, pp. 284–288.

120. Calvert, O.H., Lillehoj, E.B., Kwolek, W.F., and Zuber, M.S., Aflatoxin B_1 and G_1 production in developing *Zea mays* kernels from mixed inocula of *Aspergillus flavus* and *A. parasiticus*, *Phytopathology*, 68, 501–506, 1978.

121. Dorner, J.W., Cole, R.J., and Blankenship, P.D., Effect of inoculum rate of biological control agents on preharvest aflatoxin contamination of peanuts, *Biol. Cont.*, 12, 171–176, 1998.

122. Carter, D.A., Tran-Dinh, N., Stat, M., Kumar, S., Bui, T., and Pitt, J.I., The aflatoxins: evolution, function and prospects for control, in *Advances in Microbial Toxin Research and Its Biotechnological Exploitation*, Upadhyay, R.K., Ed., Plenum Press, New York, 2002, pp. 47–62.

123. Horn, B.W. and Dorner, J.W., Effect of competition and adverse culture conditions on aflatoxin production by *Aspergillus flavus* through successive generations, *Mycologia*, 94, 741–751, 2002.

7 The Sterigmatocystin Cluster Revisited: Lessons from a Genetic Model

Tami McDonald, Tom Hammond,
Daan Noordermeer, Yong-Qiang Zhang,
and Nancy Keller

CONTENTS

7.1 INTRODUCTION

The occurrence of turkey X disease in England in the 1960s drew attention to the health hazards of mycotoxins, specifically aflatoxins (AFs), and spurred research on these prevalent toxic and carcinogenic compounds. Since the 1960s, significant progress has been made in characterizing the biosynthesis of aflatoxin and its penultimate precursor, sterigmatocystin (ST).[1,2] Initially, advances were made in identifying the precursors and enzymatic activities of the AF/ST pathway.[2] In the 1980s and 1990s, these advances were followed by identification of genes encoding enzymatic activities of the AF/ST pathway.[1,2]

Early genetic studies of AF biosynthesis identified a cluster of AF/ST biosynthetic genes in an ~70-kb region.[3–6] Identification of the gene cluster was heralded by indications of AF gene linkage in parasexual studies.[7] Although the cluster was first viewed as an oddity, clustering of secondary metabolite synthesis genes seems to be the rule in fungi.[8,9] Fungal secondary metabolite gene clusters, including the melanin, penicillin, lovastatin, paxillin, and trichothecenes gene clusters, have been found in several genera.[9] Of these, the AF/ST cluster is perhaps the most extensively studied.

Although most enzymatic steps in the AF/ST pathway have been characterized, several steps remain unclear. Problematic areas include possible bifurcations in the pathway, the production of transitory or unstable intermediates, and the elaboration of chemically related shunt products not directly involved in AF/ST biosynthesis. Inactivation of genes in the cluster has not helped to clarify these issues. Perhaps the greatest mystery is the unexpectedly large number of genes in the ST and AF clusters that appear not to participate in the biochemical reactions required for AF/ST synthesis. In this chapter, we summarize the known biosynthetic functions in the pathway, detail problematic points, and present some hypotheses and speculation on the nature of the seemingly expendable genes.

7.2 STERIGMATOCYSTIN CLUSTER GENES INVOLVED IN STERIGMATOCYSTIN SYNTHESIS

Figure 7.1 outlines the various steps characterized in the synthesis of ST by *Aspergillus nidulans*; these are identical to those for AF production in *A. flavus* and *A. parasiticus*. Figure 7.2 presents the order of genes in the ST and AF gene cluster. Below we present the steps for protein function.

7.2.1 POLYKETIDE SYNTHASE AND FATTY ACID SYNTHASE

The AF and ST synthesis pathway is unusual in that the first step is catalyzed by a polyketide synthase (PKS) acting in concert with a fatty acid synthase (FAS). These proteins associate in a complex most likely composed of three peptides each of an α and β chain of a FAS encoded by *stcJ* and *stcK*, respectively, and one PKS encoded by *stcA*.[10] An StcJ/StcK heterodimer synthesizes hexanoyl CoA, the starter unit for StcA, which unlike most PKSs does not utilize acetyl CoA. StcA catalyzes successive

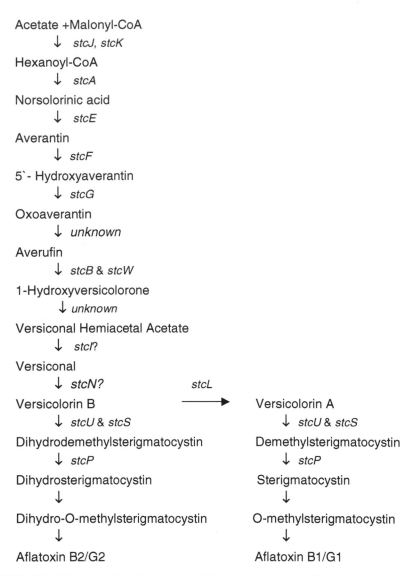

FIGURE 7.1 Aflatoxin and sterigmatocystin biosynthetic pathway. Known genes in the sterigmatocystin cluster are shown in italics, and question marks indicate postulated placement in the pathway.

rounds of malonyl CoA condensation to form the transitory polyketide noranthrone. Noranthrone is subsequently oxidized by an unknown mechanism[11] to norsolorinic acid (NOR), the first stable intermediate of the AF/ST pathway.

Brown et al.[4] disrupted both *stcJ* and *stcK* and determined that both mutants grew normally but could not produce ST. The same study also demonstrated that addition of hexanoic acid to the growth medium restored ST production in these mutants but

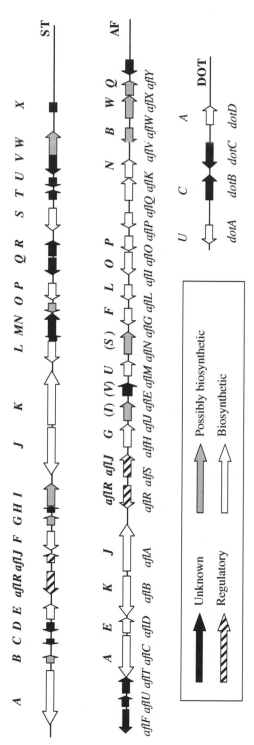

FIGURE 7.2 Order and direction of transcription of homologous genes in the sterigmatocystin (ST), aflatoxin (AF), and dothiostromin (DOT) gene clusters. Homologous genes from the ST cluster are indicated above the line; the ST homolog in parentheses indicates functional homology not yet demonstrated. The name of the gene is indicated below the line.

not in an *stcA* mutant. The genetic data supported earlier work suggesting that hexanoyl CoA was the AF/ST PKS starter unit[13] and furthermore established the existence of two distinct *Aspergillus nidulans* FASs: the ST StcJ/StcK FAS and a FasA/FasB complex required for primary metabolism. Full sequence data of *A. nidulans* (http://www-genome.wi.mit.edu/annotation/fungi/aspergillus/) suggests that the fungus has additional FAS genes, although the functions of these putative FASs are unknown.

As with disruption of *stcJ* and *stcK*, disruption of *stcA* blocks the production of ST and of all pathway intermediates but does not affect expression of other genes in the ST pathway.[14] Sequence analysis showed StcA to be an iterative type I PKS. Type I PKSs are large, multifunctional modular proteins that synthesize a polyketide chain through successive condensations of two-carbon CoA esters. As opposed to bacterial type I PKSs, which have several single-use (noniterative) modules on one protein each containing all the necessary active sites for one particular condensation and subsequent modifications, fungal iterative type I PKSs have only one module on the protein and use each active site more than once. Bacterial type II PKSs are composed of not one but several enzymes, all monofunctional, that act iteratively in a complex. Type III PKS are composed of homodimers that act directly on CoA units instead of using an acyl carrier protein (ACP) as a mediator as do type I and type II PKSs.[15]

Although PKSs vary in structure, they share common enzymatic domains. Three domains, the ketoacyl synthase (KS), acyl transferse (AT), and acyl carrier protein (ACP), are essential for PKS function and are found in all PKSs. Other domains — namely, ketoreductase (KR), dehydratase (DH), enoyl reductase (ER) and thioesterase (TE) — are present in some PKSs but not in others.[16] The ST PKS contains KS, AT, duplicated ACP, and TE domains.[14]

According to Yu and Leonard,[14] the acetyl group from hexanoyl CoA is attached to StcA via a thioester linkage. Seven malonyl–CoA units are condensed by the enzyme, with a loss of CO_2 at each condensation, to make the octaketide precurser. The octaketide is cyclicized, possibly via the activity of a dehydratase (DH), and released, possibly via the activity of a TE. Once free of the enzyme complex, the anthrone is oxidized by some non-PKS activity to the anthraquinone norsolorinic acid. Although the TE domain has been identified, Yu and Leonard found no evidence of a DH domain. The presence of such a domain is still in question, as is the mode of action of cyclization of the octaketide.

7.2.2 Monooxygenases

Monooxygenases are the most prevalent type of enzyme found in the AF and ST biosynthetic gene clusters. Although it is predicted that five monooxygenases are in the ST biosynthetic gene cluster and that five monooxygenase-mediated steps occur in ST synthesis, including one for each shift of chemical class (anthraquinone to xanthone to courmarin) and also for the desaturation of the dihydrobisfuran, not all of these functions can be assigned to an enzyme.[2] To date, three monooxygenase-mediated steps have been assigned unequivocally to an enzyme.

An inactivation strain of *stcF* was shown by Keller et al.[17] to accumulate averantin and is thus responsible for the conversion of averantin to averufin. This cytochrome P-450 monooxygenase is homologous to *avnA* (*aflG*) in *Aspergillus parasiticus*.[1,18] It has been shown that *stcL* encodes a cytochrome P-450 monoxygenase that catalyzes the desaturation of the bisfuran moiety of versicolorin B to versicolorin A; hence, *stcL* is responsible for the branchpoint of the AF/ST pathway (Figure 7.1). An inactivation strain of *stcL* accumulated versicolorin B and did not produce ST; however, feeding the mutant with versicolorin A allowed the strain to produce ST.[19] This confirmed the action of StcL after production of versicolorin B and before production of versicolorin A.

A cytochrome P-450 encoded by *stcS* is responsible for the conversion of versicolorin A to demethylsterigmatocystin and presumably dihydrodemethylsterigmatocystin. This conversion may involve an oxidation, a keto-reduction, and a decarboxylation.[20,21] StcS is responsible for the oxidation step, while StcU, a ketoreductase, reduces the keto group. Missing in this conversion of versicolorin A to ST is a decarboxylase. No gene in the ST biosynthetic pathway has been identified that is homologous to a decarboxylase, and no novel mutants have been identified that are blocked at this step. Possibly the decarboxylase is housed elsewhere in the genome, or the conversion of versicolorin A to ST proceeds in a manner that does not require a decarboxylase. No decarboxylase has been identified in the AF cluster.[21]

Activities of the two remaining monooxygenases are less straightforward. A P-450 monooxygenase encoded by *stcB* is responsible for the conversion of averufin to 1-hydroxyversicolorone; however, inactivation of *stcW*, encoding a flavin-requiring monooxygenase, results in a strain that also accumulates averufin. Thus, StcW may also catalyze the conversion of averufin to 1-hydroxyversicolorone.[17] This redundancy of function is perplexing for two reasons. First, this apparent redundancy leaves the oxidation of 1-hydroxyversicolorone to versiconal hemiacetal acetate without a catalyzing enzyme within the ST biosynthetic cluster. Second, oxidation of averufin to 1-hydroxyversicolorone should not require two enzymes, theoretically, nor does it seem likely that a dimer of the two proteins catalyzes both reactions as there is no precedent for such an action. Still, one of the enzymes may require the other for proper functioning, or 1-hydroxyversicolorone may be shunted into another biosynthetic pathway in the fungus before it can be detected.[21] Unclear results for these steps also are reported for *Aspergillus parasiticus*.[1] Elucidation of steps between the production of averufin and production of versiconal hemiacetal acetate may provide information on novel chemistry of this pathway.

7.2.3 DEHYDROGENASES

Deletion of *stcG* in *Aspergillus nidulans* results in the accumulation of 5′-hydroxyaverantin and averufanin (Sim and Keller, unpublished data). The *stcG* disruptant is leaky, however, as it still produces ST. Disruption of the *stcG* ortholog in *A. parasiticus*, *adhA* (*aflH*), resulted in accumulation of the same metabolites and also was leaky.[22] We concur with Chang et al.[22] who suggest that averufanin may be a nonenzymatic byproduct and that another dehydrogenase, AF/ST-specific or not, may be able to convert 5'-hydroxyaverantin to averufin. This could explain the leaky nature of these mutants. Evidence from *A. parasiticus* suggests that an additional step is required in the conversion of 5'-hydroxyaverantin to averufanin. Sakuno et al.[23] demonstrated that 5'-hydroxyaverantin is converted by a dehydrogenase to 5'–oxoaverantin, which is then cyclized by a cytosolically located enzyme called OAVN cyclase. 5'-hydroxyaverantin dehydrogenase is deduced to be AdhA.[22,23] The gene encoding OAVN cyclase is not reported and does not appear to be located in the AF/ST cluster.

7.2.4 KETOREDUCTASES

StcE catalyzes the keto-reduction of norsolorinic acid, a visible orange pigment, to averantin. Butchko et al.[24] disrupted the gene and used the resulting transformant to screen for mutants deficient in ST cluster regulation. StcE is orthologous to Nor-1 (AflD) in *Aspergillus parasiticus*.[1,25,26] StcU catalyzes the keto-reduction of versicolorin A to DMST. Keller et al.[27] disrupted *stcU* and demonstrated that disruption of the gene results in elimination of ST production and in the accumulation of versicolorin A. StcU is orthologous to Ver-1 (AflM) in *A. parasiticus* and Ver1 in *A. flavus*.[3,28–30] Because disruption of these genes results in straightforward phenotypes, these two mutations have become standard markers for genetic work on the ST cluster in *A. nidulans*.

7.2.5 METHYLTRANSFERASE

StcP catalyzes the methylation of demethylsterigmatocystin to ST and putatively dihydrodemethylsterigmatocystin to dihydrosterigmatocystin. Kelkar et al.[31] disrupted *stcP* and demonstrated the elimination of ST production and subsequent accumulation of demethylsterigmatocystin. The *stcP* gene is orthologous to *aflO* (formerly *dmtA* or *omtB*) in *Aspergillus flavus* and *A. parasiticus*.[1,32–34]

7.2.6 REGULATORY FACTORS AFLR AND AFLJ

AflR is a positive-acting transcription factor required for the transcription of AF/ST biosynthetic genes.[35–38] Deletion of *Aspergillus nidulans aflR* leads to the inability of the fungus to express the genes in the ST biosynthetic cluster and inability of the fungus to produce ST or any of the ST intermediates. A similar phenotype is seen in *A. flavus* and *A. parasiticus aflR* mutants.[37,39] AflR is a Cys6 zinc binuclear cluster protein of the GAL4 type in yeast.[35] These proteins have been identified in fungi only. While the *A. parasiticus* and *A. flavus aflR* genes share 95% identity,[40] the *A. nidulans* AflR protein shares only 33% identity with either *A. parasiticus* or *A. flavus* AflR. Conversely, in the zinc binuclear cluster region and in two regions in the C-terminal end, the percent similarity is as high as 71%.[41] Expression of *A. flavus aflR* in an *A. nidulans aflR* deletion strain restored transcription of genes in the ST cluster and remediated ST production, demonstrating functional homology of the proteins.

AflR recognizes binding sites in the promoter regions of ST and AF biosynthetic genes. Chang et al.[42] first proposed TTAGGCCTAA as the AflR binding site for *Aspergillus parasiticus* and *A. flavus*, but as noted in Fernandes et al.[35] this sequence is missing from the *A. nidulans* ST cluster. Work by Fernandes et al.[35] demonstrated that the AflR binding site in *A. nidulans* is 5′–TCG(N5)GCA–3′. This sequence is found in the promoter region of *stcE*, *stcF*, *stcI*, *stcJ*, *stcK*, *stcQ*, *stcS*, *stcT*, *stcU*, *stcV*, and *stcW*. Researchers determined that AflR could bind to so-called imperfect binding sites which differed from the "perfect" site described above by only one basepair.[35] Between two and nine such sites are found in the promoter region of each ST biosynthetic gene. Finally, the study by Fernandes et al.[35] suggested that AflR binding to the repeat 5′–TCG(N10)TCG–3′ may be possible. At least one intact binding site must be present for efficient transcription of a gene. Mutations in one half of the binding site cause a significant decrease in activity. Another study determined that the 5′–TCG(N5)GCA–3′ site is also recognized and necessary for AF gene expression by *A. flavus* and *A. parasiticus* AflR.[43]

Several binding sites for global regulatory proteins, including PacC (a pH regulator), CreA (carbon catabolite regulator), and AreA (nitrogen utilization regulator) are found in the *aflR* promoter (Keller, unpublished data).[44] This suggests that AF/ST gene expression can be affected by environmental factors such as pH, nitrogen, and carbon source availability.

The *aflJ* gene is located beside *aflR* and oppositely transcribed to *aflR* (Figure 7.1). Inactivation or mutation of *aflJ* gives a phenotype similar to an *aflR* deletion (i.e., a great reduction in AF or ST production) (Butchko and Keller, unpublished data).[45] Although AflJ has not been studied in *Aspergillus nidulans*, several studies have partially defined its function in *A. parasiticus*.[11,45,46] In *aflJ* deletion strains, AF production is decreased by as much as 100-fold. Transcription of genes involved at all points of the AF synthesis pathway is reduced by 5- to 20-fold. This complicated phenotype suggests that AflJ is not directly responsible for AF/ST gene transcription or for any particular enzymatic step in the pathway, but that it is in some way enhancing transcription. Chang et al.[46] demonstrated an interaction of AflJ with AflR, but not AF pathway enzymes, using a yeast two-hybrid system. It is likely that the full-length AflJ protein is required for activity, as deletion of the first 9 amino acids reduced activity of the protein by 85 to 90%, and deletion of the final 11 amino acids terminated activity. Random amino acid substitutions in the C-terminal end, however, did not affect activity. Chang et al.[46] also determined that amino acids 1 to 229 of AflR are not required for interaction with AflJ, but that two regions, one located between amino acids 230 and 238 and another at the C-terminus, are required for interaction with AflJ.[46]

Chang[11] traced the inability of the food fermentor *Aspergillus sojae*, arguably a domesticated strain of *A. parasiticus*,[46] to produce AF to a nonfunctional AflR and AflJ.[10] *A. sojae* AflR is terminated prematurely by a stop codon located 62 amino acids from the C-terminus. Truncated AflR did not interact with wild-type AflJ from either *A. parasiticus* or *A. sojae*. Similarly, the *A. sojae* wild-type AflJ, which contains only two amino acid substitutions, at amino acids 39 and 283, compared to wild-type *A. parasiticus* AflJ, could not interact with the AflR from either species.

7.3   STERIGMATOCYSTIN CLUSTER GENES WITH AMBIGUOUS OR UNASSIGNED FUNCTIONS

7.3.1   DELETED GENES WITH AMBIGUOUS PHENOTYPE

Early work on the ST cluster largely proceeded with the tacit assumption that each gene in the cluster would be responsible for one biosynthetic step, or at least for some aspect of biosynthesis; however, several gene disruptions defy this model. As noted above, some disruptions, such as those of *stcB* and *stcW*, yielded redundant phenotypes, suggesting that the pathway cannot be delineated as a "one gene, one biosynthetic" step. More puzzling are disruptions that apparently do not interrupt ST synthesis or that affect ST synthesis in an unexpected way.

7.3.1.1   *stcI* and *stcQ*

Deletions of *stcI* and *stcQ* do not affect production of ST as assayed under typical laboratory conditions. StcQ shows homology to an AF cluster gene (OrdB) that also has not been assigned a function. StcI is likely an esterase thought to be necessary in the conversion of versiconal hemiacetal acetate to versiconal (Figure 7.1). Strains carrying a disrupted *stcI* allele produce ST but also accumulate some norsolorinic acid (Keller, unpublished data). The putative *stcI* ortholog (the new *aflJ*, formerly *estA*) mediates the conversion of versiconal hemiacetal acetate to versiconal in mutants of *Aspergillus parasiticus*.[47,48] *A. nidulans* may contain another esterase capable of this bioconversion.

7.3.1.2   *stcN*

A strain of *Aspergillus nidulans* with deletion of stcN does not produce ST or accumulate ST intermediates (Keller, unpublished data); however, based on homology to the *A. parasiticus* versicolorin B synthase (AflK, formerly Vbs), stcN has tentatively been assigned a function similar to that of Vbs. Vbs catalyzes the side-chain cyclization of racemic versiconal hemiacetal to the bisfuran ring system of (–)-versicolorin B.[49] Deletion of stcN may result in instability of intermediates or processing of intermediates through another metabolic pathway in *A. nidulans*.

7.3.1.3   *stcV* and *stcC*

The dehydrogenase encoded by *stcV* is another unassigned enzyme. It is homologous to *norA* (*aflE*) in *Aspergillus parasiticus*. Disruption of *stcV* did not affect ST production (Keller, unpublished data) nor does disruption of *norA* affect AF production.[1,50] Both enzymes were once thought to be necessary in conversion of norsolorinic acid to averantin, but this activity has now been assigned to StcE in *A. nidulans* and AflD (Nor-1) in *A. parasiticus* and *A. flavus*. Both StcV and AflE have about 49% amino acid sequence similarity to an aryl alcohol dehydrogenase, an enzyme produced in the white rot fungus *Phanerochaete chrysogenum*[50] and involved in lignin degradation. Interestingly, StcC has greatest homology to chloroperoxidases, enzymes that also have been implicated in lignin degradation.[51] Like *stcV*, disruption of *stcC* does not affect ST production (data not shown). A homolog for *stcC* has not been identified in the AF gene clusters. The presence of possible ligninases in the ST and AF gene clusters is interesting to consider. Lignin deposition is commonly associated with tree growth, but lignin also is produced in certain seeds and seed coverings such as the peanut shell,[52] a substrate of *A. parasiticus*.[53]

7.3.1.4   StcT

One intriguing protein that bears additional investigation is StcT. Disruption of StcT produced a strain of *Aspergillus nidulans* with significantly less ST production than wild type (Zhang, Noordermeer, and Keller, unpublished data). Thin-layer chromatography (TLC) analysis also suggested a decrease in production of other metabolites, some possibly ST precursors. A change in pigmentation in the *stcT* deletion strain was identified with macroscopic examination. Also, spore production was approximately half that of wild type. The similarity of StcT to two proteins — translation elongation factors (EFs, e-21 to e-28) and glutathione *S*-transferases (GSTs, e-15) — was identified with sequence analysis. Although more similar to EFs, the proposed size of StcT is identical to that of GSTs but only half that of EFs. Additionally, StcT displays several conserved GST domains, so it seems that StcT may be more like a GST than an EF. The similarity between EFs and GST has been noted by others.[54]

Glutathione *S*-transferases are a family of multifunctional isozymes involved in detoxification of xenobiotics.[55,56] Interestingly, *Trypanosoma cruzi* EF exhibits similar properties, possibly via a conserved mechanism through its GST domain.[54] Mammalian GSTs are involved in detoxification of AF epoxides, the form of AF that results in DNA mutations. Mice are highly resistant to AFB_1-induced hepatocarcinogenesis because they express a particular form of GST with remarkably high catalytic activity toward the AFB_1 epoxide.[57] The GSTs constitutively expressed in human liver, the alpha class GSTs, have little to no activity toward AF epoxides; however, human mu class GSTs do have some detoxification activity toward AF epoxides, and efforts to upregulate mu GST expression through drug intervention show some promise toward achieving protection.[57] In addition to xenobiotic detoxification, GSTs conjugate reduced glutathione to plant secondary metabolites.[58] Although not proven, glutathione conjugation may protect cells from toxic effects of these secondary metabolites.

Considering the *stcT* deletion phenotype, it is interesting to speculate on the role of StcT in the context of the detoxification and protection mechanisms of GSTs. Could StcT be serving a protective role for *Aspergillus*, with loss of the protein resulting in a strain crippled in both sporulation (perhaps an indication of reduced fitness) and toxin formation? ST and AF are biotransformed into epoxides by mammalian liver P-450 monooxygenases.[57] Examination of *Aspergillus* databases (Broad Institute and TIGR) suggests that the fungi neither contain a close homolog of these P-450s nor form an epoxide. Both compounds are mutagenic toward the bread mold *Neurospora crassa*;[59,60] however, some studies have suggested that only the liver-activated form of AF — presumably AF epoxide — exhibits mutagenic activity.[61] This implies that *N. crassa* does not contain an activating P-450. This may suggest that aspergilli do not produce AF/ST epoxides and hence do not require a GST for detoxification of such a metabolite.

StcT may play a role in protection against the toxic effects of AF and ST in the fungal cell. Both compounds and several precursors are cellular toxins.[62] Although some AF/ST is secreted from the fungal cell, some remains within fungal tissue.[63] The AF/ST precursors are primarily sequestered within the cell (Keller, unpublished data). Interestingly, a homolog for StcT has not been identified in the *Aspergillus parasiticus* AF cluster, although homologs may be present outside of the cluster.

7.3.1.5 Uncharacterized ST Cluster Genes

Effects of disrupting the *stcD*, *stcH*, *stcM*, *stcO*, *stcR*, and *stcX* genes in *Aspergillus nidulans* have yet to be reported. Oxidation of 1-hydroxyversicolorone to versiconal hemiacetal acetate is catalyzed by AfII (formerly AvfA) in *A. parasiticus*.[34] Because it appears to be an *aflI* homolog, deletion of *stcO* could provide additional information on the ST synthesis pathway. Although *stcX* may be a false ORF as the putative translation product has no homology to other proteins, *stcD*, *stcH*, *stcM*, and *stcR* encode transcripts[12] (http://www.genome.ou.edu) and are considered "genuine" genes. Unfortunately, the predicted proteins from *stcD*, *stcH*, *stcM*, and *stcR* do not support a role in ST biosynthesis. Because most functions in the ST biosynthetic pathway have been assigned to cluster genes, it may be advantageous to consider nonbiosynthetic roles for the remaining genes such as those for StcC, StcV, and StcT.

7.4 MISSING FUNCTIONS IN THE STERIGMATOCYSTIN CLUSTER

Two activities thought to be important for secondary metabolite biosynthesis include toxin pumps/transporters and some form of resistance to toxin. For example, lovastatin, produced by *Aspergillus terreus*, is a potent fungicide that disrupts the function of (3*S*)-hydroxymethylglutaryl-coenzyme A (HMG-CoA) reductase that catalyzes the reduction of HMG–CoA to mevalonate during ergosterol biosynthesis. Interestingly, one of the lovastatin cluster genes encodes a putative HMG–CoA reductase[64] that may provide resistance to the fungal species containing the lovastatin cluster.[65] Among the rest of the ORFs in the lovastatin biosynthetic gene cluster, one encodes a putative resistance protein and three encode putative transporters.[64]

As described earlier, we speculate that StcT may be involved in some form of resistance to the endogenous toxic effects of ST, although neither ST nor AF may harm the producing fungi. At one point it was thought that *aflT* encoded an AF pump, but disruption of this gene in *A. parasiticus* did not affect toxin production and did not appear to have any physiological affect on the fungus.[1] Interestingly, the *stcT* homolog in the AF cluster has no *stcT* homolog and no *aflT* homolog is in the ST cluster. Again, we note that part of the deleterious effects of AF and ST on mammals is due to the AF/ST epoxide. A lack of the P-450 to generate the epoxide may be protection enough for *Aspergillus*. A caveat to this statement is our observation of a poor growing phenotype associated with an *A. nidulans* mutant that overproduces ST and ST intermediates approximately 40-fold.[66] Extreme overproduction of ST and ST intermediates could generate a poor growing phenotype for any number of reasons, including increased energy costs to the fungus, so it is not obvious if a lack of resistance mechanisms plays a role here.

7.5 PRESENCE OF THE AF/ST CLUSTER IN THE ASPERGILLI AND OTHER GENERA

Upwards of 20 species of *Aspergillus*,[67] including *A. nidulans* and *A. versicolor*, make ST. Of these, at least 6 also produce AF. Most of these species, such as *A. bombycis*,[68] *A. nomius*, *A. ochraceoroseus*,[69] and *A. pseudotamarii*[70], are comparatively rarely studied; therefore, little is known about the structure of the AF cluster in these organisms with the exception that the *A. ochraceoroseus* gene cluster is organized like the *A. nidulans* ST gene cluster.[71] The AF cluster has been sequenced extensively for the agricultural pathogens *A. parasiticus* and *A. flavus* and for the so-called "domesticated," non-aflatoxigenic clades *A. sojae* and *A. oryzae*.[72,73] AF clusters of *A. parasiticus*, *A. flavus*, *A sojae*, and *A. oryzae* are largely homologous. In general, genes in these clusters share upwards of 90% homology. This suggests a very close relationship between these species and agrees with their placement together in the *Aspergillus* section *Flavi*. Gene order also has been largely conserved between these fungi.[3,5] The ST cluster of *A. nidulans*, on the other hand, contains homologs to most of the genes found in the AF cluster, but gene order has not been conserved between *A. nidulans* and the *Flavi* species.

Interestingly, several studies indicate that the AF/ST pathway is present in a variety of genera within the filamentous ascomycetes, although no health concerns are linked with these reports. Several lichen species produce norsolorinic acid or related compounds.[74] Other ascomycetes and deuteromycetes produce various pathway intermediates — or derivatives of intermediates — as endproducts. In some cases, these metabolites are phytotoxins (e.g., dothiostromin, a versicolorin A derivative produced by *Dothiostroma pini*; the teleomorph *Mycosphaerella*).[75] With the exception of *D. pini*, the cognate cluster has not been identified in any of these fungi.

7.5.1 GENES CONVERTING STERIGMATOCYSTIN TO AFLATOXIN

An obvious difference between the AF and ST clusters is the presence of genes in the AF cluster that convert ST to AF. Yabe et al.[32] reported that two *Aspergillus parasiticus* methyltransferase activities were necessary for the conversion of demethylsterigmatocystin to AF. The first, named *omtB* (*aflO*), encodes an *O*-methyltransferase that converts demethylsterigmatocystin to ST and is orthologous to *stcP* in *A. nidulans*.[33,34] The second, an *O*-methyltransferase, named *omtA* (*aflP*), converts ST and dihydrosterigmatocystin to *O*-methylsterigmatocystin and dihydro-*O*-methylsterigmatocystin, respectively. OrdA (*A. flavus* Ord1), now AflQ, is a P-450 monooxygenase[20,76,77] that converts *O*-methylsterigmatocystin to AFB_1 and dihydro-*O*-methylsterigmatocystin to AFB_2 in *A. parasiticus* and *A. flavus*. AflQ also is required, but not sufficient, for synthesis of the G-aflatoxins in *A. parasiticus*. Additional genes in *Aspergillus parasiticus* may be responsible for the synthesis of AFG_1 and AFG_2 from AFB_1 and AFB_2, respectively. Yabe et al.[20] reported that, in addition to OrdA, an unstable microsomal enzyme and a 220-kDa cytosolic protein were required for G-aflatoxin formation. Genes encoding these proteins have not yet been identified.[20,78] Although *omtA* and *ordA* are not found in the ST cluster, proteins with significant homology to OmtA and OrdA are found in the *Aspergillus nidulans* genome (http://www-genome.wi.mit.edu/annotation/fungi/aspergillus/); however, as both methyltransferases (OmtA) and P-450 monooxygenases (OrdA) are common enzymes, it could be that these putative homologs are active in different pathways or are not expressed.

7.5.2 Unassigned Aflatoxin Cluster Genes Not Found in the *Aspergillus nidulans* ST Cluster

Aside from *aflT*, five other genes in the AF cluster have not been assigned a function. Of these, three are considered to be homologs of genes in the ST cluster in *Aspergillus nidulans*. *cypX* (*aflV*) appears to encode a P-450 monooxygenase and is orthologous to *stcB*. Another monooxygenase, *moxY* (*aflW*), is orthologous to *stcW*. Both genes have been disrupted, but no clear role in AF synthesis could be determined for either gene.[1] This pattern agrees with that established for their homologs in *A. nidulans*. OrdB (AflX) has significant homology to an oxidase similar to StcQ which, as described earlier, had no effect on ST production when disrupted. A 495-amino-acid polypeptide, encoded by *hypA* (AflY), has homology to a hypothetical protein and some homology to StcR so may be considered a fourth gene homologous to a gene in the ST cluster. One gene has no homolog in the ST cluster. Significant homology has been observed between *aflU* (*cypA*) and cytochrome P-450 monooxygenases. According to Yu et al.,[3] the *aflU* transcript is detected only under AF-inducing conditions and not under conditions unfavorable for AF production.

7.5.3 Partial Cluster Duplication in *Aspergillus parasiticus*

Some strains of *A. parasiticus* contain a partial duplicated region of the AF cluster.[79] The duplication carries copies of six genes located between *aflR* and *verA1*, as well as a copy of *omtB*, but none of the genes between *verA1* and *omtB*. Both order and direction of transcription of the genes in the partially duplicated cluster are the same as in the full cluster. Nucleic acid identity between the cognate genes is between 95 and 99%. Most of the genes are nonfunctional due to point mutations, truncation, or deletion of some segments. As vestigal transposon sequences are found at one end of the partial cluster; transposon activity may be responsible for these incongruities.[80]

Chang et al.[80] demonstrated by one-hybrid assay that AflR2 could interact with promoters of genes in the AF cluster and initiate transcription just as could AflR. Two-hybrid assays demonstrated that AflR2 interacted with AflJ at levels similar to those of AflR. Inactivation of AflR terminated accumulation of all AF precursors in the AflR disruptant, suggesting that AflR2 does not function independently. The cofunctionality of *aflR2* is due to the location of *aflR2* in the genome; however, copies of *aflR* targeted to the *trpC* locus in *Aspergillus nidulans* are functional even when the wild-type *aflR* copies are disrupted, suggesting that chromosome location is not the only factor responsible for the cofunctionality of *aflR2*.

There do not appear to be mutations in *aflJ2*. No data on its efficacy in interaction with either AflR or AflR2 are available. Point mutations causing an amino acid substitution disrupt the glycine-rich loop required for cofactor binding in the enzyme encoded by *adhA2*. Although point mutations cause eight amino acid substitutions in the EstA2 protein, Chang et al.[80] expect it to be functional. Proteins encoded by *norA2* and *verA2* both may have pretermination signals that render them nonfunctional. OmtB2 has a large portion of the N-terminal region deleted and also has a pretermination signal. Thus, it seems that only AflR2, AflJ2, and possibly EstA2 could retain some activity.

The presence of vestigal transposon sequences just outside the partially duplicated cluster region is highly suggestive of a transpositional origin for the cluster. Mutations in genes of the partial cluster suggest that this cluster is inactive or that it confers no fitness benefit to the organism. Mutational accumulation in duplicated genes that have lost function is commonplace. It is interesting, though, that AflR2, which is apparently inactive in *Aspergillus parasiticus*, should retain enough structural integrity to be active in yeast two-hybrid systems. Such activity suggests some role for AflR2 in AF gene transcription. Regardless, identifying the mechanism that interferes with AflR2-mediated transcription of AF genes could be useful in elucidating AflR mechanism.

It should be noted that many commonly used strains of *Aspergillus parasiticus*, such as CS10, do not contain a partial duplication. The partial cluster is present only from progeny or transfers of NRRL 2999 (also SU-1) isolated from Uganda[80] and also from one isolate now classified as *Aspergillus oryzae* var. *viridis* (IMI 15957, CAB Mycological Institute). Occurrence of the partial duplication is much rarer than initially proposed.[28,70]

7.6 CONCLUSIONS

Although nearly all bioconversion steps in the AF/ST pathway have been resolved and most necessary activities have been assigned to a gene located in the AF/ST gene cluster, several genes in the AF/ST cluster still have unexplained functions. These genes are transcribed under AF/ST-inducing conditions but are not transcribed under conditions that disfavor AF/ST production; therefore, these genes may influence some function of AF/ST production. However, disruption of some of these genes (*stcC*, *stcQ*, *stcI*, *stcV*) yields no apparent affect on ST production in *Aspergillus nidulans*, while disruption of others (*stcB*, *stcN*, *stcT*, *stcW*) leads to unexpected phenotypes. While some of these genes may encode redundant functions (as suggested by disruption of *stcB* and *stcW*), disruption studies have not been able to place most of these genes unequivocally at any step in the pathway. In fact, the putative activities of many of the proposed proteins (StcC, StcD, StcH, StcM, StcT) are not necessary for AF/ST biosynthesis. Clearly, the number of genes in the cluster is greater than the number of AF/ST biosynthetic processes. Perhaps it is time to broaden or shift the paradigm we use to understand this and other gene clusters.

We propose that the cluster is not just a set of genes that regulate biosynthesis of toxin but that it is a suite or package of genes that regulates several cellular activities. One component of this suite, and indeed the largest and best characterized one, is the AF/ST biosynthesis module. A second component might be cellular machinery required to protect the cell (StcT) or shuttle enzymes or transcripts around, into, or out of the cell for AF/ST synthesis. A number of the putative ST cluster proteins contain membrane-spanning regions and organelle localization signals as predicted by computer domain-finding programs, suggesting compartmentalization of the AF/ST synthesis process. Such proteins also could be involved in import of substrates and export of toxin from the cell.

Another module in the gene cluster might regulate enzymes with possible ligninase activity (StcC and StcV). Proteins associated with this molecule could degrade lignin in the seed or in other plant tissue. Such activities would not be directly related to AF/ST production but might be pathogenicity factors that allow the fungus access to substrates that are utilized in toxin formation. Toxin production, considered the reason for retaining this pathway, may be just one function from a suite of proteins encoded by this cluster. As AF/ST production is closely tied to sporulation,[81] the cluster might better be associated with fitness of the fungal pathogen and function somewhat like pathogenicity islands that contain several types of genes required for full virulence.

An interesting consideration is evolution of the AF/ST cluster. Many fungal genera, including *Bipolaris*,[82] *Cercospora*,[83] *Chaetomium*,[84] *Dothiostroma*,[85] *Farrowia*,[84] *Hypomyces*,[86] *Penicillium*,[87] *Solorina*,[74] *Lecidia*,[74] and *Xanthoria*,[74] are known to produce compounds closely related to AF/ST or AF/ST pathway intermediates. Recently, part of the dothiostromin gene cluster was sequenced. Disruption of *dotA* (= *Aspergillus nidulans* StcU and *A. parasiticus* Ver-1) resulted in a strain that accumulated versicolorin A.[85] Researchers analyzing the genomic region beside *dotA* identified three ORFs — *dotB*, *dotC*, and *dotD* — that are homologous to StcC, AflT, and a thioesterase domain of a polyketide synthase, respectively (Figure 7.2).[85] Unpublished data indicate the presence of additional biosynthetic genes that exhibit sequence similarity to AF and ST cluster genes (Figure 7.2) (Bradshaw, pers. comm.). Identification of this cluster suggests that variations of the AF/ST cluster exist in a wide distribution of genera and may provide clues toward evolution of the AF/ST gene cluster. Investigation of the function of DotB and DotC in this cluster may yield information on their homologs in *Aspergillus*. Investigation into what genes have been retained, which have been lost, and which are nonfunctional can lend insight into the ecology of these organisms, evolution of gene clusters, and ultimately perhaps control of infection and toxin production.

REFERENCES

1. Yu, J., Chang, P.K., Ehrlich, K.C., Cary, J.W, Bhatnagar, D., Cleveland, T.E., Payne, G.A., Linz, J.E., Woloshuk, C.P., and Bennett, J.W., Clustered pathway genes in aflatoxin biosynthesis, *Appl. Environ. Microbiol.*, 70, 1253–1262, 2004.
2. Hicks, J., Shimizu, K., and Keller, N.P., Genetics and biosynthesis of aflatoxins and sterigmatocystin, in *The Mycota*, Vol. XI, Kempken, F. and Bennett, J.W., Eds., Springer-Verlag, Berlin, 2002, pp. 55–70,

3. Yu, J., Chang, P.K., Cary, J.W., Wright, M., Bhatnagar, D., Cleveland, T.E., Payne, G.A., and Linz, J.E., Comparative mapping of aflatoxin pathway gene clusters in *Aspergillus parasiticus* and *Aspergillus flavus*, *Appl. Environ. Microbiol.*, 61, 2365–2371, 1995.

4. Brown, D.W., Yu, J.-H., Kelkar, H., Fernandes, M., Nesbitt, T.C., Keller, N.P., Adams, T.H., and Leonard, T.J., Twenty-five co-regulated transcripts define the sterigmatocystin gene cluster in *Aspergillus nidulans*, *Proc. Natl. Acad. Sci. USA*, 93, 1418–1422, 1996.

5. Trail, F., Mahanti, N., Rarick, M., Mehigh, R., Liang, S.H., Zhou, R., and Linz, J.E., Physical and transcriptional map of an aflatoxin gene cluster in *Aspergillus parasiticus* and functional disruption of a gene involved early in the aflatoxin pathway, *Appl. Environ. Microbiol.*, 61, 2665–2673, 1995.

6. Woloshuk, C.P. and Prieto, R., Genetic organization and function of the aflatoxin B$_1$ biosynthetic genes, *FEMS Microbiol. Lett.*, 160, 169–176, 1998.

7. Bennett, J. and Papa, K.E., The aflatoxigenic *Aspergillus* species, *Adv. Plant Pathol.*, 6, 263–280, 1988.

8. Keller, N.P. and Hohn, T.M., Metabolic pathway gene clusters in filamentous fungi, *Fungal Genet. Biol.*, 21, 17–29, 1997.

9. Zhang, Y.-Q., Wilkinson, H., Keller, N.P., and Tsitsigiannis, D., Secondary metabolite gene clusters, in *Handbook of Industrial Microbiology*, Marcel Dekker, New York, 2004.

10. Watanabe, C.M. and Townsend, C.A., Initial characterization of a type I fatty acid synthase and polyketide synthase multienzyme complex NorS in the biosynthesis of aflatoxin B$_1$, *Chem. Biol.*, 9, 981–988, 2002.

11. Chang, P.K., Lack of interaction between AFLR and AFLJ contributes to nonaflatoxigenicity of *Aspergillus sojae*, *J. Biotechnol.*, 107, 245–253, 2004.

12. Brown, D.W., Adams, T.H., and Keller, N.P., *Aspergillus* has distinct fatty acid synthases for primary and secondary metabolism, *Proc. Natl. Acad. Sci. USA*, 93, 4873–14877, 1996.

13. Brobst, S.W. and Townsend, C.A., The potential role of fatty acid initiation in the biosynthesis of the fungal aromatic polyketide aflatoxin B$_1$, *Can. J. Chem.*, 72, 200–207, 1994.

14. Yu, J.H. and Leonard, T.J., Sterigmatocystin biosynthesis in *Aspergillus nidulans* requires a novel type I polyketide synthase, *J. Bacteriol.*, 177, 4792–4800, 1995.

15. Shen, B., Polyketide biosynthesis beyond the type I, II and III polyketide synthase paradigms, *Curr. Opin. Chem. Biol.*, 7, 285–295, 2003.

16. Kroken, S., Glass, N.L., Taylor, J.W., Yoder, O.C., and Turgeon, B.G., Phylogenomic analysis of type I polyketide synthase genes in pathogenic and saprobic ascomycetes, *Proc. Natl. Acad. Sci. USA*, 100, 15670–15675, 2003.

17. Keller, N.P., Watanabe, C.M., Kelkar, H.S., Adams, T.H., and Townsend, C.A., Requirement of monooxygenase-mediated steps for sterigmatocystin biosynthesis by *Aspergillus nidulans*, *Appl. Environ. Microbiol.*, 66, 359–362, 2000.

18. Yu, J., Chang, P.K., Cary, J.W., Bhatnagar, D., and Cleveland, T.E., *avnA*, a gene encoding a cytochrome P-450 monooxygenase, is involved in the conversion of averantin to averufin in aflatoxin biosynthesis in *Aspergillus parasiticus*, *Appl. Environ. Microbiol.*, 63, 1349–1356, 1997.

19. Kelkar, H.S., Skloss, T.W., Haw, J.F., Keller, N.P., and Adams, T.H., *Aspergillus nidulans stcL* encodes a putative cytochrome P-450 monooxygenase required for bisfuran desaturation during aflatoxin/sterigmatocystin biosynthesis, *J. Biol. Chem.*, 272, 1589–1594, 1997.

20. Keller, N.P., Segner, S., Bhatnagar, D., and Adams, T.H., StcS, a putative P-450 monooxygenase, is required for the conversion of versicolorin A to sterigmatocystin in *Aspergillus nidulans*, *Appl. Environ. Microbiol.*, 61, 3628–3632, 1995.

21. Yabe, K. and Nakajima, H., Enzyme reactions and genes in aflatoxin biosynthesis, *Appl. Microbiol. Biotechnol.*, 64, 745–755, 2004.
22. Chang, P.K., Yu, J., Ehrlich, K.C., Boue, S.M., Montalbano, B.G., Bhatnagar, D., and Cleveland, T.E., AdhA in *Aspergillus parasiticus* is involved in conversion of 5′-hydroxyaverantin to averufin, *Appl. Environ. Microbiol.*, 66, 4715–4719, 2000.
23. Sakuno, E., Yabe, K., and Nakajima, H., Involvement of two cytosolic enzymes and a novel intermediate, 5′-oxoaverantin, in the pathway from 5′-hydroxyaverantin to averufin in aflatoxin biosynthesis, *Appl. Environ. Microbiol.*, 69, 6418–6426, 2003.
24. Butchko, R.A.E., Adams, T.H., and Keller, N.P., *Aspergillus nidulans* mutants defective in *stc* gene cluster regulation, *Genetics*, 153, 715–720, 1999.
25. Skory, C.D., Chang, P.K., and Linz, J.E., Regulated expression of the *nor-1* and *ver-1* genes associated with aflatoxin biosynthesis, *Appl. Environ. Microbiol.*, 59, 1642–1646, 1993.
26. Trail, F., Chang, P.K., Cary, J., and Linz, J.E., Structural and functional analysis of the *nor-1* gene involved in the biosynthesis of aflatoxins by *Aspergillus parasiticus*, *Appl. Environ. Microbiol.*, 60, 4078–4085, 1994.
27. Keller, N.P., Kantz, N.J., and Adams, T.H., *Aspergillus nidulans verA* is required for production of the mycotoxin sterigmatocystin, *Appl. Environ. Microbiol.*, 60, 1444–1450, 1994.
28. Liang, S.H., Skory, C.D., and Linz, J.E., Characterization of the function of the *ver-1A* and *ver-1B* genes involved in aflatoxin biosynthesis in *Aspergillus parasiticus*, *Appl. Environ. Microbiol.*, 62, 4568–4575, 1996.
29. Skory, C.D., Chang, P.K., Cary, J., and Linz, J.E., Isolation and characterization of a gene from *Aspergillus parasiticus* associated with the conversion of versicolorin A to sterigmatocystin in aflatoxin biosynthesis, *Appl. Environ. Microbiol.*, 58, 3527–3537, 1992.
30. Liang, S.H., Wu, T.S., Lee, R., Chu, F.S., and Linz, J.E., Analysis of mechanisms regulating expression of the *ver-1* gene, involved in aflatoxin biosynthesis, *Appl. Environ. Microbiol.*, 63, 1058–1065, 1997.
31. Kelkar, H.S., Keller, N.P., and Adams, T.H., *Aspergillus nidulans stcP* encodes an *O*-methyltransferase that is required for sterigmatocystin biosynthesis, *Appl. Environ. Microbiol.*, 62, 4296–4298, 1996.
32. Yabe, K., Ando, Y., Hashimoto, J., and Hamasaki, T., Two distinct *O*-methyltransferases in aflatoxin biosynthesis, *Appl. Environ. Microbiol.*, 55, 2172–2177, 1989.
33. Motomura, M., Chihaya, N., Shinozawa, T., Hamasaki, T., and Yabe, K., Cloning and characterization of the *O*-methyltransferase I gene (*dmtA*) from *Aspergillus parasiticus* associated with the conversions of demethylsterigmatocystin to sterigmatocystin and dihydrodemethylsterigmatocystin to dihydrosterigmatocystin in aflatoxin biosynthesis, *Appl. Environ. Microbiol.*, 65, 4987–4994, 1999.
34. Yu, J., Woloshuk, C.P., Bhatnagar, D., and Cleveland, T.E., Cloning and characterization of *avfA* and *omtB* genes involved in aflatoxin biosynthesis in three *Aspergillus* species, *Gene*, 248, 157–167, 2000.
35. Fernandes, M., Keller, N.P., and Adams, T.H., Sequence-specific binding by *Aspergillus nidulans* AflR, a C6 zinc cluster protein regulating mycotoxin biosynthesis, *Mol. Microbiol.*, 28, 1355–1365, 1998.
36. Ehrlich, K.C., Montalbano, B.G., and Cary, J.W., Binding of the C6–zinc cluster protein, AflR, to the promoters of aflatoxin pathway biosynthesis genes in *Aspergillus parasiticus*, *Gene*, 230, 249–257, 1999.
37. Woloshuk, C.P., Yousibova, G.L., Rollins, J.A., Bhatnagar, D., and Payne, G.A., Molecular characterization of the *afl-1* locus in *Aspergillus flavus*, *Appl. Environ. Microbiol.*, 61, 3019–3023, 1995.

38. Payne, G.A., Nystrom, G.J., Bhatnagar, D., Cleveland, T.E., and Woloshuk, C.P., Cloning of the *afl-2* gene involved in aflatoxin biosynthesis from *Aspergillus flavus*, *Appl. Environ. Microbiol.*, 59, 156–162, 1993.

39. Chang, P.K., Cary, J.W., Bhatnagar, D., Cleveland, T.E., Bennett, J.W., Linz, J.E., Woloshuk, C.P., and Payne, G.A., Cloning of the *Aspergillus parasiticus apa-2* gene associated with the regulation of aflatoxin biosynthesis, *Appl. Environ. Microbiol.*, 59, 3273–3279, 1993.

40. Woloshuk, C.P., Foutz, K.R., Brewer, J.F., Bhatnagar, D., Cleveland, T.E., and Payne, G.A., Molecular characterization of *aflR*, a regulatory locus for aflatoxin biosynthesis, *Appl. Environ. Microbiol.*, 60, 2408–2414, 1994.

41. Yu, J.H., Butchko, R.A., Fernandes, M., Keller, N.P., Leonard, T.J., and Adams, T.H., Conservation of structure and function of the aflatoxin regulatory gene *aflR* from *Aspergillus nidulans* and *A. flavus*, *Curr. Genet.*, 29, 549–555, 1996.

42. Chang, P.K., Ehrlich, K.C., Yu, J., Bhatnagar, D., and Cleveland, T.E., Increased expression of *Aspergillus parasiticus aflR*, encoding a sequence-specific DNA-binding protein, relieves nitrate inhibition of aflatoxin biosynthesis, *Appl. Environ. Microbiol.*, 61, 2372–2377, 1995.

43. Cary, J.W., Montalbano, B.G., and Ehrlich, K.C., Promoter elements involved in the expression of the *Aspergillus parasiticus* aflatoxin biosynthesis pathway gene *avnA*, *Biochim. Biophys. Acta*, 1491, 7–12, 2000.

44. Ehrlich, K.C., Montalbano, B.G., and Cotty, P.J., Sequence Comparison of *aflR* from different *Aspergillus* species provides evidence for variability in regulation of aflatoxin production, *Fungal Genet. Biol.*, 38, 63–74, 2003.

45. Meyers, D.M., Obrian, G., Du, W.L., Bhatnagar, D., and Payne, G.L., Characterization of *aflJ*, a gene required for conversion of pathway intermediates to aflatoxin, *Appl. Environ. Microbiol.*, 64, 3713–3717, 1998.

46. Chang, P.K., The *Aspergillus parasiticus* protein AflJ interacts with the aflatoxin pathway-specific regulator AflR, *Mol. Genet. Genomics*, 268, 711–719, 2003.

47. Chang P.-K., Yabe, K., and Yu, J., The *Aspergillus parasiticus estA*-encoded esterase converts versiconal hemiacetal acetate to versiconal and versiconol acetate to versiconol in aflatoxin biosynthesis, *Appl. Environ. Microbiol.*, 70, 3593–3599, 2004.

48. Yu, J., Chang, P.-K., Bhatnager, D., and Cleveland, T.E., Cloning and functional expression of an esterase gene in *Aspergillus parasitcus*, *Mycopathologia*, 156, 227–234, 2003.

49. Silva, J.C., Minto, R.E., Barry, III, C.E., Holland, K.A., and Townsend, C.A., Isolation and characterization of the versicolorin B synthase gene from *Aspergillus parasiticus*: expansion of the aflatoxin B$_1$ biosynthetic gene cluster, *J. Biol. Chem.*, 271, 13600–13608, 1996.

50. Cary, J.W., Wright, M., Bhatnagar, D., Lee, R., and Chu, F.S., Molecular characterization of an *Aspergillus parasiticus* dehydrogenase gene, *norA*, located on the aflatoxin biosynthesis gene cluster, *Appl. Environ. Microbiol.*, 62, 360–366, 1996.

51. Ortiz-Bermudez, P., Srebotnik, E., and Hammel, K.E., Chlorination and cleavage of lignin structures by fungal chloroperoxidases, *Appl. Environ. Microbiol.*, 69, 5015–5018, 2003.

52. Sobolev, V.S., Vanillin content in boiled peanuts, *J. Agric. Food Chem.*, 49, 3725–3727, 2001.

53. Lopez, Y., Smith, O., Sarr, B., Phillips, T., and Keller, N., Use of norsolorinic acid mutants to measure aflatoxin contamination of peanut, *Peanut Sci.*, 25, 92–99, 1999.

54. Billaut-Mulot, O., Fernandez-Gomez, R., and Ouaissi, A., Phenotype of recombinant *Trypanosoma cruzi* which overexpress elongation factor 1-gamma: possible involvement of EF-1gamma GST-like domain in the resistance to clomipramine, *Gene*, 198, 259–267, 1997.

55. Lamoureux, G.L. and Rusness, D.G., The role of glutathione and glutathione S-transferases in pesticide metabolism, selectivity, and mode of action in plants and insects, in *Coenzymes and Cofactors: Glutathione: Chemical, Biochemical, and Medical Aspects*, Part B, Vol. 3, Dolphin, D., Poulson, R., and Avramovic, O., Eds., John Wiley & Sons, New York, 1989, pp. 153–196.

56. Kreuz, K., Tommasini, R., and Martinoia, E., Old enzymes for a new job: herbicide detoxification in plants, *Plant Physiol.*, 111, 349–353, 1996.

57. Eaton, D.L., Bammler, T.K., and Kelly, E.J., Interindividual differences in response to chemoprotection against aflatoxin-induced hepatocarcinogenesis: implications for human biotransformation enzyme polymorphisms, *Adv. Exp. Med. Biol.*, 500, 559–576, 2001.

58. Marrs, K.A., The functions and regulation of glutathione S-transferases in plants, *Annu. Rev. Plant Physiol. Plant. Mol. Biol.*, 47, 127–158, 1996.

59. Ong, T.M., Mutagenic activities of aflatoxin B_1 and G_1 in *Neurospora crassa*, *Mol. Gen. Genet.*, 111, 159–170, 1971.

60. Ong, T.M. and De Serres, F.J., Mutagenicity of chemical carcinogens in *Neurospora crassa*, *Cancer Res.*, 32, 1890–1893, 1973.

61. Matzinger, P.K. and Ong, T.M., Mutation induction by rodent liver microsomal metabolites of aflatoxins B_1 and G_1 in *Neurospora crassa*, *Mutation Res.*, 37, 27–32, 1976.

62. Mori, H., Kitamura, J., Sugie, S., Kawai, K., and Hamaski, T., Genotoxicity of fungal metabolites related to aflatoxin B_1 biosynthesis, *Mutation Res.*, 143, 121–125, 1985.

63. Lawellin, D.W., Grant, D.W., and Joyce, B.K., Aflatoxin localization by the enzyme-linked immunocytochemical technique, *Appl. Environ. Microbiol.*, 34, 88–93, 1977.

64. Kennedy, J., Auclair, K., Kendrew, S.G., Park, C., Vederas, J.C., and Hutchinson, C.R., Modulation of polyketide synthase activity by accessory proteins during lovastatin biosynthesis, *Science*, 284, 1368–1372, 1999.

65. Abe,Y., Suzuki, T., Mizuno, T., Ono, C., Iwamoto, K., Hosobuchi, M., and Yoshikawa, H., Effect of increased dosage of the ML-236B (compactin) biosynthetic gene cluster on ML-236B production in *Penicillium citrinum*, *Mol. Gen. Genet.*, 268, 130–137, 2002.

66. Shimizu, K., Hicks J.K., Huang, T.P., and Keller, N.P., Pka, Ras and RGS protein interactions regulate activity of AflR, a Zn(II)2Cys6 transcription factor in *Aspergillus nidulans*, *Genetics*, 165, 1095–104, 2003.

67. Cole, R.J. and Cox, R.H., *Handbook of Toxic Fungal Metabolites*, Academic Press, New York, 1999, pp. 67–72.

68. Peterson, S.W., Ito, Y., Horn, B.W., and Goto, T., *Aspergillus bombycis*, a new aflatoxigenic species and genetic variation in its sibling species, *A. nominus*, *Mycologia*, 93, 689–703, 2001.

69. Klich, M.A., Mullaney, E.J., Daly, C.B., and Cary, J.W., Some molecular aspects of aflatoxin biosynthesis by *A. tamarii* and *A. ochraceoroseus*, *Inoculum*, 49, 28, 1998.

70. Ito, Y., Peterson, S.W., Wicklow, D.T., and Goto, T., *Aspergillus pseudotamarii*, a new aflatoxin producing species in *Aspergillus* section *Flavi*, *Mycol. Res.*, 103, 233–239, 2001.

71. Klich, M.A., Cary, J.W., Beltz, S.B., and Bennett, C.A., Phylogenetic and morphological analysis of *Aspergillus ochraceoroseus*, *Mycologia*, 95, 1252–1260, 2003.

72. Kusumoto, K.-I., Nogata, Y., and Ohta, H., Directed deletions in the aflatoxin biosynthesis gene homolog cluster of *Aspergillus oryzae*, *Curr. Genet.*, 37, 104–111, 2000.

73. Kusumoto, K., Yabe, K., Nogata, Y., and Ohta, H., *Aspergillus oryzae* with and without a homolog of aflatoxin biosynthetic gene *ver-1*, *Appl. Microbiol. Biotechnol.*, 50, 98–104, 1998.

74. Culberson, C.F., *Chemical and Botanical Guide to Lichen Products*, The University of North Carolina Press, Chapel Hill, 1969.

75. Danks, A.V. and Hodges, R., Polyhydroxyanthraquinones from *Dothiostroma pini*, *Aust. J. Chem.*, 27, 1603–1606, 1974.

76. Prieto, R. and Woloshuk, C.P., *ord1*, an oxidoreductase gene responsible for conversion of *O*-methylsterigmatocystin to aflatoxin in *Aspergillus flavus*, *Appl. Environ. Microbiol.*, 63, 1661–1666, 1997.

77. Yu, J., Chang, P.K., Ehrlich, K.C., Cary, J.W., Montalbano, B., Dyer, J.M., Bhatnagar, D., and Cleveland, T.E., Characterization of the critical amino acids of an *Aspergillus parasiticus* cytochrome P-450 monooxygenase encoded by *ordA* that is involved in the biosynthesis of aflatoxins B_1, G_1, B_2, and G_2, *Appl. Environ. Microbiol.*, 64, 4834–4841, 1998.

78. Yabe, K., Nakamura M., and Hamasaki T., Enzymatic formation of G-group aflatoxins and biosynthetic relationship between G- and B-group aflatoxins, *Appl. Environ. Microbiol.*, 65, 3867–3872, 1999.

79. Cary, J.W., Dyer, J.M, Ehrlich, K.C., Wright, M.S., Liang, S.H., and Linz, J.E., Molecular and functional characterization of a second copy of the aflatoxin regulatory gene *aflR-2* from *Aspergillus parasiticus*, *Biochim. Biophys. Acta*, 1576, 316–323, 2002.

80. Chang, P.K. and Yu, J., Characterization of a partial duplication of the aflatoxin gene cluster in *Aspergillus parasiticus* ATCC 56775, *Appl. Microbiol. Biotechnol.*, 58, 632–636, 2002.

81. Hicks, J.K., Yu, J.-H., Keller, N.P., and Adams, T.H., *Aspergillus* sporulation and mycotoxin production both require inactivation of the FadA G alpha protein-dependent signaling pathway, *EMBO J.*, 16, 4916–4923, 1997.

82. Rabie, C.J., Lubben, A., and Steyn, M., Production of sterigmatocystin by *Aspergillus versicolor* and *Biopolaris sorokiniana* on semisynthetic liquid and solid media, *Appl. Environ. Microbiol.*, 32, 206–208, 1976.

83. Assante, G., Camarda, L., Merlini, L., and Nasini, G., Dothiostromin and 2-epidothistromin from *Cercospora smilacis*, *Phytochemistry*, 16, 125–126, 1977.

84. Udagawa, S., Muroi, T., Kurata, H., Sekita, S., Yoshihira, K., Natori, S., and Umeda, M., The production of chaetoglobosins, sterigmatocystin, *O*-methylsterigmatocystin, and chaetocin by *Chaetomium* spp. and related fungi, *Can. J. Microbiol.*, 25, 170–177, 1979.

85. Bradshaw, R.E., Bhatnagar, D., Ganley, R.J., Gillman, C.J., Monahan, B.J., and Seconi, J.M., *Dothistroma pini*, a forest pathogen, contains homologs of aflatoxin biosynthetic pathway genes, *Appl. Environ. Microbiol.*, 68, 2885–2892, 2002.

86. Carey, S.T. and Nair, M.S., Metabolites of pyrenomycetes. III. Production of (+) skyrin by *Hypomyces trichothecoides*, *Lloydia*, 38, 357–358, 1975.

87. Kawai, K., Kato, T., Mori, H., Kitamura, J., and Nozawa, Y., A comparative study on cytotoxicities and biochemical properties of anthraquinone mycotoxins emodin and skyrin from *Penicillium islandicum* Sopp, *Toxicol. Lett.*, 20, 155–160, 1984.

8 Unlocking the Secrets Behind Secondary Metabolism: A Review of *Aspergillus flavus* from Pathogenicity to Functional Genomics

Kimberly A. Scheidegger and Gary A. Payne

CONTENTS

8.1   INTRODUCTION

Carcinogen. Biological weapon. Immunosuppressant. All of these terms have been used to describe aflatoxin, a toxigenic polyketide produced by the fungus *Aspergillus flavus* during secondary metabolism. In fact, the B_1 form of aflatoxin is the most potent naturally occurring carcinogen known.[1] Humans and animals can be exposed to aflatoxin by consuming food products contaminated with *A. flavus*. The fungus can colonize most food products during storage, but the pathogenic ability of *A. flavus* also enables it to infect crops such as corn, peanuts, cotton, and tree nuts long before harvest.[2] Consumption of contaminated feed by animals may result in immunosuppression, hemorrhaging, reduced weight gain, and liver cancer.[3,4] In humans, the risks associated with aflatoxin consumption have been well examined, and the International Agency for Research on Cancer (IARC) has designated aflatoxin as a human liver carcinogen.[4] As shown by epidemiological studies, the risk of developing liver cancer from aflatoxin is about 30 times higher for individuals who have had previous exposure to hepatitis B.[5] This situation often occurs in developing countries where aflatoxin concentrations in food are not regulated and where hepatitis B vaccines are not universally distributed due to economic and political complications. Biomarkers have been used to link aflatoxin to a specific G-to-T transversion in the third position of codon 249 in the p53 gene, a tumor suppressor gene that is often mutated in human cancers.[6,7] The dangers posed by aflatoxin have apparently caught the interest of Iraqi biological weapons specialists who have stockpiled concentrated aflatoxin, filling approximately 1600 liters into munitions.[8] While the use of *A. flavus* and aflatoxin in a bioweapons program may not pose any immediate dangers to human health, such a weapon would likely cause mass panic and thus be an effective psychological weapon.

Many scientists have used *Aspergillus flavus*/aflatoxin as a model for studying secondary metabolism. The biosynthetic pathway has been well characterized, and the fungus is amenable to genetic transformation and manipulation of gene expression. The epidemiology of the fungus has been described for infection of major agricultural commodities, and, recently, the phylogeny and population structure of *A. flavus* has been investigated. The effects of aflatoxin on humans and animals have been examined. Studies have even been conducted on the aflatoxin-producing ability of *A. flavus* isolates pathogenic to insects.[9] In spite of this wide body of knowledge surrounding *A. flavus*, a clear role of secondary metabolism and aflatoxin production in the ecology of the fungus has yet to be established.

The intent of this review is to examine *Aspergillus flavus* from as many different angles as possible. The classification of the fungus will be discussed as well general biology including ecology, distribution, and mycotoxin production. Classical genetic studies will be presented with an emphasis on the deduced parasexual cycle of *A. flavus*. Finally, genomic techniques and possibilities for future research directions will be revealed. It is the hope that a comprehensive review of the state of knowledge of this fungus will serve to focus new research efforts in the field of genomics such that we can obtain a better understanding of secondary metabolism in *Aspergillus*.

8.2 CLASSIFICATION OF *ASPERGILLUS FLAVUS*

8.2.1 THE GENUS *ASPERGILLUS*

The genus *Aspergillus* is classified in the Ascomycetes and includes species with no known teleomorphic stage as well as species with ascomycetous teleomorphs. Although previous classification systems have placed asexual species such as *A. flavus* into the phylum Deuteromycota, evaluation of ultrastructural, physiological, and biochemical characters as well as DNA sequence analyses have been used to place these species among their close sexual relatives.[10] Raper and Fennell[11,12] divided the genus *Aspergillus* into 18 groups which were later modified into 6 subgenera and 18 sections. These classifications were based on morphology, and recent studies have focused on comparing these traditional classification systems with molecular phylogenetic data. Peterson[13] used large subunit ribosomal RNA genes from 215 *Aspergillus* taxa including representatives of the 6 subgenera and 18 sections to examine phylogenetic relationships within the genus. The existing classification system, which contains the 6 subgenera *Aspergillus*, *Fumigati*, *Ornati*, *Clavati*, *Nidulantes*, and *Circumdati*, did not support the phylogenetic relationships identified in Peterson's study. Peterson therefore suggests a monophyletic taxonomy that places 15 sections into 3 subgenera: *Aspergillus*, *Fumigati*, or *Nidulantes*. For the purposes of this review, the classification system proposed by Peterson[13] will be used. Tamura et al.[14] conducted similar phylogenetic analyses using 18S full rDNA sequences of type strains from 6 subgenera and 18 sections of *Aspergillus*. They also found that the genus *Aspergillus* consists of three different evolutionary lines, and recommend that the current taxonomy of the genus *Aspergillus* be reconstructed to reflect the observed phylogenetic relationships. The phylogenetic relationships of selected *Aspergillus* species and their related teleomorphs as determined by 18S rDNA sequence comparisons are presented in Figure 8.1.[13] From the depicted analyses, *A. flavus* and *A. parasiticus* group together and are more closely related to *A. nidulans* than to *A. fumigatus*. It is possible to see how information such as this may be useful in genetic analyses. For example, one might predict that, based on current phylogenetic data, genes that have been found in *A. nidulans* and *A. parasiticus* will also be present in *A. flavus*.

The fungi in the genus *Aspergillus* are widespread geographically and can be either beneficial or harmful depending on the species and on the substrate being utilized. In industry, *Aspergillus* species are used for enzyme and organic acid production, foreign protein expression, and food fermentation. In nature, most members of this genus can be found in the soil, where they contribute to the degradation of nonliving substrates. *Aspergillus* species are also frequently isolated

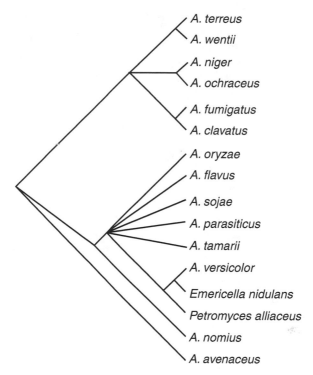

FIGURE 8.1 Molecular phylogeny of *Aspergillus* species and their related teleomorphs. Strict consensus of three trees calculated using PAUP* 4.0 (β10) in a heuristic search of 18S rDNA sequence data. The tree length is 97 steps, consistency index (CI) = 0.7010, homoplasy index (HI) = 0.2990, retention index (RI) = 0.6329, and rescaled consistency index (RC) = 0.4437. The tree was rooted using *A. avenaceus* as the outgroup species on the basis of comprehensive trees of the genus *Aspergillus*.[13] 18S rDNA sequences are available on the NCBI database (http://www.ncbi.nlm.nih.gov) under accession numbers AF516138.1, AB002063.1, D63697.1, AB002068.1, M55626.1, AB002070.1, D63698.1, D63696.1, D63700.1, D63699.1, D63701.1, AB008411.1, AB008403.1, AB002071.1, AB008404.1, and AB008395.1.

as food contaminants. Pathogenic species are the most harmful, not just through the process of infection and colonization but also because a number of pathogenic *Aspergillus* species produce toxigenic secondary metabolites on host tissue. *Aspergillus* species have been identified as pathogens on plants, insects, and animals. Some of the most important species in the genus *Aspergillus* are *A. fumigatus* (subgenus *Fumigati*, section *Fumigati*), the causal agent of aspergillosis in humans; *A. niger* (subgenus *Aspergillus*, section *Nigri*), used for citric acid production in industry; *A. oryzae* (subgenus *Aspergillus*, section *Flavi*), used for saki and soy sauce production; *A. nidulans* (teleomorph *Emericella nidulans*, subgenus *Nidulantes*, section *Nidulantes*), accepted as a model system for fungal genetics; *A. terreus* (subgenus *Aspergillus*, section *Terrei*), commonly used for biotechnological applications; and *A. flavus* (subgenus *Aspergillus*, section *Flavi*), a plant, insect, and animal pathogen and producer of aflatoxin. Of all of the groups of *Aspergillus* species, section *Flavi* in the subgenus *Aspergillus* has perhaps generated the most interest due to the impact of this group on industry, the economy, and on human and animal health. This important group of fungi will be discussed in detail in the following section.

8.2.2 ASPERGILLUS SECTION FLAVI

The diversity of ecological niches occupied by members of *Aspergillus* subgenus *Aspergillus* section *Flavi* (*A. flavus* group) and the ability of some species to produce aflatoxin make this group of fungi one of the most highly studied to date. Species in section *Flavi* occur in nature as saprophytes in the soil and on decaying plant material or as parasites on plants, insects, and animals. Nonaflatoxigenic species such as *Aspergillus oryzae* and *A. sojae* have been widely used in industry for food fermentation or for the production of enzymes.[15] In the field of agriculture, *A. flavus* and *A. parasiticus* have clearly made a mark due to their roles as plant pathogens and their ability to produce aflatoxin in infected plant parts. Studies of species in the *A. flavus* group have involved researchers with a wide range of interests including medicine, ecology, genomics, entomology, plant genetics, toxicology, economics, mycology, and plant pathology.

The classification of fungal species is often debated, and a number of characteristics have been used to determine appropriate taxonomic groupings in section *Flavi*. When the section was described by Raper and Fennell in 1965, only nine species were considered.[11] A synoptic key published in 1981 by Christensen[16] includes a taxonomic description of 14 species and 4 varieties. The key provides a thorough examination of cultural and morphological features that can be used to identify species in the *Aspergillus flavus* group and to differentiate between this group and other fungal groups with similar morphologies. The main features utilized for classification purposes were conidial head color, growth at 37°C, and dimensions of conidiophores, vesicles, and conidia.[16] In a more recent study examining evolution in the section *Flavi*, Rigo et al.[17] considered 23 species and subspecies that were either currently assigned to the section or were in closely related sections. Based on their results, they have recommended that *A. clavatoflavus* and *A. zonatus* be removed from section *Flavi*. These two species show high sequence homology to each other but appear to be unrelated to any other fungi in the *A. flavus* group. This move was also recommended in an earlier study by Peterson,[13] who found *A. clavatoflavus* and *A. zonatus* to be phylogenetically distinct from section *Flavi*. Additionally, *Petromyces alliaceus* and three fungi formerly assigned to section *Wentii*, *A. thomii*, *A. terricola*, and *A. terricola* var. *americana*, have now been moved to section *Flavi*.[18] It is likely that such revisions to the classification of species in the *Aspergillus flavus* group will continue to arise as researchers attempt to develop a clear species concept for asexual fungi. Determination of species in section *Flavi* is currently based upon morphology, mycotoxin profiles, and DNA sequence analyses.[19] These criteria can sometimes create controversy over species identification and classification and make it difficult to determine exactly how many species should be included in the section.

8.2.3 Mycotoxin Production by Species in Section *Flavi*

Perhaps the most interesting feature of *Aspergillus* section *Flavi* is the ability of some species to produce aflatoxin during secondary metabolism. Of the species classified in the section *Flavi*, only *A. flavus*, *A. parasiticus*, and *A. nomius* have been commonly recognized as producers of aflatoxin. Recent reports have since described aflatoxin production in a couple of new species classified in section *Flavi*. A report in 1996 by Goto et al.[19,20] identified aflatoxin production in *Aspergillus tamarii*. This species was found to contain both aflatoxigenic and nonaflatoxigenic isolates, thus prompting classification of the aflatoxin-producing isolates into a new species in section *Flavi*: *Aspergillus pseudotamarii*. *A. pseudotamarii* differs from *A. tamarii* based on morphology, genetics, and mycotoxin production. In 2001, *Aspergillus bombycis* was described as a new species in section *Flavi* that is most closely related to *A. nomius* on the basis of phylogenetic DNA sequence comparisons.[21] Morphologically, *A. bombycis* resembles *A. flavus*, but growth rates and mycotoxin profiles can be used to distinguish the two species. Given recent developments, a comprehensive list of aflatoxigenic species in *Aspergillus* section *Flavi* would now include *A. flavus*, *A. parasiticus*, *A. nomius*, *A. pseudotamarii*, and *A. bombycis*. Table 8.1[14,18,22,23] reflects the current knowledge of mycotoxins commonly produced by some species in section *Flavi* during secondary metabolism. The production of aflatoxin has been reported in many species, including *A. wentii*[24] and, more recently, *A. ochraceoroseus*. It is important to note that the production of mycotoxins, including aflatoxin, may not be widespread within a species. Also, a number of reports have not been confirmed or represent isolates that may have been misidentified. However, given the fact that many fungi, including those outside of the genus *Aspergillus*, produce sterigmatocystin,[25] it is easy to conceive that aflatoxin production will be confirmed in other *Aspergillus* species.

Aspergillus flavus and *A. parasiticus* are the most important toxin-producing species in the *A. flavus* group. While both of these species can accumulate mycotoxins in food products, the types of toxins they produce are somewhat different. The majority of *A. flavus* isolates produce aflatoxins B_1 and B_2 and cyclopiazonic acid (CPA), although some strains have been identified that will also produce G_1 and G_2 aflatoxins.[26,27] In contrast, *A. parasiticus* produces all four of the above aflatoxins, but does not make CPA. All of these mycotoxins are potentially dangerous if consumed by humans. Aflatoxins B_1 and B_2 have been described as carcinogenic, teratogenic, and immunosuppressive and have been linked to cirrhosis and acute liver damage. The aflatoxins G_1 and G_2 have similar effects, and the toxicity of aflatoxin G_1 is ranked just under that of B_1.[28] Dairy products from animals fed aflatoxin-contaminated feed may contain the M_1 and M_2 forms of aflatoxin. CPA also has been detected in agricultural products and is associated with gastrointestinal and neurological disorders in lab animals.[28,29] Little information is available on the accumulation of CPA and other secondary metabolites relative to the countless studies on aflatoxin levels in food products. Accordingly, the U.S. Food and Drug Administration (FDA) currently maintains regulations only on aflatoxins B_1, B_2, G_1, and G_2 in human food and animal feed at a level of 20 ng/g and on aflatoxin M_1, a metabolite of aflatoxin B_1, in milk at 0.5 ng/g. A report issued by the Food

TABLE 8.1
Production of Secondary Metabolites by Species in *Aspergillus* Section *Flavi*

Species	Aflatoxins	Other Secondary Metabolites
Aspergillus avenaceus[22]	—	Avenaciolide
Aspergillus bombycis[23]	B, G	Kojic acid
Aspergillus caelatus[22,23]	—	Kojic acid
Aspergillus flavus[22,23]	B, G	Aspergillic acid, cyclopiazonic acid, kojic acid, nominine, paspaline, paspalinine
Aspergillus lanosus[22]	—	Griseofulvin, kojic acid, met I
Aspergillus leporis[22]	—	Antibiotic Y, kojic acid, leporine, pseurotin
Aspergillus nomius[22,23]	B, G	Aspergillic acid, kojic acid, nominine, pseurotin, tenuazonic acid
Aspergillus oryzae[23]	—	Cyclopiazonic acid, kojic acid
Aspergillus parasiticus[22,23]	B, G	Aspergillic acid, kojic acid, parasiticol, parasiticolide A
Aspergillus pseudotamarii[23]	B	Cyclopiazonic acid, kojic acid
Aspergillus sojae[23]	—	Kojic acid
Aspergillus tamarii[22,23]	—	Cyclopiazonic acid, fumigaclavine A, kojic acid
Petromyces alliaceus[22]	—	Asperlicine, kojic acid, kotanins, met I, nominine, ochratoxin A and B, paspaline

Note: Secondary metabolite profiles were adapted from Samson[22] and Varga et al.[23] *Petromyces alliaceus*, the teleomorph of *Aspergillus alliaceus*, was placed in section *Flavi* on the basis of large subunit ribosomal DNA sequence analyses.[14,18]

and Agriculture Organization on worldwide mycotoxin regulations in place as of October 1, 1996, indicates that 77 countries had regulations, 13 countries had no regulations, and no data were available for 50 countries.[6,30] A report by the Food and Agriculture Organization, published in 2003, provides mycotoxin regulations for over 100 countries, including unified regulations imposed by the European Union.[6]

8.3 POPULATION BIOLOGY

It appears that wherever scientists have looked for species of *Aspergillus*, they have found them. Members of this genus have been described as ubiquitous, and this term seems to apply to substrate utilization as well as to geographic distribution. Klich et al.[31] investigated the ecology of *Aspergillus* species by compiling data from 327 individual studies on the mycoflora of soil and other substrates. They found that *A. flavus* had been isolated from all latitudes but was found at higher frequencies in desert climates and at latitudes ranging from 16 to 35°. This range of latitudes represents tropical, subtropical, and warm temperate climates. Based on the studies mentioned above, *A. flavus* appears to be able to adapt to a range of climates, habitats, and substrates. Some of the substrates that *A. flavus* has been found to colonize include avian and mammalian tissue, soils, stored grains and seeds, forages, cotton yarn, and leather. This species has also been identified as a pathogen of insects and as a contaminant in koji.[9,16,32] Other species in section *Flavi* that show high levels of diversity in temperature range and substrate utilization are *A. oryzae*, *A. parasiticus*, and *A. tamarii*.[31]

8.3.1 S and L Strain Distribution

While examining the ecology of *Aspergillus flavus* isolates, it seems appropriate to comment on some of the variation that has been observed among groups of *A. flavus* and on the distribution of these groups. Isolates have been characterized morphologically according to sclerotium size and genetically according to vegetative compatibility groups (VCGs). In morphological studies, the letters S and L have been used to describe isolates with numerous, small and few, large sclerotia, respectively. In a study conducted in West Africa, 44 different maize fields were tested for the presence of *A. flavus*. All soils contained *A. flavus*, but a greater number of L-strain isolates were found in southern regions, and a greater number of S-strain isolates were found in the north. The study also noted that only 44% of the L-strain isolates produced aflatoxins (B only), while all of the S-strain isolates produced both B and G aflatoxins.[26] Sampling of soils from a transect reaching from eastern New Mexico through Georgia to eastern Virginia revealed that most *A. flavus* isolates were from the L strain, and the highest levels of S-strain isolates were present in areas of east-central Texas and Louisiana where cotton is the main commodity.[33] Isolates from this study were not tested for aflatoxin production. Geiser et al.,[27] using isolates collected from all over the world, found some variation even within S-type strains as some of their isolates produced G aflatoxins while others did not. Thus, while separation into S and L types of strains may be a straightforward way of grouping isolates of *A. flavus*, this method of classification does not necessarily lend itself to generalizations about the toxin-producing abilities of the isolates. In regard to geographic distribution, S and L strains have been isolated from locations across the globe, but apparent differences have been noted in the frequency at which each group occurs in a given location.

8.3.2 Vegetative Compatibility Groups

Genetic classification based on VCGs has been used extensively to examine populations of *Aspergillus flavus*. VCGs are groups of isolates that are capable of forming heterokaryons through hyphal anastomosis or fusion. In fungi such as *A. flavus*, isolates belonging to the same vegetative compatibility group usually have similar morphological and physiological characteristics. There may be significant variation between VCGs, however, as researchers have determined through analysis of mycotoxin production, morphology, isozyme patterns, randomly amplified polymorphic DNA (RAPD), restriction fragment length polymorphism (RFLP), and DNA sequences.[27,34] In a study looking at morphology and mycotoxin production in VCGs of *A. flavus*, significant differences between VCGs were found with respect to general colony appearance, sclerotial morphology (number, volume, shape), and aflatoxin (B_1 + B_2), CPA, and kojic acid production.[34] Bayman and Cotty[35] also observed an association of vegetative compatibility groups with sclerotium size and aflatoxin B_1 production. Although many of the above characteristics have been shown to be statistically different among VCGs, as yet none has been used to fully assess the diversity of VCGs that exist in *Aspergillus flavus* or the evolutionary relationships between VCGs. McAlpin et al.[36] recently demonstrated the ability of a DNA probe to distinguish between VCGs based on DNA fingerprinting. While their work was limited to isolates from a single peanut field, such a technique could be used on a wider scale to assess populations of *A. flavus* from different locations worldwide.

The distribution of individual *Aspergillus flavus* vegetative compatibility groups is unknown. Studies on VCGs in this fungus have been geographically limited. What is known is that the diversity of VCGs in a given location is high and that the population of VCGs can change even over short time periods. A study by Papa[37] in 1986 identified 22 VCGs from 32 isolates collected from cornfields in Georgia. The diversity of VCGs for the study was 0.69 (number of groups/total number of isolates). Another study in 1995 examined isolates from a single peanut field in southwestern Georgia. The collection of isolates had a high diversity value (0.56), but only contained three of the original VCGs identified by Papa.[38] High levels of diversity have also been observed in Arizona, where Bayman and Cotty[39] examined populations in a single cotton field over a period of 3 years. They found 61 isolates that belonged to 13 vegetative compatibility groups in addition to 44 isolates that could not be assigned to VCGs. The profile of this population was observed to change over the course of their study. One VCG was identified in a large number of isolates during the first 2 years of the study and then was not present at all in the final year of the study. As part of the same experiment, 43 isolates were collected from other fields in Arizona. From these collections, 21 VCGs were identified, only 6 of which were also identified in the single test field.[39] All of the above studies identified high distributions of VCGs in *Aspergillus flavus*, even within areas as small as a single cotton field.

It is interesting to note that a fungus that spends much of its life in the soil growing as a saprophyte would exist in such rapidly changing populations. Observations of high levels of diversity and of rapidly shifting VCG profiles have led researchers to postulate that the airborne conidia of *Aspergillus flavus* may be responsible for the dramatic changes in population structure.[37,39] Alternatively, perhaps the diversity of *A. flavus* populations can be attributed in part to recombination events taking place beneath the soil surface. Mitotic recombination, which has thus far only been observed in the laboratory as part of the parasexual cycle, may take place in the soil between genetically similar individuals. Similarly, although no sexual stage has been identified and numerous reports support a strong clonal component in the life history of the fungus,[15,34,35,40,41] there still exists the potential for meiotic recombination. As indicated by Horn et al.,[34] it may be the dynamic and complex soil environment that imposes the greater selective pressure rather than the plant pathogenic phase of *A. flavus*'s life cycle.

8.4 ECOLOGY

8.4.1 PATHOGENICITY

Although *Aspergillus flavus* is able to grow on virtually any stored crop or resulting food product, it is of major concern on corn, cottonseed, peanuts, and tree nuts. The fungus is well known for its aggressiveness as a storage rot and its ability to produce aflatoxin in colonized seeds and grain. Most often, however, *A. flavus* infection and aflatoxin contamination is a problem long before harvest. Aflatoxin levels are closely monitored in food products, and preharvest infection even in a proportionately small amount of plant tissue can mean rejection of an entire crop. Preharvest contamination has been observed on each of the commodities listed above, but the most work on the infection process has been done with *A. flavus* ear rot on corn. Thus, the following discussion on the pathogenicity and life cycle of *A. flavus* will draw largely upon conclusions made from studies on the preharvest infection of corn.

The pathogenic ability of *Aspergillus flavus* is of great importance from an agricultural and economic standpoint but may actually be of minor importance in the ecology of the fungus.[34] *A. flavus* appears to spend most of its life growing as a saprophyte in the soil. Growth of the fungus in this habitat is supported largely by the presence of plant and animal debris. Fungal mycelium appears to be the predominant structure found in the soil, but sclerotia can be formed, thus contributing to the long-term survival of the fungus. *A. flavus* has no known sexual stage, and primary infection therefore occurs through the dissemination and germination of conidia. Figure 8.2 illustrates the possible mechanisms for the preharvest infection of peanuts, cotton, and corn by *A. flavus*.

Numerous studies have examined the survival and conidial germination of sclerotia (the production of conidiophores and conidia from sclerotia) in the soil or on infected plant parts. In an experiment looking at sclerotium production, Wicklow et al.[42] observed that *Aspergillus flavus* could produce sclerotia on corn kernels that were either artificially inoculated or were naturally infested. In a separate study, Wicklow et al.[43] found that production of conidia from sclerotia was greatly reduced by 1 to 2 years of burial in the soil, but that sclerotia remained viable even after years of burial. They also observed large numbers of propagules in the soil, such as might be present following conidial germination of the sclerotia. Earlier research by Wicklow and Donahue[44] supports this observation. They found that sclerotia of *A. flavus* produced conidia following incubation on moist sand and on field soil both with and without prior submersion under the soil surface. Additionally, a separate field study revealed that sclerotia exposed to the soil surface germinated 8 days prior to the maize silking date.[45] These studies point to the importance of sclerotia as a source of primary inoculum and provide evidence for natural selection in favor of individuals able to maintain a successful host–parasite interaction with corn.

Conidia produced by mycelium or sclerotia serve as the primary inoculum for diseases caused by *Aspergillus flavus*. Spores are carried by wind or insects to nearby plants. While insects clearly play an important role in the epidemiology of *A. flavus*,[46] Jones et al.[47] showed that *A. flavus* is able to infect corn even in an insect-free environment. The fungus will colonize silk tissue and grow down the silks to the

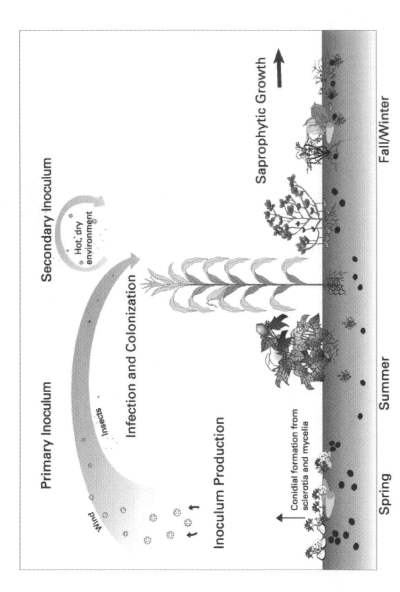

FIGURE 8.2 Diagram of the preharvest infection of cotton, corn, and peanuts by *Aspergillus flavus*. Sclerotia and conidia produced by *A. flavus* growing on crop debris and in the soil serve as primary inoculum for young plants in the spring. Later in the growing season, conidia produced on crop debris or on infected plants provide high levels of secondary inoculum when environmental conditions are conducive for disease development.

kernels where it can infect developing kernels. The exact mode of entry is still not clear. The fungus may invade thin-walled cells at the junction between the bracts and their rachillas or it may grow through the air space leading from the cob into the spikelet.[48,49] Whatever route taken, it is likely that *A. flavus* grows through the barrier that is the easiest to penetrate; therefore, while not essential for infection, wounds made by insect feeding would provide an easy mode of entry for the invading fungus. Once *Aspergillus flavus* is present in plant tissue, it can continue to grow and to produce aflatoxin, and toxin levels in improperly stored infected plant tissue can continue to increase long after harvest. While this has severe consequences for the food and feed supply, saprophytic growth is also important to consider in the life cycle of this pathogen. Infected plant tissue such as corn kernels, cobs, and leaf tissue can remain in the soil and support the fungus until the following season when newly exposed mycelium or sclerotia can give rise to conidial structures, thus producing the primary inoculum for the next infection cycle.

Although both *Aspergillus flavus* and *A. parasiticus* are able to cause disease in the field, *A. flavus* is more frequently isolated from all crops.[48] Zummo and Scott[50] compared the aggressiveness of *A. flavus* to that of *A. parasiticus* on corn and found that the two fungi were equally aggressive on inoculated ears. Where the two pathogens appeared to differ was in their ability to overwinter in the field. Uninoculated corn cobs that had been left to overwinter contained mainly *A. flavus*, and all of the sclerotia collected from these cobs were from *A. flavus*. Another important observation was that higher levels of conidia from *A. flavus* were present during ear development than were conidia from *A. parasiticus*. Although the two fungi appear to be similar in their ability to colonize host tissue, *A. flavus* is more persistent in plant debris than *A. parasiticus* and is therefore capable of producing more conidia early in the season.

8.4.2 IMPACT OF THE SURROUNDING ENVIRONMENT

Environmental conditions can play an important role in disease development. Growth of *Aspergillus flavus* is optimal when temperatures are between 36 and 38°C. At the same time, temperatures above 30°C can begin to cause heat stress in corn plants, thus leaving the invading fungus at an even greater advantage.[51] Researchers have also noted that aflatoxin contamination is greater in years with below average rainfall. Drought stress can lead to cracks in corn kernel surfaces, providing additional entry sites for hyphae of *A. flavus*.[28] It is important to note that the conditions that favor growth of *A. flavus* (high temperature, low humidity) are less than ideal for many of the microbes that would typically be present in the soil or on plant surfaces. This puts the fungus at an even greater advantage, allowing it to easily out-compete these organisms for substrates in the soil or in the plant.

The role of the environment in the incidence and severity of *Aspergillus flavus* infection of peanuts also has been examined. In a study on the effects of irrigation and drought stress on aflatoxin contamination, Cole et al.[52] found that irrigation lowered the soil temperature in the geocarposphere, thereby providing an effective control over *A. flavus* and *A. parasiticus* infection of peanuts. Corn, which is more dependent on ambient temperature than on soil temperature, did not show any significant reduction in disease levels as a result of irrigation treatments.[52] Peanut pod temperature is also an important factor in determining the extent of *A. flavus* growth. Not surprisingly, kernel colonization and aflatoxin concentrations were shown to rise as pod temperatures neared the optimum temperature for *A. flavus* growth.[53] As with corn, damage to kernels is not required for aflatoxin contamination; nevertheless, it is evident that damaged peanut kernels contain higher levels of aflatoxin.[54] Cracked kernels are easier for the fungus to penetrate and may become dehydrated, thus leading to a more favorable environment for *A. flavus*.[48]

8.5 GENETICS OF AFLATOXIN BIOSYNTHESIS

8.5.1 Genetic Analysis

Beginning with the first report of a parasexual cycle in *Aspergillus flavus*, researchers have continued to build upon previous genetic studies to learn more about aflatoxin biosynthesis and genetic, nutritional, and environmental regulation of secondary metabolism. Parasexual analyses were used to identify linkage groups and to determine gene order and centromere position. Mutant strains have been used to identify biosynthetic and regulatory genes and to determine the order of genes in the aflatoxin cluster. Resolution of individual chromosomes is now possible using pulsed-field gel electrophoresis. This technique has aided in the mapping of genes to specific chromosomes. While the biosynthetic pathway for aflatoxin has been well described, it is hoped that future genetic studies in *Aspergillus flavus* will provide additional clues into the regulatory control mechanisms used to send signals to the biosynthetic genes and/or proteins.

8.5.2 Gene Mapping

The lack of a sexual stage in *Aspergillus flavus* has complicated genetic studies in this organism. Little was known about the genetic basis for aflatoxin production until pioneering work on parasexual analysis in *Aspergillus nidulans*[55] paved the way for the discovery of a parasexual cycle in *A. flavus* by Papa in 1973. The following description of the parasexual cycle is based on original work by Papa.[56] Parasexual analysis involves the formation of heterokaryons from the haploid mycelia of two isolates followed by diploidization, mitotic recombination, and haploidization. The formation of heterokaryons is forced by plating together on minimal medium two mutants that differ in auxotrophy and conidial head color. Conidia from the heterokaryons are transferred to new plates where diploids are recovered from prototrophic colonies after 5 to 6 days. Unfortunately, the recovery of diploids is complicated by difficulties in determining the nuclear condition of *A. flavus* spores. No observable difference is apparent in conidial size between diploids and heterokaryons as was found in conidia of *A. nidulans*,[55] and, as reported in a later study by Leaich and Papa,[57] the only difference in color between diploids and heterokaryons is a uniformity of spore color in diploid conidial heads. Consequently, Papa relied upon segregation of recessive recombinants to determine ploidy levels. Plating on complete medium supplemented with *p*-fluorophenyl alanine or the fungicide benomyl is sufficient to induce the haploid condition. Segregant analysis in Papa's experiments revealed recombination between linked genes, thus indicating that mitotic crossing-over presumably occurred following the formation of diploids. This first study on parasexuality in *A. flavus* identified eight genetic loci belonging to five linkage groups.[56]

Classical genetic studies based on parasexual analysis have made possible the mapping of more than 30 genes to 8 linkage groups. These studies have utilized three classes of mutants: high aflatoxin B_2-accumulating strains, spore color and auxotrophic mutants, and mutants deficient in aflatoxin production.[58] All of the identified loci that are involved in aflatoxin production are recessive, with the exception of the *afl-1* mutant, which shows dominance in diploids but not in heterokaryons. In total, 11 aflatoxin loci have been mapped to three linkage groups. Nine loci map to linkage group VII, one locus maps to linkage group II, and the remaining locus maps to linkage group VIII.[58] Taking a closer look at linkage group VII, Papa mapped 6 of the aflatoxin mutants to the same chromosome arm in the following order: *nor* and *afl-1*, *leu*, *afl-15*, *arg-7*, *afl-17*, centromere. No crossing over was detected between *nor* and *afl-1*, and it was not possible to determine their order relative to *leu*.[59] Thus, even in these early studies, a tendency for aflatoxin genes to be clustered together was evident. The *afl-1* mutation has since been shown to be due to a deletion of the entire biosynthetic cluster.[60]

8.5.3 GENOME ORGANIZATION

The development of electrophoretic karyotype analysis has allowed researchers to go beyond the limitations imposed by parasexual analysis. As described above, classical genetics can be used to map genes to linkage groups and, in some cases, to determine gene order given the occurrence of recombination between genes. Analyses such as these are time consuming, and, if are not enough molecular markers are available, they do not reveal the actual number of chromosomes present in an organism or the chromosomal locations of the linkage groups. In the early 1980s, pulsed-field gel electrophoresis became available.[61] Using this technique, chromosomes can be separated by size and karyotype maps created. Already, a number of applications of karyotyping have been demonstrated in species of *Aspergillus*; chromosome banding patterns have been visualized, genes have been localized to specific chromosomes, copy number and chromosomal locations of transformed genes have been determined, chromosome-specific libraries have been developed, and evolutionary relationships between isolates from the same species have been examined.[61]

Karyotypes have been described for a number of species in section *Flavi*, and a karyotypic map was generated for *Aspergillus flavus*. Keller et al.[62] used contour-clamped homogeneous electric field (CHEF) gel electrophoresis to separate chromosomes in *A. flavus*, *A. parasiticus*, *A. oryzae*, *A. sojae*, *A. tamarii*, and *A. versicolor*. Due to polymorphisms in chromosome length and difficulties in the resolution of chromosomes, the exact number of chromosomes for these species could not be determined; however, it was estimated that the range in chromosome number from the species listed above ranged from five to eight. Using the molecular weight determined for individual chromosomes, one strain of *A. flavus* was estimated to have a genome size of 36 Mb.[62] Building upon previous genetic research by Papa,

Foutz et al.[63] created a karyotypic map of *Aspergillus flavus* and subsequently assigned linkage groups determined by parasexual analysis to specific chromosomes. While Keller et al.[62] reported the separation of anywhere from five to eight chromosomal bands, Foutz et al.[63] described the resolution of seven bands from both 7-day and 4-day separations. Linkage groups were assigned to six of the seven chromosomes as follows: linkage groups IV and VIII mapped to a 7-Mb chromosome, linkage group VII (containing the aflatoxin gene cluster) mapped to a 4.9-Mb chromosome, linkage group VI mapped to a 4.2-Mb chromosome, linkage group I mapped to a 3.7-Mb chromosome, linkage group II mapped to a 3.4-Mb chromosome, and no linkage groups were assigned to a 5.7-Mb chromosome. Estimation of genome size from this study was complicated by questions surrounding the 7-Mb chromosome band. The bright staining pattern combined with the data mapping two linkage groups to this band led to speculation that the band may actually represent two chromosomes. Assuming eight chromosomes, the estimated genome size would be 42.9 Mb. Assuming seven total chromosomes, the genome size was approximated at 35.9 Mb, almost identical to the 36-Mb size previously estimated.[62,63] While physical karyotyping can provide useful information about the location of specific genes and may even allow for the assignment of linkage groups to new genes without having to resort to parasexual analysis, the technique has major limitations in that it is difficult to separate chromosomes of similar size, and the resolution of chromosomal DNA is not always possible.

8.5.4 CLUSTERING OF AFLATOXIN GENES

Gene clusters, as defined by Keller and Hohn, are the linkage of two or more genes that are involved in the same metabolic or developmental pathway. Although the majority of fungal genes do not appear to be clustered, research on metabolic pathways has shown that both nutrient utilization pathways and pathways for secondary metabolism are often arranged in clusters.[64] A good example of this is the penicillin cluster, versions of which have been identified in the fungal species *Penicillium chrysogenum*,[65,66] *Cephalosporium acremonium*,[67] and *Aspergillus nidulans*.[68,69] Also, the pathway genes for the *Fusarium sporotrichiodes* trichothecene family of mycotoxins are organized into a cluster.[70–72] Despite all of these reported gene clusters, researchers have yet to understand the significance of this method of gene organization. It has been proposed that clustering of genes may allow rapid transcription of pathway genes, thus allowing the fungus to produce secondary metabolites in a short amount of time;[73] however, a regulatory role for this organization has not yet been established.[64] Another possible benefit of gene clustering is that pathway genes may be more likely to be transferred together during sexual reproduction or parasexual recombination.[64]

In *Aspergillus flavus*, the evidence for the clustering of the aflatoxin biosynthetic genes has been building ever since Papa first mapped the genetic loci of aflatoxin mutants to linkage groups using parasexual analysis. Out of the 11 aflatoxin loci that were assigned to linkage groups, 9 were mapped to linkage group VII.[74] Using electrophoretic karyotyping, Foutz et al.[63] mapped linkage group VII markers to a 4.9-Mb chromosome. These data together indicate that the aflatoxin pathway genes

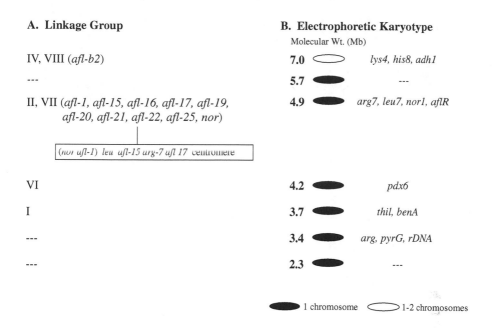

A. Linkage Group

IV, VIII (*afl-b2*)

II, VII (*afl-1, afl-15, afl-16, afl-17, afl-19, afl-20, afl-21, afl-22, afl-25, nor*)

(*nor afl-1*) *leu afl-15 arg-7 afl 17* centromere

VI

I

B. Electrophoretic Karyotype

Molecular Wt. (Mb)

7.0   *lys4, his8, adh1*

5.7   ---

4.9   *arg7, leu7, nor1, aflR*

4.2   *pdx6*

3.7   *thil, benA*

3.4   *arg, pyrG, rDNA*

2.3   ---

● 1 chromosome   ◯ 1-2 chromosomes

C. Aflatoxin Biosynthetic Cluster

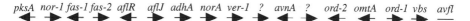

pksA   nor-1 fas-1 fas-2 aflR   aflJ adhA norA ver-1   ?   avnA   ?   ord-2 omtA ord-1 vbs   avfl
◄   ►   ◄   ►   ◄   ►   ►   ►   ►   ►   ◄   ►   ◄   ◄   ►   ►   —

FIGURE 8.3 Evidence for an aflatoxin gene cluster. (A) Most of the aflatoxin mutations studied by Papa were mapped to linkage group VII using parasexual analysis.[59,74,77] The box below linkage group VII contains the gene order of some of the mutants determined by analysis of mutant strains and recombination frequency. Mutants *nor* and *afl-1* were both distal to *leu*, but no specific order was determined for the two genes. (B) Foutz et al.[63] determined the chromosomal location of linkage group markers to chromosomes separated by size using electrophoresis.[63] The aflatoxin genes *nor-1* and *aflR* mapped to a 4.9-Mb chromosome. (C) Molecular analysis of the aflatoxin pathway has shown that the biosynthetic genes and pathway-specific regulatory genes are located in a 75-kb cluster. (The image of the aflatoxin biosynthetic cluster was adapted from Payne and Brown.[76])

are clustered together in linkage group VII, which resides on a 4.9-Mb chromosome. Prieto et al.,[75] using genetic complementation of a mutant strain (Afl-1) lacking the aflatoxin cluster, estimated the size of the cluster to be approximately 75 kb. Thus, as shown in Figure 8.3,[59,63,74,76,77] early studies using parasexual analysis provided evidence for an aflatoxin gene cluster that was later supported by electrophoretic karyotype analysis and gene mapping.

Scientists have also examined gene order in the aflatoxin/sterigmatocystin clusters of *Aspergillus parasiticus* and *A. nidulans*. The gene order found in the *A. flavus* cluster is conserved in the closely related fungus *A. parasiticus*, but the spacing between the genes shows some variation.[73] Interestingly, the order of genes in the aflatoxin cluster is very similar, but not identical, to the order in which the corresponding gene products act to convert pathway intermediates to aflatoxin.[72] Comparison to the sterigmatocystin cluster in *A. nidulans* reveals some differences in gene order and organization. The genes themselves, however, code for proteins with similar amino acid sequences.[78] Thus, even allowing for some observable differences in gene organization and order, the existence of clusters in these related fungi reveals some conservation of structure and function in the mycotoxin biosynthetic genes.

8.6 REGULATION OF AFLATOXIN BIOSYNTHESIS

8.6.1 PATHWAY-SPECIFIC AND GLOBAL REGULATION

Pathway-specific regulation of aflatoxin biosynthesis in *Aspergillus flavus* and *A. parasiticus* and of sterigmatocystin biosynthesis in *A. nidulans* is by the zinc binucleate cluster DNA binding protein AflR.[79–81] Payne et al.,[82] using genetic complementation with a wild-type cosmid library to restore aflatoxin biosynthesis in a nonproducing mutant strain of *A. flavus*, cloned the *afl-2* (*aflR*) gene and proposed a regulatory function for the gene. Overexpression of *aflR* in *A. flavus* resulted in increased pathway gene transcription and aflatoxin production.[83] Two AflR binding sites have been identified in the promoter region of the aflatoxin pathway polyketide synthase (*pksA*) gene that are required for *pksA* activity in *A. parasiticus*. These binding sites are conserved in *A. flavus*, *A. nomius*, *A. bombycis*, and *A. pseudotamarii*.[84] Research in *A. nidulans* has also demonstrated sequence-specific binding of AflR to a palindromic sequence found in the promoter of several sterigmatocystin cluster genes.[85] Thus, AflR is able to regulate the transcription of pathway genes as well as autoregulate its own transcription.[86] The observation that aflatoxin production is affected by a wide range of nutritional and environmental factors (pH, temperature, moisture, oxygen availability, carbon source, and nitrogen) indicates that other factors such as global regulators may be involved. Ehrlich et al.,[84] while examining the *pksA* promoter, located putative binding sites for the global regulatory proteins BrlA and PacC. Disruption of these sites decreased *pksA* promoter activity. Coordinated regulation of *pksA* by AflR, BrlA, and PacC could explain why aflatoxin is mainly produced in sporulating cultures that are grown at a low pH.

A number of studies have attempted to reveal what other factors might contribute to the regulation of AflR and aflatoxin biosynthesis. Liu and Chu examined *aflR* gene expression under varying environmental conditions and found that conditions previously described as not conducive for aflatoxin production were also characterized by reduced transcription of *aflR*.[87] Promoter analysis of *aflR* in *Aspergillus parasiticus* identified protein binding by AflR and another protein to a positive regulatory element at positions –100 to –118 as well as protein binding to a negative regulatory sequence further upstream. The negative regulatory binding site has homology to the consensus binding site for the pH regulatory protein PacC, thus providing evidence for PacC inhibition of aflatoxin under alkaline conditions.[88] Studies by Butchko et al.[89] and Chang et al.[90] provide evidence for putative AflR repressors in *A. nidulans* and *A. parasiticus*, respectively. Butchko et al.[89] identified three mutations not linked to the sterigmatocystin gene cluster that inhibit *aflR*

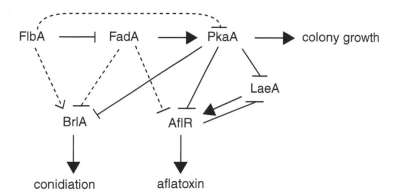

FIGURE 8.4 Model for the proposed regulation of aflatoxin biosynthesis, mediated in part through the FadA alpha subunit of a heterotrimeric G protein. Solid lines represent genetically determined regulatory events, and dashed lines indicate hypothesized activity. FadA acts through the cAMP-dependent protein kinase catalytic subunit PkaA to block transcriptional activation of sporulation and aflatoxin pathway genes by BrlA and AflR, respectively. PkaA exhibits negative control over AflR directly and indirectly by inhibition of LaeA, a protein required for AflR transcription. FadA can be partially inactivated by FlbA to restore GTPase activity and allow aflatoxin production and conidiation. (Adapted from previous models by Shimizu and Keller[93] and Calvo et al.[94])

expression. These mutations may exist in genes of *trans*-acting regulatory factors. Using an AflR carboxyl region::nitrate reductase promoter construct with no DNA binding regions to transform *A. parasiticus*, Chang et al.[90] observed high levels of aflatoxin regardless of the nitrogen source utilized. They hypothesized that the AflR carboxyl region construct might be responsible for titrating out an AflR repressor. AflR has also been shown to interact with AflJ posttranscriptionally, thus affecting the activity of the regulatory protein.[91] Recently, Jayashree et al.[92] examined calcium-mediated regulation of aflatoxin production in *A. parasiticus*. Their study provides evidence of aflatoxin regulation by calmodulin kinase phosphorylation of calcineurin (calmodulin-dependent protein phosphatase). These studies have shown that AflR is highly regulated during and after transcription and that regulation of aflatoxin production may involve calcium and pH genes.

8.6.2 G-Protein Signaling and Protein Kinase Activity

Secondary metabolism in *Aspergillus nidulans*, *A. parasiticus*, and *A. flavus* is associated with asexual reproduction, and evidence exists for a common regulatory mechanism that is mediated through a G-protein signaling pathway (Figure 8.4).[93,94] Much of the work on this pathway has been conducted in *A. nidulans*, but it is clear that the regulatory mechanisms are conserved in *A. flavus* and *A. parasiticus*.[94–96] Transcriptional and posttranscriptional regulation of BrlA (pathway-specific regulator of conidiogenesis) and AflR by pathway gene products affects fungal development and secondary metabolite production, respectively. Sporulation and mycotoxin production appear to be coordinately regulated by the activity of a *fadA* gene, encoding the alpha subunit of a heterotrimeric G-protein.[97] During vegetative growth, FadA is in its active, GTP-bound state and is unable to hydrolyze gamma-glutamyl transpeptidase (GTP). Partial inactivation of FadA by the RGS (regulator of G-protein signaling) domain protein FlbA restores GTPase activity and subsequently allows mycotoxin production and conidiation.[96–98] The discovery of a cAMP-dependent protein kinase catalytic subunit (PkaA) that was involved in sporulation and mycotoxin production provided a possible link between FadA signaling and the pathway-specific regulators BrlA and AflR. Overexpression of *pkaA* in *A. nidulans* negatively regulated AflR at both the transcriptional and posttranscriptional levels and resulted in decreased sporulation through inhibition of *brlA* gene expression. Deletion of *pkaA* in Δ*flbA* and *fadA*[G42R] (dominant, activating mutation) backgrounds partially restored conidiation.[93] These data provide evidence for mediation of FadA G-protein signaling of sporulation and mycotoxin production through PkaA.

As previously stated, PkaA appears to act both transcriptionally and posttranscriptionally to block AflR and BrlA activity. Currently, no evidence exists for the posttranscriptional regulation of BrlA, but Shimizu and Keller[93] have observed negative transcriptional regulation of *brlA* by PkaA. PkaA activity can also negatively regulate expression of *aflR*. This level of control appears to be exerted by inhibition of LaeA, a protein required for *aflR* transcription. LaeA contains two putative AflR binding sites, which may explain the inhibition of *laeA* transcription by AflR in a putative feedback circuit. Also, evidence for the posttranscriptional regulation of AflR by PkaA-directed phosphorylation has recently been found.[94] The multiple levels of control exerted by PkaA provide further evidence that secondary metabolism is highly regulated in *Aspergillus* species.

The regulation of secondary metabolism and morphological development appears to be more complex than the FlbA/FadA/PkaA model described above, however, as Shimizu and Keller[93] also hint at the involvement of a PkaA-independent mechanism for FadA signaling. For more information on regulation of secondary metabolism and fungal development in filamentous fungi, see the recent review by Calvo et al.[94]

8.6.3 Importance of Chromosomal Location

Researchers are interested in finding a link between transcriptional regulation and the chromosomal location of genes. Thus far, no evidence has been found to show that gene order in the aflatoxin cluster has any direct effect on the regulation of aflatoxin biosynthesis. Previous research has shown that, when the aflatoxin biosynthetic genes are integrated ectopically into the genome, no effect on gene expression is observed.[75,82] Recent work in *Aspergillus parasiticus*, however, has demonstrated position-dependent regulation of the aflatoxin biosynthetic gene *nor-1*. Chiou et al.[99] integrated a *nor-1*:GUS reporter construct into the *nor-1* site of the aflatoxin gene cluster and into two locations external to the cluster. Native expression levels were observed when the construct was integrated into the *nor-1* site but not when integration occurred elsewhere in the genome. Perhaps future research into this phenomenon might compare expression levels between *nor-1* promoter integration at the native *nor-1* location versus integration at other sites within the aflatoxin gene cluster.

8.7 GENOMICS

The potential applications of genomic studies in *Aspergillus* and other filamentous fungi appear limitless. Already, virulence and pathogenicity genes have been identified in some fungi that could provide novel targets for fungicides. Comparative genomics could then be used to identify a range of pathogens for which particular chemicals might have activity. Fungicide resistance that has been linked to a gene or gene mutation could be traced through populations. This could be useful in identifying areas in which certain chemicals are likely to be ineffective. Additionally, genomic studies may help to reveal the extent of recombination in a population, which could then affect disease management strategies. For example, a population that shows high levels of recombination could indicate a need for an intensive management program in which the pathogen is attacked using a range of techniques such as the use of chemicals with different modes of action as well as cultural, physical, and biological control methods.

Genomics allows scientists to use new techniques to address a number of basic research questions. In addition to the determination of gene function and synteny between species, other areas that can be addressed with comparative genomic studies include genetic redundancy, genome evolution, and speciation. Also, subsets of genes essential for particular processes can be identified by comparing species that differ in characteristics such as ecology, pathogenicity, sporulation, mating type, growth form, and substrate specificity. Yoder and Turgeon describe strategies for developing gene subsets associated with a particular characteristic using both comparative genomics and DNA hybridization.[100]

8.7.1 GENOME SEQUENCING AND COMPARATIVE GENOMICS

Comparative genomics will likely be an invaluable tool for scientists working with filamentous fungi. While the number of fungi scheduled for full-scale genome sequencing is rapidly increasing, a large number of organisms remain for which genome sequences are not likely to be available in the near future. Researchers working on a fungus with a lower sequencing priority may wish to employ existing phylogenetic data to benefit from currently available genome sequences. Closely related fungi are likely to exhibit conservation of gene order and structure. Synteny has already been observed between *Neurospora crassa* and *Magnaporthe grisea* and between *M. grisea* and *Aspergillus nidulans*, thus allowing scientists to take a comparative approach to genomics studies in these organisms.[101] Existing phylogenetic studies could be used to predict gene order in fungi that have not yet been sequenced. For example, although the complete genome sequence is not available for *A. versicolor*, this species has been shown to be closely related to *A. nidulans* on the basis of 18S ribosomal DNA sequence analysis.[14] It is likely that a good portion of the genetic information available from *A. nidulans* will be conserved in *A. versicolor*. In particular, regions of synteny that have been found between *A. nidulans* and the more distantly related fungus *M. grisea* are likely to be conserved between *A. nidulans* and *A. versicolor*.

Additionally, comparative genomics may prove useful in the task of gene function assignment. One might predict that closely related fungi would maintain some level of conservation of gene function. As hypothesized by Brendel et al.,[102] gene function may be conserved between two organisms, even if gene order is not maintained. Thus, even if further study reveals a lack of synteny between phylogenetically related organisms, the respective proteomes may still show some level of conservation. Fungi that are closely related to model organisms may therefore be able to benefit from the extensive amount of research available for these systems.

In the genus *Aspergillus*, a number of species are currently being sequenced. Comparative genomics studies between *Aspergillus* species as well as between *Aspergillus* species and other fungal genera may help researchers to identify genes that are essential for particular processes in *Aspergillus*, particularly those that function in secondary metabolism. At present, genome sequence projects are in progress for *Aspergillus nidulans*, *A. niger*, *A. oryzae*, and *A. fumigatus*. The current status of the above-listed sequencing projects can be found in the Genomes Online Database (GOLD; http://ergo.integratedgenomics.com/GOLD/). The sequencing of expressed sequence tags (ESTs) from *A. flavus* is being conducted at three different locations. Information on the *A. flavus* EST sequencing project at the University of Oklahoma can be found at the webpage listed above; information on the USDA/ARS-funded EST sequencing project underway at the Southern Regional Research Center in New Orleans, LA, can be accessed at http://www.nps.ars.usda.gov; and information on the USDA/NRI-funded research can be found at http://fungi.fgl.ncsu.edu. The sequence data generated from all of the *Aspergillus* species listed above in addition to data from other sequencing projects could be useful in determining how closely conservation of gene order matches up with existing phylogenetic trees. Given an association between evolutionary relationships and gene synteny, the finding of homologous genes in closely related fungi would be simplified by the availability of genomic sequences from a wide range of fungi.

8.7.2 Gene Expression Analysis

Of course, the study of genomics goes far beyond genome sequencing and sequence comparisons. Many of the open reading frames in newly released sequences are novel[103] and therefore cannot be functionally classified through comparative genomics. Other methods must be employed to provide some insight into the functions of the resulting proteins. Many techniques have been developed for large-scale gene expression analysis. Some of the more common techniques include EST sequencing, serial analysis of gene expression (SAGE), differential display, and microarray analysis. As suggested by Yoder and Turgeon,[100] results obtained from genomic techniques such as those listed above should be further supported by methods such as gene disruption, deletion, or silencing.

A recent report on microarray analysis in *Aspergillus flavus* and *A. parasiticus* provides an example of how gene expression analysis can be used to identify genes involved in the regulation of aflatoxin biosynthesis.[104] Microarrays were made by spotting polymerase chain reaction (PCR) products of ESTs of genes temporally differentially expressed with respect to aflatoxin production on glass slides. The 753

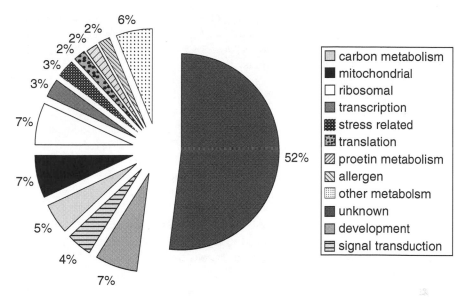

FIGURE 8.5 Metabolic classification of *Aspergillus flavus* genes used for microarray analysis of gene expression during aflatoxin production. 753 ESTs were assigned functional groups based on their putative cellular functions determined from blastn and blastx analyses against the NCBI database (http://www.ncbi.nlm.nih.gov/BLAST/). (Adapted from work described by O'Brian et al.[104])

ESTs represented genes from a wide variety of functional categories (Figure 8.5),[104] including the aflatoxin biosynthetic genes *ver-1*, *omtA*, *nor-1*, and *pksA*. The largest category (52%) was composed of genes of unknown function. Although these genes were differentially expressed between a time point before the initiation of aflatoxin biosynthesis and a second time point taken during aflatoxin accumulation, the differences in transcript levels may not be related to aflatoxin production. Many other cellular processes are transcriptionally regulated and may be active in an older culture and not in a younger culture or vice versa. This point is demonstrated by the high number of genes in Figure 8.5 that appear to be involved in primary metabolism. Aflatoxin is a secondary metabolite and is therefore made after primary metabolic activities have slowed or stopped. Differential expression of genes involved in primary metabolism would be expected between time points taken before and then during aflatoxin biosynthesis. The list of temporally differentially expressed genes included on the microarray slides could be narrowed by microarray experiments in which the ESTs are hybridized to cDNA from aflatoxin-producing and nonproducing cultures maintained under similar growth conditions. Genes that are consistently differentially expressed under a variety of conditions affecting aflatoxin production are likely to have some function related to aflatoxin. A number of different conditions are currently being examined by microarray analysis, including carbon and nitrogen source, temperature, pH, and genetic mutation. One microarray experiment comparing a wild-type strain to a FadA mutant strain of *Aspergillus flavus*, identified 165 genes with higher levels of transcription in the wild-type strain. From this subset, genes of interest, including some of unknown function, are being disrupted to screen for phenotypes associated with the regulation or biosynthesis of aflatoxin.[105] In this way, genomic strategies such as microarray analysis can be used to screen large numbers of genes for putative functions.

8.8 SUMMARY

The genus *Aspergillus* presents many advantages to addressing the questions surrounding secondary metabolism in fungi. A number of fungal species within the genus share the ability to produce aflatoxin or sterigmatocystin. This allows scientists to work with a number of different systems to address similar questions. While the discovery of parasexual cycles in *Aspergillus flavus* and *A. parasiticus* has greatly advanced genetic studies in these organisms, the presence of a sexual cycle in *A. nidulans* makes this fungus readily amenable to mutant development. The use of *A. nidulans* as a model system in combination with studies in the aflatoxigenic species will be essential to answering the many questions that still surround the regulation and ecological significance of secondary metabolism.

ACKNOWLEDGMENTS

We thank Ignazio Carbone, Ahmad Fakhoury, Greg O'Brian, and Sandy Smith for their assistance with the construction of images for this review.

REFERENCES

1. Squire, R.A., Ranking animal carcinogens: a proposed regulatory approach, *Science*, 214, 887–891, 1989.
2. Brown, M.P., Brown-Jenco, C.S., and Payne, G.A., Genetic and molecular analysis of aflatoxin biosynthesis, *Fungal Genet. Biol.*, 26(2), 81–98, 1999.
3. Miller, D.M. and Wilson, D.M., Veterinary diseases related to aflatoxins, in *The Toxicology of Aflatoxins*, Eaton, D.L. and Groopman, J.D., Eds., Academic Press, San Diego, CA, 1994, pp. 347–364.
4. Wogan, G.N., Impacts of chemicals on liver cancer risk, *Semin. Cancer Biol.*, 10(3), 201–210, 2000.
5. Henry, S.H., Bosch, R.X., Troxell, R.C., and Bolger, P.M., Public health: reducing liver cancer — global control of aflatoxin, *Science*, 286, 2453–2454, 1999.
6. CAST, *Mycotoxins: Risks in Plant, Animal, and Human Systems*, Richards, J. L., and Payne, G. A., Eds., Task Force Report 139, Council for Agricultural Science and Technology, Washington, D.C., 2003.
7. Scholl, P. and Groopman, J.D., Epidemiology of human aflatoxin exposures and its relationship to liver cancer, in *Molecular Approaches to Food Safety: Issues Involving Toxic Microorganisms*, Eklund, M., Richard, J. L., and Mise, K., Eds., Alaken, Fort Collins, CO, 1995, pp. 169–182.
8. Stone, R., Biodefense: peering into the shadows — Iraq's bioweapons program, *Science*, 297(5584), 1110–1112, 2002.
9. Gupta, A. and Gopal, M., Aflatoxin production by *Aspergillus flavus* isolates pathogenic to coconut insect pests, *World J. Microbiol. Biotechnol.*, 18(4), 325–331, 2002.

10. Alexopoulos, C.J., Mims, C.W., and Blackwell, M., *Introductory Mycology*, 4th ed., John Wiley & Sons, New York, 1996.

11. Raper, K. B. and Fennell, D.I., *The Genus Aspergillus*, Williams & Wilkins, Baltimore, MD, 1965.

12. Gams, W., Christensen, M., Onions, A. H., Pitt, J.I., and Samson, R.A., Infrageneric taxa of *Aspergillus*, in *Advances in Penicillium and Aspergillus Systematics*, Samson, R.A. and Pitt, J.I., Eds., Plenum Press, New York, 1985, pp. 55–62.

13. Peterson, S.W., Phylogenetic relationships in *Aspergillus* based on rDNA sequence analysis, in *Integration of Modern Taxonomic Methods for Penicillium and Aspergillus Classification*, Samson, R.A. and Pitt, J.I., Eds., Harwood Academic, Singapore, 2000, pp. 323–355.

14. Tamura, M., Kawahara, K., and Sugiyama, J., Molecular phylogeny of *Aspergillus* and associated teleomorphs in the Trichocomaceae (Eurotiales), in *Integration of Modern Taxonomic Methods for Penicillium and Aspergillus Classification*, Samson, R.A. and Pitt, J.I., Eds., Harwood Academic, Singapore, 2000, pp. 357–372.

15. Geiser, D.M., Pitt, J.I., and Taylor, J.W., Cryptic speciation and recombination in the aflatoxin-producing fungus *Aspergillus flavus*, *Proc. Natl. Acad. Sci. USA*, 95(1), 388–393, 1998.

16. Christensen, M., A synoptic key and evaluation of species in the *Aspergillus flavus* group, *Mycologia*, 73(6), 1056–1084, 1981.

17. Rigo, K., Varga, J., Toth, B., Teren, J., Mesterhazy, A., and Kozakiewicz, Z., Evolutionary relationships within *Aspergillus* section *Flavi* based on sequences of the intergenic transcribed spacer regions and the 5.8S rRNA gene, *J. Gen. Appl. Microbiol.*, 48(1), 9–16, 2002.

18. Peterson, S.W., Phylogenetic analysis of *Aspergillus* sections *Cremei* and *Wentii*, based on ribosomal DNA sequences, *Mycol. Res.*, 99, 1349–1355, 1995.

19. Ito, Y., Peterson, S.W., Wicklow, D.T., and Goto, T., *Aspergillus pseudotamarii*, a new aflatoxin producing species in *Aspergillus* section *Flavi*, *Mycol. Res.*, 105, 233–239, 2001.

20. Goto, T., Wicklow, D.T., and Ito, Y., Aflatoxin and cyclopiazonic acid production by a sclerotium-producing *Aspergillus tamarii* strain, *Appl. Environ. Microbiol.*, 62, 4036–4038, 1996.

21. Peterson, S.W., Ito, Y., Horn, B.W., and Goto, T., *Aspergillus bombycis*, a new aflatoxigenic species and genetic variation in its sibling species, *A. nomius*, *Mycologia*, 93(4), 689–703, 2001.

22. Samson, R.A., Current fungal taxonomy and mycotoxins, in *Mycotoxins and Phycotoxins in Perspective at the Turn of the Millennium*, de Koe, W.J. et al., Eds., Ponsen & Looyen, Wageningen, The Netherlands, 2001.

23. Varga, J., Rigo, K., Toth, B., Teren, J., Kozakiewicz, Z., Evolutionary relationships among *Aspergillus* species producing economically important mycotoxins, *Food Technol. Biotechnol.*, 41(1), 29–36, 2003.

24. Schroeder, H.W. and Verrett, M.J., Production of aflatoxin by *Aspergillus wentii* Wehmer, *Can. J. Microbiol.*, 15, 895–898, 1969.

25. Barnes, S.E., Dola, T.P., Bennett, J.W., and Bhatnagar, D., Synthesis of sterigmatocystin on a chemically defined medium by species of *Aspergillus* and *Chaetomium*, *Mycopathologia*, 125, 173–178, 1994.

26. Cardwell, K.F. and Cotty, P.J., Distribution of *Aspergillus* section *Flavi* among field soils from the four agroecological zones of the Republic of Benin, West Africa, *Plant Dis.*, 86(4), 434–439, 2002.

27. Geiser, D.M., Dorner, J.W., Horn, B.W., and Taylor, J.W., The phylogenetics of myc-
    otoxin and sclerotium production in *Aspergillus flavus* and *Aspergillus oryzae*, *Fungal
    Genet. Biol.*, 31(3), 169–179, 2000.
28. Bhatnagar, D., Cleveland, T.E., and Payne, G.A., *Aspergillus flavus*, in *Encyclopedia of
    Food Microbiology*, Robinson, R.K., Batt, C.A., and Patel, P.D., Eds., Academic Press,
    London, 2000, pp. 72–79.
29. Bryden, W.I., Occurrence and biological effects of cyclopiazonic acid, in *Emerging
    Food Safety Problems Resulting from Microbial Contamination: Proceedings of the
    Seventh International Symposium on Toxic Microorganisms*, Mise, K. and Richard, J.L.,
    Eds., UJNR, Tokyo, 1991, pp. 127–147,
30. FAO, *Worldwide Regulations for Mycotoxins 1995: A Compendium*, Food and Nutrition
    Paper 64, Food and Agriculture Organization, United Nations, Rome, Italy, 1997.
31. Klich, M.A., Tiffany, L.H., and Knaphus, G., Ecology of the aspergilli of soils and litter,
    in *Aspergillus: Biology and Industrial Applications*, Bennett, J.W. and Klich, M.A.,
    Eds., Butterworth-Heinemann, Boston, MA, 1992, pp. 329–353.
32. St. Leger, R.J., Screen, S.E., and Shams-Pirzadeh, B., Lack of host specialization in
    Aspergillus flavus, *Appl. Environ. Microbiol.*, 66(1), 320–324, 2000.
33. Horn, B.W. and Dorner, J.W., Soil populations of *Aspergillus* species from section *Flavi*
    along a transect through peanut-growing regions of the United States, *Mycologia*, 90(5),
    767–776, 1998.
34. Horn, B.W., Greene, R.L., Sobolev, V.S., Dorner, J.W., Powell, J.H., and Layton, R.C.,
    Association of morphology and mycotoxin production with vegetative compatibility
    groups in *Aspergillus flavus*, *A. parasiticus*, and *A. tamarii*, *Mycologia*, 88(4), 574–587,
    1996.
35. Bayman, P. and Cotty, P.J., Genetic diversity in *Aspergillus flavus*: association with
    aflatoxin production and morphology, *Can. J. Bot. Revue Canadienne De Botanique*,
    71(1), 23–31, 1993.
36. McAlpin, C.E., Wicklow, D.T., and Horn, B.W., DNA fingerprinting analysis of vege-
    tative compatibility groups in *Aspergillus flavus* from a peanut field in Georgia, *Plant
    Dis.*, 86(3), 254–258, 2002.
37. Papa, K.E., Heterokaryon incompatibility in *Aspergillus flavus*, *Mycologia*, 78(1),
    98–101, 1986.
38. Horn, B.W. and Greene, R.L., Vegetative compatibility within populations of *Aspergillus
    flavus*, *Aspergillus parasiticus*, and *A. tamarii* from a peanut field, *Mycologia*, 87(3),
    324–332, 1995.
39. Bayman, P. and Cotty, P.J., Vegetative compatibility and genetic diversity in the *Aspergil-
    lus flavus* population of a single field, *Can. J. Bot. (Revue Canadienne De Botanique)*,
    69(8), 1707–1711, 1991.
40. Croft, J.H., Genetic variation and evolution in *Aspergillus*, in *Evolutionary Biology of
    the Fungi*, Rayner, A.D.M., Brasier, C.M., and Moore, D., Eds., Academic Press,
    London, 1987, pp. 311–323.
41. Novas, M.V. and Cabral, D., Association of mycotoxin and sclerotia production with
    compatibility groups in *Aspergillus flavus* from peanut in Argentina, *Plant Dis.*, 86(3),
    215–219, 2002.
42. Wicklow, D.T., Horn, B.W., and Cole, R.J., Sclerotium production by *Aspergillus flavus*
    on corn kernels, *Mycologia*, 74(3), 398–403, 1982.
43. Wicklow, D.T., Wilson, D.M., and Nelsen, T.C., Survival of *Aspergillus flavus* sclerotia
    and conidia buried in soil in Illinois or Georgia, *Phytopathology*, 83(11), 1141–1147,
    1993.

44. Wicklow, D.T. and Donahue, J.E., Sporogenic germination of sclerotia in *Aspergillus flavus* and *Aspergillus parasiticus*, *Trans. Br. Mycol. Soc.*, 82, 621–624, 1984.

45. Wicklow, D.T. and Wilson, D.M., Germination of *Aspergillus flavus* sclerotia in a Georgia maize field, *Trans. Br. Mycol. Soc.*, 87(4), 651–653, 1986.

46. Widstrom, N.W., The aflatoxin problem with corn grain, in *Advances in Agronomy*, Sparks, D.L., Ed., Academic Press, New York, 1996, pp. 219–280.

47. Jones, R.K., Duncan, H.E., Payne, G.A., and Leonard, K.J., Factors influencing infection by *Aspergillus flavus* in silk-inoculated corn, *Plant Dis.*, 64, 859, 1980.

48. Payne, G.A., Process of contamination by aflatoxin-producing fungi and their impact on crops, in *Mycotoxins in Agriculture and Food Safety*, Sinha, K.K. and Bhatnagar, D., Eds, Marcel Dekker, New York, 1998, pp. 279–306.

49. Smart, M.G., Wicklow, D.T., and Caldwell, R.W., Pathogenesis in *Aspergillus* ear rot of maize: light microscopy of fungal spread from wounds, *Phytopathology*, 80(12), 1287–1294, 1990.

50. Zummo, N. and Scott, G.E., Relative aggressiveness of *Aspergillus flavus* and *A. parasiticus* on maize in Mississippi, *Plant Dis.*, 74, 978–981, 1990.

51. Payne, G.A., Aflatoxin in maize, *CRC Crit. Rev. Plant Sci.*, 10(5), 423–440, 1992.

52. Cole, R.J., Hill, R.A., Blankenship, P.D., Sanders, T.H., and Garren, K.H., Influence of irrigation and drought stress on invasion by *Aspergillus flavus* of corn kernels and peanut pods, *Dev. Ind. Microbiol.*, 23, 229–236, 1982.

53. Sanders, T.H., Blankenship, P.D., Cole, R.J., and Hill, R.A., Effect of soil temperature and drought on peanut pod and stem temperatures relative to *Aspergillus flavus* invasion and aflatoxin contamination, *Mycopathologia*, 86, 51–54, 1984.

54. Blankenship, P.D., Cole, R.J., Sanders, T.H., and Hill, R.A., Effect of geocarposphere temperature on pre-harvest colonization of drought-stressed peanuts by *Aspergillus flavus* and subsequent aflatoxin contamination, *Mycopathologia*, 85, 69–74, 1984.

55. Pontecorvo, G., Roper, J.A., Hemmons, L.M., MacDonald, K.D., and Bufton, A.W.J., The genetics of *Aspergillus nidulans*, *Adv. Genet.*, 5, 141–238, 1953.

56. Papa, K.E., Parasexual cycle in *Aspergillus flavus*, *Mycologia*, 65(5), 1201–1205, 1973.

57. Leaich, L.L. and Papa, K.E., Identification of diploids of *Aspergillus flavus* by the nuclear condition of the conidia, *Mycologia*, 67, 674–678, 1975.

58. Bennett, J.W. and Papa, K.E., The aflatoxigenic *Aspergillus* spp., in *Genetics of Plant Pathogenic Fungi*, Ingram, D.S. and Williams, P.A., Eds., Academic Press, London, 1988, pp. 263–280.

59. Papa, K.E., Genetics of *Aspergillus flavus*: linkage of aflatoxin mutants, *Can. J. Microbiol.*, 30(1), 68–73, 1984.

60. Woloshuk, C.P., Yousibova, G.L., Rollins, J.A., Bhatnagar, D., and Payne, G.A., Molecular characterization of the *afl-1* locus in *Aspergillus flavus*, *Appl. Environ. Microbiol.*, 61, 3019–3023, 1995.

61. Swart, K., Debets, A.J.M., Holub, E.F., Bos, C.J., and Hoekstra, R.F., Physical karyotyping: genetic and taxonomic applications in aspergilli, in *The Genus Aspergillus*, Powell, K.A., Renwick, A., and Peberdy, J.F., Eds., Plenum Press, New York, 1994, pp. 233–240.

62. Keller, N.P., Cleveland, T.E., and Bhatnagar, D., Variable electrophoretic karyotypes of members of *Aspergillus* section *Flavi*, *Curr. Genet.*, 21(4–5), 371–375, 1992.

63. Foutz, K.R., Woloshuk, C.P., and Payne, G.A., Cloning and assignment of linkage group loci to a karyotypic map of the filamentous fungus *Aspergillus flavus*, *Mycologia*, 87(6), 787–794, 1995.

64. Keller, N.P. and Hohn, T.M., Metabolic pathway gene clusters in filamentous fungi, *Fungal Genet. Biol.*, 21(1), 17–29, 1997.

65. Diez, B., Gutierrez, S., Barredo, J.L., Vansolingen, P., Vandervoort, L.H.M., and Martin, J.F., The cluster of penicillin biosynthetic genes: identification and characterization of the *Pcbab* gene encoding the alpha-aminoadipyl–cysteinyl–valine synthetase and linkage to the *Pcbc* and *Pende* genes, *J. Biol. Chem.*, 265(27), 16358–16365, 1990.

66. Smith, D.J., Burnham, M.K.R., Edwards, J., Earl, A.J., and Turner, G., Cloning and heterologous expression of the penicillin biosynthetic gene cluster from *Penicillium chrysogenum*, *Bio-Technology*, 8(1), 39–41, 1990.

67. Gutierrez, S., Diez, B., Montenegro, E., and Martin, J.F., Characterization of the *Cephalosporium–Acremonium Pcbab* gene encoding alpha-aminoadipyl–cysteinyl–valine synthetase, a large multidomain peptide synthetase: linkage to the *Pcbc* gene as a cluster of early cephalosporin biosynthetic genes and evidence of multiple functional domains, *J. Bacteriol.*, 173(7), 2354–2365, 1991.

68. Maccabe, A.P., Riach, M.B.R., Unkles, S.E., and Kinghorn, J.R., The *Aspergillus nidulans Npea* locus consists of 3 contiguous genes required for penicillin biosynthesis, *EMBO J.*, 9(1), 279–287, 1990.

69. Maccabe, A.P., Vanliempt, H., Palissa, H., Unkles, S.E., Riach, M.B.R., Pfeifer, E., Vondohren, H., and Kinghorn, J.R., Delta-(L-alpha-aminoadipyl)-L-cysteinyl-D-valine synthetase from *Aspergillus nidulans*: molecular characterization of the *Acva* gene encoding the 1st enzyme of the penicillin biosynthetic-pathway, *J. Biol. Chem.*, 266(19), 12646–12654, 1991.

70. Hohn, T.M., McCormick, S.P., and Desjardins, A.E., Evidence for a gene cluster involving trichothecene-pathway biosynthetic genes in *Fusarium sporotrichioides*, *Curr. Genet.*, 24(4), 291–295, 1993.

71. McCormick, S.P., Hohn, T.M., and Desjardins, A.E., Isolation and characterization of *Tri 3*, a gene encoding 15-*O*-acetyltransferase from *Fusarium sporotrichioides*, *Appl. Environ. Microbiol.*, 62, 353–359, 1996.

72. Sweeney, M.J. and Dobson, A.D.W., Molecular biology of mycotoxin biosynthesis, *FEMS Microbiol. Lett.*, 175, 149–163, 1999.

73. Yu, J.J., Chang, P.K., Cary, J.W., Wright, M., Bhatnagar, D., Cleveland, T.E., Payne, G.A., and Linz, J.E., Comparative mapping of aflatoxin pathway gene clusters in *Aspergillus parasiticus* and *Aspergillus flavus*, *Appl. Environ. Microbiol.*, 61(6), 2365–2371, 1995.

74. Papa, K.E., Genetics of *Aspergillus flavus*: complementation and mapping of aflatoxin mutants, *Genet. Res.*, 34(1), 1–9, 1979.

75. Prieto, R., Yousibova, G.L., and Woloshuk, C.P., Identification of aflatoxin biosynthesis genes by genetic complementation in an *Aspergillus flavus* mutant lacking the aflatoxin gene cluster, *Appl. Environ. Microbiol.*, 62(10), 3567–3571, 1996.

76. Payne, G.A. and Brown, M.P., Genetics and physiology of aflatoxin biosynthesis, *Annu. Rev. Phytopathol.*, 36, 329–362, 1998.

77. Papa, K.E., Norsolorinic acid mutant of *Aspergillus flavus*, *J. Gen. Microbiol.*, 128, 1345–1348, 1982.

78. Woloshuk, C.P. and Prieto, R., Genetic organization and function of the aflatoxin B_1 biosynthetic genes, *FEMS Microbiol. Lett.*, 160(2), 169–176, 1998.

79. Chang, P.K., Cary, J.W., Bhatnagar, D., Cleveland, T.E., Bennett, J.W., Linz, J.E., Woloshuk, C.P., and Payne, G.A., Cloning of the *Aspergillus parasiticus apa-2* gene associated with the regulation of aflatoxin biosynthesis, *Appl. Environ. Microbiol.*, 59(10), 3273–3279, 1993.

80. Woloshuk, C.P., Foutz, K.R., Brewer, J.F., Bhatnagar, D., Cleveland, T.E., and Payne, G.A., Molecular characterization of *aflR*, a regulatory locus for aflatoxin biosynthesis, *Appl. Environ. Microbiol.*, 60(7), 2408–2414, 1994.

81. Yu, J.H., Butchko, R.A.E., Fernandes, M., Keller, N.P., Leonard, T.J., and Adams, T.H., Conservation of structure and function of the aflatoxin regulatory gene *aflR* from *Aspergillus nidulans* and *A. flavus*, *Curr. Genet.*, 29(6), 549–555, 1996.

82. Payne, G.A., Nystrom, G.J., Bhatnagar, D., Cleveland, T.E., and Woloshuk, C.P., Cloning of the *afl-2* gene involved in aflatoxin biosynthesis from *Aspergillus flavus*, *Appl. Environ. Microbiol.*, 59(1), 156–162, 1993.

83. Flaherty, J.E. and Payne, G.A., Overexpression of *aflR* leads to upregulation of pathway gene transcription and increased aflatoxin production in *Aspergillus flavus*, *Appl. Environ. Microbiol.*, 63(10), 3995–4000, 1997.

84. Ehrlich, K.C., Montalbano, B.G., Cary, J.W., and Cotty, P.J., Promoter elements in the aflatoxin pathway polyketide synthase gene, *Biochim. Biophys. Acta*, 1576, 171–175, 2002.

85. Fernandes, M., Keller, N.P., and Adams, T.H., Sequence-specific binding by *Aspergillus nidulans* AflR, a C-6 zinc cluster protein regulating mycotoxin biosynthesis, *Molec. Microbiol.*, 28(6), 1355–1365, 1998.

86. Chang, P.K., Ehrlich, K.C., Yu, J.J., Bhatnagar, D., and Cleveland, T.E., Increased expression of *Aspergillus parasiticus aflR*, encoding a sequence-specific DNA-binding protein, relieves nitrate inhibition of aflatoxin biosynthesis, *Appl. Environ. Microbiol.*, 61(6), 2372–2377, 1995.

87. Liu, B.H. and Chu, F.S., Regulation of *aflR* and its product, AflR, associated with aflatoxin biosynthesis, *Appl. Environ. Microbiol.*, 64(10), 3718–3723, 1998.

88. Ehrlich, K.C., Cary, J.W., and Montalbano, B.G., Characterization of the promoter for the gene encoding the aflatoxin biosynthetic pathway regulatory protein AflR, *Biochim. Biophys. Acta*, 1444(3), 412–417, 1999.

89. Butchko, R.A.E., Adams, T.H., and Keller, N.P., *Aspergillus nidulans* mutants defective in Stc gene cluster regulation, *Genetics*, 153(2), 715–720, 1999.

90. Chang, P.K., Yu, J.J., Bhatnagar, D., Cleveland, T.E., Repressor-AflR interaction modulates aflatoxin biosynthesis in *Aspergillus parasiticus*, *Mycopathologia*, 147(2), 105–112, 1999.

91. Chang, P.K. and Yu, J., Characterization of a partial duplication of the aflatoxin gene cluster in *Aspergillus parasiticus* ATCC 56775, *Appl. Microbiol. Biotechnol.*, 58, 632–636, 2002.

92. Jayashree, T., Rao, J.P., and Subramanyam, C., Regulation of aflatoxin production by Ca^{2+}/calmodulin-dependent protein phosphorylation and dephosphorylation, *FEMS Microbiol. Lett.*, 183(2), 215–219, 2000.

93. Shimizu, K. and Keller, N.P., Genetic involvement of a cAMP-dependent protein kinase in a G protein signaling pathway regulating morphological and chemical transitions in *Aspergillus nidulans*, *Genetics*, 157(2), 591–600, 2001.

94. Calvo, A.M., Wilson, R.A., Bok, J.W., and Keller, N.P., Relationship between secondary metabolism and fungal development, *Microbiol. Mol. Biol. Rev.*, 66(3), 447–459, 2002.

95. Guzmán-de-Peña, D. and Ruiz-Herrera, J., Relationship between aflatoxin biosynthesis and sporulation in *Aspergillus parasiticus*, *Fungal Genet. Biol.*, 21(2), 198–205, 1997.

96. Hicks, J.K., Yu, J.H., Keller, N.P., and Adams, T.H., *Aspergillus* sporulation and mycotoxin production both require inactivation of the FadA G alpha protein-dependent signaling pathway, *EMBO J.*, 16(16), 4916–4923, 1997.

97. Yu, J.H., Wieser, J., and Adams, T.H., The *Aspergillus* FlbA RGS domain protein antagonizes G protein signaling to block proliferation and allow development, *EMBO J.*, 15(19), 5184–5190, 1996.

98. Lee, B.N. and Adams, T.H., Overexpression of *flbA*, an early regulator of *Aspergillus* asexual sporulation, leads to activation of *brlA* and premature initiation of development, *Molec. Microbiol.*, 14(2), 323–334, 1994.

99. Chiou, C.H., Miller, M., Wilson, D.L., Trail, F., and Linz, J.E., Chromosomal location plays a role in regulation of aflatoxin gene expression in *Aspergillus parasiticus*, *Appl. Environ. Microbiol.*, 68(1), 306–315, 2002.

100. Yoder, O.C. and Turgeon, B.G., Fungal genomics and pathogenicity, *Curr. Opin. Plant Biol.*, 4(4), 315–321, 2001.

101. Jeong, J.S. and Dean, R.A., Comparative studies of gene organization between *Magnaporthe grisea* and other fungal species, in *Proc. XXI Fungal Genetics Conference*, Pacific Grove, CA, March 13–18, 2001.

102. Brendel, V., Kurtz, S., and Walbot, V., Comparative genomics of *Arabidopsis* and maize: prospects and limitations, *Genome Biol.*, 3(3), 1005.1–1005.6, 2002.

103. Bennett, J.W., White paper: genomics for filamentous fungi, *Fungal Genet. Biol.*, 21(1), 3–7, 1997.

104. O'Brian, G.R., Fakhoury, A.M., and Payne, G.A., Identification of genes differentially expressed during aflatoxin biosynthesis in *Aspergillus flavus* and *Aspergillus parasiticus*, *Fungal Genet. Biol.*, 39, 118–127, 2003.

105. Scheidegger, K.A., O'Brian, G.R., Keller, N.P., and Payne, G.A., Gene expression analysis in a wild type and FadA mutant of *Aspergillus flavus*, *Phytopathology*, 92, S73, 2002.

9 Progress in Elucidating the Molecular Basis of the Host Plant– *Aspergillus flavus* Interaction: A Basis for Devising Strategies to Reduce Aflatoxin Contamination in Crops

Thomas E. Cleveland, Jiujiang Yu,
Deepak Bhatnagar, Zhi-Yuan Chen,
Robert L. Brown, Perng-Kuang Chang,
and Jeffrey W. Cary

CONTENTS

9.1   INTRODUCTION

No completely effective control strategies are available to prevent aflatoxin accumulation in the field when conditions are favorable for the fungus.[1] A complete understanding of the host plant–*Aspergillus flavus* interaction and aflatoxin contamination process will help in the development of new control strategies aimed at interrupting the mechanisms responsible for preharvest aflatoxin contamination with the goal of producing a safer, economically viable food and feed supply.[2] Numerous investigations, as reviewed in this article, have attempted to gain a better understanding of the relationship between the host plant and the invading fungus, *A. flavus*, because this relationship affects the aflatoxin contamination process. It is now hypothesized that several host plant and fungal genes are probably involved in determining the degree of aflatoxin contamination of the crop.

For example, as will be discussed later, proteomic analysis has identified several proteins in corn kernels for which the level of expression can be correlated with resistance to aflatoxin contamination. The corn model provides the best genetically characterized crop for studying the biochemistry of "natural" seed-based resistance to aflatoxin contamination because of the availability of a wide range in levels of resistance and susceptibility to aflatoxin contamination in varieties of this crop which provides a very useful system for conducting differential biochemical comparisons of these varieties. *Aspergillus flavus* hydrolases produced during invasion of the host plant are probably necessary for the establishment and production of aflatoxin in host tissues. In addition, a gene cluster and regulatory genes (e.g., *aflR*) governing aflatoxin biosynthesis have been characterized in the fungus.

Many of the early investigations were limited to the study of only one gene or gene product from either the fungus or the plant at a time and could thus be characterized as more targeted genomics studies. The need for the use of genomics and proteomics technologies to study global expression of genes has become more obvious as researchers have discovered that a complex array of multiple fungal and host plant genes probably govern aflatoxin contamination of crops. In fact, despite the extensive literature on plant and fungal factors that may regulate the aflatoxin contamination process, it is likely that several genes governing the host plant–*Aspergillus flavus* interaction and aflatoxin biosynthesis have not yet been identified. These earlier studies provided valuable insights into which categories of fungal and host plant traits are most important in governing the plant–fungus interaction, thus facilitating the search for additional genes and proteins in expressed sequence tag (EST) or protein databases, respectively.

Aspergillus flavus genomics and proteomics of seed- and kernel-based resistance are investigative tools for simultaneous discovery and analysis of the biochemical function and genetic regulation of the critical genes governing the plant–fungal interaction and aflatoxin biosynthesis. *A. flavus* ESTs and microarray technology may allow rapid identification of the majority, if not all, of the genes expressed in the fungal genome and help to understand better the coordinated regulation of gene expression. The *A. flavus* EST and corn kernel proteomics programs at the U.S. Department of Agriculture (USDA) Agricultural Research Service (ARS) Southern Regional Research Center (SRRC)[1] are aimed at understanding the genetic control and regulation of aflatoxin biosynthesis by potential regulators upstream of *aflR*,[2] the mechanism of aflatoxin production in response to internal and external factors,[3] the relationship between primary and secondary metabolism,[4] the basis of fungal pathogenicity, and the mechanism of seed-based resistance to fungal invasion and aflatoxin contamination in corn.[5] Current plans in the Food and Feed Safety Program at the SRRC are to construct a microarray containing *A. flavus* EST sequences to detect simultaneously an entire set of genes expressed under specific and variable conditions of plant–fungal interactions. By applying fungal EST/microarray and complementary seed proteomics technologies, those genes that may be responsible for or related to aflatoxin production, signal transduction, plant–microbe interactions, and fungal development and pathogenicity can be characterized, thus leading to development of strategies to enhance host plant resistance to aflatoxin contamination through the use of marker-assisted breeding and gene insertion technologies.

9.2 KNOWN *ASPERGILLUS FLAVUS* GENES INVOLVED IN CROP INVASION AND AFLATOXIN FORMATION

9.2.1 Fungal Virulence Genes

Though well known for its ability to cause aflatoxin contamination in crops such as corn, peanut, cottonseed, and tree nuts, *Aspergillus flavus* is generally regarded as saprophytic in nature, but, like many *Aspergillus* species, it is also considered to be an opportunistic pathogen. *A. flavus* requires wounds or otherwise weakened hosts for successful colonization,[3,4] but like other plant pathogenic fungi it employs hydrolytic enzymes such as pectinases, proteases, and amylases for successful invasion and utilization of host plant tissues. Characterizing and understanding the relative contribution of these hydrolases in fungal pathogenicity would benefit efforts to target invasive enzymes for inhibition, perhaps through use of technologies to enhance expression of hydrolase inhibitors in the host plant.

9.2.1.1 Pectinases

Pectin is a major constituent of plant cell walls, and a number of enzymes collectively termed pectinases are the first cell-wall-degrading hydrolases produced by fungal pathogens during the infection process. Isolates of *Aspergillus flavus* have been found to produce three distinct pectinases designated P1, P3, and P2c,[5] as well as the pectin methylesterase.[6] P1 and P3 are produced by both low- and high-virulence *A. flavus* strains isolated from the field, while P2c is produced by only highly virulent field strains.[7] The ability of isolates of *A. flavus* to damage and spread between cotton boll locules was shown to be at least partially related to variations in the production of P2c.[8] Strains lacking P2c did not cause as much damage to intercarpillary walls, thus limiting their spread throughout the cotton boll. Interestingly, P2c was the only pectinase produced by *A. flavus* that was not subject to catabolite repression in culture by simple sugars commonly found in developing cotton bolls. The gene encoding P2c, designated *pecA*, has been cloned and characterized in both *A. flavus* and *A. parasiticus*.[9,10] Gene replacement following introduction of a disrupted version of the gene encoding P2c into a highly virulent strain of *A. flavus* resulted in transformants with a significant reduction in aggressiveness upon inoculation in cotton bolls.[11] Conversely, when *pecA* was introduced into a low-virulence strain that lacked P2c, the ability of the transformant to invade and spread in bolls was significantly increased. Although studies have demonstrated a correlation between the aggressiveness of *A. flavus* and P2c activity, other factors also appear to be involved in overall virulence. The fact that *A. flavus* strains lacking P2c are still capable of causing disease indicates that multiple factors, including other cell-wall-degrading enzymes, are likely to be involved. Regulation of *pecA* expression is probably very important in pathogenesis. Insensitivity of *pecA* to glucose repression allows for a constitutive level of P2c production, thus facilitating the initial stages of fungal infection. It is conceivable that pectic fragments generated by P2c digestion of the plant cell wall may then induce expression of other pectinases and cell-wall-degrading enzymes that further promote fungal invasion and spread.

9.2.1.2 Proteases

A number of studies have demonstrated the production of proteases by *Aspergillus flavus* isolates during growth on various natural and synthetic substrates;[12–16] however, none of these studies was able to find a direct correlation between protease production and fungal virulence. Isoelectric focusing (IEF) analysis of *A. flavus* strains isolated from humans, plants, and insects demonstrated very similar patterns of protease isozymes when cultured on 1% horse-lung polymer medium.[14] Quantitative differences in protease levels between isolates did not correlate with their ability to colonize insects. Two *A. flavus* isolates — AF12, displaying low virulence and lacking pectinase P2c, and AF13, displaying high virulence and producing P2c — were compared for production of nonpectinolytic hydrolases after growth on 10%

potato dextrose broth.[15] AF13 produced higher levels of protease than AF12 but isoform differences between the two isolates was inconclusive. Similar results were obtained when AF12 and AF13 were inoculated into cotton bolls as no discernable difference in production of nonpectinolytic hydrolase isoforms in the two *A. flavus* isolates was detected.[17] The best evidence to date for a role of proteases in fungal virulence was reported in results obtained during corn kernel infection assays.[16] During infection of corn kernels by *A. flavus*, the major protease produced was identified as an alkaline protease that demonstrated significant homology to the alkaline protease of *A. oryzae*. A mutant expressing high levels of this alkaline protease caused kernel rot symptoms more severe than seen with the wild-type strain.

9.2.1.3 Amylases

A number of studies have provided evidence that amylases produced by *Aspergillus flavus* during growth on synthetic medium or on corn kernels play a role in the growth of the fungus and its ability to produce aflatoxin. Indirect evidence for the importance of amylase production on fungal growth and toxin production was provided from studies on the identification of resistance factors in corn kernels.[18,19] A 14-kDa corn trypsin inhibitor (TI) protein associated with host resistance to *A. flavus* was found to inhibit fungal production of extracellular α-amylase, as well as reduce the activity of the amylase. Purified TI overexpressed in *Escherichia coli* was also found to inhibit the ability of *A. flavus* spores to germinate and to inhibit hyphal growth.[18] The *amy1* gene of *A. flavus* encoding α-amylase has been cloned and *amy1* knockout mutants have been constructed.[20] *A. flavus* mutants with a disrupted *amy1* gene did not make extracellular α-amylase and reduced growth on starch medium by 55% of that observed for the wild-type. Results of wounded and nonwounded corn kernel growth and toxin production assays indicated that α-amylase facilitates the growth of *A. flavus* from a wound in the endosperm to the embryo and is important for aflatoxin production.[19] It was also shown that the bifunctional 14-kDa TI/α-amylase inhibitor protein from corn was capable of inhibiting the α-amylase from the *A. flavus* strain used in these studies.

In an effort to identify more potent inhibitors of α-amylase activity in *Aspergillus flavus*, a study was performed in which extracts of over 200 different plant species were screened for their ability to inhibit *A. flavus* α-amylase.[21] A 36-kDa bifunctional lectin-arcelin-α-amylase inhibitor (AILP) from *Lablab purpureus* was identified that inhibited *A. flavus* α-amylase as well as spore germination and hyphal growth. AILP was found to be about 30 times more active than the 14-kDa corn TI/α-amylase inhibitor against *A. flavus* α-amylase. AILP was determined to be a competitive inhibitor with starch for the α-amylase from *A. flavus*, and its associated lectin activity was believed to be responsible in large part for inhibition of fungal growth. Growth of low-virulent (AF12) and high-virulent (AF13) strains of *A. flavus* on 10% potato dextrose broth (PDB) resulted in amylase activity being significantly higher in AF13 than AF12.[15] It was shown that AF13 produced two amylase isoforms and AF12 apparently produced only one. It was hypothesized that the differences in amylase isoforms may account for the observed differences in aggressiveness of the two *A. flavus* strains, though this has yet to be proven.

9.2.1.4 Other Hydrolases

In addition to the aforementioned enzyme activities, *Aspergillus flavus* has been shown to produce cellulases, xylanases, chitinases, lipases, and cutinases during growth on media containing inducers of these enzymes or approximating major substrates found in plant tissues. Analysis of xylanases and cellulases produced by *A. flavus* strains AF12 and AF13 during growth on 10% PDB detected no cellulase activity and no significant difference in xylanase activity.[15] Cellulase, xylanase, chitinase, and cutinase activity was detected for *A. flavus* growing on minimal medium supplemented with carboxymethyl cellulose, birchwood xylan, colloidal chitin, and polycaprolactone, respectively.[13] Lipases also appear to play a role in fungal growth and toxin production. Time-course studies of substrate utilization by *A. flavus* in medium simulating corn kernels showed that hydrolysis of starch and triglycerides occurred simultaneously.[22] A similar study of media simulating cotton-seed reserve materials demonstrated that sugars were utilized for initial growth and upon exhaustion triglycerides were then hydrolyzed.[23] Removal of lipids from ground whole cottonseed resulted in a reduction in aflatoxin production by *A. flavus* of approximately three orders of magnitude. Cloning of the *A. flavus* lipase gene has opened the door to research to gain a better understanding of the role of this enzyme in fungal growth and toxin synthesis through the use of gene expression or disruption analyses, for example.

Due to its broad host range and apparent lack of host specificity, *Aspergillus flavus* has evolved a wide array of hydrolases to utilize the numerous substrates that constitute its ecological niche. With the exception of pectinase P2c, no hydrolase has been identified that plays a definitive role in the observed differences in aggressiveness of *A. flavus* strains with respect to infection and toxin production. While some of the hydrolases (pectinases and proteases) may contribute to the ability of the fungus to spread in plant tissues due to disruption of natural structural barriers, the function of the other hydrolases is probably limited to nutrient acquisition, induction of aflatoxin synthesis, and overall vigor of the fungus. Many hydrolases appear to be present as isoforms in the fungus. The presence of isoforms has been demonstrated in the case of some of these hydrolases, and this may be due to the presence of gene families encoding a particular class of hydrolase or perhaps post-translational modifications to the protein. The possibility exists that the presence of a unique isoform or even differences in expression of genes within a hydrolase gene family may be responsible for observed differences in levels of virulence between fungal isolates; therefore, analysis of the regulation of expression of single genes (or multiple genes using microarray technology) within a hydrolytic gene family or production of unique isoforms due to posttranslational modifications may provide clues as to the observed level of virulence in *A. flavus*.

9.2.2 Nutrient Utilization Genes

Expression of nutrient utilization genes in the fungus is critical in processing plant products into forms that are conducive for aflatoxin formation. Knowledge of these processes could suggest strategies to interrupt the contamination process. Mateles and Adye[24] examined 17 carbon compounds used by *Aspergillus flavus* and reported that sucrose, fructose, and glucose were the best carbon sources for aflatoxin production. Starch, mannitol, sorbitol, and galactose yielded intermediate amounts of aflatoxin. Davis and Diener[25] concluded from their study of *A. parasiticus* that the majority of carbon compounds that are normally oxidized through both the hexose monophosphate shunt and the glycolytic pathway supported growth and aflatoxin production. Despite the fact that carbon source is one of the most important determinants of aflatoxin biosynthesis, relatively few genes associated with carbon utilization and regulation have been isolated and characterized. Extracellular α-amylase and glucoamylase have been purified from *A. flavus*,[26] but their association with starch degradation and aflatoxin production has not been examined.

Plant pectins also provide a nutrient source for the fungus, which can produce pectinases for the utilization of pectic substrates. Two genes, *pecA* and *pecB*, encoding endopolyglacturonases were cloned from a highly aggressive strain of *Aspergillus flavus*. The *pecA* product, P2c, produced in certain *A. flavus* strains, promotes more fungal damage and spread in cotton bolls compared to *A. flavus* isolates that do not produce P2c.[11]

Yu et al.[27] isolated four genes that constitute a gene cluster related to sugar utilization in *Aspergillus parasiticus*. The *nadA*, *hxtA*, *glcA*, and *sugR* genes show homology to genes encoding a NADH oxidase, a hexose transporter protein, 1,4- or -1,6-glucosidases, and a Cys6-type transcription factor, respectively. Real-time (RT)-PCR analysis demonstrated that the *hxtA* gene was expressed concurrently with the aflatoxin biosynthetic gene *omtA*. A link between this sugar utilization gene cluster and induction of aflatoxin biosynthesis by simple sugars has been suggested. Most recently, three sugar utilization gene clusters have been identified from *A. oryzae*, a species of industrial importance and phylogenetically closely related to *A. flavus* and *A. parasiticus*. Takizawa et al.,[28] using an *A. oryzae* EST clone homologous to the yeast maltase gene (*MAL62*) to screen an *A. oryzae* genomic library, isolated two different gene clusters. The cluster involved in maltose utilization consists of *malT*, a *MAL62* homolog; *malP*, a gene homologous to the yeast maltose permease gene *MAL61*; and *malR*, which encodes a putative nonfunctional GAL4-type zinc cluster transcriptional regulator because of a truncation in its carboxy-terminal-coding region. The second sugar gene cluster in *A. oryzae* consists of four genes homologous to the four *A. parasiticus* genes *nadA*, *hexA*, *glcA*, and *sugR* in the same gene order. The *nadA* gene homolog has a deletion in its coding region and likely is nonfunctional (Gomi, pers. comm.; accession no. AB072433).

A third identified gene cluster is involved in starch degradation and consists of *amyR* encoding a zinc cluster transcriptional activator, *agdA* encoding an α-glucosidase, and *amyA* encoding Taka-amylase A.[29] *amyR* disruptants grew poorly on a starch medium and produced low amounts of amylolytic enzymes, including α-amylase and glucoamylase; however, the *amyR* disruptants grew normally on a maltose medium, indicating that *amyR* does not regulate maltose utilization genes. These observations strongly support the notion that the sugar utilization gene cluster identified in *A. parasiticus* is not related to starch degradation but more likely is related to the utilization of simple sugars. The ESTs homologous to *nadA* and *hxtA* were found in the authors' *A. flavus* EST library (USDA/ARS/SRRC, New Orleans, LA). An additional *A. flavus* hexose transporter (HXT) gene homologous to *A.*

parasiticus hxt1 (accession no. AF010145), also was well expressed in another *A. flavus* EST library, and several *hxt1*-related ESTs were identified. Whether expression of the genes in the identified sugar utilization gene cluster is only induced in the presence of a particular saccharide remains to be investigated. Ongoing efforts to obtain a complete *A. flavus* EST database and future microarray work at the SRRC in New Orleans should provide insights into the relationship of the physically linked sugar utilization and aflatoxin gene clusters.

Nitrogen sources also play an important role in aflatoxin biosynthesis. Good nitrogen-containing amino acids that promote aflatoxin production include glutamate, aspartate, asparagine, alanine, methionine, histidine, and proline.[30] How genes responsible for the utilization of these amino acids and their regulation relate to aflatoxin biosynthesis is not clear. Other nitrogen sources, such as peptone and nitrate, have been shown to inhibit aflatoxin production. It is interesting to note that most fungi cannot carry out nitrification (the conversion of nitrogenous compounds, whether inorganic ammonia or organic amino acids, from a reduced to a more oxidized state), but *Aspergillus flavus* and *A. parasiticus* can. White and Johnson[31] have established a correlation between nitrification and aflatoxin production. Of 51 *A. flavus* isolates, 46 oxidized peptone in a nitrification medium, producing an average of 90 mg of the NO_3 form of nitrogen per liter. In contrast, only 2 out of 27 isolates representing 9 other *Aspergillus* groups (*A. wentii*, *A. ochraceus*, *A. glauces*, *A. niger*, *A. nidulans*, *A. flavipes*, *A. fumigatus*, *A. versicolor*, and *A. candidus*) formed nitrate, and the quantity was nearly an order of magnitude lower. Thus, peptone suppression of aflatoxin biosynthesis is most probably due to the nitrification process, but the molecular mechanisms involved are still not clear. Kachholz and Demain[32] reported that nitrate (40 to 340 mM) reduced aflatoxin yields by 75% in aflatoxin-producing and averufin-producing *A. parasiticus* strains. They excluded the ambient pH and the increased energy cost of reducing nitrate to ammonia as causes of the nitrate effect. This inhibition appears not to act on the biosynthetic enzymes involved but probably acts on formation of aflatoxin pathway enzymes by an unknown mechanism. Niehaus and Jiang[33] proposed that inhibition of aflatoxin production by nitrate is due to an increased cytoplasmic NADPH/NADP ratio resulting from the induction of the mannitol cycle, which favors biosynthetic reduction, promoting utilization of malonyl coenzyme A and NADPH for fatty acid synthesis rather than for polyketide synthesis. They also showed increased activity of glucose-6-phosphate dehydrogenase of the pentose phosphate pathway (for NADPH generation) and the mannitol cycle enzymes mannitol dehydrogenase and mannitol-1-phosphate dehydrogenase in the presence of nitrate. In contrast with their view, an interesting observation is that production of sterigmatocystin, a toxin penultimate to aflatoxin in *A. nidulans*, is promoted by nitrate but inhibited by ammonium.[34] Singh et al.[35] showed that the maximal specific activities of the mannitol cycle enzymes hexokinase, mannitol-1-phosphate dehydrogenase, mannitol-1-phosphate phosphatase, and mannitol dehydrogense in extracts of *A. nidulans* mycelia grown on glucose plus ammonium or urea as the nitrogen sources increased two- to threefold as compared with those using nitrate as the nitrogen source. This finding suggests that nitrate promotes polyketide (sterigmatocystin) synthesis in *A. nidulans* through an increased NADPH/NADP ratio, a striking reverse relationship to that reported for *A. parasiticus*.

Chang et al.[36] examined transcript profiles of *nor-1*, *ver-1*, and *omtA* activated by the introduction of an additional copy of the aflatoxin pathway specific regulatory gene *aflR* in *Aspergillus parasiticus* strains. They showed that, in nitrate medium, transcripts for the above aflatoxin genes were absent over a wide range of time points but present in the transformed strains at later time points. Consistent with this observation, overexpression of the carboxy-coding portion of *aflR* (*aflRC*) alleviated the nitrate inhibition. Chang et al.[37] proposed that additional copies of *aflR* or *aflRC* might result in elevated basal levels of the transcription activator AFLR, which could overcome the inhibitory effect of nitrate, possibly through interaction with a negative regulator (repressor) in the nitrogen control circuit on aflatoxin pathway gene transcription. Variability in AREA-binding sites in the *aflR* promoter of various *A. flavus* groups has been suggested to be associated with different levels of aflatoxin production (Ehrlich, pers. comm.). The *A. parasiticus* major nitrogen regulator AREA fusion protein has been shown to bind several GATA elements clustered in the 0.7-kb intergenic region of *aflR* and the *aflJ* coactivator gene.[38] Whether an interaction between AFLR and AREA exists and affects aflatoxin biosynthesis remains to be investigated. Flaherty and Payne,[39] using *aflR* driven by the *A. nidulans gpdA* promoter, also observed elevated levels of aflatoxin pathway gene transcripts and aflatoxin production in *A. flavus* on sucrose low-salts media (SLS); however, a greater than 90% reduction in aflatoxin production is common for *A. flavus* and *A. parasiticus* on SLS media amended with nitrate as the nitrogen source. In buffered medium, West African *A. flavus* S_{GB} isolates were more sensitive to nitrate repression of aflatoxin biosynthesis than were North American S_B isolates;[40] thus, other unknown genetic and physiological factors may play an important role in this complex phenomenon of nitrate inhibition of aflatoxin production.

9.2.3 AFLATOXIN BIOSYNTHETIC PATHWAY AND REGULATORY GENES

It is known that plant metabolites affect the expression of the aflatoxin pathway during the host plant–fungus interaction, but until genes governing aflatoxin formation are fully characterized and their regulation established, the molecular basis of aflatoxin production in the plant cannot be investigated.

9.2.3.1 Aflatoxin Pathway Genes

Aflatoxin biosynthesis is a multiple enzyme process involving over a dozen bioconversion steps (Figure 9.1). In an effort to understand the biosynthetic process of aflatoxin formation, significant progress has been made in the last decade in discovering the genes and their enzymes involved in each step of the aflatoxin biosynthetic pathway. After establishment of the aflatoxin pathway gene cluster in *Aspergillus parasiticus* and *A. flavus*,[41,42] almost all of the genes involved in aflatoxin formation have been identified.[43–55] At least 24 genes, including the regulatory genes, *aflR* and *aflJ*, were identified or characterized within the approximately 70-kb DNA regions

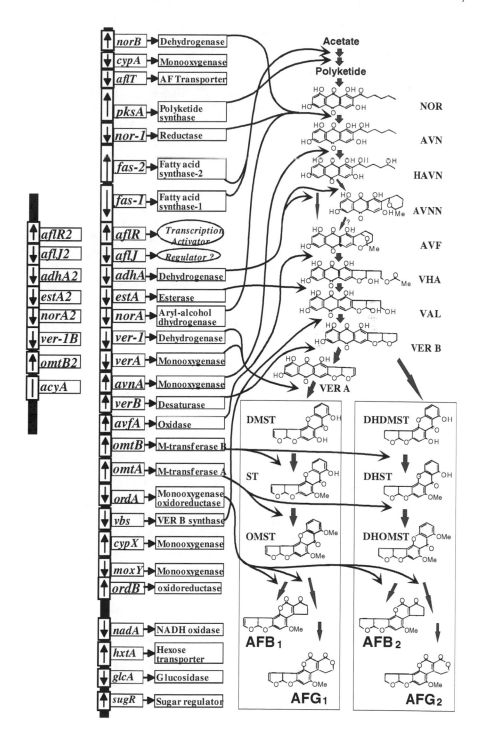

in the *A. parasiticus* and *A. flavus* chromosomes.[41,53,56,57] The *cypX, moxY*[53], and *ordB* defined one end of the aflatoxin pathway gene cluster, and the *norB, cypA,* and *aflT* might possibly mark the other end of this cluster (Figure 9.1) (Yu et al. and Chang et al., unpublished data).

In *Aspergillus parasiticus*, duplication of aflatoxin genes *ver-1* and *aflR* was first suggested by Mehigh et al. and Liang and Linz (unpublished data) and then reported by Liang et al.[58] This partial duplicated aflatoxin gene cluster consisting of seven duplicated genes, *aflR2, aflJ2, adhA2, estA2, norA2, ver-1B,* and *omtB2*, has been cloned and characterized by Chang and Yu.[46] The genes within this partially dupli-cated cluster, due possibly to the chromosome location (Yu et al., unpublished data), were found to be nonfunctional under normal conditions even though no apparent defects were identified in some of these genes (*aflR2, aflJ2, adhA2, estA2*).[59]

In the early steps of aflatoxin biosynthesis, the conversion from acetate to polyketide and to norsolorinic acid (NOR) involves at least two fatty acid synthases (FASs) and a polyketide synthase (PKS).[60–63] The genes for these enzymes are cloned. The genes *fas-1* and *fas-2* encode fatty acid synthase 1 (FASα) and fatty acid synthase 2 (FASβ), respectively,[64] and the gene *pksA* encodes a PKS for the synthesis of polyketide in *Aspergillus parasiticus*.[44,47] Norsolorinic acid is the first stable inter-mediate in the pathway.[65,66] The conversion of NOR to averantin (AVN) involves a reductase that is encoded by the *nor-1* gene.[67,68] The *norA* gene encoding an aryl-alcohol dehydrogenase[43] and the gene *norB*, which was found to be homologous to the *nor-1* and *norA* genes (Yu et al., unpublished data), might also be involved in the conversion from NOR to AVN. The *avnA* gene was identified and characterized[51] to encode a cytochrome P-450-type monooxygenase for conversion of AVN to 5′-hydroxyaverantin (HAVN) in *A. parasiticus*. The gene, *adhA*, encoding for an alcohol dehydrogenase in *A. parasiticus* for the conversion of 5′-hydroxyaverantin to aver-ufanin (AVNN) and averufin (AVF), was cloned and characterized.[45] The *avfA* gene cloned from both *A. parasiticus* and an AVF-accumulating *A. flavus* strain as well

---

FIGURE 9.1 Proposed and generally accepted pathway for aflatoxin B_1, B_2, G_1, and G_2 biosynthesis and the corresponding genes and their enzymes. The aflatoxin biosynthetic path-way gene cluster in *Aspergillus parasiticus* and *A. flavus* and the nonfunctional, partially duplicated aflatoxin gene cluster in *A. parasiticus* are shown. The gene names are labeled on the side of the cluster. Arrows indicate the direction of gene transcription. The homologous genes between the sterigmatocystin pathway gene cluster in *A. nidulans* and aflatoxin pathway gene cluster in *A. parasiticus* and *A. flavus* are connected by a line. The four sugar utilization genes linked to the aflatoxin pathway gene cluster and separated by a 5-kb spacer are on the bottom of panel A. Abbreviations for the intermediates: norsolorinic acid (NOR), averantin (AVN), 5′-hydroxyaverantin (HAVN), averufanin (AVNN), averufin (AVF), versiconal hemi-acetal acetate (VHA), versiconal (VAL), versicolorin B (VER B), versicolorin A (VER A), demethylsterigmatocystin (DMST), sterigmatocystin (ST), *O*-methylsterigmatocystin (OMST), aflatoxin B_1 (AFB_1), aflatoxin G_1 (AFG_1), demethyldihydrosterigmatocystin (DMDHST), dihy-drosterigmatocystin (DHST), dihydro-*O*-methylsterigmatocystin (DHOMST), aflatoxin B_2 (AFB_2), aflatoxin G_2 (AFG_2), and methyltransferase (M-transferase).

as *A. sojae* strain[54] encodes an enzyme homologous to an oxidase that is responsible for the conversion from AVF to versiconal hemiacetal acetate (VHA). The *estA*[69] encoding an esterase could be the gene responsible for the conversion of VHA to versiconal (VAL) in aflatoxin biosynthesis.[70–75] Silva and Townsend[50] and McGuire et al.[76] cloned, characterized, and expressed the *vbs* gene in the aflatoxin pathway gene cluster for the conversion from VAL to versicolorin B (VER B) in *A. parasiticus*. This is a key step in the aflatoxin biosynthesis, as it closes the bisfuran ring of aflatoxin for binding to DNA.

In the later steps of the aflatoxin biosynthetic pathway, VER B is a critical branch point[77] leading to either aflatoxin B_1 (AFB$_1$) and aflatoxin G_1 (AFG$_1$) or aflatoxin B_2 (AFB$_2$) and aflatoxin G_2 (AFG$_2$). The *verB* gene encoding a P-450 monooxygenase/desaturase (Bhatnagar et al., unpublished data) might be responsible for the conversion of VER B to versicolorin A (VER A) because it is homologous to *Aspergillus nidulans stcL*, which was demonstrated to be required for the conversion of VER B to VER A in *A. nidulans*.[78] The *ver-1* gene[79] is another cloned gene involved in a key step in aflatoxin synthesis that is required for the conversion of VER A to demethylsterigmatocystin (DMST) in *A. parasiticus*. The *verA* gene (Yu, unpublished data) in *A. parasiticus* might also be involved in this reaction because it is homologous to *stcS*,[80,81] which encodes a P-450 monooxygenase involved in the conversion of VER A to DMST in *A. nidulans*.[82] The genes responsible for the conversion of DMST to sterigmatocystin (ST) and demethyldihydrosterigmatocystin (DMDHST) to dihydrosterigmatocystin (DHST) were concurrently cloned in *A. parasiticus* by Motomura et al.[83] (*dmtA*, for *O*-methyltransferase I) and in *A. parasiticus*, *A. flavus*, and *A. sojae* by Yu et al.[54] (*omtB*, for *O*-methyltransferase B). The gene for the conversion of ST to *O*-methylsterigmatocystin (OMST) and DMST to dihydro-*O*-methylsterigmatocystin (DHOMST) was cloned by Yu et al.[84,85] The enzyme was expressed in *Escherichia coli* and its activity to convert ST to OMST was demonstrated by substrate feeding studies.[84] Prieto et al.[86] and Prieto and Woloshuk[87] reported in *A. flavus* that a P-450 monooxygenase gene, *ord-1*, is required for the conversion of OMST to AFB$_1$ and AFG$_1$ and DMDHST to AFB$_2$ and AFG$_2$. Yu et al.[52] cloned the P-450 monooxygenase gene *ordA* from *A. parasiticus* and an *A. flavus* mutant strain. By *in vitro* expression and substrate feeding study in a yeast system, it was demonstrated that this gene is responsible for this reaction.

9.2.3.2 Aflatoxin Pathway Regulatory Genes

As was postulated,[88] a positive regulatory gene in the aflatoxin pathway gene cluster *aflR* activates pathway gene transcription. The *aflR* gene, coding for a sequence-specific, Gal 4-type zinc-binuclear DNA-binding protein of 47 kDa, has been shown to be required for transcriptional activation of most, if not all, the structural genes[36,37,39,89–94] by binding to the promoter of the structural genes in *A. parasiticus*, *A. flavus*, and *A. nidulans*.[95–97] Adjacent to the *aflR* gene in the aflatoxin gene cluster, a divergently transcribed gene, *aflJ*, was also found to be involved in the regulation of transcription (Chang, unpublished data).[98] The exact mechanism by which *aflJ* modulates transcription of these pathway genes in concert with *aflR* remains to be determined. The gene *aflT*, encoding a predicted membrane-bound protein (Chang and Yu, unpublished data; accession no. AF268071) might be involved in aflatoxin secretion. Other than the genetic factors, nutritional and environmental factors are also important in the regulation of aflatoxin formation. The nutritional factors are discussed separately in this chapter.

9.3 REGULATION OF FUNGAL INVASION AND AFLATOXIN CONTAMINATION BY HOST PLANT FACTORS THROUGH INTERFERENCE OR INHIBITION OF FUNGAL VIRULENCE, GROWTH, AND TOXIN BIOSYNTHESIS

9.3.1 INTERFERENCE WITH FUNGAL VIRULENCE OR GROWTH BY HOST FACTORS

Plants rely on a variety of mechanisms to protect themselves from pathogen attacks. These mechanisms include synthesis of inhibitory compounds such as phenols, melanins, tannins, or phytoalexins, as well as accumulation of proteins that can directly inhibit fungal growth.[99] Much of the work on elucidation of plant defense mechanisms against *Aspergillus flavus* has been done using corn as a model system. Corn kernels, for example, have a number of potential resistance factors that could be useful in enhancing resistance to fungal invasion and aflatoxin contamination through marker-selective breeding. The use of proteomics to compare differentially resistant corn varieties has revealed several kernel proteins correlating in their levels in the kernel with resistance to aflatoxin contamination. Having extensive information on fungal genes (through the *A. flavus* EST project) critical in fungal survival, development, virulence, and aflatoxin formation could lead to more educated decisions with regard to selection of the most effective resistance factors in corn (and other crops) inhibitory to *A. flavus* for use in marker-selective breeding or gene insertion technologies.

9.3.1.1 Corn Kernel Waxes and Phenolic Compounds

Studies by Guo et al.[100] indicated that wax and cutin from corn kernel pericarps of genotype GT-MAS:gk can reduce aflatoxin accumulation, probably through reduction of infection and growth of the fungus. GT-MAS:gk wax was found to be chemically different from, and present in greater amounts than, wax from kernels of susceptible hybrids.[101] Further investigation by Gembeh et al.[102] discovered that GT-MAS:gk wax contained phenolic compounds, such as alkylresorcinols, in higher amounts than did susceptible genotypes, and these compounds demonstrated *in vitro* inhibition of *Aspergillus flavus* growth.

9.3.1.2 Corn Kernel Proteins/Enzymes

The expression of proteins and enzymes in plants, whether constitutive or induced, can have direct or indirect action on the course of pathogenesis. These proteins and enzymes, as discussed below, include cell-wall-degrading activities, proteins with antimicrobial properties, and lytic enzymes.

9.3.1.2.1   Chitinases and Beta-1,3-Glucanases

The antifungal activity of corn chitinases was first reported by Roberts and Selitrennikoff.[103] The growth of *Trichoderma reesei* and *Phycomyces blakesleeanus* was inhibited at concentrations as low as 1 and 3 µg per filter disc, respectively.[103,104] In another study, two 28-kDa chitinases isolated from corn were shown to inhibit *T. reesei*, *Alternaria solani*, and *Fusarium oxysporum*.[105] Wu et al.[106] reported that the expression of two chitinase genes was induced by *Aspergillus flavus* in aleurone layers and embryos. Cordero et al.[107] observed a coordinated induction of one beta-1,3-glucanase and three chitinase isoforms in corn seedlings in response to infection by *Fusarium moniliforme*. A recent study by Lozovaya et al.[108] reported that the growth of *A. flavus* was inhibited more by callus of a resistant corn genotype (Tex 6 × Mo17) than by a sensitive genotype (Pa91). This inhibition correlated with the activity levels of beta-1,3-glucanase in the callus and in the culture medium.

9.3.1.2.2   Proteinase/Alpha-Amylase Inhibitors/Zeamatin

The most extensively studied proteinase inhibitor is trypsin inhibitor (TI). Among these inhibitors, some have been found to have activity against both trypsin and α-amylase.[109] So far, TIs have been isolated from many plants, and antifungal activities have been reported for TI proteins from barley,[110] corn,[111] cabbage,[112] and pearl millet.[113] Thus far, three proteinase inhibitors have been isolated from corn. One is the 7-kDa TI protein,[114] for which no antifungal activity has been reported. Another is the 22-kDa TI/α-amylase inhibitor,[115] which shares over 97% homology with a 22-kDa antifungal protein[99] and zeamatin.[116] The latter has demonstrated *in vitro* antifungal properties at low concentrations against *Candida albicans*, *Neurospora crassa*, *Trichoderma reesei*,[116] and *Aspergillus flavus*[117] by causing a rapid release of cytoplasmic material from these fungi.[116] The third one is the 14-kDa TI protein, which shares no homology to the 22-kDa TI and belongs to the cereal proteinase inhibitor family.[115] This inhibitor was also reported to be an α-amylase inhibitor of insects, as well.[109] Antifungal activities of the 14-kDa TI were first reported by Chen et al.[111] *In vitro* studies using overexpressed TI purified from *Escherichia coli* demonstrated inhibition of both conidia germination and hyphal growth of nine plant pathogenic fungi, including *A. flavus*, *A. parasiticus*, and *Fusarium moniliforme*.[18] TI is constitutively present at high levels in corn genotypes normally resistant to *A. flavus* infection and aflatoxin contamination, but at low or undetectable levels in susceptible genotypes.[111]

9.3.1.2.3   Ribosome-Inactivating Proteins

Ribosome-inactivating proteins (RIPs), ubiquitously present at high concentrations in plant tissues, are actually RNA *N*-glycosidases that catalyze the removal of a specific adenine residue from a conserved 28S rRNA loop required for elongation factor 1 alpha binding; therefore, RIPs are remarkably potent catalytic inactivators of eukaryotic protein synthesis. The purified corn RIP, which is also known as albumin b-32,[118] inhibited the hyphal development of *Aspergillus flavus in vitro*.[117] Purified barley RIPs exhibited antifungal activity *in vitro* against *Alternaria alternata*, *Phycomyces blakesleeanus*, and *Trichoderma reesei*.[103]

9.3.2 Stress-Responsive Proteins and Their Possible Role in Inhibiting Fungal Invasion

To enhance the identification of resistance-associated proteins (RAPs), a proteomics approach was recently employed.[119,120] Endosperm and embryo proteins of several resistant and susceptible genotypes have been compared using large-format, two-dimensional gel electrophoresis, and over a dozen constitutively expressed proteins, either unique or fivefold upregulated in resistant genotypes, were identified. These RAPs can be grouped into three categories: storage proteins (globulins [GLBs], late embryogenesis abundant proteins [LEAs]), stress-related proteins (heat shock proteins [HSPs], water stress inducible proteins [WSI18s], cold-regulated proteins [CORs], aldose reductase [ALD], glyoxalase I [GLX1], and peroxredoxin antioxdant [PER1]), and antifungal proteins (14-kDa TI, pathogenesis-related protein 10 [PR10]). Both GLB and LEA contain high levels of glycine (6 to 9%) and are highly hydrophilic. The expression of GLB1 and LEA3 has been reported to be stress responsive and ABA dependent.[121] Transgenic rice overexpressing a barley LEA3 protein HVA1 in leaves and roots showed significantly increased tolerance to water deficit and salinity and improved recovery upon the removal of stress conditions;[122] therefore, LEA genes may hold considerable potential for use as molecular tools for genetic crop improvement toward stress tolerance.[122] ALD has been reported to be involved in the synthesis of an osmolyte, sorbitol.[123] Its expression in barley embryos is temporally correlated with the acquisition of desiccation tolerance (ability to function while dehydrated).[124] Recently, it was found that an NADPH-dependent alfalfa ALD protects transgenic tobacco plants against lipid peroxidation under chemical (paraquat and heavy metal) and drought stresses.[125]

Glyoxalase I is believed to be involved in the detoxification of methylglyoxal produced from triosephosphates and during glycolysis. Methylglyoxal is a potent cytotoxic compound known to arrest growth and react with DNA and protein[126] and it increases sister chromatid exchanges.[127] The expression of glyoxalase I was found to be upregulated in response to salt and water stresses in *Brassica juncea*[128] and tomato.[129] Transgenic tobacco plants overexpressing *Brassica juncea* glyoxalase I showed significant tolerance to methylglyoxal and high salt.[128] Plant small HSPs possess molecular chaperone activity *in vitro*.[130] A recent study by Wehmeyer and Vierling[131] found that the level of HSP17.4 protein correlates with desiccation tolerance and suggests that HSPs have a general protective role throughout seed development; however, the physiological functions of other RAPs (COR, PER1, and PR10) have not been well studied. Although the proteomics approach was initiated to enhance identification of resistance-associated proteins among the thousands of kernel proteins present, stress-related proteins were not intentionally targeted in these studies.

The repeated association between stress-related protein expression and aflatoxin-resistance may be important discoveries, as drought is known to dramatically increase aflatoxin levels in corn.[132] Studies from other laboratories have demonstrated that LEA3,[122] small HSPs,[131] ALD[125], and GLX1[128] are involved in host plant drought, salt-stress, or desiccation tolerances. Possession of unique or higher levels of stress-related proteins, constitutively expressed, may put resistant lines in an advantageous position over susceptible ones in the ability to synthesize proteins and defend against pathogens under stress conditions. Results of these studies indicate that the necessary requirements for developing commercially useful yet aflatoxin-resistant corn lines may require inclusion of these proteins, in addition to the high-level expression of antifungal proteins.

9.3.3 Interference with Aflatoxin Biosynthesis and Related Genes by Host Plant Factors and Natural Products

Several plant-derived inhibitors of aflatoxin synthesis exist, and this subject has been reviewed extensively.[133,134] Examples of natural products that may have potential in augmenting host plant resistance against *Aspergillus flavus* infection are certain plant-derived volatile compounds. Results have shown that aflatoxigenic strains of *A. flavus* and *A. parasiticus* when grown *in vitro* in the presence of specific cotton-leaf or maize volatiles exhibit alterations in aflatoxin production accompanied by variations in growth of the fungi.[135–138] These earlier studies showed that plant volatile compounds can alter *Aspergillus* growth and, consequently, aflatoxin production. In some cases, both fungal growth and toxin production were inhibited; in others, growth was not significantly affected while aflatoxin synthesis was markedly inhibited or growth and toxin production were enhanced. Recent studies have measured the effect of specific volatile compounds not only on fungal growth and toxin production but also on fungal morphology.[139,140] In one study,[139] two alcohols, 3-methyl-1-butanol (3-MB) and nonanol, and two terpenes, camphene and limonene, were chosen as representative cotton-leaf volatiles based on the effects they had on fungal growth or aflatoxin production in previous investigations. The 3-MB-treated samples exhibited a decrease in fungal radial growth that was directly proportional to the volatile dosage. Additionally, 3-MB treatment resulted in loss of mycelial pigmentation and a decrease in sporulation. Limonene and camphene yielded negligible results, but nonanol inhibited radial growth and induced uniquely aerial hyphae. In comparison to an unexposed control, aflatoxin production increased in cultures exposed to 3-MB but decreased when exposed to the other three volatiles studied. Another study[140] measured the effects on *A. parasiticus* of three corn-derived volatile compounds, *n*-decyl aldehyde, hexanol, and octanol. These three compounds were previously found to be variably expressed in five *Aspergillus*-resistant maize varieties and three susceptible varieties. It was found that all three volatile compounds reduced radial growth but only *n*-decyl aldehyde significantly inhibited aflatoxin biosynthesis in *A. parasiticus*; octanol, on the other hand, stimulated toxin production. While the volatile compound *n*-decyl aldehyde had less of an effect on radial growth than the other volatiles, the *n*-decyl treated colonies had a predominance of uniquely aerial hyphae and significantly fewer condiophores than the control and other aldehyde treatment groups.

In future research, it may be possible to use plant lipoxygenase (LOX) activities as molecular markers in breeding crops for resistance to aflatoxin contamination, as most of the volatile compounds identified (see above examples) and also hydroperoxy fatty acids (precursors to some of the volatiles) are LOX pathway products and can have inhibitory activities against fungal growth and/or aflatoxin biosynthesis.[141–143]

Several additional compounds from corn, peanuts, and walnuts have been identified that have significant effects on aflatoxin production. For example, 4-acetyl-benzoxazolin-2-one (ABOA), anthocyanins, and related flavonoids and carotenoids containing an α-ionone type ring (from maize) were found to be effective inhibitors of aflatoxin production.[144–147] Beta-carotenes from corn rather than from peanuts were more effective in over 90% reduction of aflatoxin production at concentrations of 50 μg/mL.[148] Naphthoquinones routinely found in walnut husks were found to be inhibitory to spore germination and growth of *Aspergillus flavus* as well as aflatoxin production by the fungus.[149] Interestingly, several natural compounds (anthroquinones, conmarins, and flavone-type flavonoids) isolated from various plants were shown to be potent inhibitors of aflatoxin B_1-8,9-epoxide formation.[150]

9.4 USE OF FUNGAL GENOMICS AND SEED/KERNEL PROTEOMICS TO INVESTIGATE MECHANISMS REGULATING *A. FLAVUS* INVASION AND AFLATOXIN CONTAMINATION OF CROPS DURING PLANT–FUNGUS INTERACTIONS

Investigation of the biochemical function and genetic regulation of the genes in a fungal system on a genomic scale will aid in gaining a better understanding of the complex host plant–fungus interaction, which influences aflatoxin contamination, and in devising strategies to interrupt the contamination process. Extensive progress has been made in identifying resistance markers through proteomic comparisons of differentially resistant corn varieties, thus indicating protein markers that could be used in breeding or gene insertion technologies to enhance resistance in crops to aflatoxin contamination.[120] In addition, *Aspergillus flavus* EST technology[151] will allow rapid identification of the majority, if not all, of the genes expressed in the fungal genome and promote a better understanding of their functions, regulation, coordination of gene expression in response to internal and external factors, relationships between primary and secondary metabolism, plant–fungal interactions, and fungal pathogenicity, as well as evolutionary biology. Microarrays made from the EST sequences can be used to detect a whole set of genes expressed under specific environmental conditions, for example. This technology allows us to study a complete set of fungal genes, simultaneously, that are responsible for, or related to, toxin production. Microarray technology is expected to provide valuable information on factors that are responsible for turning on and off aflatoxin production during the fungal-plant interaction.

An *Aspergillus flavus* EST/microarray project is currently underway.[151] A normalized cDNA library was made from combined mycelia of *A. flavus* wild-type strain NRRL3357 grown under several medium conditions. Sequencing of the cDNA clones was contracted to The Institute for Genomic Research (TIGR). Preliminary results of a blast search indicated that 7214 expressed unique genes would be identified within 22,000 cDNA sequences obtained. Among the genes identified, many are rare copy genes potentially involved in secondary metabolism and gene regulation. ESTs for several hydrolases (possible fungal virulence factors), regulatory and pathway enzyme proteins governing aflatoxin biosynthesis, factors possibly involved in signal transduction, and factors possibly involved in fungal development (e.g., sporulation) have been identified.[151]

REFERENCES

1. Bhatnagar, D., Lillehoj, E.B., and Arora, D.K., Eds., *Handbook of Applied Mycology*, Vol. 5, Plenum Press, New York, 1992, 443 pp.
2. Bhatnagar, D., Cotty, P.J., and Cleveland, T.E., Genetic and biological control of aflatoxigenic fungi, in *Microbial Food Contamination*, Wilson, C.L. and Droby, S., Eds., CRC Press, Boca Raton, FL, 2001, pp. 207–240.
3. Raper, K.B. and Fennell, D.I., *The Genus* Aspergillus, Williams & Wilkins, Baltimore, MD, 1965.
4. Watkins, G.M., *Compendium of Cotton Diseases*, American Phytopathological Press, St. Paul, MN, 1981.
5. Cleveland, T.E. and McCormick, S.P., Identification of pectinases produced in cotton bolls infected with *Aspergillus flavus*, *Phytopathology*, 77, 1498–1503, 1987.
6. Cotty, P.J., Cleveland, T.E., Brown, R.L., and Mellon, J.E., Variation in polygalacturonase production among *Aspergillus flavus* isolates, *Appl. Environ. Microbiol.*, 56, 3885–3887, 1990.
7. Cleveland, T.E. and Cotty, P.J., Invasiveness of *Aspergillus flavus* isolates in wounded cotton bolls is associated with production of a specific fungal polygalacturonase, *Phytopathology*, 81, 155–158, 1991.
8. Brown, R.L., Cleveland, T.E., Cotty, P.J., and Mellon, J.E., Spread of *Aspergillus flavus* in cotton bolls, decay of intercapillary membranes, and production of fungal pectinases, *Phytopathology*, 82, 462–467, 1992.
9. Cary, J.W., Brown, R.L., Cleveland, T.E., Whitehead, M., and Dean, R.A., Cloning and characterization of a novel polygalacturonase-encoding gene from *Aspergillus parasiticus*, *Gene*, 153, 129–133, 1995.
10. Whitehead, M.P., Shieh, M.T., Cleveland, T.E., Cary, J.W., and Dean, R.A., Isolation and characterization of polygalacturonase genes (*pecA* and *pecB*) from *Aspergillus flavus*, *Appl. Environ. Microbiol.*, 61, 3316–3322, 1995.
11. Shieh, M.T., Brown, R.L., Whitehead, M.P., Cary, J.W., Cotty, P.J., Cleveland, T.E., and Dean, R.A., Molecular genetic evidence for the involvement of a specific polygalacturonase, P2c, in the invasion and spread of *Aspergillus flavus* in cotton bolls, *Appl. Environ. Microbiol.*, 63, 3548–3552, 1997.
12. Mellon, J.E. and Cotty, P.J., Expression of elastinolytic activity among isolates in *Aspergillus* section *Flavi*, *Mycopathologia*, 131, 115–120, 1995.
13. St. Leger, R.J., Joshi, L., and Roberts, D.W., Adaptation of proteases and carbohydrases of saprophytic, phytopathogenic and entomopathogenic fungi to the requirements of their ecological niches, *Microbiology*, 143, 1983–1992, 1997.
14. St. Leger, R.J., Screen S.E., and Shams-Pirzadeh, B., Lack of host specialization in *Aspergillus flavus*, *Appl. Environ. Microbiol.*, 66, 320–324, 2000.
15. Brown, R.L., Chen, Z.-Y., Cleveland, T.E., Cotty, P.J., and Cary, J.W., Variation in *in vitro* alpha-amylase and protease activity is related to the virulence of *Aspergillus flavus* isolates, *J. Food Protect.*, 64, 401–404, 2001.

16. Chen, Z.-Y., Brown, R.L., Damann, K.E., and Cleveland, T.E., Characterization of an alkaline protease excreted by *Aspergillus flavus* and its function in fungal infection of corn kernels, *Phytopathology*, 89, S15, 1999.

17. Brown, R.L., Chen, Z.-Y., and Cleveland, T.E., The production of hydrolytic enzymes by *Aspergillus flavus* isolates differing in invasive ability in cotton bolls, *Phytopathology*, 88, S11, 1998.

18. Chen Z.-Y., Brown, R.L., Lax, A.R., Cleveland, T.E., and Russin, J.S., Inhibition of plant-pathogenic fungi by a corn trypsin inhibitor overexpressed in *Escherichia coli*, *Appl. Environ. Microbiol.*, 65, 1320–1324, 1999.

19. Chen, Z.-Y., Brown, R.L., Russin, J.S., Lax, A.R., and Cleveland, T.E., A corn trypsin inhibitor with antifungal activity inhibits *Aspergillus flavus* α-amylase, *Phytopathology*, 89, 902–907, 1999.

20. Fakhoury, A.M. and Woloshuk, C.P., Amy1, the α-amylase gene of *Aspergillus flavus*: involvement in aflatoxin biosynthesis in maize kernels, *Phytopathology*, 89, 908–914, 1999.

21. Fakhoury, A.M. and Woloshuk, C.P., Inhibition of growth of *Aspergillus flavus* and fungal alpha-amylases by a lectin-like protein from *Lablab purpureus*, *Mol. Plant Microbe Interact.*, 14, 955–961, 2001.

22. Mellon, J.E., Dowd, M.K., and Cotty, P.J., Time course study of substrate utilization by *Aspergillus flavus* in medium simulating corn (*Zea mays*) kernels, *J. Agr. Food Chem.*, 50, 648–652, 2002.

23. Mellon, J.E., Cotty, P.J., and Dowd, M.K., Influence of lipids with and without other cottonseed reserve materials on aflatoxin B(1) production by *Aspergillus flavus*, *J. Agr. Food Chem.*, 48, 3611–3615, 2000.

24. Mateles, R.I. and Adye, J.C., Production of aflatoxins in submerged culture, *Appl. Microbiol.*, 13, 208–221, 1965.

25. Davis, N. and Diener, U.L., Growth and aflatoxin production by *Aspergillus parasiticus* from various carbon sources, *Appl. Microbiol.*, 16, 158–159, 1968.

26. Abou-Zeid, A.M., Production, purification and characterization of an extracellular alpha-amylase enzyme isolated from *Aspergillus flavus*, *Microbios*, 89, 55–66, 1997.

27. Yu, J., Chang, P.-K., Bhatnagar, D., and Cleveland, T.E., Cloning of a sugar utilization gene cluster in *Aspergillus parasiticus*, *Biochim. Biophys. Acta*, 1493, 211–214, 2000.

28. Takizawa, M., Akao, T., Akita, O., and Gomi, K., Structural Features of Maltose Utilization Gene Clusters in *Aspergillus oryzae*, paper presented at the Fungal Genetics Conference, Asilomar, CA, 2001.

29. Gomi, K., Akeno, T., Minetoki, T., Ozeki, K., Kumagai, C., Okazaki, N., and Iimura, Y., Molecular cloning and characterization of a transcriptional activator gene, *amyR*, involved in the amylolytic gene expression in *Aspergillus oryzae*, *Biosci. Biotech. Biochem.*, 64, 816–827, 2000.

30. Maggon, K.K., Gupta, S.K., and Venkitasubramanian, T.A., Biosynthesis of aflatoxins, *Bacteriol. Rev.*, 41, 822–855, 1977.

31. White, J.P. and Johnson, G.T., Aflatoxin production correlated with nitrification in *Aspergillus flavus* group species, *Mycologia*, 74, 718–723, 1982.

32. Kachholz, T. and Demain, A.L., Nitrate repression of averufin and aflatoxin biosynthesis, *J. Nat. Prod.*, 46, 499–506, 1983.

33. Niehaus, G.W. and Jiang, W., Nitrate induces enzymes of the mannitol cycle and suppresses versicolorin synthesis in *Aspergillus parasiticus*, *Mycopathologia*, 107, 131–137, 1989.

34. Feng, G.H. and Leonard, T.J., Culture conditions control expression of the genes for aflatoxin and sterigmatocystin biosynthesis in *Aspergillus parasiticus* and *A. nidulans*, *Appl. Environ. Microbiol.*, 64, 2275–2277, 1998.

35. Singh, M., Scrutton, N.S., and Scrutton, M.C., NADPH generation in *Aspergillus nidulans*: is the mannitol cycle involved?, *J. Gen. Microbiol.*, 134, 643–654, 1988.

36. Chang, P.-K., Ehrlich, K.C., Yu, J., Bhatnagar, D., and Cleveland, T.E., Increased expression of *Aspergillus parasiticus aflR*, encoding a sequence-specific DNA binding protein, relieves nitrate inhibition of aflatoxin biosynthesis, *Appl. Environ. Microbiol.*, 61, 2372–2377, 1995.

37. Chang, P.-K., Yu, J., Bhatnagar, D., and Cleveland, T.E., Repressor–AFLR interaction modulates aflatoxin biosynthesis in *Aspergillus parasiticus*, *Mycopathologia*, 147, 105–112, 1999.

38. Chang, P.-K., Yu, J., Bhatnagar, D., and Cleveland, T.E., Characterization of the *Aspergillus parasiticus* major nitrogen regulatory gene, *areA*, *Biochim. Biophys. Acta*, 1491, 263–266, 2000.

39. Flaherty, J.E. and Payne, G.A., Overexpression of *aflR* leads to upregulation of pathway gene expression and increased aflatoxin production in *Aspergillus flavus*, *Appl. Environ. Microbiol.*, 63, 3995–4000, 1997.

40. Cotty, P.J. and Cardwell, K.F., Divergence of West African and North American communities of *Aspergillus* section *Flavi*, *Appl. Environ. Microbiol.*, 65, 2264–2266, 1999.

41. Yu, J., Chang, P.-K., Cary, J.W., Wright, M., Bhatnagar, D., Cleveland, T.E., Payne, G.A., and Linz, J.E., Comparative mapping of aflatoxin pathway gene clusters in *Aspergillus parasiticus* and *Aspergillus flavus*, *Appl. Environ. Microbiol.*, 61, 2365–2371, 1995.

42. Trail, F., Mahanti, N., Rarick, M., Mehigh, R., Liang, S.H., Zhou, R., and Linz, J.E., Physical and transcriptional map of an aflatoxin gene cluster in *Aspergillus parasiticus* and functional disruption of a gene involved early in the aflatoxin pathway, *Appl. Environ. Microbiol.*, 61, 2665–2673, 1995.

43. Cary, J.W., Wright, M., Bhatnagar, D., Lee, R., and Chu, F.S., Molecular characterization of an *Aspergillus parasiticus* dehydrogenase gene, *norA*, located on the aflatoxin biosynthesis gene cluster, *Appl. Environ. Microbiol.*, 62, 360–366, 1996.

44. Chang, P.-K., Cary, J.W., Yu, J., Bhatnagar, D., and Cleveland, T.E., *Aspergillus parasiticus* polyketide synthase gene, *pksA*, a homolog of *Aspergillus nidulans wA*, is required for aflatoxin B_1, *Mol. Genet. Genom.*, 248, 270–277, 1995.

45. Chang, P.-K., Yu, J., Ehrlich, K.C., Boue, S.M., Montalbano, B.G., Bhatnagar, D., and Cleveland, T.E., The aflatoxin biosynthesis gene *adhA* in *Aspergillus parasiticus* is involved in conversion of 5′-hydroxyaverantin to averufin, *Appl. Environ. Microbiol.*, 66, 4715– 4719, 2000.

46. Chang, P.-K. and Yu, J., Characterization of a partial duplication of the aflatoxin gene cluster in *Aspergillus parasiticus* ATCC 56775, *Appl. Microbiol. Biotechnol.*, 58, 632–636, 2002.

47. Feng, G.H. and Leonard, T.J., Characterization of the polyketide synthase gene (*pksL1*) required for aflatoxin biosynthesis in *Aspergillus parasiticus*, *J. Bacteriol.*, 177, 6246–5624, 1995.

48. Mahanti, N., Bhatnagar, D., Cary, J.W., Joubran, J., and Linz, J.E., Structure and function of *fas-1A*, a gene encoding a putative fatty acid synthetase directly involved in aflatoxin biosynthesis in *Aspergillus parasiticus*, *Appl. Environ. Microbiol.*, 62, 191–195, 1996.

49. Silva, J.C., Minto, R.E., Barry, C.E., Holland, K.A., and Townsend, C.A., Isolation and characterization of the versicolorin B Synthase gene from *Aspergillus parasiticus*: expansion of the aflatoxin B_1 biosynthetic cluster, *J. Biol. Chem.*, 271, 13600–13608, 1996.

50. Silva, J.C. and Townsend, C.A., Heterologous expression, isolation, and characterization of versicolorin B synthase from *Aspergillus parasiticus*, *J. Biol. Chem.*, 272, 804–813, 1996.

51. Yu, J., Chang, P.-K., Cary, J.W., Bhatnagar, D., and Cleveland, T.E., *avnA*, a gene encoding a cytochrome P-450 monooxygenase is involved in the conversion of averantin to averufin in aflatoxin biosynthesis in *Aspergillus parasiticus*, *Appl. Environ. Microbiol.*, 63, 1349–1356, 1997.

52. Yu, J., Chang, P.-K., Cary, J.W., Ehrlich, K.C., Montalbano, B., Dyer, J.M., Bhatnagar, D., and Cleveland, T.E., Characterization of the critical amino acids of an *Aspergillus parasiticus* cytochrome P450 monooxygenase encoded by *Orda* involved in aflatoxin B_1, G_1, B_2, and G_2 biosynthesis, *Appl. Environ. Microbiol.*, 64, 4834–4841, 1998.

53. Yu, J., Chang, P.-K., Bhatnagar, D., and Cleveland, T.E., Genes encoding cytochrome P-450 and monooxigenase enzymes define one end of the aflatoxin pathway gene cluster in *Aspergillus parasiticus*, *Appl. Microbiol. Biotechnol.*, 53, 583–590, 2000.

54. Yu, J., Woloshuk, C.P., Bhatnagar, D., and Cleveland, T.E., Cloning and characterization of *avfA* and *omtB* genes involved in aflatoxin biosynthesis in three *Aspergillus* species, *Gene*, 248, 157–167, 2000.

55. Yu, J., Chang, P.-K., Bhatnagar, D., and Cleveland, T.E., Cloning of sugar utilization gene cluster in *Aspergillus parasiticus*, *Biochim. Biophys. Acta*, 1493, 211–214, 2000.

56. Cleveland, T.E., Cary, J.W., Brown, R.L., Bhatnagar, D., Yu, J., Chang, P.K., Chlan, C.A., and Rajasekaran, K., Use of biotechnology to eliminate aflatoxin in preharvest crops, *Bull Inst. Compr. Agr. Sci. Kinki Univ.*, 5, 75–90, 1997.

57. Yu, J., Genetics and biochemistry of mycotoxin synthesis, in *Handbook of Fungal Biotechnology*, Arora, D.K., Bridge, P.D., and Bhatnagar, D., Eds., Marcel Dekker, New York, 2002.

58. Liang, S.-H., Skory, C.D., and Linz, J.E., Characterization of the function of the *ver-1A and ver-1B* genes, involved in aflatoxin biosynthesis in *Aspergillus parasiticus*, *Appl. Environ. Microbiol.*, 62, 4568–4575, 1996.

59. Chiou, C.H., Miller, M., Wilson, D.L., Trail, F., and Linz, J.E., Chromosomal location plays a role in regulation of aflatoxin gene expression in *Aspergillus parasiticus*, *Appl. Environ. Microbiol.*, 68, 306–315, 2002.

60. Townsend, C.A., Christensen, S.B., and Trautwein, K., Hexanoate as a starter unit in polyketide synthesis, *J. Am. Chem. Soc.*, 106, 3868–3869, 1984.

61. Bhatnagar, D., Ehrlich, K.C., and Cleveland, T.E., Oxidation-reduction reactions in biosynthesis of secondary metabolites, in *Handbook of Applied Mycology: Mycotoxins in Ecological Systems*, Bhatnagar, D., Lillehoj, E.B., and Arora, D.K., Eds., Marcel Dekker, New York, 255–286, 1992.

62. Trail, F., Nibedita, M., and Linz, J., Molecular biology of aflatoxin biosynthesis, *Microbiology*, 141, 755–765, 1995.

63. Brown, D.W., Adams, T.H., and Keller, N.P., *Aspergillus* has distinct fatty acid synthases for primary and secondary metabolism, *Proc. Natl. Acad. Sci. USA*, 14873–14877, 1996.

64. Payne, G.A. and Brown, M.P., Genetics and physiology of aflatoxin biosynthesis, *Annu. Rev. Phytopathol.*, 36, 329–362, 1998.

65. Bennett, J.W., Chang, P.K., and Bhatnagar, D., One gene to whole pathway: the role of norsolorinic acid in aflatoxin research, *Adv. Appl. Microbiol.*, 45, 1–15, 1997.

66. Papa, K.E., Norsolorinic acid mutant of *Aspergillus flavus*, *J. Gen. Microbiol.*, 128, 1345–1348, 1982.

67. Chang, P.-K., Skory, C.D., and Linz, J.E., Cloning of a gene associated with aflatoxin biosynthesis in *Aspergillus parasiticus*, *Curr. Genet.*, 21, 231–233, 1992.

68. Trail, F., Chang, P.-K., Cary, J., and Linz, J.E., Structural and functional analysis of the nor-1 gene involved in the biosynthesis of aflatoxins by Aspergillus parasiticus, Appl. Environ. Microbiol., 60, 4078–4085, 1994.

69. Yu, J., Chang, P.-K., Bhatnagar, D., and Cleveland, T.E., Cloning and functional expression of an esterase gene in Aspergillus parasiticus, Mycopathologia, 156, 227–234, 2002.

70. Yao, R.C. and Hsieh, D.P.H., Step of dichlorvos inhibition in the pathway of aflatoxin biosynthesis, Appl. Microbiol., 28, 52–57, 1974.

71. Schroeder, H.W., Cole, R.S., Grigsby, R.D., and Hein, H.J., Inhibition of aflatoxin production and tentative identification of an aflatoxin intermediate "versicolor acetate" from treatment with dichlorvos, Appl. Microbiol., 27, 394–399, 1974.

72. Bennett, J.W., Lee, L.S., and Cucullu, A.F., Effect of dichlorvos on aflatoxin and versicolorin A production in Aspergillus parasiticus, Bot. Gaz., 137, 318–324, 1976.

73. Fitzell, D.L., Singh, R., Hsieh, D.P.H., and Motell, E.L., Nuclear magnetic resonance identification of versicolor hemiacetal acetate as an intermediate in aflatoxin biosynthesis, Agric. Food Chem., 25, 1193–1197, 1977.

74. Yabe, K, Ando, Y., and Hamasaki, T., A metabolic grid among versiconal hemiacetal acetate, versiconol acetate, versiconol and versiconal during aflatoxin biosynthesis, J. Gen. Microbiol., 137, 2469–2475, 1991.

75. Yabe, K., Nakamura, Y., Nakajima, H., Ando, Y., and Hamasaki, T., Enzymatic conversion of norsolinic acid to averufin in aflatoxin biosynthesis, Appl. Environ. Microbiol., 57, 1340–1345, 1991.

76. McGuire, S.M., Silva, J.C., Casillas, E.G., and Townsend, C.A., Purification and characterization of versicolorin B synthase from Aspergillus parasiticus: catalysis of the stereodifferentiating cyclization in aflatoxin biosynthesis essential to DNA interaction, Biochemistry, 35, 11470–11486, 1996.

77. Bhatnagar, D., Cleveland, T.E., and Kingston, D.G.I., Enzymological evidence for separate pathways for aflatoxin B_1 and B_2, Biosyn. Biochem., 30, 4343–4350, 1991.

78. Kelkar, H.S., Hernant, S., Skloss, T.W., Haw, J.F., Keller, N.P., and Adams, T.H., Aspergillus nidulans stcL encodes a putative cytochrome P-450 monooxygenase required for bisfuran desaturation during aflatoxin/sterigmatocystin biosynthesis, J. Biol. Chem., 272, 1589–1594, 1997.

79. Skory, C.D., Chang, P.-K., Cary, J., and Linz, J.E., Isolation and characterization of a gene from Aspergillus parasiticus associated with the conversion of versicolorin A to sterigmatocystin in aflatoxin biosynthesis, Appl. Environ. Microbiol., 58, 3527–3537, 1992.

80. Keller, N.P., Segner, S., Bhatnagar, D., and Adams, T.H., stcS, a putative P-450 monooxygenase, is required for the conversion of versicolorin A to sterigmatocystin in Aspergillus nidulans, Appl. Environ. Microbiol., 61, 3628–3632, 1995.

81. Keller, N.P., Brown, D., Butchko, R.A.E., Fernandes, M., Kelkar, H., Nesbitt, C., Segner, S., Bhatnagar, D., Cleveland, T.E., and Adams, T.H., A conserved polyketide mycotoxin gene cluster in Aspergillus nidulans, in Molecular Approaches to Food Safety Issues Involving Toxic Microorganisms, Richard, J.L., Ed., Alaken, Fort Collins, CO, 1995, pp. 263–277.

82. Brown, D.W., Yu, J.-H., Kelkar, H.S., Fernandes, M., Nesbitt, T.C., Keller, N.P., Adams, T.H., and Leonard, T.J., Twenty-five coregulated transcripts define a sterigmatocystin gene cluster in Aspergillus nidulans, Proc. Natl. Acad. Sci. USA, 93, 1418–1422, 1996.

83. Motomura, M., Chihaya, N., Shinozawa, T., Hamasaki, T., and Yabe, K., Cloning and characterization of the *O*-methyltransferase I gene (*dmtA*) from *Aspergillus parasiticus* associated with the conversions of demethylsterigmatocystin to sterigmatocystin and dihydrodemethylsterigmatocystin to dihydrosterigmatocystin in aflatoxin biosynthesis, *Appl. Environ. Microbiol.*, 65, 4987–4994, 1999.

84. Yu, J., Cary, J.W., Bhatnagar, D., Cleveland, T.E., Keller, N.P., and Chu, F.S., Cloning and characterization of a cDNA from *Aspergillus parasiticus* encoding an *O*-methyltransferase involved in aflatoxin biosynthesis, *Appl. Environ. Microbiol.*, 59, 3564–3571, 1993.

85. Yu, J., Chang, P.-K., Payne, G.A., Cary, J.W., Bhatnagar, D., and Cleveland, T.E., Comparison of the *omtA* genes encoding *O*-methyltransferases involved in aflatoxin biosynthesis from *Aspergillus parasiticus* and *A. flavus*, *Gene*, 163, 121–125, 1995.

86. Prieto, R., Yousibova, G.L., and Woloshuk, C.P., Identification of aflatoxin biosynthesis genes by genetic complementation in an *Aspergillus flavus* mutant lacking the aflatoxin gene cluster, *Appl. Environ. Microbiol.*, 62(10), 3567–3571, 1996.

87. Prieto, R. and Woloshuk, C.P., *ord1*, an oxidoreductase gene responsible for conversion of *O*-methylsterigmatocystin to aflatoxin in *Aspergillus flavus*, *Appl. Environ. Microbiol.*, 63, 1661–1666, 1997.

88. Cleveland, T.E. and Bhatnagar, D., Molecular regulation of aflatoxin biosynthesis, in *Pennington Center Nutrition Series*, Vol. 1, *Mycotoxins, Cancer and Health*, Bray, G.A. and Ryan, D.H., Eds., Louisiana State University Press, Baton Rouge, 1991, pp. 270–287.

89. Chang, P.-K., Cary, J.W., Bhatnagar, D., Cleveland, T.E., Bennett, J.W., Linz, J.E., Woloshuk, C.P., and Payne, G.A., Cloning of the *Aspergillus parasiticus apa*-2 gene associated with the regulation of aflatoxin biosynthesis, *Appl. Environ. Microbiol.*, 59, 3273–3279, 1993.

90. Chang, P.-K., Yu, J., Bhatnagar, D., and Cleveland, T.E., The carboxy-terminal portion of the aflatoxin pathway regulatory protein *AFLR* of *Aspergillus parasiticus* activates *GAL1:lacZ* gene expression in *Saccharomyces cerevisiae*, *Appl. Environ. Microbiol.*, 65, 2058–2512, 1999.

91. Ehrlich, K.C., Montalbano, B.G., Bhatnagar, D., and Cleveland, T.E., Alteration of different domains in AFLR affects aflatoxin pathway metabolism in *Aspergillus parasiticus* transformants, *Fungal Genet. Biol.*, 23, 279–287, 1998.

92. Payne, G.A., Nystrom, G.J., Bhatnagar, D., Cleveland, T.E., and Woloshuk, C.P., Cloning of the *afl*-2 gene involved in aflatoxin biosynthesis from *Aspergillus flavus*, *Appl. Environ. Microbiol.*, 59, 156–162, 1993.

93. Woloshuk, C.P., Foutz, K.R., Brewer, J.F., Bhatnagar, D., Cleveland, T.E., and Payne, G.A., Molecular characterization of *aflR*, a regulatory locus for aflatoxin biosynthesis, *Appl. Environ. Microbiol.*, 60, 240814, 1994.

94. Yu, J.-H., Butchko, R.A., Fernandes, M., Keller, N.P., Leonard, T.J., and Adams, T.H., Conservation of structure and function of the aflatoxin regulatory gene *aflR* from *Aspergillus nidulans* and *A. flavus*, *Curr. Genet.*, 29, 549–555, 1996.

95. Ehrlich, K.C., Cary, J.W., and Montalbano, B.G., Characterization of the promoter for the gene encoding the aflatoxin biosynthetic pathway regulatory protein AFLR, *Biochim. Biophys. Acta*, 1444, 412–417, 1999.

96. Ehrlich, K.C., Montalbano, B.G., and Cary, J.W., Binding of the C6–zinc cluster protein, AFLR, to the promoters of aflatoxin pathway biosynthesis genes in *Aspergillus parasiticus*, *Gene*, 230, 249–257, 1999.

97. Fernandes, M., Keller, N.P., and Adams, T.H., Sequence-specific binding by *Aspergillus nidulans AflR*, a C6 zinc cluster protein regulating mycotoxin biosynthesis, *Mol. Microbiol.*, 28, 1355–1365, 1998.

98. Meyers, D.M., Obrian, G., Du, W.L., Bhatnagar, D., and Payne, G.A., Characterization of *aflJ*, a gene required for conversion of pathway intermediates to aflatoxin, *Appl. Environ. Microbiol.*, 64, 3713–3717, 1998.

99. Huynh, Q.K., Borgmeyer, J.R., and Zobel, J.F., Isolation and characterization of a 22 kDa protein with antifungal properties from maize seeds, *Biochem. Biophys. Res. Commun.*, 182, 1–5, 1992.

100. Guo, B.-Z., Russin, J.S., Cleveland, T.E., Brown, R.L., and Widstrom, N.W., Wax and cutin layers in maize kernels associated with resistance to aflatoxin production by *Aspergillus flavus*, *J. Food Protect.*, 58, 296–300, 1995.

101. Russin, J.S., Guo, B.Z., Tubajika, K.M., Brown, R.L., Cleveland, T.E., and Widstrom, N.W., Comparison of kernel wax from corn genotypes resistant or susceptible to *Aspergillus flavus*, *Phytopathology*, 87, 529–533, 1997.

102. Gembeh, S.V., Brown, R.L., Grimm, C., and Cleveland, T.E., Identification of chemical components of corn kernel pericarp wax associated with resistance to *Aspergillus flavus* infection and aflatoxin production, *J. Agr. Food Chem.*, 49, 4635–4641, 2001.

103. Roberts, W.K. and Selitrennikoff, C.P., Isolation and partial characterization of two antifungal proteins from barley, *Biochim. Biophys. Acta*, 880, 161–170, 1986.

104. Roberts, W.K. and Selitrennikoff, C.P., Plant and bacterial chitinases differ in antifungal activity, *J. Gen. Microbiol.*, 134, 169–176, 1988.

105. Huynh, Q.K., Hironaka, C.M., Levine, E.B., Smith, C. E., Borgmeyer, J.R., and Shah, D.M., Antifungal proteins from plants: purification, molecular cloning, and antifungal properties of chitinases from maize seed, *J. Biol. Chem.*, 267, 6635–6640, 1992.

106. Wu, S., Kriz, A.L., and Widholm, J.M., Molecular analysis of two cDNA clones encoding acidic class I chitinase in maize, *Plant Physiol.*, 105, 1097–1105, 1994.

107. Cordero, M.J., Raventos, D., and San Segundo, B., Differential expression and induction of chitinases and β-1,3-glucanases in response to fungal infection during germination of maize seeds, *Mol. Plant Microbe Interact.*, 7, 23–31, 1994.

108. Lozovaya, V.V., Waranyuwat, A., and Widholm, J.M., β-1,3-glucanase and resistance to *Aspergillus flavus* infection in maize, *Crop Sci.*, 38, 1255–1260, 1998.

109. Chen, M.-S., Feng, G., Zen, K.C., Richardson, M., Valdes-Rodriguez, S., Reeck, G.R., and Kramer, K.J., α-Amylases from three species of stored grain *Coleoptera* and their inhibition by wheat and corn proteinaceous inhibitors, *Insect Biochem. Molec.* 22, 261–268, 1992.

110. Terras, F.R.G., Schoofs, H.M.E., Thevissen, K., Osborn, R.W., Vanderleyden, J., Cammue, B.P.A., and Broekaert, W.F., Synergistic enhancement of the antifungal activity of wheat and barley thionins by radish and oilseed rape 2S albumins and by barley trypsin inhibitors, *Plant Physiol.*, 103, 1311–1319, 1993.

111. Chen, Z.-Y., Brown, R.L., Lax, A.R., Guo, B.Z., Cleveland, T.E., and Russin, J.S., Resistance to *Aspergillus flavus* in corn kernels is associated with a 14 kDa protein, *Phytopathology*, 88, 276–281, 1998.

112. Lorito, M., Broadway, R.M., Hayes, C.K., Woo, S.L., Noviello, C., Williams, D.L., and Harman, G.E., Proteinase inhibitors from plants as a novel class of fungicides, *Mol. Plant Microbe Interact.*, 7, 525–527, 1994.

113. Joshi, B.N., Sainani, M.N., Bastawade, K.B., Gupta, V.S., and Ranjekar, P.K., Cysteine protease inhibitor from pearl millet: a new class of antifungal protein, *Biochem. Biophys. Res. Commun.*, 246, 382–387, 1998.

114. Hochstrasser, K., Illchmann, K., and Werle E., Plant protease inhibitors. VII. The amino acid sequence of the specific trypsin inhibitor from maize seeds and the characterization of the polymer, *Hoppe Seyler's Z. Physiol. Chem.*, 351, 721–728, 1970.

115. Richardson, M., Seed storage proteins: the enzyme inhibitors, *Methods Plant Biochem.*, 5, 259–305, 1991.

116. Roberts, W.K. and Selitrennikoff, C.P., Zeamatin, an antifungal protein from maize with membrane-permeabilizing activity, *J. Gen. Microbiol.*, 136, 1771–1778, 1990.

117. Guo, B.-Z., Chen, Z.-Y., Brown, R.L., Lax, A.R., Cleveland, T.E., Russin, J.S., Mehta, A.D., Selitrennikoff, C.P., and Widstrom, N.W., Germination induces accumulation of specific proteins and antifungal activities in corn kernels, *Phytopathology*, 87, 1174–1178, 1997.

118. Hey, T.D., Hartley, M., and Walsh, T.A., Maize ribosome-inactivating protein (b-32): homologs in related species, effects on maize ribosomes, and modulation of activity by pro-peptide deletions, *Plant Physiol.*, 107, 1323–1332, 1995.

119. Chen, Z.-Y., Brown, R.L., Damann, K.E., and Cleveland, T.E., Proteome comparisons of corn kernels resistant or susceptible to *Aspergillus flavus* infection, *Phytopathology*, 90, S14, 2000.

120. Chen, Z.-Y., Brown, R.L., Damann, K.E., and Cleveland, T.E., Identification of unique or elevated levels of kernel proteins in aflatoxin-resistant maize genotypes through proteome analysis. *Phytopathology*, 92, 1084–1094, 2002.

121. Thomann, E.B., Sollinger, J., White, C., and Rivin, C.J., Accumulation of group 3 late embryogenesis abundant proteins in *Zea mays* embryos, *Plant Physiol.*, 99, 607–614, 1992.

122. Xu, D., Duan, X., Wang, B., Hong, B., Ho, T.H.D., and Wu, R., Expression of a late embryogenesis abundant protein gene HVA1, from barley confers tolerance to water deficit and salt stress in transgenic rice, *Plant Physiol.*, 110, 249–257, 1996.

123. Bartels, D., Engelhardt, K., Roncarati, R., Schneider, K., Rotter, M., and Salamini, F., An ABA and GA modulated gene expressed in the barley embryo encodes an aldose reductase related protein, *EMBO J.*, 10, 1037–1043, 1991.

124. Roncarati, R., Salamini, F., and Bartels, D., An aldose reductase homologous gene from barley: regulation and function, *Plant J.*, 7, 809–822, 1995.

125. Oberschall A., Deak, M., Torok, K., Sass, L., Vass, I., Kovacs, I., Feher, A., Dudits, D., and Horvath, G.V., A novel aldose/aldehyde reductase protects transgenic plants against lipid peroxidation under chemical and drought stresses, *Plant J.*, 24, 437–446, 2000.

126. Papoulis, A., Al-Abed, Y., and Bucala, R., Identification of N2-(-1-carboxylethyl) guanine (CEG) as a guanine advanced glycosylation endproduct, *Biochemistry*, 34, 648–655, 1995.

127. Thornalley, P.J., The glyoxalase system: new developments towards functional characterization of metabolic pathways fundamental to biological life, *Biochem. J.*, 269, 1–11, 1990.

128. Veena, Reddy, V.S. and Sopory, S.K., Glyoxalase I from *Brassica juncea*: molecular cloning, regulation and its over-expression confer tolerance in transgenic tobacco under stress, *Plant J.*, 17, 385–395, 1999.

129. Espartero, J., Sanchez-Aguayo, I., and Pardo, J.M., Molecular characterization of glyoxalase-i from a higher plant, upregulation by stress, *Plant Mol. Biol.*, 29, 1223–1233, 1996.

130. Lee, G.J., Roseman, A.M., Saibil, H.R., and Vierling, E., A small heat shock protein stably binds heat-denatured model substrates and can maintain a substrate in a folding-competent state, *EMBO J.*, 16, 59–671, 1997.

131. Wehmeyer, N. and Vierling, E., The expression of small heat shock proteins in seeds responds to discrete developmental signals and suggests a general protective role in desiccation tolerance, *Plant Physiol.*, 122, 1099–1108, 2000.

132. Payne, G.A., Process of contamination by aflatoxin-producing fungi and their impact on crops, in *Mycotoxins in Agriculture and Food Safety*, Sinha, K.K. and Bhatnagar, D., Eds., Marcel Dekker, New York, 1998, pp. 279–306.

133. Zaika, L.L. and Buchanan, R.L., Review of compounds affecting biosynthesis or bioregulation of aflatoxins, *J. Food Protect.*, 50, 681–708, 1987.

134. Bhatnagar, D., Cleveland, T.E., Brown, R.L., Cary, J.W., Yu, J., and Chang, P.-K., Preharvest aflatoxin contamination: elimination through biotechnology, in *Ecological Agriculture and Sustainable Development*, Vol. 1, Dhaliwal, G.S. et al., Eds., Chapman Enterprises, New Delhi, India, 1998, pp. 100–129.

135. Wilson, D.M., Gueddner, R.C., McKinney, J.K., Lievsay, R.H., Evans, B.D., and Hill, R.A., Effect of α-ionone on *Aspergillus flavus* and *Aspergillus parasiticus* growth, sporulation, morphology and aflatoxin production, *J. AOCS*, 58, 582A, 1981.

136. Zeringue, Jr., H.J. and McCormick, S.P., Relationships between cotton leaf-derived volatiles and growth of *Aspergillus flavus*, *J. AOCS*, 66, 581–585, 1989.

137. Zeringue, Jr., H.J., Effects of $C_6–C_{10}$ alkenals and alkanals eliciting a defense response in the developing cotton boll, *Phytochemistry*, 31, 2305–2308, 1992.

138. Zeringue, Jr., H.J., Brown, R.L., Neucere, J.N., and Cleveland, T.E., Relationship between $C_6–C_{12}$ alkanal and alkenal volatile contents and resistance of maize genotypes to *Aspergillus flavus* and aflatoxin production, *J. Agric. Chem.*, 44, 403–404, 1996.

139. Greene-McDowelle, D.M., Ingber, B.F., Wright, M.S., Zeringue, Jr., H.J., Bhatnagar, D., and Cleveland, T.E., The effects of selected cotton-leaf volatiles on growth, development and aflatoxin production of *Aspergillus parasiticus*, *Toxicon*, 37, 883–893, 1999.

140. Wright, M.S., Greene-McDowelle, D.M., Zeringue, Jr., H.J., Bhatnagar, D., and Cleveland, T.E., Effect of volatile aldehydes from *Aspergillus*-resistant varieties of corn on *Aspergillus parasiticus* growth and aflatoxin production, *Toxicon*, 38, 1215–1223, 2000.

141. Wilson, R.A., Gardner, H.W., and Keller, N.P., Cultivar-dependent expression of a maize lipoxygenase responsive to seed infesting fungi, *J. Biol. Chem.*, 276, 25766–25774, 2001.

142. Burow, G.B., Garnder, J.W., and Keller, N.P., A peanut seed lipoxygenase responsive to *Aspergillus* colonization, *Plant Mol. Biol.*, 42, 689–701, 2002.

143. Zeringue, Jr., H.J., Possible involvement of lipoxygenase in a defense response in aflatoxigenic *Aspergillus*–cotton plant interactions, *Can. J. Botany*, 74, 98–102, 1996.

144. Miller, J.D., Fiedler, D.A., Dowd, P.F., Norton, R.A., and Collins, F.W., Isolation of 4-acetyl-benzoxazolin-2-one (4–ABOA) and diferuloylputricine from an extract of *Gibberella* ear rot-resistant corn that blocks mycotoxin biosynthesis and the insect toxicity of 4-ABOA and related compounds, *Biochem. Syst. Ecol.*, 24, 647–658, 1996.

145. Norton, R.A. and Dowd, P.F., Effect of steryl cinnamic acid derivatives from corn bran on *Aspergillus flavus*, corn earworm larvae, and dried fruit beetle larvae and adults, *J. Agr. Food Chem.*, 44, 2412–2416, 1996.

146. Norton, R.A., Effect of carotenoids on aflatoxin B_1 synthesis by *Aspergillus flavus*, *Phytopathology*, 87, 814–821, 1997.

147. Norton, R.A., Inhibition of aflatoxin B_1 biosynthesis by *Aspergillus flavus* by anthocyanidins and related flavonoids, *J. Agr. Food Chem.*, 47, 1230–1235, 1999.

148. Wicklow, D.T., Norton, R.A., and McAlpin, C.E., B-carotene inhibition of aflatoxin biosynthesis among *Aspergillus flavus* genotypes from Illinois corn, *Myoscience*, 39, 167–172, 1998.

149. Mahoney, N., Molyneux, R.J., and Campbell, B.C., Regulation of aflatoxin production by naphthoquinones of walnut (*Jinglans regia*), *J. Agr. Food Chem.*, 48, 4418–4421, 2000.

150. Lee, S.E., Campbell, B.C., Molyneux, R.J., Hasegarva, S., and Lee, H.S., Inhibitory effects of naturally occurring compounds on aflatoxin B(1) biotransformation, *J. Agr. Food Chem.*, 49, 5171–5177, 2001.

151. Yu, J., Bhatnagar, D., Whitelaw, C.A., Cleveland, T.E., and Nierman, W.C., Report on *Aspergillus flavus* EST project: A tool for eliminating aflatoxin contamination, in *Proc. of the Second Fungal Genomics Workshop*, San Antonio, TX, October 23–25, 2002, National Corn Growers Association, St. Louis, MO, 2002, p. 27.

10 Epidemiology of Aflatoxin Exposure and Human Liver Cancer

Jia-Sheng Wang and Lili Tang

CONTENTS

10.1 INTRODUCTION

Aflatoxins (AF), mainly produced by *Aspergillus flavus* and *A. parasiticus*, are a group of naturally occurring fungal metabolites that have long been recognized as significant environmental contaminants.[1,2] Aflatoxin B_1 (AFB_1) is the most common mycotoxin found in human food and animal feed.[2,3] AFB_1 is a potent hepatocarcinogen that can induce tumors in many species of animals, including rodents, nonhuman primates, and fish.[3,4] While the liver is the major target organ, under certain circumstances, significant numbers of tumors have been found in lung, kidney, and colon.[5]

Primary liver cancer, mainly hepatocellular carcinoma (HCC), is one of the most common human diseases in Asia and Africa and among populations of Asian– and Hispanic–Americans.[4,6,7] The poor prognosis of this malignancy results in its being the third leading cause of cancer deaths in the world.[2,6] In the People's Republic of China (PRC), HCC is the second leading cause of cancer mortality with at least 350,000 deaths per year.[8] The PRC has several endemic regions in which HCC is the number one cause of cancer death, and the annual incidence rate is usually higher than 50/100,000.[2,9] Fusui County in Guangxi Zhuang Autonomous Region and Qidong city in Jiangsu Province are two of these high-risk areas that have the highest HCC incidence and mortality rates in the PRC. In Fusui, HCC not only constitutes over 65% of total cancer deaths[10] but also usually strikes people at an earlier age.

195

The median age of onset of this malignancy is between 35 and 45 years in this high-risk area. In Qidong, liver cancer accounts for 10% of all adult deaths in several townships.[11] Because effective treatment is unavailable for patients suffering from this cancer, the mortality of HCC is almost equal to its incidence in these endemic areas. In contrast, the annual incidence of HCC in the United States is about 1.5/100,000.[12] Clearly, the incidence of liver cancer varies worldwide by at least 100-fold.

Over the past 40 years extensive efforts have been made to investigate the association between aflatoxin (AF) exposure and human liver cancer. These studies were hindered in earlier years by a lack of adequate biomarkers and dosimetry data on AF intake, excretion, and metabolism in humans, as well as by the general poor quality of worldwide cancer morbidity and mortality statistics.[13] Many studies carried out in the past decade have been incorporated with the molecular analysis of the cancer gene targets and AF-specific molecular biomarkers, which have spurred the efforts to assess AF exposure and human liver cancer risks. These molecular epidemiological studies eventually led to the reclassification of naturally occurring AF to a group 1 human carcinogen by the International Agency for Research on Cancer (IARC) in 1993,[14] and the evaluation was reaffirmed in 2002.[15]

Chronic infection with hepatitis B virus (HBV) is another major risk factor for HCC.[16] About 80% of the cases of HCC are associated with chronic HBV infection. Epidemiological studies have found that carriers of HBV are more likely to develop HCC than noncarriers. The absolute lifetime risks of HCC for individual HBV carriers range from 20 to 25% based on studies in some special populations.[17,18] IARC classified HBV as a group I known human carcinogen in 1994. HBV infection is also one of the major risk factors for HCC in the Guangxi region of the PRC. A cohort study[20] in southern Guangxi, including Fusui, found that approximately one quarter of the male population tested HBsAg positive. Over 90% of subsequent HCC cases tested HBsAg positive at recruitment, and the incidence of HCC among HBsAg carriers was more than 1% annually. On the other hand, this region has a very low prevalence of hepatitis C virus (HCV) infection among HCC cases and population controls.[21]

Multiple risk factors, in addition to dietary AF exposure and chronic infection with HBV/HCV, were identified to determine the etiology of liver cancer in different populations and geographic regions; these factors included excessive alcoholic consumption, drinking water contamination, nutritional factors, and occupational carcinogen exposure. This chapter focuses only on the relationship between AF exposure and liver cancer although the synergistic effects of AF exposure and HBV infection are also mentioned. Excellent recent reviews have been published to address the toxicology of AF as a public health concern[22] and the modulation of AF biomarkers for liver cancer prevention.[23]

10.2 ECOLOGICAL AND CROSS-SECTIONAL STUDIES

Since the discovery of aflatoxin in the early 1960s, many ecological or cross-sectional studies have been conducted in different parts of the world to explore the possible linkage of AF to human liver cancer risk.[4,14] Most of these investigations suffered from a lack of good data on AF exposure and poor-quality information on cancer incidence. In addition, studies carried out before 1980 also suffered from the inability to accurately test cases for hepatitis B virus status, another major risk factor for human liver cancer. Nevertheless, these studies revealed that areas with the highest presumed AF intake also had the highest liver cancer rates; for example, increased AF ingestion from 3 to 222 ng per kg body weight per day corresponded to increased liver cancer incidence values extending from a minimum of 2.0 to a maximum of 35.0/100,000 per year.[13]

Thirteen ecological and cross-sectional epidemiological studies were summarized by the IARC.[15] In one of these studies, Van Rensburg et al.[24,25] studied the occurrence and potential etiologies of HCC for the period from 1968 to 1974 in the Province of Inhambane, Mozambique. These incidence rates were compared with those observed in South Africa among mineworkers migrating from Inhambane. Food samples were randomly collected and AF content determined in six districts of Inhambane as well as from Manhica-Magude, a region of lower liver cancer incidence. A third set of food samples was taken in Transkei, where an even lower incidence of liver cancer had been recorded. When all of the calculations were completed, the mean AF dietary intake values were significantly correlated to the varied liver cancer rates.

Peers et al.[26,27] extended the database for Africa and published a study conducted in Swaziland. The data collected were analyzed for the relationship between AF exposure, HBV infection, and the incidence of liver cancer. The levels of AF intake were evaluated in dietary samples from households across the country and in crop samples taken from farms. The prevalence of HBV markers was estimated from the serum of blood donors. Liver cancer incidence was recorded for the years 1979 to 1983 through a national system of cancer registration. Across four broad geographic regions, more than a fivefold variation occurred in the estimated daily intake of AF, ranging from 3.1 to 17.5 µg. The proportion of HBV-exposed males was very high but varied relatively little by geographic region; however, liver cancer incidence varied over a fivefold range and was strongly associated with estimated levels of AF. In an analysis involving ten smaller subregions, AF exposure emerged as a more important determinant of the variation in liver cancer incidence than the prevalence of hepatitis infection.

Hatch et al.[28] conducted a study in eight areas of Taiwan with a wide range of rates of mortality from HCC. In order to estimate AF levels in these areas, a representative sample of 250 adult residents in total was selected. Participants were interviewed and were asked to provide both morning urine and blood specimens. Serum was used for detecting HBsAg and urine was used for detecting AF and metabolites. Measured AF values ranged from 0.7 to 511.7 pg equivalents of AFB_1/mL urine. Mean levels were similar in men and women and in HBV carriers and noncarriers. The primary analyses were carried out utilizing individual measurements of AFB_1 equivalents and HBsAg status with the HCC rate (sex-specific, age-adjusted) of the entire area in which the individual resided. The mean levels of AF and HBsAg correlated with the HCC rates. The univariate correlations between HCC and AF at the ecological level were 0.83 ($p = 0.01$) in men and 0.49 ($p = 0.22$) in women. The correlations were much lower, albeit statistically significant, when analyzed at the individual level: 0.29 ($p = 0.002$) in men and 0.17 ($p = 0.047$) in women. In the multivariate regression analysis, HCC was significantly associated with AF levels, after adjusting for age, sex, and HBsAg. Adjustments for smoking and alcohol consumption in a subset of 190 subjects with available interview data and the inclusion of interaction terms did not materially affect the findings. Thus, the very different types of analyses all pointed to an association between urinary AF and HCC.

Omer et al.[29] carried out a comparison of AF contamination of peanut products in two areas of Sudan. The study was carried out in 1995 and involved the selection of peanut butter samples from local markets using a staged sampling approach to identify markets in the two study areas. Samples were characterized as to how they had been stored and were analyzed for AFB_1 by high-performance liquid chromatography (HPLC). Mean AFB_1 levels were much higher in "high-risk" western Sudan (87.4 ± 197.3 µg/kg) than in central Sudan (8.5 ± 6.8 µg/kg). Also, dietary questionnaires among people recruited for a small case-control study indicated that residents in western Sudan consumed more peanut butter than residents in central Sudan.

While most of these published studies cited above found a positive association between AF exposure and liver cancer, several studies have not. A cross-sectional study by Campbell et al.[30] that took samples from 48 widely scattered counties in the PRC revealed no association between composite AF metabolites in human bladder and liver cancer mortality rates. Also, another study carried out in five selected areas of Thailand did not find significant correlation between AF exposure and liver cancer rates.[31]

10.3 CASE-CONTROL STUDIES

Many hospital-based case-control studies have been reported and summarized by the IARC.[14,15] Bulatao-Jayme et al.[32] compared the dietary intakes of confirmed primary liver cancer cases in the Philippines against age- and sex-matched controls. By using dietary recall, the frequency and amounts of food items consumed were calculated into units of AF load per day. These calculations revealed that the mean AF load per day of the liver cancer cases was 4.5 times higher than the controls. Alcohol intake as a risk factor was also analyzed by stratifying the cases into heavy and light AF exposure groups. These researchers combined AF load and alcohol intake and identified a synergistic and statistically significant effect on relative risk with AF exposure and alcohol intake.

Olubuyide et al.[33,34] carried out a small case-control study in Nigeria to assess the role of HBV and AF in primary HCC. The cases included 22 patients at a university hospital in Ibadan in 1988. Controls were 22 patients from the gastroenterology ward of the same hospital with acid peptic disease unrelated to liver diseases who were matched for sex and age. Blood samples were collected after the patients were on the hospital diet for a week and were analyzed for HBsAg, a number of AFs (B_1, B_2, M_1, M_2, G_1, and G_2), and aflatoxicol. HBsAg was detected in 16 cases and 8 controls. Elevated levels of AF were detected in 5 (23%) cases and 1 (5%) control, the difference being significant ($p < 0.05$).

In a population-based case-control study carried out in Haimen City, Jiangsu Province, PRC, MacGlynn et al.[35] found that genetic variation in two AFB_1 detoxification genes, epoxide hydrolase (EPHX) and glutathione S-transferase M_1 (GSTM1), was correlated with the presence of serum AFB_1–albumin adducts and the presence of HCC, as well as with TP53 codon 249 mutations.

Mandishona et al.[36] carried out a small case-control study in South Africa aimed primarily at determining the role of dietary iron overload in the etiology of HCC. They also collected information on exposure to AFB_1. The cases included 24 consecutive patients with HCC in two hospitals of one province of South Africa. Two control series were assembled. A matched (sex, age, race) series of 48 (2 controls per case) was selected from patients hospitalized primarily with trauma or infection. In addition, 75 relatives and family members of the patients with HCC constituted a second control series. Interviews were conducted and blood samples taken. Laboratory analyses included measurement of serum AFB_1–albumin adducts, iron overload, HBsAg, anti-HCV, and other biochemical parameters. The median level of AFB_1–albumin adducts (pg/mg) was lower among the patients with HCC (7.3; range, 2.4 to 91.2) than among the hospital controls (21.7; range, 0 to 45.6) and family controls (8.7; range, 0.7 to 82.1). Several other parameters (e.g., HBsAg, serum ferritin) were higher among the cases than the controls.

Omer et al.[37] conducted a case-control study in Sudan to assess the association between peanut butter intake as a source of AF and the GSTM1 genotype in the etiology of HCC. The cases included 150 patients with HCC who were diagnosed in five out of six hospitals of Khartoum. The controls were 205 residents selected from the same areas by a two-stage process. Data collection involved a questionnaire that included a particularly detailed history of peanut butter consumption and information on potential confounders. The peanut butter history was transformed into a quantitative cumulative index. Usable blood samples were analyzed for HBsAg and anti-HCV (115 cases and 199 controls) and genotyped for GSTM1 (110 cases and 189 controls). The patients with HCC consumed more peanut butter than did the controls. A clear dose–response relationship was observed between average peanut butter consumption and risk for HCC. In the highest quartile of consumption, the odds ratio (OR) ranged from 3.4 to 4.0 depending on the covariates included in the model, and all were statistically significant. The pattern of risk differed by region. Peanut butter consumption represented no increased risk in central Sudan but a very high risk in western Sudan (OR in the highest quartile, 8.7). AF contamination of peanut butter was found to be a much greater problem in western Sudan than in central Sudan.[29] The authors also noted, however, that residents of the two regions are ethnically different, so effect modification by unmeasured genetic or environmental factors cannot be excluded. While GSTM1 genotype was not a risk factor for HCC, it was a strong effect modifier. The excess risk due to peanut butter consumption was restricted to cases with GSTM1-null genotype; the OR in the highest quartile of peanut butter exposure among GSTM1-null cases was 17 (95% confidence interval [CI]; range, 2.7 to 105)..

McGlynn et al.[38] recently reported a study to explore susceptibility to AFB_1-related primary HCC in humans. The study genotyped 11 loci in 2 families of AFB_1 detoxification genes: GSTs and EPHX in samples from 231 HCC cases and 256 controls. After adjustment for multiple comparisons, only one polymorphism in the EPHX family 2 locus remained significantly associated with HCC (OR = 2.06, 95% CI; range, 1.13 to 3.12).

Although strong evidence suggests an association between dietary AF exposure and HCC incidence in the above case-control studies, several investigations do not support this positive association.[14] In a case-control study in Thailand,[39] a positive correlation with HBsAg status was found but no increase in risk with recent AF exposure estimated by dietary intake and measurement of AF-albumin adducts in serum. A recently reported case-control study[40] in Haimen, China, investigated the impact of multiple factors in a total of 248 HCC cases and 248 sex-, age-, and residence-matched controls. HBV/HCV infection was found to be significantly correlated to the HCC (OR = 9.75, 95% CI; range, 4.7–20.2) and no association with peanut intake (one of AF sources). No AF biomarkers were measured in this study.

10.4 COHORT STUDIES

In general, the most rigorous test of an association between an agent and disease outcome is found in prospective epidemiological studies, in which healthy people are recruited, questionnaires and biological samples taken, and the cohort followed until significant numbers of cases are obtained. A nested study within the cohort can then be designed to match cases and controls. Because the controls were recruited at the same time and with the same health status as the cases, they are better matched than in traditional case-control studies.

Studies by Yeh et al.[41,42] on the epidemiology of HCC in the Guangxi Autonomous Region, PRC, investigated the interaction between HBV infection and dietary AF exposure. The staple food of people living in this region during the 1960s and 1970s was corn, which was often contaminated with high levels of AFB_1. In some heavily contaminated areas, AFB_1 content ranged from 53.8 to 303 ppb, while the lightly contaminated regions showed AFB_1 levels in grains of less than 5 ppb. After 5 to 8 years of follow-up, HCC incidence was determined for these two regions of heavy and light aflatoxin contamination. Those individuals who were HBV surface antigen (HBsAg) positive and found to have heavy aflatoxin exposure had a HCC incidence of 649 cases per 100,000 compared with 66 cases per 100,000 in lightly contaminated aflatoxin areas. Those people who were HBsAg negative and eating heavily contaminated aflatoxin diets had a HCC rate of 99 per 100,000 compared with no cases detected in the lightly contaminated area.[20]

Qian et al.[43] updated a cohort study previously described by Ross et al.[44] of 18,244 male residents of Shanghai, PRC. The cohort was established between January 1986 and September 1989, and participants were recruited by invitation from four geographically defined areas and responded to questionnaires administered by nurses, usually in their homes, on lifestyle (including smoking and alcohol consumption) and on food frequency. Blood and urine specimens were collected. The men were followed up by identification of death records in district vital statistics units and through linkage with the Shanghai Cancer Registry (estimated to be 85% complete). The cohort was followed to February 1992, resulting in 69,393 person-years of follow-up. Of 364 cancer cases identified, 55 were diagnosed as HCC, 9 of which were confirmed by biopsy. The reported diet history based on a frequency checklist of 45 food items usually consumed as an adult was combined with a set of independently measured AF levels in various local foods to derive a quantitative measure of dietary AF exposure. In a cohort-type analysis, using the lowest tertile of aflatoxin exposure as reference, the middle tertile had a relative risk (RR), adjusted for age and smoking, of 1.6 (95% CI; range, 0.8–3.1; 25 cases) and the highest tertile had an OR of 0.9 (95% CI; range, 0.4 to 1.9; 16 cases).

To assess the risks in relation to biomarkers of AF exposure, a nested case-control study was conducted using 50 of the cases.[43] Controls were selected from among people who had no history of liver cancer on the date of cancer diagnosis of the index cases and were matched to cases in ratios ranging from 10:1 to 3:1, yielding a total of 267 controls. For each case and control, urine samples were analyzed for AFB_1, P_1, M_1, Q_1, G_1, and AFB_1–N^7-guanine adducts. HBsAg was measured by radioimmunoassay. Out of 50 cases, 32 were HBsAG positive, and 31 out of 267 controls were HBsAg positive. Each of the six biomarkers of AF exposure was more frequently present among cases than controls. For 36 of the 50 liver cancer cases and 109 of 267 controls, results were positive in at least one of the four assays analyzed for the full set of cases and controls (adjusted RR, 5.0; 95% CI; range, 2.1 to 12). The highest risks were found among subjects with AFB_1–N^7-guanine adducts. Compared with subjects who had no AF biomarkers and were HBsAg negative, the interaction of the two factors was supramultiplicative, with RRs as follows: AF biomarker only, 3.4 (95% CI; range, 1.1 to 10); HBsAg only, 7.3 (95% CI; range, 2.2 to 24); both factors, 59 (95% CI; range, 17 to 212). These results show a causal relationship between the presence of two specific biomarkers (AF and HBsAg) and HCC risk.

Another nested case-control study[45] within a cohort established in Qidong, PRC, has followed 804 healthy HBsAg-positive individuals (728 male, 76 female) ages 30 to 65 years. From 1993 to 1995, 38 of these individuals developed HCC, and the age, gender, residence, and time of sampling matched serum samples from 34 of these cases to 170 controls. AFB_1–albumin adduct levels were determined by radio-immunoassay. The RR for HCC cases among AFB_1–albumin-positive individuals was 2.4 (95% CI; range, 1.2 to 4.7).

Several cohort studies were performed in Penghu and Taiwan, China, to explore the relationship of AF and HBV exposure and liver cancer in the past decade. A prospective cohort study reported by Chen et al.[46] enrolled 4691 men and 1796 women, ages 30 to 65 years. The subjects were selected from a housing register maintained by the local administration. Participants were interviewed on a variety of sociodemographic, dietary, and medical history topics. Blood samples were collected and stored frozen. A two-stage screening process for HCC was undertaken which included serological markers and clinical assessments with ultrasonography. Subjects were further followed up with annual examinations. A total of 33 cases of HCC were diagnosed by December 1993, of whom 2 were negative for HBsAg. A total of 123 controls were selected from within the cohort among unaffected subjects and matched with cases for age, sex, village, and date of blood collection. Blood samples from cases and controls were analyzed for HBsAg, anti-hepatitis C virus (HCV) antibodies, and AFB_1–albumin adducts, although samples for adduct analysis were usable for only 20 cases and 86 controls. Using logistic regression, with age and sex adjustment and a detection limit for albumin adducts of 0.01 pmol/mg as the cutoff value, the OR for an association between the presence of AFB_1–albumin adducts and HCC was 3.2 (13 cases; 95% CI; range, 1.1 to 8.9). When the statistical model also included several other covariates (HBsAg, anti-HCV, family history of liver cancer or cirrhosis), the OR for AFB_1–albumin adducts rose to 5.5 (95% CI; range, 1.2 to 2.5). Also, an extremely high risk was associated with positive HBsAg status (OR, 129; 95% CI; range, 25 to 659). The authors surmised that peanut contamination was a major source of AF in this population.

A cohort study was carried out by Wang et al.[47] in seven townships of Taiwan, China, including three on the Penghu Islets and four on Taiwan Island. Of the total population of 89,342 eligible subjects selected from local housing office records and mailed an invitation to a cancer screening project, 25,618 (29%) volunteered to participate. Among participants, 47% were men, and enrollment occurred from July 1990 to June 1992. Participants were interviewed to elicit information on sociodemographic characteristics, alcohol and smoking habits, and medical history. Fasting blood and spot urine specimens were collected and stored frozen. Serum samples were assayed for HBsAg and α-fetoprotein (α-FP), anti-HCV, and various markers of liver function. Abdominal ultrasonography was carried out among a subgroup of high-risk persons from two Penghu Islets. All participants were recontacted by invitation to local research centers or by telephone interviews between 1992 and 1994. Periodic searches for death certificates from local housing offices and through linkage with the national death and cancer registries were carried out. The overall follow-up rate was >98%. Between February 1991 and June 1995, 56 HCC cases were identified in the cohort, of which 22 were histologically or cytologically confirmed. For each case, 4 controls were selected among cohort members who were free of liver cancer or cirrhosis at the time of identification and who were matched for age, sex, township, and recruitment date. Altogether, 56 HCC cases and 220 controls were studied. Serum specimens (52 cases and 168 controls) and urine specimens (38 cases and 137 controls) were available for analysis. Urinary AF metabolites were determined using a monoclonal antibody with high affinity to AFB_1 and significant cross-reactivity to AFB_2, M_1, G_1, and P_1. Serum AF–albumin adducts was measured. Using conditional logistic regression, the OR for liver cancer corresponding to detectable levels of AF–albumin adducts was 4.6 (95% CI; range, 2.0 to 10) before adjustment for HBsAg and 1.6 (95% CI; range, 0.4 to 5.5) after adjustment. For high levels of urinary aflatoxin metabolites, the OR was 3.3 (95% CI; range, 1.4 to 7.7) before adjustment for HBsAg and 3.8 (95% CI; range, 1.1 to 13) after adjustment. Although little or no effect of AF biomarkers on HCC was observed among HBsAg-negative subjects, quite strong effects were seen among HBsAg-positive subjects, especially in the analysis using AF metabolites as the exposure.

Sun et al.[48] recently reported the results from a nested case-control study of an extended follow-up of the cohort previously described by Wang et al.[47] Seventy-nine HBsAg-positive cases of HCC were identified between 1991 and 1997 and matched for age, gender, residence, and date of recruitment with controls, as well as several randomly selected HBsAg-positive controls (total of 149). Blood samples were collected and analyzed for HBV and HCV, for AFB_1–albumin adducts, and for

GSTM1 and T1 genotypes. In a conditional logistic regression analysis, a significant relationship was observed between HCC risk and AFB_1–albumin adducts (OR = 2.0; 95% CI; range, 1.1 to 3.7). GSTM1- and GSTT1-null genotypes were associated with a decreased risk for HCC (GSTM1-null: OR = 0.4; 95% CI; range, 0.2 to 0.7; GSTT1-null: OR = 0.5; 95% CI; range, 0.2 to 0.9). A statistically significant $p = 0.03$) interaction was found between AFB_1–albumin adducts and GSTT1 genotype, indicating a more pronounced risk among those who were GSTT1-null genotype (OR = 3.7; 95% CI; range, 1.5 to 9.3) and no risk among those who had the non-null genotype (OR = 0.9; 95% CI; range, 0.3 to 2.4).

Yu et al.[49] also carried out a cohort study in Taiwan to study the role of AF in the etiology of HCC. A cohort of 4841 male asymptomatic HBsAg carriers and 2501 male noncarriers, ages 30 to 65 years, was recruited from the Government Employee Central Clinics and the Liver Unit of a hospital in Taipei from 1988 to 1992. At entry into the study, each participant was interviewed to obtain information on demographic characteristics, habits of cigarette smoking and alcohol consumption, and diet (including the frequency of consuming peanuts and fermented bean products, which are thought to be the major AF-contaminated foodstuffs in Taiwan), as well as personal and family histories of major chronic diseases. Urine and blood samples from study subjects were stored frozen. All HBsAg carriers in this study had both ultrasonography and α-FP measurements taken every 6 to 12 months. Follow-up of HBsAg-negative people was carried out by annual examination that included a serum α-FP test. The response rate to the periodic follow-up examinations was approximately 72% for HBsAg carriers and 80% for HBsAg-negative people. Information on HCC occurrence and the vital status of study subjects who did not participate in the follow-up examinations was obtained form both computerized data files of the national death certification and the cancer registry. By the end of 1994, 34,579 person-years of follow-up had been accumulated, an average of 4.7 years per person. During the follow-up period, 50 HCC cases were identified. All HCC cases were diagnosed on the basis of either pathological and cytological examinations or an elevated α-FP level combined with at least one positive image.

To investigate the role of AF, a nested case-control comparison was carried out, in which two separate matched controls per case were selected, one who was HBsAg positive and one who was HBsAg negative. Levels of AF metabolites in urine were analyzed by reverse-phase HPLC, allowing measurement of AFM_1, AFP_1, AFB_1, AFG_1, and AFB_1–N^7-guanine. Most subjects were also tested for anti-HCV. After exclusion of subjects with missing specimens, analyses were available on 43 matched case-control sets. Among all the HCC cases, only one occurred in the HBsAg-negative subcohort, and that one was positive for anti-HCV. All study subjects were positive for AFM_1, 81% for AFP_1, 43% for AFB_1–N^7-guanine adducts, 28% for AFB_1, and 12% for AFG_1. A significant correlation ($r = 0.35$) was found between reported dietary intake of various foods thought to contain AF and levels of urinary AFM_1. No significant correlations with other AF metabolites were observed. The main analyses, using conditional logistic regression, were carried out among cases and controls who were HBsAg carriers. Four of the five AF biomarkers, but not AFG_1, were associated with an elevated risk for HCC among subjects in the highest tertile of exposure, although only for AFM_1 was this significant. The OR in the highest tertile of AFM_1 exposure, after adjustment for education, ethnicity, alcohol use, and smoking, was 6.0 (23 cases; 95% CI; range, 1.2 to 29). When pairs of these AF biomarkers were examined, certain combinations were found to be associated with particularly high risk: subjects with detectable AFB_1–N^7-guanine, and high levels of AFM_1 had an OR of 12 (16 cases; 95% CI; range, 1.2 to 117).

To investigate the role of HBV and AF in the etiology of liver cancer, Lu et al.[50] carried out a nested case-control analysis within a cohort of 737 male HBsAg carriers and 699 HBsAg noncarriers in Qidong, China (follow-up was from 1987 to 1997). Among the HBsAg carriers, 30 cases of liver cancer were matched for age and place of residence with 150 non-cases from the cohort. Level of AFB_1–albumin adducts were significantly higher among cases than among controls, both in proportion and in concentration. The crude OR was 3.5 (95% CI; 1.3 to 10).

Sun et al.[51] reported studies on 145 men with chronic hepatitis B infection in a cohort. These HBV-positive men had been detected in a prevalence survey carried out from 1981 to 1982 in two townships in Qidong, China. They were recruited for the follow-up study from 1987 to 1998. At recruitment, they were interviewed and examined; eight urine samples were obtained at monthly intervals and blood was drawn periodically throughout the follow-up period. The urine samples for each individual were pooled and AFM_1 was measured in the pooled sample. No patients were lost to follow-up. The mean age of the cohort was 39 years in 1998. Over the period of follow-up, 22 of the 145 subjects were diagnosed with liver cancer, of which 10 had pathological confirmation. Anti-HCV-positive subjects had an increased risk for HCC compared with subjects who were anti-HCV-negative, and subjects with a family history of HCC had an increased risk compared with subjects who did not have a family history of HCC. The median concentration of AFM_1 in urine was 9.6 ng/L, and the highest concentration was 243 ng/L. Using 3.6 ng/L as the cutoff point in the Cox proportional hazard model, the RR for HCC among subjects with high AFM_1 compared with those having low AFM_1 was 3.3 (95% CI; range, 1.2 to 8.9). When anti-HCV status and family history of HCC were also included in the model, the RR for HCC associated with AFM_1 was 4.5 (95% CI; range, 1.6 to 13).

Taken together, these epidemiological results provide the scientific basis for the reclassification of AF as a known human carcinogen. Biologically, the indication that hepatitis viruses and AF can act in a concerted fashion to increase cancer risk has been clearly shown; however, AF exposure in the absence of chronic HBV infection is also etiologically associated with liver cancer. These findings provide a compelling reason for increasing efforts both in HBV immunization programs and in the development of concerted programs to lower dietary AF exposure as means of lowering human cancer risk.

10.5 AFLATOXIN EXPOSURE AND MUTATIONS IN THE P53 TUMOR SUPPRESSOR GENE

The relationship between AF exposure and development of HCC is further high-lighted by the molecular target studies of the p53 tumor suppressor gene (TP53), the most common mutated gene detected in human cancers. Initial results came from two independent studies of TP53 mutations in HCC occurring in populations exposed to high levels of dietary AF and indicate high frequencies of G → T transversion, with clustering at codon 249.[52,53] In contrast, studies of TP53 mutations in HCCs from Japan and Western countries with little exposure to AF found no mutations at codon 249.[54] These studies provide a circumstantial linkage between this signature mutation of p53 and AF exposure in HCC from China and Southern Africa.

Since these early findings, numerous investigations to determine the frequency of TP53 mutations, in particular the prevalence of G → T transitions at codon 249, in populations with high and low levels of aflatoxin exposure have been conducted. Li et al.[55] analyzed samples from two areas of China and found that 9/20 (45%) HCCs from Qidong, an area of high AFB_1 exposure, had TP53 mutations, and all of these were codon 249 mutations. In contrast, in HCCs from Shanghai, an area of intermediate aflatoxin exposure, 3/18 (17%) cases had a TP53 mutation and only 1/3 (33%) was located in codon 249. All but one of the TP53 mutations determined in this study was in found cases positive for HBV infection. A recent study of the HCC cases from the same regions found 7/14 (50%) and 5/10 (50%) samples from Qidong and Shanghai, respectively, to have a TP53 mutation. Of these, 100% (7/7) and 60% (3/5), respectively, were codon 249 transversions.[56] Similar results have been reported for the TP53 mutation in liver tumors from Guangxi Province in China.[57] The observation of the codon 249 mutation in TP53 with AF exposure is not limited to only China. Senegal is another country that has an extremely high incidence of liver cancer and in which there is a high exposure to dietary aflatoxin. A study conducted on 15 HCC samples from this country detected 10 (67%) cases with a mutation at codon 249 of the TP53 gene, the highest frequency reported to date.[58]

Fujimoto et al.[59] examined HCC tissues obtained from two different areas in China: Qidong, where exposure to HBV and AFB_1 is high, and Beijing, where exposure to HBV is high but that of AFB_1 is low. They analyzed these tumor tissues for mutations in the TP53 gene and loss of heterozygosity for the TP53, Rb, and APC genes. The frequencies of mutation, loss, and aberration of the TP53 gene in 25 HCC specimens from Qidong were 60, 58, and 80%, respectively. The frequencies in 9 HCC specimens from Beijing were 56, 57, and 78%; however, the frequencies of G → T transversion at codon 249 in HCCs from Qidong and Beijing were 52 and 0%, respectively. These data show distinct differences in the pattern of TP53 mutations at codon 249 between HCCs in Qidong and Beijing and suggest that AFB_1 and/or other environmental carcinogens may contribute to this difference.

Aguilar et al.[60] examined the role of AFB_1 and TP53 mutations in HCCs and in normal liver samples from the United States, Thailand, and Qidong, China, where AFB_1 exposures are negligible, low, and high, respectively. The frequency of the AGG to AGT mutation at codon 249 parallels the level of AFB_1 exposure, which further supports the hypothesis that AF has a causative and probably early role in human hepatocarcinogenesis.

Results from experimental studies have also linked AF as a causative agent in the described TP53 mutations. As previously mentioned, AFB_1 exposure causes G → T transversion in bacteria and human cells. Puisieux et al.[61] found that AFB_1–epoxide can bind to the particular codon 249 of TP53 in a plasmid *in vitro*. Further study[62] examined the mutagenesis of codons 247 to 250 of the TP53 gene by rat liver microsome-activated AFB_1 in human HepG2 cells and found that AFB_1 preferentially induced the transversion of G → T in the third position of codon 249; however, AFB_1 also induced G → T and C → A transversion into adjacent codons, albeit at lower frequencies. Cerutti et al.[63] studied the mutability of codons 247 to 250 of TP53 with AFB_1 in human hepatocytes using the same strategy and found that AFB_1 preferentially induced the transversion of G → T in the third position of codon 249, generating the same mutation that is found in a large fraction of HCCs from regions of the world with AFB_1-contaminated food. These experimental results support a role for AFB_1 as an etiological factor for HCCs in heavily AFB_1-contaminated areas. Using the human TP53 gene in an *in vitro* assay, codon 249 has been shown to be a preferential site for formation of AFB_1–N^7-guanine adducts,[61] evidence consistent with a role for AF in the mutations seen in human tumors.

While the evidence for a role of AF in the incidence of codon 249 mutations in TP53 from the above studies is persuasive, the level of exposure to AF has been classified by factors such as geographic residence rather than measurement of AF exposure at the individual level. The limitations of this approach have been reviewed by Lasky and Magde.[64] Only a few studies have been conducted to date that measure both AF adduct levels and TP53 mutational status in HCC cases. The largest and most recent study to assess the relationship between the presences of AFB_1 adducts, HBV status and TP53 mutations was reported by Lunn and coworkers,[65] who investigated 105 HCC cases in Taiwan. Mutations in the TP53 gene were detected in 28% (29/105) of cases by single-strand conformation polymorphism and DNA sequencing, revealed that 12 of these were specific codon 249 mutations. Mutant TP53 protein was detected in 35% (37/105) of HCC cases by immunohistochemistry. AFB_1–DNA adducts were detected in 66% (69/105) of tumor tissues and were associated with TP53 DNA (OR = 2.9; $p = 0.082$) and protein mutations (OR = 2.9; $p = 0.054$) with only borderline significance. No statistically significant association between AFB_1–DNA adducts and codon 249 mutations was observed. All of the codon 249 mutations ($n = 12$) occurred in HBsAg-seropositive carriers, resulting in an OR of 10.0 ($p < 0.05$), suggesting that HBV may be involved in the selection of these mutations.

In a recent report, Jackson et al.[66] described the prospective detection of codon 249 mutations of TP53 in plasma of HCC patients using short oligonucleotide mass analysis. From a prospective cohort of 1638 high-risk individuals in Qidong, China, 16 liver cancer cases, diagnosed between 1997 and 2001, were selected on the basis of available annual plasma samples spanning the years before and after diagnosis. The codon 249 mutation was detected in plasma samples obtained after diagnosis in 7 of 15 cases (46.7%). The mutation was also detected in the plasma of 4 of 8 cases positive at the time of diagnosis at least 1 year and in one case 5 years prior to the diagnosis. The authors suggested that specific TP53 mutation measured in plasma may serve as early detection (prediagnosis) biomarkers for HCC.

In summary, studies of the prevalence of codon 249 mutations in HCC cases from patients in areas of high or low exposure to AF suggest that a G → T transition at the third base is associated with AF exposure, and *in vitro* data would seem to support this hypothesis. A majority of codon 249 mutations are found in patients with an HBV infection implicating an association. However, in comparisons of codon

249 mutations in regions of high HBV infection but varying levels of AFB_1 exposure, the mutation only occurs in areas of high AFB_1 exposure. HBV evidently plays an important role in mutagenesis, perhaps by causing preferential selection of cells harboring the mutation. The use of the codon 249 mutation as a marker of exposure to AF must be done with caution until evidence has been obtained from studies measuring both AFB_1 adducts and mutations in the same individual.

10.6 SUMMARY

Many epidemiological studies carried out in the past 20 years have been incorporated with the molecular analysis of the cancer gene targets, such as the p53 tumor suppressor gene, and AF-specific biomarkers, such as AFB_1–albumin adducts in serum and AFB_1–N^7–guanine and AFM_1 in urine. These studies have spurred the efforts to assess AF exposure and human liver cancer risks. Evidence drawn from these molecular epidemiological studies led to the classification of naturally occurring AF, as well as AFB_1, as group I human carcinogens by the IARC in 1993, a finding reaffirmed in 2002 based on the latest research data.

REFERENCES

1. Busby, Jr., W.F. and Wogan, G.N., Aflatoxins, in *Chemical Carcinogens*, 2nd ed., Searle, C.E., Ed., American Chemical Society, Washington, D.C., 1985, pp. 945–1136.
2. Wang, J.-S., Kensler, T.W., and Groopman, J.D., Toxicants in food: fungal contaminants, in *Nutrition and Chemical Toxicity*, Ioannides, C., Ed., John Wiley & Sons, New York, 1998, pp. 29–57.
3. Eaton, D.L. and Groopman, J.D., *The Toxicology of Aflatoxins: Human Health, Veterinary and Agricultural Significance*, Academic Press, New York, 1994, 544 pp.
4. Wogan, G.N., Aflatoxins as risk factors for hepatocellular carcinoma in humans, *Cancer Res.*, 52, 2114s–2118s, 1992.
5. Wang, J.-S. and Groopman, J.D., DNA damage by mycotoxins, *Mutation Res.*, 424, 167–181, 1999.
6. ACS, *Cancer Facts and Figures*, American Cancer Society, Atlanta, GA, 1995–2004.
7. Parkin, D., Pisani, P., and Ferlay, J., Estimates of the worldwide incidence of 18 major cancers in 1985, *Int. J. Cancer*, 54, 594–606, 1993.
8. Li, N.-D., Lu, F.-Z., Zhang, S.-W., Mo, R., and Sun, X.-D., Trends and prediction in malignant tumors mortality in past 20 years in China, *Chin J. Oncol.*, 19, 3–9, 1997.
9. Yu, S.Z., Primary prevention of hepatocellular carcinoma, *J. Gastroenterol. Hepatol.*, 10, 674–682, 1995.
10. Wang, J.-S., Huang, T., Su, J., Liang, F., Wei, Z., Liang, Y., Luo, H., Kuang, S.Y., Qian, G.S., Sun, G., He, X., Kensler, T.W., and Groopman, J.D., Hepatocellular carcinoma and aflatoxin exposure in Zhuqing village, Fusui County, People's Republic of China, *Cancer Epidemiol Biomarkers Prev.*, 10, 143–146, 2001.
11. Wang, J.-S., Qian, G.-S., Zarba, A., He, X., Zhu, Y.-R., Zhang, B.-C., Jacobson, L., Gange, S. J., Munoz, A., Kensler, T.W., and Groopman, J.D., Temporal patterns of aflatoxin–albumin adducts in hepatitis B surface antigen-positive and antigen-negative residents of Daxin, Qidong County, People's Republic of China, *Cancer Epidemiol. Biomarkers Prev.*, 5, 253–261, 1996.

12. Stoloff, L., Aflatoxin as a cause of primary liver-cell cancer in the United States: a probability study, *Nutr. Cancer*, 5, 165–186, 1983.

13. Groopman, J.D., Wang, J.-S., and Scholl, P.F., Molecular biomarkers for aflatoxin: from adducts to gene mutations to human liver cancer, *Can. J. Physiol. Pharmacol.*, 74, 203–209, 1996.

14. International Agency for Research on Cancer, Some naturally occurring substances: food items and constituents, heterocyclic aromatic amines and mycotoxins, in *Monographs on the Evaluation of Carcinogenic Risks to Humans*, Vol. 56, IARC Press, Lyon, 1993, pp. 245–395.

15. International Agency for Research on Cancer, Some traditional herbal medicines: mycotoxins, naphthalene and styrene, in *Monographs on the Evaluation of Carcinogenic Risks to Humans*, Vol. 82, IARC Press, Lyon, 2002, pp. 171–274.

16. Beasley, R., Hepatitis B virus: the major etiology of hepatocellular carcinoma, *Cancer (Phila.)*, 61, 1942–1956, 1988.

17. London, W.T., Evans, A.A., McGlynn, K., Buetow, K., An, P., Gao, L.-L., Lustbader, E., Ross, E., Chen, G.-C., and Shen, F.-M., Viral, host and environmental risk factors for hepatocellular carcinoma: a prospective study in Haimen City, China, *Intervirology*, 38, 155–161, 1995.

18. Evans, A.A., O'Connell, A.P., Pugh, J. C., Mason, W.S., Shen, F.-M., Chen, G.-C., Lin, W.-Y., Dia, A., M'Boup, S., Drame, B., and London, W.T., Geographic variation in viral load among hepatitis B carriers with differing risk of hepatocellular carcinoma, *Cancer Epidemiol. Biomarkers Prev.*, 7, 559–565, 1998.

19. International Agency for Research on Cancer, Hepatitis viruses, in *Monographs on the Evaluation of Carcinogenic Risks to Humans*, Vol. 59, IARC Press, Lyon., 1994, pp. 45–221.

20. Yeh, F.S., Yu, M.C., Mo, C.C., Luo, S., Tong, M.J., and Henderson, B.E., Hepatitis B virus, aflatoxins, and hepatocellular carcinoma in southern Guangxi, China, *Cancer Res.*, 49, 2506–2509, 1989.

21. Yuan, J.-M., Govindarajan, S., Henderson, B.E., and Yu, M.C., Low prevalence of hepatitis C infection in hepatocellular carcinoma (HCC) cases and population controls in Guangxi, a hyperendemic region for HCC in the People's Republic of China, *Br. J. Cancer*, 74, 491–493, 1996.

22. Wild, C.P. and Turner, P.C., The toxicology of aflatoxins as a basis for public health decisions, *Mutagenesis*, 17, 471–481, 2002.

23. Kensler, T.W., Qian, G.-S., Chen, J.-G., and Groopman, J.D., Translational strategies for cancer prevention in liver, *Nat. Rev. Cancer*, 3, 321–329, 2003.

24. Van Rensburg, S.J., Cook-Mozaffari, P., Van Schalkwyk, D.J., Van der Watt, J.J., Vincent, T.J., and Purchase, I.F., Hepatocellular carcinoma and dietary aflatoxin in Mozambique and Transkei, *Br. J. Cancer*, 51, 713–726, 1985.

25. Van Rensburg, S.J., Van Schalkwyk, G.C., and Van Schalkwyk, D.J., Primary liver cancer and aflatoxin intake in Transkei, *J. Environ. Pathol. Toxicol. Oncol.*, 10, 11–16, 1990.

26. Peers, F.G., Gilman, G.A., and Linsell, C.A., Dietary aflatoxins and human liver cancer: a study in Swaziland, *Int. J. Cancer*, 17, 167–176, 1976.

27. Peers, F., Bosch, X., Kaldor, J., Linsell, A., and Pluijmen, M., Aflatoxin exposure, hepatitis B virus infection and liver cancer in Swaziland, *Int. J. Cancer*, 39, 545–553, 1987.

28. Hatch, M.C., Chen, C.J., Levin, B., Ji, B.T., Yang, G.Y., Hsu, S.W., Wang, L.W., Hsieh, L.L., and Santella, R.M., Urinary aflatoxin levels, hepatitis B virus infection and hepatocellular carcinoma in Taiwan, *Int. J. Cancer*, 54, 931–934, 1993.

29. Omer, R.E., Bakker, M.I., Van't Veer, P., Hoogenboom, R.L.A.P., Polman, T.H.G., Alink, G.M., Idris, M.O., Kadaru, A.M.Y., and Kok, F.J., Aflatoxin and liver cancer in Sudan, *Nutr. Cancer*, 32, 174–180, 1998.

30. Campbell, T.C., Chen, J., Liu, C., Li, J., and Parpia, B., Nonassociation of aflatoxin with primary liver cancer in a cross-sectional ecological survey in the People's Republic of China, *Cancer Res.*, 50, 6881–6893, 1990.

31. Srivatanakul, P., Parkin, D.M., Jiang, Y.Z., Khlat, M., Kao-Ian, U.T., Sontipong, S., and Wild, C.P., The role of infection by *Opisthorchis viverrini*, hepatitis B virus, and aflatoxin exposure in the etiology of liver cancer in Thailand: a correlation study, *Cancer*, 68, 2411–2417, 1991.

32. Bulata-Jayme, J., Almero, E.M., Castro, C.A., Jardeleza, T.R., and Salamat, L., A case-control dietary study of primary liver cancer risk from aflatoxin exposure, *Int. J. Epidemiol.*, 11, 112–119, 1982.

33. Olubuyide, I.O., Maxwell, S.M., Hood, H., Neal, G.E, and Hendrickse, R.G., HBsAg, aflatoxins and primary hepatoxellular carcinoma, *Afr. J. Med. Med Sci.*, 22, 89–91, 1993.

34. Olubuyide, I.O., Maxwell, S.M., Akinyinka, O.O., Hart, C.A., Neal, G.E., and Hendrickse, R.G., HBsAg and aflatoxins in sera of rural (Igbo-Ora) and urban (Ibadan) populations in Nigeria, *Afr. J. Med. Med Sci.*, 22, 77–80, 1993.

35. McGlycnn, K.A., Rosvold, E.A., Lustbader, E.D., Hu, Y., Clapper, M.L., Zhou, T., Wild, C.P., Xia, X.-L., Baffoe-Bonnie, A., Ofori-Adjei, D., Chen, G.-C., London, W.T., Shen, F.-M., and Buetow, K.H., Susceptibility to hepatocellular carcinoma is associated with genetic variation in the enzymatic detoxification of aflatoxin B_1, *Proc. Natl. Acad. Sci. USA*, 92, 2384–2387, 1995.

36. Mandishona, E., MacPhail, A.P., Gordeuk, V.R., Kedda, M.A., Paterson, A.C., Rouault, T.A., and Kew, M.C., Dietary iron overload as risk factor for hepatocellular carcinoma in black Africans, *Hepatology*, 27, 1563–1566, 1998.

37. Omer, R.E., Verhoef, L., Van't Veer, P., Idris, M.O., Kadaru, A.M.Y., Kampaman, E., Bunschoten, A., and Kok, F.J., Peanut butter intake, GSTM1 genotype and hepatocellular carcinoma: a case-control study in Sudan, *Cancer Causes Control*, 12, 23–32, 2001.

38. McGlynn, K.A., Hunter, K., LeVoyer, T., Roush, J., Wise, P., Michielli, R.A., Shen, F.M., Evans, A.A., London, W.T., and Buetow, K.H., Susceptibility of aflatoxin B_1-related primary hepatocellular carcinoma in mice and humans, *Cancer Res.*, 63, 4594–4601, 2003.

39. Srivatanakul, P., Parkin, D.M., Khlat, M., Chenvidhya, D., Chotiwan, P., Insiriposng, S., L'Abbe, K.A., and Wild, C.P., Liver cancer in Thailand: a case control study of hepatocellular carcinoma, *Int. J. Cancer*, 48, 329–332, 1991.

40. Yu, S.Z., Huang, X.E., Koide, T., Cheng, G., Chen, G.C., Harada, K., Ueno, Y., Sueoka, E., Oda, H., Tashiro, F., Mizokami, M., Ohno, T., Xiang, J., and Tokudome, S., Hepatitis B and C virus infection, lifestyle and genetic polymorphisms as risk factors for hepatocellular carcinoma in Haimen, China, *Jpn. J. Cancer Res.*, 93, 1287–1292, 2002.

41. Yeh, F.S., Mo, C.C., and Yen, R.C., Risk factors for hepatocellular carcinoma in Guangxi, People's Republic of China, *Natl. Cancer Inst. Monogr.*, 69, 47–48, 1985.

42. Yeh, F.S. and Shen, K.N., Epidemiology and early diagnosis of primary liver cancer in China, *Adv. Cancer Res.*, 47, 297–329, 1986.

43. Qian, G.S., Yu, M.C., Ross, R., Yuan, J.M., Gao, Y.T., Wogan, G.N., and Groopman, J.D., A follow-up study of urinary markers of aflatoxin exposure and liver cancer risk in Shanghai, P.R.C., *Cancer Epidemiol. Biomarkers Prev.*, 3, 3–11, 1994.

44. Ross, R., Yuan, J.M., Yu, M., Wogan, G.N., Qian, G.S., Tu, J.T., Groopman, J.D., Gao, Y.T., and Henderson, B.E., Urinary aflatoxin biomarkers and risk of hepatocellular carcinoma, *Lancet*, 339, 943–946, 1992.

45. Kuang, S.-Y., Fang, X., Lu, P.-X., Zhang, Q.-N., Wu, Y., Wang, J., Zhu, Y.-R., Groopman, J.D., Kensler, T.W., and Qian, G.-S., Aflatoxin-albumin adducts and risk of hepatocellular carcinoma in residents of Qidong, People's Republic of China, *Proc. AACR*, 37, 1714, 1996.

46. Chen, C.J., Wang, L.Y., Lu, S.N., Wu, M.H., You, S.L., Zhang, Y.L., Wang, L.W., and Santella, R.M., Elevated aflatoxin exposure and increased risk of hepatocellular carcinoma, *Hepatology*, 24, 38–42, 1996.

47. Wang, L.Y., Hatch, M., Chen, C.J., Levin, B., You, S.L., Lu, S.N., Wu, M.H., Wu, W.P., Wang, L.W., Wang, Q., Huang, G.T., Yang, P.M., Lee, H.S., and Santella, R.M., Aflatoxin exposure and risk of hepatocellular carcinoma in Taiwan, *Int. J. Cancer*, 67, 620–625, 1996.

48. Sun, C.A., Wang, L.Y., Chen, C.J., Lu, S.N., You, S.L., Wang, L.W., Wang, Q., Wu, D.M., and Santella, R.M., Genetic polymorphisms of glutathione S-transferases M_1 and T_1 associated with susceptibility to aflatoxin-related hepatocarcinogenesis among chronic hepatitis B carriers: a nested case-control study in Taiwan, *Carcinogenesis*, 22, 1289–1294, 2001.

49. Yu, M.W., Lien, J.P., Chiu, Y.H., Santella, R.M., Liaw, Y.F., and Chen, C.J., Effect of aflatoxin metabolism and DNA adduct formation on hepatocellular carcinoma among chronic hepatitis B carriers in Taiwan, *J. Hepatol.*, 27, 320–330, 1997.

50. Lu, P., Kuang, S., Wang, J., Fang, X., Zhang, Q.N., Wu, Y., Lu, Z.H., and Qian, G.S., Hepatitis B virus infection and aflatoxin exposure in the development of primary liver cancer, *Zhonghua Yi Xue Za Zhi (Nat. Med. J. China)*, 78, 340–342, 1998.

51. Sun, Z., Lu, P., Cail, M.H., Pee, D., Zhang, Q., Ming, L., Wang, J., Wu, Y., Liu, G., Wu, Y., and Zhu, Y., Increased risk of hepatocellular carcinoma in male hepatitis B surface antigen carriers with chronic hepatitis who have detectable urinary aflatoxin metabolite M_1, *Hepatology*, 30, 379–383, 1999.

52. Bressac, B., Kew, M., Wands, J., and Ozturk, M., Selective G to T mutations of p53 gene in hepatocellular carcinoma from Southern Africa, *Nature*, 350, 429–431, 1991.

53. Hsu, I.C., Metcalf, R.A., Sun, T., Wesh, J.A., Wang, N.J., and Harris, C.C., Mutational hotspot in the p53 gene in human hepatocellular carcinomas, *Nature*, 350, 427–428, 1991.

54. Ozturk, M., P53 mutation in hepatocellular carcinoma after aflatoxin exposure, *Lancet*, 338, 1356–1359, 1991.

55. Li, D., Cao, Y., He, L., Wang, N.J., and Gu, J., Aberrations of p53 gene in human hepatocellular carcinoma from China, *Carcinogenesis*, 14, 169–173, 1993.

56. Rashid, A., Wang, J.-S., Qian, G.-S., Lu, P.-X., Hamilton, S.R., and Groopman, J.D., Genetic alteration in hepatocellular carcinomas: association between loss of chromosome 4q and p53 gene mutations, *Br. J. Cancer*, 80, 59–66, 1999.

57. Stern, M.C., Umbach, D.M., Yu, M.C., London, S.J., Zhang, Z.-Q., and Taylor, J.A., Hepatitis B, aflatoxin B_1, and p53 codon 249 mutation in hepatocellular carcinomas from Guangxi, People's Republic of China, and a meta-analysis of existing studies, *Cancer Epidemiol. Biomarkers Prev.*, 10, 617–625, 2001.

58. Coursaget, P., Depril, N., Chabaud, M., Nandi, R., Mayelo, V., LeCann, P., and Yvonnet, B., High prevalence of mutations at codon 249 of p53 gene in hepatocellular carcinomas from Senegal, *Br. J. Cancer*, 67, 1395–1397, 1993.

59. Fujimoto, Y., Hampton, L.L., Wirth, P.J., Wand, N.J., Xie, J.P., and Thorgeirsso, S.S., Alterations of tumor suppressor genes and allelic losses in human hepatocellular carcinomas in China, *Cancer Res.*, 54, 281–285, 1994.

60. Aguilar, F., Harris, C.C., Sun, T., Hollstein, M., and Cerutti, P., Geographic variation of p53 mutational profile in nonmalignant human liver, *Science*, 264, 1317–1319, 1994.

61. Puisieux, A., Lim, S., Groopman, J.D., and Ozturk, M., Selective targeting of p53 gene mutational hotspots in human cancers by etiologically defined carcinogens, *Cancer Res.*, 51, 6185–6189, 1991.
62. Aguilar, F., Hussain, S.P., and Cerutti, P., Aflatoxin B_1 induces the transversion of G → T in codon 249 of the *p*53 tumor suppressor gene in human hepatocytes, *Proc. Natl. Acad. Sci. USA*, 90, 8586–8590, 1993.
63. Cerutti, P., Hussain, P., Pourzand, C., and Aguilar, F., Mutagenesis of the H-ras protooncogene and the p53 tumor suppressor gene, *Cancer Res.*, 54, 1934s–1938s, 1994.
64. Lasky, T. and Magder, L., Hepatocellular carcinoma p53 G → T transversions at codon 249: the fingerprint of aflatoxin exposure?, *Environ. Health Perspect.*, 105, 392–397, 1997.
65. Lunn, R.M., Langlois, R.G., Hsieh, L.L., Thompson, C.L., and Bell, D.A., XRCC1 polymorphisms: effects on aflatoxin B_1–DNA adducts and glycophorin A variant frequency, *Cancer Res.*, 59, 2557–2561, 1999.
66. Jackson, P.E., Kuang, S.-Y., Wang, J.-B., Strickland, P.T., Munoz, A., Kensler, T.W., Qian, G.-S., Groopman, J.D., Prospective detection of codon 249 mutations in plasma of hepatocellular carcinoma patients, *Carcinogenesis*, 24, 1657–1663, 2003.

11 Risk of Exposure to and Mitigation of Effects of Aflatoxin on Human Health: A West African Example

Kitty F. Cardwell and Sara H. Henry

CONTENTS

11.1 INTRODUCTION

The purpose of this chapter is to examine the relative risk of exposure of different human populations to foodborne aflatoxins, the types of health impact that may be incurred by dietary exposure to aflatoxins, and possible strategies likely to mitigate risks to human health. Risk of exposure is examined in a global context comparing the risk of toxin exposure by levels of national socioeconomic development. The risk of exposure is then reexamined in the context of agroecology, distribution of toxigenicity of *Aspergillus flavus*, and social factors that influence food management practices. The effects of aflatoxin exposure on human health are explored in three sections: human disease and nutritional status, carcinogenicity, and child growth and development. The section concerning mitigation of the effects of aflatoxin on human health contrasts efficacy of regulation, food basket modification, and production-side agriculture intervention. It is concluded that the risk of hepatocellular carcinoma in developing countries, such as West Africa, may be addressed by vaccination for hepatitis B virus and other public health options. Young children in West Africa who are chronically exposed to aflatoxin in foods and who consume nutritionally deficient diets have been shown to be stunted and underweight, as measured by World Health Organization z-scores.

11.2 FACTORS INVOLVED IN HUMAN EXPOSURE TO AFLATOXIN

11.2.1 GLOBAL DISTRIBUTION: DEVELOPED vs. DEVELOPINg COUNTRIES

In developed countries, infrastructure exists for monitoring contaminant levels in foods and feeds. In developing countries and in poor rural agricultural communities, exposure to aflatoxins has been shown to occur as shown in Table 11.1.[24,22] Developed countries tend to have diverse and abundant food supplies and can divert aflatoxin-contaminated food or feed to other uses; for example, aflatoxin-contaminated corn can be fed to beef cows within the limits set by the U.S. Food and Drug Administration (FDA).[21] Developing countries may not have the choice of diverting contaminated foods away from human consumption, and the overall food-basket diversity tends to be low. When aflatoxin-vulnerable foods are the primary staple, the chance of chronic and deleterious exposure is much higher.[19] Developed country farmers have more options to adopt agronomic practices that reduce aflatoxin contamination in crops including choice of crop variety, possible crop rotation, planting density, weed control, nitrogen fertilization, insect control, irrigation to minimize drought stress, use of mechanized drying as opposed to field drying, and provision of dry, pest-free crop storage facilities.[3] Regardless of the economic status of a country, aflatoxin contamination varies markedly with seasons due to climatic conditions, and when ideal conditions occur even advanced management techniques may not suffice to prevent contamination.

Estimating population exposure to aflatoxins is difficult. Classical methods of measuring food consumption include short-term-recall, daily recording of food items

TABLE 11.1
Estimated Population Exposures Based on Analysis of Aflatoxins in Food

Country	Sampling Period	Food Source[a]	Range of Estimated Aflatoxin Exposure ($\mu g/kg/day$)[b]	Ref.
Kenya	1969–1970	H	3.5–14.8	51
Swaziland	1972–1973	H	5.1–43.1	40
	1982–1983	H	11.4–159	52
Mozambique	1969–1974	P	38.6–183.7	64
Transkei	1976–1977	P	16.5	64
The Gambia	1988	P	4–115	68
China (southern Guangxi)	1978–1984	M	6.5–53	59
Thailand	1969–1970	P	66.5–53	59

[a] H, uncooked food samples from the home; P, samples of cooked food; M, samples from the market.
[b] AFB_1, except Kenya (B_1 and B_2) and The Gambia (B_1, B_2, G_1, G_2).

consumed; food-frequency questionnaires; and analysis of food intake by weighing food before consumption. These are then combined with laboratory analyses of levels of mycotoxins in food samples to ascertain relative exposure rates for individuals. These methods are not easy to apply even in developed countries but are particularly difficult to utilize in poor, rural agricultural communities.[24] In general, more data on human exposure to aflatoxins are available from developed than from developing countries. Hall and Wild[28] summarized estimates of population exposure to aflatoxins based on analysis of food from several developing countries (Table 11.1).

In most developed countries, aflatoxin levels in human food are regulated at a low parts-per-billion ($\mu g/kg$) range because of concerns about the potent hepato-carcinogenicity of aflatoxin B_1.[53,37] In developing countries, although Codex standards are statutory laws in most countries, mechanisms to effect compliance are not in place. Except in developing countries where public awareness programs are attempted, consumers may be unaware that they are being exposed to high levels of mycotoxins in their staple diets.[8]

11.2.2 REGIONAL DISTRIBUTION: AGROECOSYSTEM INFLUENCE

Climatic and edaphic factors, agricultural management systems, insect pest pressure, and food processing customs are all factors in risk of aflatoxin accumulation in foods. The most vulnerable crops are maize (*Zea mays*), groundnut (*Arachid hypogaea*), and tree nuts The risk of aflatoxin contamination is a function of several factors, including:

- Presence of toxigenic fungus in the soil[9,10,14–16]
- Soil infertility[26,41,63]
- Drought stress
- *Striga*, a parasitic weed; crop diseases, particularly vascular disease[41]

- Insect damage[27,41,57,58]
- Excessive heat during kernel development[48]
- Delayed harvest[26,63]
- Harvest and postharvest damage to kernel or grain[41]
- Sanitation and management of harvested produce[26,63]
- Dry down and moisture in storage[26,27]
- Postharvest insect feeding[27]

In agroecosystems with one or more of the risk factors, crops are likely to contain aflatoxin, increasing the potential for human exposure.

11.2.2.1 Temperate Zones

In cool temperate zones, including Canada and much of Europe, the risk of aflatoxin contamination of indigenous food supplies is very low.[37] *Aspergillus flavus* grows with higher temperatures and less available water than most other fungi,[35] making it more competitive in these conditions than other fungi.[38] In cooler climates and mid-altitudes, other fungi such as *Fusarium* spp. are more likely to occur than *Aspergillus* spp.[47] In warm, drought-prone zones of the United States, such as the Southeast, Arkansas, Texas, and Oklahoma, problems of aflatoxin contamination sporadically occur in maize, groundnut, and pistachio nut (*Pistacio vera*), primarily in drought years (Table 11.2). Maize is particularly severely affected in the southern United States when nighttime temperatures are high and kernel integrity is breached.[48] As can be seen in Table 11.2, which is based on FDA data, levels of aflatoxins in shelled maize designated for human consumption that is grown in the Corn Belt or elsewhere in the United States generally are lower than levels in maize grown in the Southeast, Arkansas, Texas, or Oklahoma.

Table 11.2
Aflatoxins in Shelled Maize Designated for Human Consumption in Differing Geographic Regions of the United States[70–73]

Area	Year	Total Number of Products Examined	Percent of Products >1 µg/g Aflatoxins (%)	Percent of Products >20 µg/g Aflatoxins (%)	Maximum Value (µg/g)
Southeast	1992	53	20.7	11.3	82
Corn belt		114	12.3	0.0	17
Arizona, Oklahoma, and Texas		35	17.1	5.7	77
Rest of United States		37	2.7	2.7	34
Southeast	1995	23	8.7	0.0	4
Corn belt		113	0.9	0.0	8
Arizona, Oklahoma, and Texas		44	20.4	4.5	681
Rest of United States		18	0.0	0.0	0

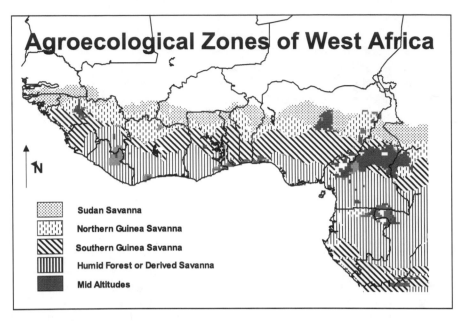

FIGURE 11.1 Agroecological zones of West Africa. West and central Africa are characterized by a range of agroecologies. Starting at the coast there is either humid forest or derived savanna mosaic with high rainfall. Progressing north, rainfall decreases gradually, giving rise to the Southern Guinea Savanna (moist savanna) and the Northern Guinea savanna (moist to dry savanna). Above the northern Guinea savanna, the transition to the Sahara is a very dry zone called the Sudan savanna. Maize is produced in all of these zones. We asked the question: "Is the maize in any agroecological zone more predisposed to aflatoxin contamination?"

Africa typifies the risk factors for aflatoxin that occur in different agroecologies in the tropics (Figure 11.1). Across all of sub-Saharan Africa is a range of ecologies, from desert to deep, humid tropics and cool mid-altitudes. West and central Africa have a gradient of agroecologies ranging from very humid forest and coastal savanna in the south to arid savannas bordering the Sahara desert in the north, with mid-altitude highlands regions of Nigeria and Cameroon.[26,47,63] These agroecosystems have a range of climatic conditions, cropping systems, storage practices, and food consumption patterns.[8,19,23,26,47,63] The risk of aflatoxin contamination and human exposure through consumption of contaminated foods is different in each of these agroecosystems. The conditions for risk of commodity contamination can be extrapolated to other tropical regions, while crop management practices, food processing, and consumption patterns may vary when taken on a larger geographic scale.

11.2.2.2 Humid Tropics

The humid coastal savanna and humid forested areas of West and central Africa are characterized by a bimodal rainfall distributed over 9 months and the possibility of multiple growing cycles in a year. Maize is the dominant crop, and some groundnuts are produced. Several factors in these ecologies could lead to high toxin levels;

however, in several studies,[19,26,47,63] this has not been the case. Very low amounts of aflatoxin were found in stored maize in Nigeria,[63] Benin,[26] and Cameroon.[47] In Benin, this finding was confirmed in a study of blood albumin–aflatoxin adducts in young children. Some of the lowest exposure levels seen were in the humid coastal savannas of those countries.[22,67,68] In the contiguous countries of Cameroon, Nigeria, Benin, Togo, and Ghana, humid-zone maize is sown with the first rains (first season); it is generally harvested early and eaten as "green" maize. What little mature maize is harvested is eaten as quickly as possible because storing the crop safely is very difficult. It is rare for maize to be planted in the second cropping season because lepidopteran stem borers increase to the point where yield losses are too high to make maize worthwhile to plant.[5,63]

In most countries, groundnuts are not grown in coastal and forest areas, although some nongovernmental organization programs promote them as a source of dietary protein. In Benin and Togo, people in the humid coastal savannas eat groundnuts on average 1.4 days a week.[19] In these regions, alternate foods, particularly plantain (*Plantago major* L.), root, and tuberous crops, are the locally produced primary staples. It is also possible that adequate rainfall in these zones makes crops less susceptible to invasion by *Aspergillus flavus*, but they are more likely to be infected with *Fusarium* mycotoxins.[47]

Southern Guinea Savanna (SGS) is moist grassland or derived forest, also with a 9-month rainy season. In the SGS, continuous maize planting is common, beginning with the first rains in May until mid-September. Soil fertility levels are typically low, and pre- and postharvest insect pressure is high.[27,57] The first harvest often falls within a short but unpredictable break in the rains in August. It is common for maize in this zone to be harvested with a 20-μg/g grain moisture and then be put in storage structures designed to facilitate grain drying.[27,63] These structures are traditionally constructed of woven natural materials on conical raised platforms and covered with a thatched roof. They provide good natural aeration that allows the grain to dry to about 14 μg/g.[26] Insect feeding and concomitant rehumidification of the grain are common in these structures.[27,58] Aflatoxin has been detected in up to 50% of grain samples drawn from these stores, with AFB_1 concentrations ranging from 0 to 500 μg/kg.[26] Egal et al.[19] found that 93% of household maize samples in Benin and Togo were infested with an average of over 1000 colony-forming units of *Aspergillus flavus*. In that study, aflatoxin–albumin blood levels in children in the SGS of Benin and Togo were the highest levels seen across the agroecological zones. Maize was consumed on average 6.6 days a week, while groundnut was consumed as a snack 4.5 days of the week.[19] In this type of agroecology, the risk of chronic dietary exposure to aflatoxin is high.

Rainfall in Northern Guinea Savanna (NGS), extending from 9° latitude north, begins in June and ends in November. Maize and groundnut are prevalent in the cropping systems. In Nigeria, this zone is the most developed for agriculture, where maize hybrid seed technology and fertilizer use are highest. Udoh et al.[63] found the maize aflatoxin levels in this zone in Nigeria to be low; however, in Benin and Togo, where crop management systems are less developed, this zone was similar to the SGS in grain aflatoxin concentration[10,26] and frequency and CFU levels of *Aspergillus flavus* found in foods.[19] In the NGS, farmers have the problem of fitting maize production into a 6-month rainy season. Most tropical lowland maize cultivars mature in 100 to 120 days, so multiple plantings are possible, although drying of early harvests is very difficult. It is common to find maize, groundnuts, and cotton inter-cropped and rotated on the same land. This zone also is subject to insect pressure in the field and in storage.[27,57] Maize is consumed 5.6 days a week, groundnuts 2.6 days. In this zone, it was found that wealthier households had higher blood aflatoxin albumin adduct levels. These were associated with more purchase and consumption of groundnut as a snack;[19] therefore, this type of agroecology also has conditions conducive to chronic foodborne aflatoxin exposure.

Sudan savanna (SS) typifies arid tropical and subdesert savannas where maize is intercropped with sorghum (*Sorghum bicolor*) and millet (*Pennisetum glaucum*) and where the majority of groundnuts are grown. This zone is characterized by a short rainfall period lasting from July to September and high temperatures. Generally one crop a year can be grown, making storage and commerce of cereal and legume grains practical. Stored crops must last from one harvest to the next. Although the storage conditions are dry and subject to low insect pressure, growing conditions are often poor, with temperature and drought stress common. Drought stress is one of the most important factors in aflatoxin formation in both maize and groundnuts.[66] The condition of the crop going into storage and the general condition of the bin itself are critical for maintaining good food quality.[26] In this zone in some countries, farmers shock maize and dry it in sheaves in the field. Hell et al.[26] and Udoh et al.[63] found that field-dried maize was of poorer quality and had more insect damage and a higher risk of aflatoxin contamination. A common practice in West Africa is to thresh maize in the field, thereby letting it come directly into contact with the soil. Weathered and exposed grain goes into clay bins covered by thatched roofs for up to 12 months. Even a slight wetting will result in mold growth and toxin production. High toxin levels can be found in foods in this zone.[8,10] Maize is consumed 5.7 days a week, groundnuts 4.8 days.[19]

11.2.2.3 Mid-Altitudes

Agroecological zones 800 m and more above sea level tend to have very low aflatoxin contamination in maize.[47,63] This is presumably because of cooler climate and less stressful conditions during production and storage; however, *Fusarium* species and associated toxins have been shown to be prevalent under these conditions.[47]

In summary, in parts of sub-Saharan Africa and similar agroecologies in other parts of the world where food basket options are limited, the chances for chronic dietary exposure to unsafe levels of aflatoxin are high. Figure 11.2 shows the zones in Africa that are at high risk of aflatoxin exposure, as well as the zones in which greater exposure to *Fusarium* toxins would be expected.

11.2.3 DISTRIBUTION OF *ASPERGILLUS FLAVUS* STRAINS

Diversity in the population of *Aspergillus flavus* exists with respect to toxin produc-tion and sclerotial size.[1,14] S-strain (those producing small sclerotia) isolates in the United States produce high amounts of aflatoxin B only, while S strains from Africa

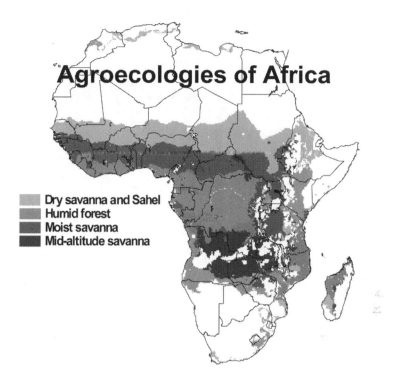

FIGURE 11.2 Agroecologies of Africa. The agroecological zones that are most predisposed to aflatoxin contamination are the moist and dry savannas. Cool areas and mid-altitudes are more likely to see *Fusarium* toxins than aflatoxins. International Institute of Tropical Agriculture (IITA) stations show where sampling has been conducted. A large part of sub-Saharan Africa is comprised of moist to dry savannas that have the right conditions for the development of aflatoxins.

and Thailand produce both aflatoxins B and G consistently in high amounts.[15,29] L strains (with large sclerotia) on both continents produce a range of aflatoxin B from none to very high. In both the United States and West Africa, S-strain isolates are relatively more likely to be found in dryer ecologies.[11,16] In West Africa, as agroecology transitions from wetter to dryer from south to north, S-strain *A. flavus* became more prevalent relative to the L strain in field soils[9,11] and in maize and groundnuts.[19] Although most white maize samples were infested with *A. flavus*, the percentage of samples containing *A. flavus* CFUs decreased significantly from north to south for both L and S strains. The average sample in the north contained more S-strain CFUs than in the south, while samples in the center contained more L-strain CFUs than samples in the north and south.[11,16]

11.2.4 SOCIAL SYSTEM AND FOOD BASKET

Social factors such as education and access to disposable income determine food sanitation and the variety of foods in the household diet. One aspect of developed

TABLE 11.3
U.S. Peanut Butter and Tree Nuts Examined for Aflatoxins[70–73]

Product	Year	Total Number of Products Examined	Percent of Products >1 µg/kg Aflatoxins (%)	Percent of Products >20 µg/kg Aflatoxins (%)	Maximum Value (µg/kg)
Peanut butter	1992	82	22.0	0.0	9
	1995	70	41.0	0.0	18
Peanuts, shelled, roasted	1992	89	9.0	2.2	31
	1995	82	7.3	0.0	5
Peanuts, in-shell, roasted	1992	19	0	0.0	0
	1995	5	0.0	0.0	0
Almonds	1992	55	1.8	0.0	11
	1995	36	5.6	0.0	3
Pecan	1992	66	1.5	0.0	2
	1995	55	7.3	0.0	15
Pistachio	1992	18	5.5	0.0	2
	1995	11	9.0	0.0	5
Walnut	1992	51	5.9	2.0	87
	1995	44	15.9	6.8	44

Note: FDA action levels for total aflatoxins are 20 µg/kg in all products, except milk designated for humans, and 0.5 µg/kg AFM_1 in milk and milk products. In animal feeds, the levels are 20 µg/kg in corn and peanut products for immature animals and dairy cattle; 100 µg/kg in corn and peanut products for breeding beef cattle, swine, and nature poultry; 200 µg/kg in corn and peanut products for finishing swine; 300 µg/kg in corn and peanut products for finishing beef cattle, 300 µg/kg of cottonseed meal as a feed ingredient; and 20 µg/kg for all other feedstuffs.

economies is access to a broad array of consumer options. In these social systems, an inexpensive, abundant, and safe food supply is considered a human right. Food safety is a public concern and is managed through regulation and consumer education. Monitoring of vulnerable commodities in the United States shows that these foods are not highly contaminated; therefore, even frequent consumers are not exposed to high levels of aflatoxin (Table 11.3).

In developing countries, public sector management of food safety issues is not a given, leaving the majority of food-related issues to individual consumer and farmer awareness. Access to a broader array of foods is also lacking, leaving the majority of the caloric intake of the population coming from one or two principal staples. Presumably, protective food preparation would be a learned behavior and therefore might be expected to be practiced by people with greater access to information and education. Also, in developing countries, it would be expected that households with higher economic status might have more access to a variety of foods and greater tolerance for removing and disposing of damaged grain, thereby lowering the overall aflatoxin exposure levels relative to less well-off neighbors. These hypotheses were tested in a series of villages in West Africa by Egal et al.[19]

In West Africa within ecozones the consumption frequency of maize was stable across socioeconomic lines, consumed at a comparable frequency by rich and poor, educated and illiterate. The association between maize consumption and aflatoxin exposure in this study by Egal et al.[19] was especially strong. Aflatoxin exposure was assessed by measuring aflatoxin–albumin (AF-alb) adducts in peripheral blood; these adducts reflect consumption of toxin over the preceding 2 to 3 months. AF-alb blood adducts increased in children as parts per billion of aflatoxin ($\mu g/kg$) and CFU levels of *Aspergillus flavus* in the household stores of maize and groundnuts rose. An increasing frequency of consumption correlated to increased AF-alb adduct levels in children under 5. In Benin, the average child consumed maize 6.2 days a week preceding the survey. Children in the southern half of Benin and Togo (CS and SGS) had a higher consumption frequency than children in the north (NGS and SS). The traditional diet in the SS includes millet and sorghum as cereal staples, with maize being produced for market, but maize is the most important crop under cultivation in the other zones. In the SS, where maize consumption frequency was low relative to the other zones, children of educated mothers consumed less maize, perhaps because other foods might be more preferred by well-educated mothers.

In the study by Egal et al.,[19] the importance of groundnut consumption as a source of aflatoxin exposure was less obvious. Great variation in the frequency of consumption of groundnuts was seen. Groundnuts were consumed fresh, as roasted nuts, as cookies, and as groundnut oil used to prepare food. In the week preceding the survey, the average child consumed groundnuts 3.4 days a week. Regional differences were considerable; the average consumption frequency in the SS and SGS was threefold higher than in the coastal savanna, where climate is unfavorable for groundnut production (respectively, 4.7 and 1.4 days a week). With the exception of the SS, the frequency of consumption increased as household and maternal economic status went up. The bulk of production of groundnuts takes place in the SS; in this area, it appears that disposable income is not as important a factor in influencing consumption. In the SGS, maternal education was another factor causing variation in frequency of intake. Maternal education was associated with more frequent consumption of groundnuts among children in this region, where nongovernmental organizations have promoted groundnut consumption as an inexpensive and effective way to reduce protein energy malnutrition (kwashiorkor). It is possible that educated mothers have put this message to practice more than uneducated mothers.

11.2.5 ASSOCIATION OF AFLATOXIN EXPOSURE WITH DISEASES AND DISORDERS

11.2.5.1 Human Disease and Nutritional Status

Extensive reviews of the effects of aflatoxin exposure on human health have been published.[69] Maize consumption had already been identified as a health hazard in earlier studies focusing on the outbreak of hepatitis associated with the consumption of high levels of aflatoxin in India and Kenya,[36,46] and numerous studies have linked consumption of contaminated groundnuts to liver cancer.[32]

11.2.5.2 Carcinogenicity

Aflatoxins are among the most potent mutagenic and carcinogenic substances known in sensitive species. The acute toxicity of aflatoxin B_1, the most toxic of the aflatoxins, varies from a LD_{50} of 0.34 μg/kg in 1-day-old Pekin ducklings to >150 μg/kg in the CFW Swiss mouse. Chronic exposure to aflatoxins is an efficient method of inducing hepatocellular cancer (HCC); in the sensitive species F344 rats, two cycles each of 5 days' duration with administration of 25 μg AFB_1 each day to young (approximately 100-g) rats produced preneoplastic foci 2 to 3 months after dosing. Hepatic cancers arose after about 1 year, and a small incidence (about 12%) arose about 23 months after dosing.[55]

Because the metabolism and toxicokinetics of aflatoxins are not clearly understood, sensitivity differences between species to the effects of aflatoxins cannot be fully explained. Differences in P-450 isoform activities, due either to genetic polymorphisms or to environmental alteration in expression, may be important contributors. Glutathione S-transferase detoxification is a crucial factor in susceptibility to AFB_1 toxicity.[42]

Human hepatocarcinomas (HCC) are common in some developing countries, particularly China, Southeast Asia, and sub-Saharan Africa, and are relatively common in Japan and some Mediterranean Basin countries. HCC is rare in the Americas and Northern Europe. Pockets of high-risk populations have been described in the Amazonian basin, among Eskimos, and in special populations such as renal transplant patients. The incidence of HCC is two to three times higher in men than in women.[28,33]

A growing body of evidence points to a synergistic relationship between aflatoxins and hepatitis B (and possibly C) virus in the etiology of human HCC (Table 11.4). Most of the available epidemiological studies, including data on aflatoxin exposure, have been done in high-risk countries, where both HBV and aflatoxin are prevalent. Because the nature of the interaction between low doses of aflatoxin and HBV is not understood, extrapolation of human HCC risks from these areas to those where both HBV and aflatoxin exposures are less common is very difficult.[28,33] Although Table 11.4 may be regarded as a simplification of complex epidemiologic data, it is clear that risk factors for human liver cancer vary between Europe and the United States and Africa and Asia; hence, considerations of the risks of liver cancer in these areas must necessarily be different, as will be discussed later.

11.2.6 Growth Suppression/Immunotoxicity

11.2.6.1 Growth and Immune Suppression in Animals

Several studies have shown aflatoxins to be immunomodulatory in domestic and laboratory animals at doses in the mg/kg range.[4,24] Cell-mediated immunity (CMI) is suppressed, and delayed-type hypersensitivity is impaired. In addition, nonspecific humoral substances are suppressed, antibody formation is reduced, allograft rejection is suppressed, phagocytic activity is decreased, and blastogenic response to mitogens is decreased.[43] Maternal dietary exposure to AFB_1 during gestation and lactation

TABLE 11.4
Liver Cancer Etiology: Attributable Fractions
in Europe/United States and Africa/Asia

Risk Factor	Europe and United States	Africa and Asia
Hepatitis B	<15% (4–50%)	60% (40–90%)
Hepatitis C	60% (12–64%)	<10%
Aflatoxin	Limited or none	Not quantified
Tobacco	<15%	Not estimated
Alcohol	<12%	29% (one study)
Oral contraceptives	10–50%	Not estimated
Others including hemochromatosis	<5%	<5%

Source: JECFA, *Safety Evaluation of Certain Food Additives*, WHO Food Additive Series 40, Joint FAO/WHO Expert Committee on Food Additives, International Program on Chemical Safety, World Health Organization, Geneva, 1998.

affected the immune system of developing pigs.[60] Because aflatoxins impair both cellular and humoral immune systems, sensitive animals are more susceptible to bacterial, viral, fungal, and parasitic diseases.[43] Studies in poultry have indicated that immune competence is compromised when feeds contain about 100 μg/kg aflatoxin.[17] By comparison, the levels shown to be affecting the immune system in poultry are similar to those levels in the food of 30% of Gambian children.[61]

11.2.6.2 Growth Suppression in Humans

In a cross-sectional study of 480 children in West Africa (Benin and Togo), Gong et al.[22] showed a highly significant relationship between AF-alb serum adducts and growth faltering in children under 5. Aflatoxin was detected in 99% of the children sampled. Children with stunting or who were underweight had 30 to 40% higher mean AF-alb concentrations. The negative correlation between individual AF-alb concentration and each of the three growth parameters (height for age z-score, weight for age z-score, and weight for height z-score) was highly significant. A clear dose–response relationship was observed between AF-alb concentration and height for age and weight for age z-scores. The effect was most acute at the time of weaning children from breast milk onto solid foods (primarily maize porridge).[23] It could not be determined from the cross-sectional design of the study whether the mechanism of interaction between aflatoxin exposure and impaired growth was the result of aflatoxin toxicity or reflected consumption of fungus-affected food of poor nutritional quality. Underweight children are more susceptible to chronic disease and are more likely to die early.[31]

In Gambia, season of birth has been associated with altered morbidity and mortality (frequently infection-related) in adulthood.[44] Aflatoxins are prevalent in the population's food supply, but seasonal variations occur in the level of food contamination and exposure to aflatoxin. These interactions were further studied by

Turner et al.[62] In this study, 472 Gambian children ages 6 to 9 years born during a 5-year maternal dietary supplementation trial were the subjects. In rural Gambia, season can strongly influence both adult's and children's nutritional status. Weight loss occurs in pregnant and lactating women and birth weight is reduced 200 to 300 g during the annual wet season from July to November (the hungry season) relative to other seasons. Maternal dietary supplementation can reduce this difference. Turner et al.[62] studied levels of AF-alb, micronutrients levels, and a number of immune tests reflecting T-cell, B-cell, and mucosal secretion as measured by the CMI test, vaccine response, and level of secreted immunoglobulin A (IgA) in the saliva of these children. AF-alb was detected in 93% of the children, and the level was strongly associated with month of sampling. sIgA was markedly lower in children with detectable AF-alb levels compared with those with nondetectable levels. Antibody response to one of four pneumococcal serotypes, but not rabies vaccine, was weakly associated with high levels of AF-alb. No association between CMI response to test antigens and AF-alb was found. Seasonal variations in a number of micronutrients, such as vitamin C, alpha- and beta-carotene, and lycopene were observed. These variations reflected periods from January to May, when citrus fruits and mangos were available, and from September to October, when more green leafy vegetables were available. The only association with AF-alb was a negative correlation with vitamin C. A weak association between adduct level and wasting was observed, but none for stunting or being underweight. These children were older than those observed in the Gong et al.[22] study; younger children may be more sensitive to the growth-inhibitory effects of aflatoxin. Also, levels of AF-alb were higher in the children in Benin and Togo. These studies emphasize the need to further investigate the relationships among growth, immunocompetence, and aflatoxin exposure, especially in highly aflatoxin-exposed populations of children.

11.3 RISK MITIGATION

11.3.1 EFFICACY OF SAMPLING PROTOCOLS AND REGULATORY ACTION LEVELS

One method of reducing risk of exposure to foodborne aflatoxin is effective monitoring and exclusion of contaminated lots; however, sampling objectives differ. The level of accuracy and precision and the risk of sampling error within a sampling protocol must be defined and understood. The highest precision is required if one is expecting to consistently detect low μg/kg occurrence in a large lot of commodity for regulatory purposes. The degree of accuracy should not depend on the contamination level. The same accuracy can be maintained by sampling asymptotically more units from a sampling universe as the contamination level decreases. This is especially true for aggregated problems such as *Aspergillus flavus* toxins. The distribution of aflatoxin in stored grains is not uniform, and only a small portion of the grains may contain very high quantities of the toxin.[12] The U.S. Department of Agriculture recommends 24 kg of peanut and 2- to 5-kg samples of maize, sorghum, and other grains to determine the average aflatoxin distribution in a lot.[65] Coker[12] compared various sampling procedures used in the United States, United Kingdom, and The Netherlands. These plans are based upon the probability of rejection of a lot or sample using operating curves predicated on probability of positive detection with increased concentration of toxin per commodity. In the large-scale market operating paradigm, the use of statistics weighing the mean/variance ratio guides the size and number of samples required to minimize false-positive and -negative results.

In small-scale traditional agriculture systems, sampling procedures or sample analysis limitations for aflatoxin are problematic. To obtain a 10-pound sample from a village granary, small-scale marketer, or household food basket is often impossible in developing countries. Coker[12] presents a sampling plan for problematic commodities based on a Weibull function with an acceptable level of aflatoxin as the driving function variable. This procedure would still require the collection of 6 1-kg samples, and 3 to 6 sample analyses per sample. In addition to the physical limitation on sample size, most developing country laboratories have very limited operational budgets, so the number of sample analyses will be restricted. These limitations require consideration if the intent is to protect the consumer by monitoring vulnerable foods in dispersed, small-scale systems. This is where an honest assessment is required as to what levels of exposure are important and are especially crucial if low contamination levels are important.

To assess the risk of exposure in African villages, Egal et al.[19] were able to collect 100-g samples of maize and groundnut from the family larder. Predictably, the detection of aflatoxin-positive samples was low in these small samples; however, in this work, the amount of aflatoxin (µg/kg) and CFUs of *Aspergillus flavus* in the food were highly correlated with blood toxin levels in children from the household where the sample was taken. Although detection of aflatoxin contamination of maize and groundnuts was infrequent (less than 10%), up to 90% of the maize and 58% of the groundnut samples were infested with *A. flavus*. Presence of the fungus may be a more reliable indicator for risk assessments of foodborne exposure. It also may be possible to turn the equations around so an estimate of exposure could be calculated from a limited sample size and number, based on the likelihood of presence of toxin when the fungus is present. It would not be an exact measure, as is required for market regulation, but it would help to understand public health impact.

Another aspect of the sampling and standards question is illustrated by the work of Otsuki et al.[49] at the World Bank. He attempted to quantify the impact of a European Union aflatoxin standard of 2 µg/kg on food exports from Africa. This case, as discussed below, is a good example of the trade-offs between acceptable levels of risk, relationships between international trading partners, and perspectives of developed vs. developing countries.

In 1998, the Joint FAO/WHO Expert Committee on Food Additives (JECFA) estimated that implementing a 10-µg/kg standard (total aflatoxin) would lead to a risk of 39 cancer deaths per year per billion people, with an uncertainty range between 7 and 164 people. This estimate assumed a European population with 1% carriers of hepatitis B and an aflatoxin carcinogenic potency equal to 0.3 death per year per 100,000 carriers of HBV and 0.01 cancer death per year per 100,000 population among noncarriers.

The Middle East and Africa export many of their products to Western Europe; hence, these areas are likely to be significantly affected by regulations set in European import markets. Based on the JECFA analysis, Otsuki et al.[49] estimated that the proposed EU standard would impose a considerable loss of export revenue from cereals, edible nuts, and dried and preserved fruits in African countries. Maximum allowable aflatoxin levels in Europe range from 1 to 20 $\mu g/kg$, while in Africa the average is 44 $\mu g/kg$. African export revenue was estimated to decrease by 59% for cereals and 47% for dried and preserved fruits and edible nuts. This is a difference of approximately US$400 million. Otsuki et al.[49] illustrated the burden of the cost of compliance with WTO obligations in the least developed countries by noting that these costs can exceed total government budgets for all expenditures.

A risk reduction of 2.3 deaths per billion per year would be achieved in the European Union under the proposed 2-$\mu g/kg$ aflatoxin standard, according to the estimates of Otsuki et al. This estimated reduction of liver cancer is small compared to the total number of deaths of liver cancer in the European Union. The World Health Organization has estimated that about 33,000 people die from liver cancer every year in the European Union (population of .5 billion). Epidemiological studies would not even be able to measure reliably this small reduction in liver cancer cases.

11.3.2 CANCER RISK REDUCTION

An overwhelming body of data across species has demonstrated the potency of AFB_1 as a carcinogen and mutagen.[32] The best evidence indicating an interaction between hepatitis B virus (HBV) and aflatoxin in human liver cancer has come from a cohort study in Shanghai, China, involving more than 18,000 men.[54,56,74] Assays for urinary AFB_1, its metabolites AFP_1 and AFM_1, DNA adducts, and hepatitis B surface antigen (HBsAg) status have been undertaken. Subjects with liver cancer were significantly more likely than controls to have detectable concentrations of the aflatoxin compounds. Positivity for HBsAg was strongly associated with liver cancer risk. Thus, aflatoxin exposure in the presence of a persistent HBV infection increases the risk of human liver cancer.[28]

Such factors as unknown genetic and host response interactions may play a role in the liver cancer/HBV/AFB interaction.[28,33] Evans et al.[20] compared three independent cohorts of male HBsAg carriers in Senegal, in Haimen City, China, and among HBsAg carriers in the United States (largely Asian origin). The risk of liver cancer in China (878 per 100,000 person-years [py]) was dramatically higher than in Senegal (68 per 100,000 py) or among United States HBV carriers (330 per 100,000 py). The prevalence of HBsAg was only moderately higher in Senegal (20% vs. 16%) than in China, and the level of aflatoxin exposure was expected to be higher in the African setting.

Vaccination for HBV has been shown to drastically reduce liver cancer risk in some populations. JECFA[34] has recommended that vaccination for HBV must take high priority in preventing HCC. There are many HBV carriers (approximately 360 million worldwide). In addition, about 110,000 cases of HCC cases yearly worldwide have been attributed to hepatitis C virus infection (HCV). Access to HBV vaccine is incomplete, especially in developing countries; no vaccine is available for HCV as yet.

The experience of Korea in reducing adult liver cancer by vaccination for HBV is an excellent example of vaccination importance. The prevalence of HBV infection and HCC is high (about 21 per 100,000); aflatoxin contamination is relatively high. In 370,000 males followed for more than 3 years, HBV vaccination drastically reduced HCC (incidence of 215 cases/100,000 vs. 8 cases/100,000).[39] This reduction in HCC cases was accomplished without any additional resources being expended on reducing aflatoxins in the food supply and without any change in aflatoxin regulations.

In Taiwan, an area of hyperendemic infection and moderate to high aflatoxin exposure, the immunization program against HBV reduced the rate of liver cancer in children 6 to 14 years of age from 0.7 per 100,000 between 1981 and 1986 to 0.57 between 1986 and 1989, and then to 0.36 from 1990 to 1994[33]. Because the incidence of liver cancer peaks in the sixth decade of life in Taiwan, at least 40 years may be required to see an overall decrease in the rate of liver cancer as a result of the vaccination program.

Both these populations should be followed in future years to further elucidate the relationship among aflatoxin, liver cancer, and HBV. These studies lend support to the hypothesis that the carcinogenic potency of aflatoxin may be reduced in humans by vaccination for HBV, as pointed out by JECFA.[33] The possibility should be considered that in the case of liver cancer scarce public health resources in developing countries may better be used for HBV vaccination programs (and thereby reduce incidence of liver cancer) than to lower aflatoxin levels to those required in the European Union. However, the effects of chronic exposure to relatively high levels of aflatoxins on growth and development of children should also be considered, and cost-effective methods to monitor and mitigate this exposure are needed.

11.3.3 AGRICULTURAL MANAGEMENT

The best way to avoid the negative effects of aflatoxin on public health and economies, is to limit or reduce the contamination of foods in the first place. Numerous intervention points exist in the process of food production, from preharvest through harvest and storage to food processing and preparation. Crop and harvest management have been extensively treated in many fora.[26,27,41,63] Some effective management practices, such as efficient drying, can reduce toxic contamination of foods wherever they are deployed. Other management practices are more specific to small-scale production systems. For example, in northern Nigeria, maize is shocked, dried, and thrashed to shell the ears in the field, bringing grain in direct contact with soils.[63] It was shown that this practice considerably increased the chance of aflatoxin contamination. Changing this practice could lower the risk, but no single practice can reduce aflatoxin-contamination risk to zero. The extent to which effective management modifications can be implemented is determined by agroecology and economies of scale. Technologies such as host plant resistance and biological control can be scale neutral. The following is not an exhaustive treatment of all possible intervention strategies, but presents some possibilities of biological control and host plant resistance technologies that have not yet been extensively deployed.

In the United States, biological control has been used to reduce aflatoxin contamination in various crops such as cotton,[14] groundnut,[13] and maize.[6,18] This technique involves the application to soil of a non-aflatoxigenic biological control strain of *Aspergillus flavus* or *A. parasiticus,* resulting in a high population density that allows the biological control strain to effectively compete with the native aflatoxigenic strains during invasion under conditions favorable for aflatoxin contamination. Invasion of a seed in soil (e.g., groundnut) solely by the biological control agent would be expected because of its high density relative to the wild-type strain in the soil. This would result in less aflatoxin contamination. For maize and cottonseed, the high population of the non-aflatoxigenic biological control strain in soil produces abundant spores on the soil surface that become airborne to infect grains and seeds.[30]

The potential to reduce aflatoxin contamination in maize using the biological control tactics mentioned above has been evaluated in Benin, where 90% of the aspergilli are *A. flavus*.[11] The non-aflatoxigenic strains of *A. flavus* (BN22 from Benin and AF36 from the United States) were tested against aflatoxigenic strains of *A. flavus* (BN40 from Benin and AF13 from the United States) and *A. parasiticus* (BN48) *in vitro*.[2,9] All non-aflatoxigenic isolates significantly reduced toxin production by the African *A. parasiticus* isolate BN48. *In vitro*, the American non-aflatoxigenic isolate AF36 was effective against the American aflatoxigenic isolate AF13 but not the aflatoxigenic African S-strain BN40, suggesting that there may be specificity of action of some non-aflatoxigenic strains. The African non-aflatoxigenic L-strain BN30 was the only isolate that reduced toxin production by the highly aflatoxigenic African S-strain BN40. BN30 was also very effective in reducing the amount of toxin produced in maize in the field when coinoculated with the highly toxic S strain.[2] Selected non-aflatoxigenic strains specific for different agroecozones need to be identified and tested in large areas.

This technology has a potential to remove aflatoxin from foods grown in high-risk environments. The additional benefit of this technology is that it would reduce aflatoxin levels in maize, groundnuts, and cotton, where these crops are intercropped and rotated. It would not eliminate the causal fungi from the commodities but would only reduce direct impact by toxic contamination. Additionally, the logistics of deployment are a challenge, requiring a concerted effort by governments, industry, and the international development sector.[21]

Host resistance and genetic engineering are the technologies that would give the most easily deployable solution if and when aflatoxin or fungal resistances are found. Plant breeders have been using traditional techniques for over 25 years to try to develop plant cultivars that are resistant to aflatoxin. Progress has been made in maize,[6] but it is open to discussion as to whether traditional plant breeding will ever provide sufficient resistance to be a solution in and of itself.

New genetic tools, however, may provide important new advances in plant genetic engineering for resistance. Engineering of maize and cotton to reduce lepidopteran damage is expected to bring concomitant parallel benefits of reduced mycotoxin contamination;[45] however, insect vectoring is not the only mechanism of ingress of the fungus, so insect control is only one factor in reducing contamination levels.[7,50]

It may eventually be possible to engineer plants for reduced fungal ingress and survival by inserting genes for antifungal compounds or aflatoxin blockers. A West

African inbred maize line was found to support fungal infection, but with little aflatoxin formation.[6] Other resistance mechanisms such as resistance to the infection process and resistance to environmental stresses[66] may be available to build into maize to reduce aflatoxin development in the field.

In the case of developing countries where maize is a primary staple food, with few options for food-basket diversification, it may be necessary to rethink the paradigm of how to breed for increased resistance. Often, to increase yield, breeders have selected for increased kernel size.[7] This tends to increase susceptibility to silk-cut[48] and other types of pericarp and testa breaks, facilitating ingress of *Aspergillus flavus*. An alternative strategy, particularly for tropical agroecologies, would be to increase yield by increasing kernel density and number but not kernel size. The advantage of this would be improved postharvest process, reduced damage during shelling, quicker drying, increased postharvest insect resistance, etc. The importance of reducing susceptibility in food crops cannot be overstated.

11.4 CONCLUSIONS

Codex standards for aflatoxins in foods were put in place because of the possible carcinogenicity of aflatoxins as observed in animal models and in geographic correlations of risk of liver cancer with probability of foodborne exposure. The most recent epidemiology has cast some doubt on the relative importance of aflatoxin as an independent causal factor in human liver cancer. Reducing aflatoxin levels in foods by regulation may not be the most effective means to reduce risk of human liver cancer. In a 1998 analysis of liver cancer, aflatoxin, and hepatitis B, JECFA stated, "The carcinogenic potency of aflatoxin in HbsAg-negative individuals is substantially higher than the potency in HBsAg-positive individuals. Thus, reduction of the intake of aflatoxin in populations with a high prevalence of HbsAg-negative individuals will have greater impact on reducing liver cancer rates than reduction in populations with a low prevalence of HBsAg-negative individuals." This study further indicated that "populations with a low prevalence of HbsAg-positive individuals and/or with a low mean intake of aflatoxin (less than 1 μg/kg bw) are unlikely to exhibit detectable differences in population risks for standards in the range of 10 to 20 μg/kg." Therefore, JECFA has recommended that developing countries could effectively lower liver cancer incidence by vaccinating for HBV. The development of a global alliance for vaccines and immunization is a hopeful beginning.[24]

The macroeconomic consequence of high child morbidity and mortality on a country more than overshadows the costs of surveillance and crop management practices to reduce risk of exposure to aflatoxins. Child survivorship and developmental health are cornerstones of stable population growth and economic development. The studies by Gong et al.[22,23] revealed a striking association between exposure to aflatoxin and both stunting and being underweight in children in West Africa. Given the immunotoxicity of aflatoxin in animal models,[53] aflatoxin may have the potential to suppress immune system development in human children as well. In the West African study, 99% of the children tested were positive for serum–aflatoxin adducts. These observations emphasize the need to develop strategies to monitor for and reduce exposure to aflatoxin, possibly involving interventions targeted at the postweaning period in African children.[22,23]

Given the exposure risk in much of Africa and given the effect of exposure on human health, particularly child development, the risk mitigation options must be carefully weighed. The bottom line is that liver cancer may not be the only important public health effect of aflatoxin. Evidence is accumulating that aflatoxin effects on child growth in developing countries, such as West Africa, in populations chronically exposed to high levels of aflatoxin may be equally important to overall public health. Regulatory standards for aflatoxins are justified and should be extended to countries not currently in compliance, but these must be accompanied by the research and development in the agricultural sector to ensure a food supply that is not contaminated. The protection offered by the regulatory standards in developing countries has to be balanced against the loss of contaminated crops to human food and the loss of export income.

Current regulatory action levels for aflatoxins in developed countries are offering adequate protection from liver cancer as a well as protecting child development and growth. If current regulatory standards are lowered in developed countries, the impact of this action on developing countries should be considered in the context of global public health and the global economy. The high cost of the current regulatory monitoring methods is the single most important factor driving noncompliance in Africa. The result is not only loss in trade but also the inability to monitor exposure risk and target appropriate policy and management solutions. Research is needed to develop inexpensive, scale-adjusted monitoring protocols.

REFERENCES

1. Bayman, P. and Cotty, P.J., Genetic diversity in *Aspergillus* flavus: association with aflatoxin production and morphology, *Can. J. Botany*, 71, 23–24, 1993.
2. Bandyopadhyay, R. and Cardwell, K.F., Species of *Trichoderma* and *Aspergillus* as biological control agents against plant diseases in Africa, in *Biological Control in Integrated Pest Management Systems in Africa*, Neuenschwander, P., Borgemeister, C., and Langewald, J., Eds., CAB International, Wallingford, 2003.
3. Bilgrami, K.S. and Choudhary, A.K., Mycotoxins in preharvest contamination of agricultural crops, in *Mycotoxins in Agriculture and Food Safety*, Sinha, K.K. and Bhatnagar, D., Eds., Marcel Dekker, New York, 1998, pp. 1–43.
4. Bondy, G.S. and Pestka, J.J., Immmunomodulation by fungal toxins, *J. Toxicol. Environ. Health*, 83, 109–143, 2000.
5. Bosque-Pérez, N.A. and Schulthess, F., Maize: West and Central Africa, in *African Cereal Stem Borer: Economic Importance, Taxonomy, Natural Enemies and Control*, Polaszek, A., Ed., CAB International, Wallingford, 1998, pp. 11–24.
6. Brown, R.L., Chen, Z.-Y., Menkir, A., Cleveland, T.E., Cardwell, K., Kling, J., and White, D.G., Resistance to aflatoxin accumulation in kernels of maize inbreds selected for ear rot resistance in west and central Africa. *J. Food Prot.*, 64, 396–400, 2001.
7. Cardwell, K.F., Kling, J.G., Maziya-Dixon, B., and Bosque-Perez, N., Interactions between *Fusarium verticillioides*, *Aspergillus flavus* and insects in improved maize populations in lowland Africa, *Phytopathology*, 90, 276–284, 2000.

8. Cardwell, K.F., Mycotoxin contamination in foods in Africa: antinutritional factors, *Food Nutr. Bull.*, 21, 488–493, 2000.

9. Cardwell, K.F. and Cotty, P.J., Interactions among U.S. and African *Aspergillus* spp. strains: influence on aflatoxin production, *Phytopathology*, 90, 11, 2000.

10. Cardwell, K.F., Desjardins, A.E., Henry, S.M., Munkvold, G., and Robens, J., Mycotoxins: the cost of achieving food security and food quality, APSNet, August 2001 (http://www.apsnet.org/online/feature/mycotoxin/top.html).

11. Cardwell, K.F. and Cotty, P.J., Distribution of *Aspergillus* section *Flavi* among field soils from the four agroecological zones of the Republic of Benin, West Africa, *Plant Dis.*, 86, 434–439, 2002.

12. Coker, R.D., Design of sampling plans for determination of mycotoxins in foods and feeds, in *Mycotoxins in Agriculture and Food Safety*, Sinha, K.K. and Bhatnagar, D., Eds., Marcel Dekker, New York, 1998, pp. 1-43109–1-43133.

13. Cole, R. and Dorner, J.W., Biological control of aflatoxin and cyclopiazonic acid contamination of peanuts, in *Mycotoxin Contamination: Health Risk and Prevention Project*, Kumagai, S. et al., Eds., Japanese Association of Mycotoxicology, Tokyo, 2000, pp. 70–73.

14. Cotty, P.J., Bayman, P., Egel, D.S., and Elias, K.S., Agriculture, aflatoxins, and *Aspergillus*, in *The Genus Aspergillus: From Taxonomy and Genetics to Industrial Applications*, FEMS Symposium No. 69, Powell, K.A., Renwick, A., and Peabody, J.F., Eds., Plenum Press, New York, 1994, pp. 1–27.

15. Cotty, P.J. and Cardwell, K.F., Divergence of West African and North American communities of *Aspergillus* section *Flavi*, *Appl. Environ. Microbiol.*, 65, 2264–2266, 1999.

16. Cotty, P.J., Aflatoxin-producing potential of communities of *Aspergillus* section *Flavi* from cotton producing areas in the United States, *Mycol. Res.*, 101, 698–704, 1997.

17. Coulombe, R.A., Non-hepatic disposition and effects of aflatoxin B_1, in *The Toxicology of Aflatoxins: Human Health, Veterinary and Agricultural Significance*, Eaton, D.A. and Groopman, J.D., Eds., Academic Press, San Diego, CA, 1993, pp. 89–98.

18. Dorner, J.W., Cole, R.J., and Wicklow, D.T., Aflatoxin reduction in corn through field application of competitive fungi, *J. Food Prot.*, 62, 650–656, 1999.

19. Egal, S., Hounsa, A., Gong, Y.Y., Turner, P.C., Wild, C.P., Hall, A.J., and Cardwell, K.F., Dietary exposure to aflatoxin from maize and groundnut in young children from Benin and Togo, West Africa, *Int. J. Food Microbiol.*, 2005 (in press).

20. Evans, A.A., O'Connell, A.P., Puch, J.C., Mason, W.S., Shen, F., Chen, B.-C., Lin, W.-Y., Dia, A., M'Boup, S., Dramé, B., and London, W.T., Geographic variation in viral load among hepatitis B carriers with differing risks of hepatocellular carcinoma, *Cancer Epidemiol. Biomarkers Prev.*, 7, 559–565, 1998.

21. FDA, *Action Levels for Aflatoxin in Animal Feeds*, Compliance Policy Guides (CPG) 7126.33 (section 683.100), CPG 7106.10 (section 527.400), CPG 7120.26 (section 555.400), U.S. Food and Drug Administration, Rockville, MD, 1996.

22. Gong, Y.Y., Cardwell, K.F., Hounsa, A., Egal, S., Turner, P.C., Hall, A.J., and Wild, C.P., Dietary aflatoxin exposure and impaired growth in young children from Benin and Togo: cross-sectional study, *Br. Med. J.*, 325, 20–21, 2002.

23. Gong, Y.Y., Hounsa, A., Egal, S., Turner, P.C., Hall, A.J., Cardwell, K., and Wild, C.P., Determinants of aflatoxin exposure in young children from Benin and Togo, West Africa: the critical role of weaning, *Int. J. Epidemiol.*, 35, 566–562, 2003.

24. Hall, A.J. and Wild, C.P., Epidemiology of alfatoxin related disease, in *The Toxicology of Aflatoxins*, Eaton, D.L. and Groopman J.D., Eds., Academic Press, San Diego, CA, 1994, pp. 233–258.

25. Hall, A.J. and Wild, C.P., Liver cancer in low and middle income countries [editorial], *Br. Med. J.*, 326, 994–995, 2003.

26. Hell, K., Cardwell, K.F., Setamou, M., and Poehling, H.-M., The influence of storage practices on aflatoxin contamination of maize in four agroecological zones of Benin, west Africa, *J. Stored Products Res.*, 36, 365–382, 2000.

27. Hell, K., Cardwell, K.F., Setamou, M., and Schulthess, F., Influence of insect infestation on aflatoxin contamination of stored maize in four agroecological regions in Benin, *Afr. Entomol.*, 8, 169–177, 2000.

28. Henry, S.H. and Bosch, F.X., Foodborne disease and mycotoxin epidemiology, in *Foodborne Disease Handbook*, 2nd ed., Hui, Y.H., Smith, R.A., and Spoerke, Jr., D.G., Eds., Marcel Dekker, New York, 2001.

29. Hesseltine, C.S., Shotwell, O., Smith, M., Ellis, J.J., Vandegraft, E., and Shannon, G., Production of various aflatoxins by strains of the *Aspergillus flavus* series, in *Proc. U.S.–Japan Conference on Toxic Microorganisms*, M. Herzberg, Ed., U.S. Government Printing Office, Washington, D.C., 1970. pp 202–210.

30. Horn, B.W., Greene, R.L., Sorensen, R.B., Blankenship, P.D., and Dorner, J.W., Conidial movement of nontoxigenic *Aspergillus flavus* and *A. parasiticus* in peanut fields following application to soil, *Mycopathologia*, 151, 81–92, 2001.

31. Hunt, J., Agricultural research as a public investment, *Food Nutr. Bull.*, 21, 562, 2000.

32. IARC, Some naturally occurring substances: food items and constituents, heterocyclic aromatic amines and mycotoxins, in *IARC Monographs on the Evaluation of Carcinogenic Risks of Chemicals to Humans*, No. 56, International Agency for Research on Cancer, Lyon, 1993, pp. 245–395.

33. JECFA, *Safety Evaluation of Certain Food Additives*, WHO Food Additive Series 40, Joint FAO/WHO Expert Committee on Food Additives, International Program on Chemical Safety, World Health Organization, Geneva, 1998.

34. JEFCA, *Evaluation of Certain Mycotoxins in Food: Estimates of M_1 in Diet in Various Parts of the World*, Joint FAO/WHO Expert Committee on Food Additives, International Program on Chemical Safety, World Health Organization, 2002, pp. 1–54.

35. Klich, M.A., Tiffany, L.H., and Knaphus, G., Ecology of the aspergilli of soils and litter, in Aspergillus: *Biology and Industrial Applications*, Bennett, J.W. and Klich, M.A., Eds., Butterworth-Heineman, Stoneham, MA, 1992, pp. 327–351.

36. Krishnamachari, K.A., Bhat, R.V., Nagarajan, V., and Tilak, T.B.G., Hepatitis due to aflatoxicosis: an outbreak in western India, *Lancet*, i, 1061–1063, 1975.

37. Kuiper-Goodman, T., Prevention of human mycotoxicoses through risk assessment and risk management, in *Mycotoxins in Grains: Compounds Other Than Aflatoxin*, Miller, J.D. and Trenholm, H.L., Eds., Eagan Press, St. Paul, MN, 1994, pp. 439–469.

38. Lacey, J., Aspergilli in feeds and seeds, in *The Genus* Aspergillus: *From Taxonomy and Genetics Industrial Applications*, Powell, K.A., Renwick, A., and Peberdy, J.F, Eds., Plenum Press, New York, 1994, pp. 73–92.

39. Lee, M.-S., Kim, D.-H., Kim, H.-S., Kim, C.-Y., Park, T.-S., Yoo, K.-Y., Park, B.-J., and Ahn, Y.-O., Hepatitis B vaccination and reduced risk of primary liver cancer among male adults: a cohort study in Korea, *Int. J. Epidemiol.*, 27, 316, 1998.

40. Linsell, C.A. and Peers, F.G., Aflatoxin and liver cell cancer, *Trans. R. Soc. Trop. Med. Hyg.*, 71, 471–473, 1977.

41. Lopez-Garcia, R. and Park, D.L., Effectiveness of postharvest procedures in management of mycotoxin hazards, in *Mycotoxins in Agriculture and Food Safety*, Sinha, K.K. and Bhatnagar, D., Eds., Marcel Dekker, New York, 1998, pp. 407–435.

42. Massey, T.E., Stewart, R.K., Daniels, J.M., and Liu, L., Biochemical and molecular aspects of mammalian susceptibility to aflatoxin B_1 carcinogenesis, *Proc. Soc. Exp. Biol. Med.*, 208, 213–227, 1995.

43. Miller, D.M. and Wilson, D.M., Veterinary diseases related to aflatoxins, in *The Toxicology of Aflatoxins: Human Health, Veterinary, and Agricultural*, Eaton, D. and Groopman, J., Eds., Academic Press, San Diego, CA, 1994, pp. 347–367.

44. Moore, S.E., Cole, T.J., Collinson, A.C., Poskitt, E.M.E., McGregor, I.A., and Prentice, A.M., Prenatal or early postnatal events predict infectious deaths in young adulthood in rural Africa, *Int. J. Epidemiol.*, 28, 1088–1095, 1999.

45. Munkvold, G.P., Mycotoxins in corn: occurrence, impacts, and management, in *Corn Chemistry and Technology*, 2nd ed., White, P. and Johnson, L., Eds., American Association of Cereal Chemists, St. Paul, MN, 2003.

46. Nagindu, A., Johnson, B.K., Kenya, P.R., Ngira, J.A., Ooheng, D.M., Nandwa, H., Omunid, T.N., Jansen, A.J., Ngare, W., Kaviti, J.N., Gatei, D., and Siongok, T.A., Outbreak of acute hepatitis caused by aflatoxin poisoning in Kenya, *Lancet*, i, 1346–1348, 1982.

47. Ngoko, Z., Marasas, W.F.O., Rheeder, J.P., Shephard, G.S., Wingfield, M.J., and Cardwell, K.F., Fungal infection and mycotoxin contamination of maize in the humid forest and the western highlands of Cameroon, *Phytoparasitica*, 29, 352–360, 2001.

48. Odvody, G.N., Spencer, N., and Remers, J.A., Description of silk cut, a stress-related loss of kernel integrity in preharvest maize, *Plant Dis.*, 81, 439–444, 1997.

49. Otsuki, T., Wilson, J.S., and Sewadeh, M., Saving two in a billion: quantifying the trade effect of European food safety standards on African exports, *Food Policy*, 26, 495–514, 2001.

50. Payne, G., Process of contamination by aflatoxin-producing fungi and their impact on crops, in *Mycotoxins in Agriculture and Food Safety*, Sinha, K.K. and Bhatnagar, D., Eds., Marcel Dekker, New York, 1998, pp. 270–307.

51. Peers, F. and Linsell, A., Dietary aflatoxins and liver cancer, *Br. J. Cancer*, 27, 473–484, 1973.

52. Peers, F., Bosch, X., Kaldor, J., Linsell, A., and Pluijment, M., Aflatoxin exposure, hepatitis B virus infection, and liver cancer in Swaziland, *Int. J. Cancer*, 39, 545–553, 1987.

53. Pestka, J.J. and Bondy, G.S., Immunotoxic effects of mycotoxins, in *Mycotoxins in Grains: Compounds Other Than Aflatoxin*, Miller, J.D. and Trenholm, H.L., Eds., Eagan Press, St. Paul, MN, 1994, pp 339–359.

54. Qian, G.-S., Ross, R.K., Yu, M.C., Yuan, J.-M., Gao, Y.-T., Henderson, B.E., Wogan, G.N., and Groopman, J.D., A follow-up study of urinary markers of aflatoxin exposure and liver cancer in Shanghai, People's Republic of China, *Cancer Epidemiol. Biomarkers Prev.*, 3, 3–10, 1994.

55. Roebuck, B.D. and Maxuitenko, Y.Y., Biochemical mechanisms and biological implications for the toxicity of aflatoxin as related to aflatoxin carcinogenesis, in *The Toxicology of Aflatoxins*, Eaton, D.L. and Groopman, J.D., Eds., Academic Press, San Diego, CA, 1994, p. 529.

56. Ross, R.K., Yuan, J.-M., Yu, M.C., Wogan, G.N., Qian, G.-S., Tu, J.T., Groopman, J.D., Gao, Y.-T., and Henderson, B.E., Urinary aflatoxin biomarkers and risk of hepatocellular carcinoma, *Lancet*, 339, 943–946, 1992.

57. Setamou, M., Cardwell, K.F., Schulthess, F., and Hell, K., *Aspergillus flavus* infection and aflatoxin contamination of preharvest maize in Benin, *Plant Dis.*, 81, 1323–1327, 1997.

58. Setamou, M., Cardwell, K.F., Schulthess, F., and Hell, K., Effect of insect damage to maize ears, with special reference to *Mussidia nigrivenella* on *Aspergillus flavus* infection and aflatoxin production in maize before harvest in the Republic of Benin, *J. Econ. Entomol.*, 91, 433–438, 1998.

59. Shank, R.C., Gordon, J.E., Wogan, G.N., Nondasuta, A., and Subhamani, B., Dietary aflatoxins and human liver cancer. III. Field survey of rural Thai families for ingested aflatoxins, *Food Cosmet. Toxicol.*, 10, 501–507, 1972.

60. Silvotti, L., Petterino, C., Bonomi, A., and Cabassi, E., Immunotoxicological effects of maternal aflatoxin exposure in weaned piglets, *Vet. Rec.*, 141, 469–472, 1997.

61. Turner, P.C., Mendy, M., Whittle, H., Fortuin, M., Hall, A.J., and Wild, C.P., Hepatitis B infection and aflatoxin biomarker levels in Gambian children, *Trop. Med. Int. Health*, 5, 837–841, 2000.

62. Turner, P.C., Moore, S.E., Hall, A.J., Prentice, A.M., and Wild, C.P., Modification of immune function through exposure to dietary aflatoxin in Gambian children, *Environ. Health Perspect.*, 111(2), 217–220, 2003.

63. Udoh, J.M., Ikotun, I.O., and Cardwell, K.F., Storage structures and aflatoxin content of maize in five agroecological zones of Nigeria, *J. Stored Products Res.*, 36, 187–201, 2000.

64. Van Rensburg, S.J., Cook-Mozaffari, P., Van Schalkwyk, D.J., Van der Watt, J.J., Vincent, T.J., and Purchase, I.F., Hepatocellular carcinoma and dietary aflatoxin in Mozambique and Transkei, *Br. J. Cancer*, 51, 713–726, 1985.

65. Whitaker, T.B., Dickens, J.W., and Monroe, R.J., Variability associated with testing corn for aflatoxin, *J. AOCS*, 56, 789–794. 1979.

66. Wicklow, D.T., Preharvest origins of toxigenic fungi in stored grain, in *Proc. 6th Int. Working Conf. on Stored Product Protection, Canberra, Australia*, Highley, E., Wright, E.J., Banks, H.J., and Champ, B.R., Eds., CAB International, Wallingford, 1994, pp. 1075–1081.

67. Wild, C.P., Jiang, Y.Z., Sabbioni, G., Chapot, B., and Montesano, R., Evaluation of methods for quantitation of aflatoxin–albumin adducts and their application to human exposure assessment, *Cancer Res.*, 50, 245–251, 1990.

68. Wild, C.P., Hudson, G.J., Sabbiono, G., Chapot, B., Hall, A.J., Wogan, G.N., Whittle, H., Montesano, R., and Groopman, J.D., Dietary intake of aflatoxins and the level of albumin-bound aflatoxin in peripheral blood in The Gambia, West Africa, *Cancer Epidemiol. Biomarkers Prev.*, 1, 299–234, 1992.

69. Wild, C.P. and Hall, A.J., Epidemiology of mycotoxin-related disease, in *The Mycota. VI. Human and Animal Relationships*, Miller, H., Ed., Springer-Verlag, Berlin, 1996, pp. 213–225.

70. Wood, G.E., Aflatoxins in domestic and imported foods and feeds, *J. Assoc. Off. Anal. Chem.*, 72, 543, 1989.

71. Wood, G.E., Mycotoxins in foods and their safety ramifications, in *Food Safety Assessment*, Finley, J.W., Robinson, S.F., and Armstrong, D.J., Eds., ACS Symp. Series 484, American Chemical Society, Washington, D.C., 1992, p. 261.

72. Wood, G.E., Mycotoxins in foods and feeds in the United States, *J. Animal Sci.*, 70, 3941, 1992.

73. Wood, G.E. and Trucksess, M.W., Regulatory control programs for mycotoxin-contaminated food, in *Mycotoxins in Agriculture and Food Safety*, Sinha, K.K. and Bhatnagar, D., Eds., Marcel Dekker, New York, 1998, pp. 459–481.

74. Yuan, J.M., Ross, R.K., Stanczyk, F.Z., Govindaragan, S., and Gao, Y.-T., A cohort study of serum testosterone and hepatocellular carcinoma in Shanghai, China, *Int. J. Cancer*, 6, 4991–4493, 1995.

12 Advances in Sampling and Analysis for Aflatoxins in Food and Animal Feed

John Gilbert and Eugenia A. Vargas

CONTENTS

12.1 INTRODUCTION

The analysis of aflatoxins was first carried out more than 30 years ago using thin-layer chromatography (TLC). Despite significant advances in instrumentation, particularly the use of high-performance liquid chromatography (HPLC) for aflatoxin analysis, for many laboratories TLC still remains attractive. TLC is a simple, low-cost, and robust technique and is still routinely used by those in developing countries. The imposition of regulations for aflatoxins in foods and feed has provided the drive to improve analytical methods and extend validation, particularly in the European Union,[1,2] where strict controls have been introduced for aflatoxin B_1 at low ng/g levels in cereals, nuts, dried fruit, and spices and for aflatoxin M_1 at 0.05 ng/L in milk. At the same time, much innovation has occurred in terms of developing rapid methods for monitoring commodities at various stages in agricultural production which are required if preventative measure are to be successfully implemented.

A number of recent reviews have covered analytical methodology for determining aflatoxins in foods[3] and more specifically rapid methods,[4] TLC methods,[5] and HPLC with fluorescence detection.[6] Some reviews have specifically dealt with formal validation of analytical methods for mycotoxins in foods and feeds.[7] In this review, we have tried to take a holistic approach to assessing advances in determining aflatoxins. The review thus includes instrumental methods, rapid screening approaches, and confirmatory techniques and also covers sampling, which cannot be separated from the analytical determinations. We have compiled recent information on methods for determining aflatoxins in a wide variety of matrices and have not only assessed performance from the standpoint of formal validation but also included information on in-house validation. This review is limited to papers that have been published from 1995 onward, although where appropriate some earlier reviews are referenced.

12.2 SAMPLING PLANS AND SAMPLING DEVICES

The importance of sampling is generally recognized, as is the fact that meaningful results can only be obtained if representative samples are taken and properly homogenized prior to subsampling for analysis. Despite this recognition, sampling is still much neglected; often, in the drive to develop rapid methods because sampling and sample preparation are very time consuming (with no shortcuts), proper sampling is frequently overlooked. Whitaker[8] has recently reviewed approaches to sampling. The importance of sampling as a contribution to total variability has been well recognized for many years. It has been shown that variability increases as aflatoxin concentration increases,[9] and this holds true for each step of the test procedure. For example, in testing a lot of peanuts using 1.1-kg samples and 50-g subsamples, the overall variance, subsampling variance, sample preparation variance, and variance in the analytical determinative step were 82.9, 73.1, 37.5, and 10.7%, respectively.

Sampling has been featured on the agendas of such international organizations as Codex Alimentarius and has become an integral part of aflatoxin regulations. For example, the European Union directive covering aflatoxins in nuts, dried fruit, cereals, and spices stipulates in detail the sampling regime to be followed depending on lot size.[10] For a specified lot size of a commodity the directive specifies the number of incremental samples to be taken and the total aggregate sample weight. The directive specifies that the aggregate sample (30 kg in most cases) should be divided into three 10-kg subsamples. Each 10-kg subsample must be separately ground finely and mixed thoroughly to complete homogenization. Exactly how this should be undertaken is not specified although the directive does state that grinding and mixing should be carried out using a process "that has been demonstrated to achieve complete homogenization." Finally, the action in terms of acceptance/rejection of the lot is specified depending on the analytical results obtained for the subsamples.

The sampling plan specified in the European Union directive has the major advantage that it is absolutely clear as to how the sample should be taken;[10] thus, the way in which the regulatory limit is to be applied is unequivocal to both producers and importers. It is not clear, however, how the sampling plan was derived nor have the operating characteristic curves associated with this plan been published. Thus, producers and importers do not know the "producer risk" associated with operating this plan, nor is it clear to those concerned with food safety what the "consumer risks" are. In all probability the sampling plans, which cover a range of commodities of very different particle sizes and for which in many instances little is known about aflatoxin distribution, have all been derived by extrapolation from work on aflatoxin distributions in lots of peanuts, the most studied commodity. When an examination was carried out of ten different theoretical distributions to simulate aflatoxin distribution of contaminated peanut lots,[11] it was shown that the negative binomial, log normal, and compound-gamma distribution with a shape parameter = 0.5[12] provided the greatest number of acceptance fits. The negative binomial distribution provided the highest percentage of statistically acceptable best fits, and this supports the widespread use of this distribution function in design of sampling plans.[12]

A useful comparison has been made of the performance of sampling plans used in the United States, United Kingdom, and The Netherlands to test raw shelled peanuts for aflatoxins.[13] The plans are very different in terms of the intended operating levels of 15, 10, and 3 ng/g of aflatoxin in peanuts and the numbers of sampling units and sample sizes of 3 (21.8 kg), 1 (10 kg), and 4 (7.5 kg) for the United States, United Kingdom, and The Netherlands, respectively. Clearly, using smaller sample sizes and smaller numbers of samples for analysis offers practical advantages, but performance is compromised. Of the three plans, the overall assessment was that the U.S. plan accepts the highest number of lots and the Dutch plan rejects the greatest number of lots, whereas the U.K. plan is somewhere in-between. However, the Dutch plan accepts the lowest number of bad lots, and the U.K. plan accepts the greatest number of bad lots. In a subsequent paper,[14] six sampling plans were devised to show the effects of sample size (5, 10, and 20 kg) and sample acceptance levels (10, 20, and 30 ng/g) on misclassification of lots. In a study on cottonseed examining 100-tonne piles of commodity it was shown that when three pneumatic probe samplers were evaluated, they had little influence on the variance of the test results.[15] The fact that the performance of a sampling plan is a function of the level of contamination at which the plan is applied[16] has led to a method by which the plan performance can be predicted by linking it to the aflatoxin distribution in the crop.

The sampling plan in the European Union regulations[10] was based to a large extent on the Dutch plan, although elements were drawn from the U.K. and other sampling regimes, which in part explains why it is not well described in terms of its performance. Animal feedstuffs are totally different in terms of aflatoxin distribution due to the mixing effects during processing, and a normal distribution curve applies in this situation.[17] This means that precise sampling plans for commodities such as copra meal pellets, copra cake, and palm kernel cake can be developed which consist of low sample weights and small numbers of incremental samples.

Perhaps one of the most important observations coming out of sampling is the ability to identify a lot associated with the highest risk of contamination. For peanut lots, it was found that when examining sound mature kernels plus sound splits, other kernels, loose shelled kernels, and damaged kernels, the last three were associated with highest risk.[18] This information was subsequently employed to evaluate the performance of an aflatoxin sampling plan based on preferential analysis of sorted fractions.[19] This approach is attractive in that it offers the possibilities of remedial action through sorting at an early stage.

12.3 SCREENING METHODS

In the framework of this chapter, screening is taken to include not only rapid methods that might be employed for laboratory analysis of samples but also techniques that might be used in the field or *in situ* in storage or processing areas to assess whether aflatoxins are present. Two problems must be overcome when devising effective rapid screening techniques. First is the requirement to handle solid matrices such as nuts and grain, and second is the need to achieve very high sensitivity (ng/g levels). The matrix problem is clearly less of an issue with respect to testing for aflatoxin M_1 in milk than the sensitivity requirement (European Commission limit of 0.05 ng/mL). If screening methods for solid samples necessitate sample homogenization and then solvent extraction, the rapidity of the technique becomes less of a factor, as the speed advantage of the detection stage is effectively canceled out by the overall time demands of preliminary sample preparation.

A number of innovative ideas for novel detection of aflatoxins have been published, but none has as yet really been pursued to the point of becoming a viable practical screening technique. DNA electrochemical biosensors are based on the binding of certain toxins to calf thymus DNA, which can be immobilized on an electrode surface.[20,21] In principle, the approach can be demonstrated to work for detection but lacks specificity as the sensor will respond to any substance that has DNA-binding affinity. The sensors were proposed for use in monitoring wastewater, which is not really relevant to our situation, and the sensors are not sufficiently sensitive to meet regulatory requirements.[21] In contrast, a modular separation-based fiberoptic sensor has been proposed[22] that seems to have adequate sensitivity (0.005 ng/mL for aflatoxin B_1 in buffer) but is still limited to handling only liquid matrices. This type of device could, however, find application in monitoring liquid streams; for example, during the wet milling of corn aflatoxins can be transferred to corn-steep liquor during processing, or, if developed for aflatoxin M_1, it could find application in the dairy sector.

Aflatoxin M_1 can interact with bilayer lipid membranes, and this interaction can be used for direct electrochemical sensing.[23,24] Although this appears to be attractive in terms of specificity and speed of response, unfortunately the initial detection limit of 750 mg/mL was far too high to be of practical use; however, stabilized systems of filter-supported membranes have been shown to be capable of achieving significantly improved sensitivity.[25] These kinds of membranes have been proposed for use in detecting aflatoxin M_1 in cheese,[26] but in this case single-strand DNA oligomers are incorporated into the membranes to control surface electrostatic properties. This incorporation has led to achievement of a sensitivity that is much closer to regulatory limits, and with the ability to analyze four cheese samples per minute, the technique appears to be viable for *in situ* testing.

Antibodies have for some time played a significant part in the development of rapid screening techniques. One approach has been to develop a fully automated system based on immunoaffinity column chromatography[27] using online fluorescence detection of aflatoxins. A prototype hand-held device was shown to be sensitive to 0.1 ng/g of aflatoxin (although it is not clear whether it is specific to B_1 or intended to measure total aflatoxins) and to be very rapid, giving a result in 2 minutes. The technique of surface plasmon resonance is based on detection of refractive index changes (measured as a resonance angle) between an antibody and toxin solution flowing continuously over the surface of a sensor chip. This approach has been used for aflatoxin B_1 detection,[28] and when incorporated into a commercial system (BIA-CORE®) has shown good reproducibility in the range of 3.9 to 98.0 ng/mL aflatoxin B_1 in solution. A different approach has been proposed utilizing antibodies, this time coated onto polymethylmethacrylate beads and packed into a flow cell.[29] Determinations of levels of aflatoxin B_1 were made by direct measurement of the fluorescence emission from the beads after excitation from a lamp. Good recovery for aflatoxin B_1 was demonstrated, and sensitivity at low ng/g levels was achieved after extraction from naturally contaminated matrices. Yet another variation involves production of an optrode that contains an immobilized reagent that reacts with the analyte and quickly indicates its concentration.[30] Such a fluorescence-based optrode for aflatoxin B_1 was shown to be sensitive to 0.05 to 1.0 ng/mL of aflatoxin B_1 in an extract from naturally contaminated nuts. Unfortunately, however, for all of these devices, solid samples would require significant sample preparation, and if proper sampling was not undertaken these time-consuming grinding and extraction processes would tend to negate the advantage of speed and thus the attractiveness of *in situ* testing.

A huge variety of commercially available antibody-based test kits for aflatoxins is available. The AOAC International website (http://www.aoac.org/testkits) lists some 11 different formats of test kits offered by ten different companies. The kits for aflatoxin B_1, total aflatoxins, and aflatoxin M_1 utilize antibodies coated variously onto cups, enzyme-linked immunosorbent assay (ELISA) plates, columns, cards, and tubes, with different approaches being used for the read-out devices. Although in each case the manufacturers have made extensive claims as to the performance of these kits, only one has been performance tested by the AOAC, and only one other has been validated by a full interlaboratory collaborative study. Despite the ready availability of commercial kits and notwithstanding it was more than 20 years ago when papers were first published describing the use of antibody-based methods for aflatoxins, new publications are still appearing,[31,32] although apparently offering little novelty or advantage. Indirect ELISAs have been developed based on using commercially available reagents including commercially available antibodies.[33] Apart from some cost-saving, this approach appears to offer little advantage, compared to using commercial test kits. A novel signal-amplification technology, termed super-CARD and based on catalyzed reporter deposition, has been reported.[34] It offers fast determination of aflatoxin B_1, although the reported sensitivity in picograms per well is difficult to relate to more usually reported ng/g regulatory limits. Where indirect ELISAs have been employed in surveillance work, such as for monitoring aflatoxins in chilies[32] and aflatoxin M_1 in milk[35] and infant formula and yogurt,[36] generally good agreement has been achieved when samples were analyzed in duplicate and compared with HPLC results.

Although as indicated above, many very sophisticated developments utilize antibody and sensor technology, one should not lose sight of equally effective screening methods based on simpler approaches. A rapid, quantitative, and inexpensive method has been reported for determining aflatoxins in corn, cornmeal, popcorn, rice, wheat, cottonseed, and peanuts.[37] The approach involves solid-phase extraction on a proprietary column followed by elution and fluorescence determination directly in the eluted solution after bromination. Individual analyses can be conducted in less than 5 minutes, and the method has been shown to be sensitive to 5 ng/g for total aflatoxins in the above matrices. Refinements have also been made to the original minicolumn approach to screening for aflatoxins.[38] A minicolumn has been developed that incorporates *lahar*, a material indigenous to the Philippines, as a substitute for silica gel in one of the layers.[38] It is possible to produce a more intense blue fluorescent band than with a minicolumn without *lahar*, and this design has improved the detection limit for aflatoxins to around 15 ng/g. This minicolumn was demonstrated to be accurate for screening copra meal, in addition to being simple, economical, and rapid in that tests could be performed in 15 minutes.

12.4   ADVANCES IN SAMPLE CLEAN-UP

A major problem associated with most analytical methods for the determination of aflatoxins is the presence of coextractives with the potential to interfere in the analysis, requiring a good clean-up step to remove these coextractives before quantification. In the period covered by this review, a variety of clean-up procedures have been used to assess aflatoxin contamination in a great number of different and complex matrices either by TLC or LC, including, respectively, HPTLC and HPLC (Table 12.1). At the turn of the millennium, conventional clean-up such as liquid–liquid partition is still extensively employed alone or in combination with solid-phase extraction, particularly in combination with the laborious silica gel column chromatography.[39] Other conventional solid-phase materials have also been employed, such as surface-modified bonded silica (e.g., C_{18}, C_8, C_2^6, and Florisil®).[40,41]

Attempts have been made to improve the sensitivity, selectivity, and safety of aflatoxin methods by employing more efficient solid-phase products. Special attention has been given to the reduction of the use of chlorinated solvents by the employment of alternative extractants and as a consequence the development of new solid-phase clean-up procedures such as the multimode columns,[42–44] Romer multifunctional columns,[44] and immunosorbents;[45,46] however, notwithstanding these changes, the long-established AOAC contamination branch (CB) method and its variation are still largely employed and continue to be recommended by AOAC International.[39] Substitution of the highly toxic benzene with toluene for the preparation of aflatoxin standard solutions has been accomplished with the calculation of molar absortivities in toluene–acetonitrile (9+1, v/v), which has led to the modification of AOAC method 971.22.[47]

Recently, great improvements have been achieved in aflatoxin analysis with the use of immunoaffinity solid-phase extraction (SPE) sorbents.[109] So-called immunosorbents, through improved selectivity in the SPE step,[48] have allowed the development of highly selective methods with detection limits as low as 0.02 ng/g.[46] Immunoaffinity column clean-up has been shown to be a robust technique for the purification, separation, and concentration of aflatoxin M_1 in milk[49,50] and dairy products,[51] aflatoxin B_1 in a large variety of complex matrices such as baby food and infant formula,[46] and aflatoxin B_1–N^7-guanine adducts and aflatoxicol in urine.[52] Particularly interesting is the use of immunoaffinity columns for matrices such as chili powder that generally give low recovery of aflatoxin B_1 due probably to occlusion of the mycotoxin by chili components.[53]

Usually, better performance, especially in terms of sensitivity and accuracy, has been achieved using immunoaffinity-based methods when compared to conventional solid-phase extraction, including AOAC methods (Table 12.1), with few exceptions. A method comparison study for the determination of aflatoxins in groundnut cake using a phenyl cartridge compared to the CB method has shown comparable precision data for the two methods.[54] A phenyl-bonded, solid-phase-based, clean-up method has also been compared with four immunoaffinity methods for the analysis of sorghum and maize. The phenyl-bonded phase showed better precision (1.7 to 3.7%) and better recoveries (92 to 111.4%) than the immunoaffinity-column-based methods, which showed recoveries and precision varying from 67 to 105% and 3.0 to 10.8%, respectively.[55] A method using solid-phase extraction (silica Sep-Pak® Plus) has also been reported to give better performance when compared to immunoaffinity clean-up in the determination of aflatoxin B_1 in olive oil.[56] A column-switching HPLC method has been developed for aflatoxin M_1 in milk and urine that uses four ionic exchangers as the stationary phase; it does not require a clean-up step prior to injection onto the HPLC. A low detection limit was achieved (ng/L), and the method performance was in agreement with an immunoaffinity method, with the latter showing lower recovery and greater background interference.[57]

A disadvantage of the newest solid-phase immunoaffinity and multifunctional columns is the cost; however, the immunoaffinity columns can be reused.[58] Immunoaffinity column clean-up is quite straightforward and can be easily automated, making possible a high throughput of samples per run of analysis. The time saved during daily routine analysis counts as a distinct advantage over multifunctional columns and even a number of commercially available SPE columns.

An inexpensive and cost-effective basic aluminum oxide minicolumn has also been reported as a suitable fast and low-cost alternative for the usually costly commercial minicolumns.[59] This column has been used for the analysis of groundnuts, peanuts, cottonseed, and corn meal with recoveries on the order of 73% and relative standard deviation (RSD) varying from 0.0 to 5.9%.[59] Reverse-direction phase in overpressured layer chromatography (OPLC) has also been shown to be an inexpensive alternative clean-up step, albeit not straightforward, for the determination of aflatoxins in wheat.[60]

Associated with the accuracy of analytical methods for aflatoxins is the need to also investigate the suitability of various extractants for the aflatoxin determination. Acetone has been shown to increase recovery of aflatoxin B_1 in maize and sorghum under the same analytical conditions when compared to acetonitrile;[55] however, higher recoveries of aflatoxin B_1 from dry materials such as infant formula, animal feed, and paprika have been reported with the use of aqueous acetonitrile, aqueous acetone, and aqueous methanol. Differences in the recoveries are assumed to be due to different absorption of water by dry materials or solvent layer separation, making MeOH–H_2O more suitable for the extraction of aflatoxin B_1 compared to MeCN–H_2O and acetone–H_2O.[61] Recovery experiments for aflatoxin B_1 from groundnut cake have shown that acetone–H_2O is more efficient as an extractant than chloroform when the sample is prepared as a slurry and when using a different clean-up procedure (phenyl-bonded

TABLE 12.1
Methods for the Determination of Total Aflatoxins and Aflatoxin B_1 in Food and Feed

Sample Type (Country of Origin)	Clean–Up	Chromatography	Limit of Detection (ng/g B_1)	Recovery (%)	Validation (RSD %)	Authors	Ref.
Medicinal herbs and plant extracts (Germany)	Immunoaffinity column	HPLC–fluorescence postcolumn derivatization with electrochemical bromination	0.05	66.4–99.4	In-house (5.1)	Reif and Metzger (1995)	108
Peanut meal (Italy)	Liquid–liquid partition and silica gel column chromatography	LC/MS	1.5	Not given	Not given	Cappiello et al. (1995)	94
Milk (AFM_1) (Cyprus)	Immunoaffinity column	HPLC–fluorescence	10 (ng/L)	79.3–98.7	In-house (5.8–8.8)	Ioannou-Kakouri et al. (1995)	110
Airborne dust (Sweden)	Immunoaffinity column	HPLC–fluorescence postcolumn derivatization with electrochemical bromination	3.1	97	In-house (4–10)	Kussak et al. (1995)	111
Groundnut cake (United Kingdom)	Phenyl-bonded cartridge	HPLC–fluorescence postcolumn derivatization with iodine	2.7	81–87	In-house (0.8–13.2)	Roch et al. (1995)	54
Indian sorghum and Pakistani maize (United Kingdom)	Immunoaffinity columns (four procedures) Phenyl-bonded cartridge	TLC–fluorescence densitometry	Not given	67.4–105.1 92.0–111.4	In-house (3.0–12.5) In-house (1.7–3.7)	Bradburn et al. (1995)	55

Matrix	Cleanup	Detection	Detection limit	Recovery (%)	Validation	Reference	Ref.
Urine (Sweden)	Immunoaffinity column	HPLC–fluorescence postcolumn derivatization with electrochemical bromination	6.8 pg/mL	97–102	In-house (1–5)	Kussak et al. (1995)	85
Copra meal (Philippines)	Liquid–liquid partition and silica gel column chromatography	Two-dimensional TLC ultraviolet light TFA derivative	5.0	100–122 61–122 82–100	In-house AOAC (15.7) AOCS (10.8) EC (8.0)	Arim et al. (1995)	113
Cheese (France)	Immunoaffinity column Silica Sep-Pak®–SPE	HPLC–fluorescence	0.010	70 60–65	In-house (9–29) (not given)	Dragacci et al. (1995)	114
Nuts (peanuts, cashews, pistachios, almonds, corn) (Japan)	Isolute multimode column	HPLC–fluorescence TFA derivative	0.01	87.2–97.4 —	In-house (not given)	Akyama et al. (1996)	42
Melon seeds (United States)	Liquid–liquid partition and silica gel column chromatography Liquid–liquid partition and silica gel column chromatography Liquid–liquid partition	TLC	8.0	75–100	In-house CD method (modified) (13.2) CB RCS (modified) (13.1) BF method (15.2)	DiProssimo and Malek (1996)	115
Peanuts and peanut butter (United States)	Liquid–liquid partition	Two-dimensional imaging HPTLC–CCD	4.5 pg	97.8	In-house (2.6)	Liang et al. (1996)	78
Pistachio kernels and shells (The Netherlands)	Octadecil SPE	HPLC–fluorescence postcolumn derivatization with electrochemical bromination	0.8	92	In house (13)	Scholten and Spanjer (1996)	116

TABLE 12.1 (cont.)
Methods for the Determination of Total Aflatoxins and Aflatoxin B_1 in Food and Feed

Sample Type (Country of Origin)	Clean–Up	Chromatography	Limit of Detection (ng/g B_1)	Recovery (%)	Validation (RSD %)	Authors	Ref.
Corn, food matrices, and milk (United States)	Immunoaffinity column	Automated HPLC fluorescence	—	61–107 71–83 (AFM_1)	In-house (15) (16–20) (AFM_1)	Carman et al. (1996)	71
Nuts, dried vegetables, cereals, seeds, spices, medicinal plants, and herbs (Egypt)	Liquid–liquid partition and silica gel column chromatography	HPLC–ultraviolet detection and ffluorescence	2 ng	95	None	Selim et al. (1996)	117
Corn and peanut meal (United States)	Liquid–liquid partition	FITC-based optrode	0.05–1.0 ng/mL	Not given	AOAC 979.18	Carter et al. (1997)	30
Liquor (Taiwan)	Immunoaffinity column	Fluorometry HPLC–fluorescence	1 0.5	23.3–96.2 30.6–97.5	(1.0–56.7) (1.3–21.9)	Lin and Fu (1997)	118
Corn (India)	—	TLC TFA derivative	>5.0	Not given	AOAC 1984	Bhat et al. (1997)	119
Green coffee beans from Africa/Asia (Japan)	Florisil + affinity column	HPLC–fluorescence–TFA derivative	2.0	76	Not given	Nakajima et al. (1997)	121
Nut puree, peanut butter, and pistachio nut (United Kingdom)	Centrifugation	Automated particle-based immunosensor	4	103–136	In-house (0.06–0.7)	Strachan et al. (1997)	29
Milk (AFM_1) (Greece)	C_{18} Sep-Pak®	ELISA HPLC–fluorescence–TFA derivative	5 ng/L 0.15 ng/L	83.7–115.5	In-house (0.08–0.1) (mean)	Markati and Melissari (1997)	35

Sample	Cleanup	Determination	Detection limit	Recovery (%)	Reference material	Reference	No.
Poultry and pig feeds (grain sorghum, maize, processed soy bean, rice meal, cottonseed meal, poultry and pig feed) (Colombia)	Mycosep #224	HPLC–fluorescence–TFA derivative	1.0	82–109	In-house (0.8–27.1)	Céspedes and Diaz (1997)	81
Beer (Canada)	Immunoaffinity column	HPLC–fluorescence–TFA derivative	20 ng/L	90–104	In-house (not given)	Scott and Lawrence (1997)	80
Milk and urine (AFM$_1$) (France)	HPLC cation and anionic exchange precolumn	Column-switching HPLC fluorescence	2.5 ng/L	94.8–98.7	In-house (<10)	Simon et al. (1998)	57
Figs, peanuts, and spices (Denmark)	Liquid–liquid partition and column chromatography	LC/MS	0.1	42–276	Not given	Vahl and Jørgensen (1998)	122
Corn (Hungary)	Reversed-phase OPLC	OPLC densitometry	None	None	None	Otta et al. (1998)	75
Urine (aflatoxicol) (United Kingdom)	Immunoaffinity column	HPLC–fluorescence postcolumn electrochemical bromination	1 pg/mL	96–101	In-house (not given)	Kussak et al. (1998)	52
Snack and confectionary peanut and corn products from Malasya and Philippines (Japan)	ISOLUTE® multimode column	HPLC–fluorescence–TFA derivative	1.0	79–135	Not given	Ali et al. (1999)	43
Fish (Hungary)	Immunoaffinity column Liquid–liquid partition and silica gel chromatography Predevelopment OPLC	HPLC–fluorescence–TFA derivative HPLC ultraviolet OPLC densitometry	None	56–99 58–67 84.7–94.1	In-house (not given)	Papp et al. (1999)	74

TABLE 12.1 (cont.)
Methods for the Determination of Total Aflatoxins and Aflatoxin B$_1$ in Food and Feed

Sample Type (Country of Origin)	Clean–Up	Chromatography	Limit of Detection (ng/g B$_1$)	Recovery (%)	Validation (RSD %)	Authors	Ref.
Peanuts (China)	Multifunctional column	HPTLC densitometry	0.5	96.3–99.0	In-house (5.5)	Peng et al. (1999)	65
Copra meal (Philippines)	Liquid-liquid partition and salt precipitation	Aflatoxin band fluorescence ultraviolet light	15	–	In-house (qualitative)	Arim et al. (1999)	123
Peanut butter, pistachio paste, dried fig paste, and paprika powder (European Union)	Immunoaffinity column	HPLC–fluorescence postcolumn derivatization–PBPB or electrochemical bromination with Kobra cell (PCD$_{EC}$)	1 0.1 (pistachio paste)	82–109	AOAC 999.07 RSD$_r$ (3.1–20.0) RSD$_R$ (9.1–32.2)	Stroka et al. (2000)	45
Food matrices (paprika powder, peanut butter, pistachios, corn flour)	Immunoaffinity column	One-dimensional TLC–fluorodensitometry	0.2–0.6	76–87	In-house (1.4–8.9)	Stroka et al. (2000)	69
Paprika (Italy)	Immunoaffinity column	One-dimensional TLC–fluorodensitometry	1.2	None	AOAC 999.07	Stroka and Anklam (2000)	77
Human urine (Czech Republic)	Immunoaffinity column	ELISA HPTLC–fluorescence detection/ densitometric analysis	5 ng/L (AFM$_1$)	75–85	In-house (6.6–10.1)	Skarkova and Ostry (2000)	70

Peanuts (China)	Immunoaffinity column	HPLC–fluorescence postcolumn derivatization–electrochemical bromination with Kobra cell (PCD_{EC})	0.1	74.8–97.3 (total aflatoxins)	In-house (9.2–15)	Zhang et al. (2000)	83
Wheat (Hungary)	Predevelopment of TLC in the reverse direction	OPLC (densitometry)	0.14 ng (0.5)	85.4–111.5	In-house (<5.1)	Papp et al (2000)	76
Dairy products (AFM_1) (Korea)	C_{18} Sep-Pak®	ELISA / HPLC	0.002 ng/mL / 0.01 ng/mL	84–106.5 / 87–120	In-house (3.9–8.2) / In-house (2.5–6.6)	Kim et al. (2000)	36
Maize imported into United Kingdom (United Kingdom)	Silica Sep-Pak®	HPLC–fluorescence postcolumn derivatization–electrochemical bromination	0.1	86–95	(6.1)	Scudamore and Patel (2000)	82
Fish, corn, and wheat (Hungary)	Liquid–liquid partition (fish) / Predevelopment of TLC in the reverse direction	OPLC (densitometry)	None	84.9–94.1	In-house (7.7–10.3)	Otta et al. (2000)	60
Corn (Venezuela)	Immunoaffinity column	TLC with ultraviolet light / Visual analysis	2	96–98	Not given	Medina-Martinez and Martinez (2000)	125
Triticale, wheat, and rye artificially contaminated with aflatoxin fungi *A. parasiticus* NRRL 2999 (Argentina)	—	TLV visual analysis	20	86.6–93.3	In-house AOAC 49209 (9.0–19.4)	Bilotti et al. (2000)	124

TABLE 12.1 (cont.)
Methods for the Determination of Total Aflatoxins and Aflatoxin B_1 in Food and Feed

Sample Type (Country of Origin)	Clean–Up	Chromatography	Limit of Detection (ng/g B_1)	Recovery (%)	Validation (RSD %)	Authors	Ref.
Olive oil (Greece)	Liquid–liquid partition and silica Sep-Pak® cartridge (method A) Centrifugation and IAC (method B)	Prederivatization with TFA	0.0028 0.056	87.2 (method A) 84.8 (method B)	In-house (6.8) (method A) (17.8) (method B)	Daradimos et al. (2000)	56
Cereal grains (yellow corn, maize, gluten, soybean meal) (Egypt)	Liquid–liquid partition	TLC–fluorescence densitometry Confirmation by two-dimensional TLC	5	79–97	AOAC 1995 BF Method (1–13)	El-Tahan et al. (2000)	120
Baby food (infant formula) (European Union)	Immunoaffinity column	HPLC–fluorescence Postcolumn derivatization–PBPB or electrochemical bromination with Kobra cell (PCD_{EC})	0.02	92–101	AOAC 2000.16 RSD_r (3.5–14) RSD_R (9–23)	Stroka et al. (2001)	46
Milk (European Union)	Immunoaffinity column	HPLC–fluorescence	0.02 ng/mL (AFM_1)	74–107	AOAC 2000.08 RSD_r (8–18) RSD_R (21–31)	Dragacci et al. (2001)	50
Telemes cheese (Greece)	Immunoaffinity column	HPLC–spectrofluorometer	None	80–89	In-house	Govaris et al. (2001)	51

Biological materials (AFB$_1$–lysine adduct)	—	TLC fluorodensitometer HPLC–fluorescence	None	62–72 87–99	Not given	Sujatha et al. (2001)	112
Corn (Brazil)	Florisil® cartridge	TLC densitometry	0.2	94.2	16.2	Castro and Vargas (2001)	63
Corn (Brazil)	Florisil® cartridge	TLC densitometry	0.2	94	15	Vargas et al. (2001)	64
Chilli pods and powder (India)	Liquid–liquid partition	Indirect ELISA	1.0	67–112	In house (<10)	Reddy et al. (2001)	32
Peanuts, pistachios nuts, almond, maize, nutmeg, and red pepper (Japan)	Autoprep MF-A and Multisep #228	LC–fluorescence–TFA derivative LCMS/ESI	1	None	(0.32–4.18) (4.34)	Tanaka et al. (2002)	44
Spices (pepper, black pepper, nutmeg, allspice, thyme, cinnamon, paprika, cumin) (Japan)	Isolute® multimode column	Two-dimensional HPLC (ODS and Diol columns)–fluorescence –TFA derivative	5.0 (0.5 with 250-µL injection)	Not given	Not given	Onji et al. (2002)	79
Food and feed matrices (corn, pistachio paste, peanut butter, fig paste, animal feed) (Italy, European Union)	Immunoaffinity column	HPLC–fluorescence Electrochemical bromination (PCD$_{BC}$) and ultraviolet (PCD$_{UV1}$ and PCD$_{UV2}$)	Not given	Not given	In-house (0.3–1.8) (PCD$_{UV1}$) (0.8–1.3) (PCD$_{UV2}$) (0.9–2.0) (PCD$_{BC}$)	Papadopoulou–Bouraoui et al. (2002)	86
Corn, cottonseed, almonds, Brazil nuts, pistachios, walnuts, corn meal, and raw peanuts (United States)	Aluminum oxide minicolumn	HPLC–photochemical reactor–fluorescence	1.0	72.3–103.7 80–87	In-house (0.1–15.8)	Sobolev and Dorner (2002)	59

TABLE 12.1 (cont.)
Methods for the Determination of Total Aflatoxins and Aflatoxin B$_1$ in Food and Feed

Sample Type (Country of Origin)	Clean–Up	Chromatography	Limit of Detection (ng/g B$_1$)	Recovery (%)	Validation (RSD %)	Authors	Ref.
Dried oil palm front and oil palm front base feed (Japan)	MycoSep #226 or #228 columns	TLC or HPLC	0.5 (OPF) 5.0 (cubes and pellets; HPLC) 10 (TLC)	>75	In-house (9.7)	Goto et al. (2002)	66

Note: CCD, charge-coupled device; EC, electrochemical; ELISA, enzyme-linked immunosorbent assay; ESI, electrospray ionization; FITC, fluorescein isothiocyanate; HPLC, high-performance liquid chromatography; HPTLC, high-performance, thin-layer chromatography; IAC, immunoaffinity column; LC/MS, liquid chromatography/mass spectrometry; MS, mass spectrometry; OPLC, overpressured liquid chromatography; PBPB, pyridinium hydrobromide perbromide; PCD, postcolumn derivatization; SPE, solid-phase extraction; TFA, trifluoroacetic acid; TLC, thin-layer chromatography; UV, ultraviolet.

cartridges and silica gel chromatography).[54] It is important to consider that the interaction of aflatoxin and silica is very weak and low recoveries due to loss of aflatoxin in the chromatographic stage can be caused by the presence of ethanol in the chloroform.[62,63]

12.5 TLC AND HPTLC METHODOLOGY

Thin-layer chromatography has been the most widely used and established separation and quantification technique since its development in the early 1960s. Low cost is the main advantage associated with TLC-based procedures, and its advantages have recently been demonstrated and emphasized by IDF/IUPAC/IAEA collaborative studies to validate TLC-based methods.[49] Visual TLC has been the method of choice in many countries producing agricultural commodities but lacking in expensive instrumentation, thus TLC is the only technique available for official control of aflatoxins in products that are usually exported to countries where strict regulations have been laid down.[1,2] Some of the factors affecting the acceptance of TLC as a quantitative method, such as its lack of resolution and poor sensitivity, have been overcome in recent years; however, quantification is still a limiting factor due to the high cost of commercial fluorodensitometers that could otherwise decrease the variability associated with the ability of individual analysts to quantify aflatoxins by visual TLC analysis (Vargas et al., 2001, unpublished results).

In recent years, the performance and simplicity of TLC methods have also been improved to some extent with the application of solid-phase extraction cartridge clean-up prior to the TLC step, followed by either by visual or densitometric determination. Acceptable recoveries (>75%) and RSDs (<20%) have been achieved with TLC following clean-up using phenyl-bonded cartridges and immunoaffinity column,[55] Florisil® cartridges,[64] and multifunctional columns[65,66] with densitometric quantification. The use of more advanced clean-up procedures has also favored the use of more precise and efficient planar chromatography such as the HPTLC.[67] Detection limits as low as 0.2 ng/g for aflatoxin B_1 and method performance characteristics meeting standards required by international organizations[68] have been achieved with Florisil®-based clean-up and one-dimensional TLC with densitometric quantification for corn.[63] Promising analytical approaches include the combination of robust immunoaffinity column clean-up with low-cost TLC for the analysis of aflatoxins in paprika powder, peanut butter, and pistachios,[69] or HPTLC for the analysis of aflatoxin M_1 in urine.[70] Improved clean-up techniques have dramatically changed the analytical perspective for aflatoxin determination by providing sample extracts free of major matrix interferences and suitable for one-dimensional TLC analysis, making the TLC method more straightforward and amenable to automation. An automated robotic procedure for the analysis of aflatoxins in grains, nuts, and milk using immunoaffinity clean-up has been developed and validated against the official AOAC CB method, with mean recovery of 86% for AB_1 and an overall coefficient of variation (CV) of 15%, thus demonstrating advantages such speediness and precision.[71]

Usually, two-dimensional (2-D) TLC has been used for sample extracts that contain interferences. One important aspect related to separation and quantification of aflatoxins by 2-D TLC is that this technique causes elongation of sample spots when compared to aflatoxin standards. Additionally, different fluorescence is produced as a consequence of the use of different development solvents. Both factors increase the variability of 2-D TLC, whether associated with the abilities of individual analysts in visual TLC or with the densitometry (Vargas et al., 2001, unpublished results). However, TLC should always be considered as an important tool as it is fast and cost effective and can be used in routine applications (such as crude extract analysis); it offers versatility in the use of different solvent systems and can be applied to different visualization system using the same sample extract.[77] TLC allows those in developing countries to assess aflatoxin contamination irrespective of the purpose of the assessment, whether qualitative or quantitative; however, greater analytical variability in the determination of aflatoxins, within and among laboratories, is associated with TLC compared to HPLC.[73]

Overpressured layer chromatography, a planar-based chromatography technique, has been reported to be a rapid, reproducible, and cost-effective technique for quantitative determination of aflatoxins in fish[60,74] and corn.[60,75] Recovery results (75 to 94%) for aflatoxin B_1 in fish were higher than those achieved by HPLC with fluorescence (56 to 99%) and ultraviolet detection (58 to 67%). Robustness of the OPLC procedure with regard to separation has been demonstrated to be largely dependent on the type of plate used (TLC or HPTLC) in the analysis of wheat.[76]

Attempts have been made to develop alternatives to expensive commercial TLC densitometers. These developments could be extremely helpful in building the ability to analyze aflatoxins in developing countries, especially if the densitometers could be available on a semicommercial scale. A simple, inexpensive, and reliable device for densitometric quantification (SeBaDeC) is based on the measurement of fluorescence reflection. Comparable correlation coefficients (>0.99) were achieved for a commercial scanner (CAS) and SeBaDeC for all aflatoxins except for aflatoxin G_2, where CAS gave lower detection and quantification limits.[77] An operated charge-coupled imaging system (2-D) that has been evaluated for the quantitative determination of aflatoxins by HPTLC demonstrated low sensitivity (4.5 pg) and recovery from 90 to 100% (RSD < 3%). This system is claimed to be faster than a slit scanner densitometer.[78]

12.6 HPLC METHODS

Separation and detection of aflatoxins have been accomplished by reversed-phase (RP) and normal-phase (NP) liquid chromatography (LC), including high-performance liquid chromatography (HPLC) with fluorescence detection, reversed-flow micellar eletrokinetic chromatography (RF-MEKC), capillary electrokinetic chromatography (CEKC) with multiphoton excited (MPE) fluorescence detection, and HPLC and µHPLC with near-ultraviolet, laser-induced fluorescence (near-UV LIF) detection. A number of arrangements in the separation stage for HPLC have been proposed to provide less expensive alternatives for increasing the sensitivity of the technique. Two-dimensional liquid chromatography employing both ODS and DIOL columns has been used as a precolumn for the analysis of a number of spices (pepper, black pepper, nutmeg allspice, thyme, cinnamon, paprika, and cumin) with detection limits of 0.5 µg/kg and linearity of 0.99 when a volume of up to 250 µL is injected in the system.[79] A column-switching HPLC method has been developed for aflatoxin M_1 in milk and urine that uses four ionic exchangers as the stationary phase, does not require a clean-up step prior to injection into the HPLC, and has a detection level on the order of ng/g.[57]

The sensitivity of RP-HPLC for detection of aflatoxins has been improved by the enhancement of the least fluorescent aflatoxin B_1 and aflatoxin G_1 to the levels of aflatoxin B_2 and aflatoxin G_2 in aqueous solution through postcolumn derivatization (PCD) with iodine, bromine, or electrochemical bromination. Prederivatization, although the simplest method and largely used in the last decade for the analysis of several foods[43,80] and feed,[81] has been replaced due to the instability of B_{2a} and G_{2a} compounds and the fact that it introduces an additional step in the analysis. PCD with iodine, although being used for the assessment of aflatoxins and adopted by AOAC,[39] presents many experimental problems such as corrosion and deterioration of the equipment (pumps and connections), instability of the iodine solution (thus requiring daily preparation), and stability of the mobile phase. These drawbacks are minimized when bromine generated from pyridinium hydrobromide (PBPB) or electrochemically generated bromine is used, although the latter is not broadly accepted due to the Kobra cell being a proprietary product that is not always readily available. Regardless, a number of studies have been undertaken using PCD with bromine or electrochemical bromination for the analysis of aflatoxin B_1 in matrices such as maize,[82] groundnuts,[59] peanuts,[83] dried fruits,[84] and aflatoxins B_1, B_2, G_1, G_2, M_1, and Q_1 in urine[85] with improved method sensitivity. The combination of immunoaffinity column clean-up with PCD (PBPB) or an electrochemical cell (Kobra cell) has been shown to increase the sensitivity of HPLC methods for aflatoxin B_1, such as in baby food, with detection limits as low as 0.02 ng/g being achieved.[46]

Commercially available devices for PCD techniques using electrochemical (EC) bromination and ultraviolet irradiation, PCD_{UV1} or PCD_{UV2}, have been compared, with both systems showing good performance for aflatoxin determinations in corn, pistachio paste, peanut butter, fig paste, and animal feed, with RSDs ranging from 0.3 to 1.8% for PCD_{UV1}, 0.8 to 1.3% for PCD_{UV2}, and 0.9 to 2.0% for PCD_{EC}. Response ratios for the PCD_{UV1}/PCD_{EC} for both ultraviolet systems were higher than 0.8 for aflatoxin B_1.[86]

A nondestructive PCD for RP-HPLC has been proposed using cyclodextrin compounds (CyDs) such as 2,6-*ortho*-dimethyl-β-CyD (DMβ–CyD) to form inclusion complexes which lead to increased fluorescence of aflatoxin B_1 and G_1. The β–cyclodextrin (β–CyD) complex resulted in a more stable signal than the DMβ–CyD complex; the limit of detection achieved for DMβ–CyD was 4 mg/L and for β–CyD it was 9 mg/L.[87] The viability of the application of the CyDs as fluorosphores has extended to the analysis of aflatoxin P_1, M_1, and Q_1.[6] The use of anionic β–CyD derivatives as a pseudostationary phase in the separation buffer has been reported to improve quantum yields of aflatoxins.

The viability of using a near-UV LIF detector equipped with a He–Cd laser with µHPLC or HPLC and an output capillary of 320 µm has been demonstrated for the analysis of very low concentrations of aflatoxins B_1 and G_1 (0.1 ng/g), with sensitivity levels as low as 1.2 pg for aflatoxins G_2 and B_2 (signal/noise > 20).[89]

Evaluation of the possibility of applying voltammetric detection (−1.25 V vs. Ag/AgCl) for the determination of aflatoxin by HPLC was carried out with different sample extracts (melon seeds, corn meal, corn flakes, mixed nuts) extracted by the AOAC CB method. The sensitivity of the HPLC method was sufficient to detect only aflatoxin B_1 (2.5 ng/g), with good agreement achieved compared to the AOAC CB method,[91] indicating that clean-up may not be enough to provide higher sensitivity. Based on the ability of aflatoxin molecules to undergo electrochemical oxidation (Glassy carbon eletrode, −1.4 V, $LiClO_4$), Elizalde-González et al.[92] proposed a method for the amperometric detection of aflatoxins by HPLC with sensitivity less than 10 ng for all aflatoxins. Studies on the rate of oxidation demonstrated that aflatoxin G_1 is less stable to ultraviolet irradiation when compared to aflatoxin B_2, indicating that special care should be taken with ultraviolet light or irradiation when analyzing aflatoxins.

12.7   OTHER CHROMATOGRAPHIC APPROACHES

Some published papers describe alternative chromatographic methods, although the benefits of such approaches are not always clear. Capillary electrophoresis has the advantage that it avoids the use of organic solvents, although the technique is not widely available as an alternative in many laboratories routinely conducting HPLC. It has been demonstrated[90] that aflatoxin B_1 can be determined in corn by capillary electrophoresis (CEKC) with laser-induced fluorescence detection at 0.5 ng/g in 15 minutes after clean-up comparable to that required for HPLC. Comparable average recovery results have been reported for capillary electrophoresis (CE)–LIF (85.2%) and HPLC (89%), and good correlation between these two methods ($r^2 > 0.9$) with the AOAC CB method was shown in the analysis of corn. The combination of immunoaffinity column clean-up with CE–LIF has been evaluated and, although giving a limit of detection of 1 ng/g, which is twice the level using the AOAC CB method,[90] it seems promising when improvements in HPLC condition (micro-HPLC) and in the detection such as proposed by Siméon et al.[89] can be implemented.

For electrophoresis, derivatization of aflatoxin is not required, which arguably also makes the approach more straightforward than HPLC where postcolumn iodination or bromination or precolumn derivatization is necessary. Sensitivity can be further improved by using multiphoton excitation with CEKC, and detection at levels 10^4 better than previously achieved by capillary separation in less than 90 seconds have demonstrated the potential of this technique.[88] Micellar electrokinetic chromatography (MEKC) is conducted in polyacrylamide-coated capillaries under almost complete suppression of electroosmotic flow,[93] and when small amounts of organic solvents are used in the buffer system good separation of aflatoxins was achieved; however, only standards were analyzed in this paper and no indications were given as to applicability to real samples or the advantages compared to HPLC.

12.8   CONFIRMATORY METHODS

For pesticides and veterinary drug residues and for other food contaminants, confirmation of positive results by mass spectrometry is now taken as the norm, and in some cases is mandatory; however for aflatoxins, the specificity incurred by their fluorescence has historically been thought adequate confirmation. The low levels at which monitoring of aflatoxins is carried out has also precluded the use of mass spectrometry. The use of particle-beam liquid chromatography/mass spectrometry (LC/MS) has been advocated for confirmation,[94] which has the advantage from a mass-spectrometry perspective of producing spectra with characteristic fragmentation patterns. Detection limits at the nanogram level are inadequate for confirmation at most regulatory limits, however. Electrospray ionization produces simpler spectra and with better sensitivity than particle beam ionization and has been successfully used to analyze aflatoxins in dust samples of contaminated commodities.[95] Sensitivity in the low picogram range was demonstrated for selected ion monitoring and for multiple reaction monitoring (in tandem MS mode). With this sensitivity and with relative standard deviations of a few percent the electrospray approach is comparable to fluorescence HPLC detection. It thus seems to be viable as a rigorous confirmation for real samples where enfringement of regulatory limits is suspected. This approach has been extended by others[44] applying electrospray LC/MS to the detection of aflatoxins in peanuts, pistachios, almonds, maize, nutmeg, and red peppers at levels down to 1 ng/g and with a RSD of 4.3%. Confirmation of identification has also been achieved from full-scan atmospheric pressure chemical ionization (APCI) spectra using LC/MS[96] where aflatoxins were detected in samples of incaprina (a high-protein food supplement based on corn and cottonseed flour) intended for children on protein-deficient diets.

12.9 VALIDATION OF ANALYTICAL METHODS FOR AFLATOXINS

A vast literature is comprised of either proposed methods for determining aflatoxins (which in many instances have only had limited testing on real samples) or customized methods that have been employed but little is known about their performance; however, the methods that have actually been fully validated by an interlaboratory collaborative study are much fewer, and when one is seeking a method for a particular commodity and to meet a target regulatory limit the literature is quite sparse. The process of method validation has been recently described,[97] and a well-established harmonized protocol for conducting collaborative studies is accepted internationally.[98] A recent review[7] has tabulated the performance characteristics of methods for aflatoxin B_1, total aflatoxins, and aflatoxin M_1 from 38 publications dating from 1968 to 2001. These methods cover commodities such as almonds, Brazil nuts, coconut, copra, corn, cottonseed, fig paste, paprika, peanut butter, soybeans, animal feed, eggs, ginger, liquid milk, cheese, milk powder, butter, and liver. If these methods are further sorted by eliminating those with applicability ranges higher than current regulatory limits and removing those with unacceptably high RSD_r and RSD_R values, actually only a very small number of methods meet the needs of official laboratories in the European Union[68] or those testing commodities who wish to ensure compliance for export to the European Union. Most of the methods that meet these requirements were validated though the European Union Standards, Measurements, and Testing (SMT) Programme and are based on immunoaffinity column clean-up and HPLC with fluorescence detection for aflatoxin B_1 and total aflatoxins in peanut butter, pistachio paste, fig paste, and paprika[45] and for aflatoxin M_1 in liquid milk.[50] A method has also been validated for determining aflatoxin B_1 in baby food (infant formula) at the very low target level of 0.1 ng/g,[46] which was anticipated as being the likely future regulatory limit for this commodity.

Validation of methods through full interlaboratory collaborative studies is expensive to undertake and is a time-consuming process. Validation has thus tended to focus on the requirements of developed countries, and in recent years it has been almost only sophisticated methods such as HPLC that have been validated to meet the needs for official methods for enforcement. Where demanding standards for aflatoxins have to be met by countries exporting to the European Union and elsewhere, equipment such as HPLC is not always available so there is a real need for more appropriate methods, such as those based on TLC. Most TLC methods that were validated many years ago employed clean-up methods that have subsequently been vastly improved. Extracts prepared using immunoaffinity columns are far cleaner than those obtained by more conventional solid-phase clean-up and if combined with TLC can make the whole process a more attractive option for analysis of aflatoxins. A joint IDF/IUPAC/IAEA project has recently been carried out for the validation of a TLC method for liquid and powdered milk[49] with immunoaffinity column clean-up. The RSD_r values ranged from 26 to 39% and the RSD_R values ranged from 34 to 53%, which, although a little disappointing, were comparable to those of other TLC studies for aflatoxin M_1, but the levels of contamination were lower than previously studied by TLC. Interestingly, the performance of the TLC method was best ($RSD_r = 26\%$; $RSD_R = 34\%$) at the level of contamination of 0.14 ng/mL of aflatoxin M_1 in liquid milk, which was the lowest level studied. This compares with values of $RSD_r = 8\%$ and $RSD_R = 21\%$ for a recently studied HPLC method[50] using an immunoaffinity column clean-up for liquid milk containing 0.103 ng/mL of aflatoxin M_1. European regulations for aflatoxins do not stipulate specific methods but indicate that any method can be employed that meets certain minimum performance standards. These have been specified as minimum performance parameters that are required for methods to be considered as CEN standards,[68] which for levels of 0.1 to 0.5 ng/mL are RSD_r 30% and RSD_R 50%. These parameters have been met by the immunoaffinity column TLC method.[49]

12.10 PROFICIENCY TESTING

In terms of the total number of samples determined per annum worldwide, aflatoxins must be one of the most frequently analyzed class of chemical contaminants found in food and feedstuffs. The overall cost of making these determinations together with the considerable health and economic impact of getting the "wrong" result should command the need for ensuring that determinations are meaningful. The use of validated methods, implementation of accreditation of laboratories, and participation in proficiency testing have all been advocated as essential quality assurance measures for mycotoxin analysis.[99] Of these, proficiency testing gives the best indication of performance both of individual laboratories as well as the more general performance of the analytical community in a specific sector. Data from the international proficiency testing scheme, FAPAS, from 1990 to 1996 showed that, of some 4766 determinations of aflatoxins, 91% of laboratories who reported results demonstrated satisfactory performance as exemplified by their z-scores.[100] This assessment was based on z-scoring using σ values obtained from the Horwitz equation,[101,126] which was subsequently shown to be rather generous at low levels of determination.[102] For a typical round of aflatoxin analysis in peanut meal containing 25 ng/g total aflatoxins,[103] it was shown that when using σ-values from the Horwitz equation, 84% of laboratories were satisfactory but based on σ-values achievable through "best practices" this measurement fell to 71%. Although the percentage of laboratories performing well does not seem to be very impressive, this figure was based on "satisfactory" results falling in the range of 15.8 to 35.1 ng/g for a true value of 25 ng/g, which by perception seems in fact to be quite generous. One also needs to take into account that this is probably not a true reflection of the overall position for those undertaking aflatoxin analysis, as it tends to be the better laboratories, who are striving to achieve good quality results, who take part in proficiency testing. For a smaller cohort of laboratories (21 in total) in Thailand, 68% performed satisfactorily for determining aflatoxins in contaminated corn, but only 48% were satisfactory for determining aflatoxins in peanuts.[104] In this case, the laboratories were using ELISA, TLC, and minicolumn screening which is probably why the overall satisfactory percentage was lower than the FAPAS data, which had a high proportion of laboratories using HPLC. With regard to a group of laboratories largely weighted toward Eastern and Central Europe who took part in proficiency testing in 1996,[105] of 34 laboratories taking part, only 6 were rated unsatisfactory or questionable (17%) when determining aflatoxin B_1 in an animal feed containing 31 ng/g. While these snapshots provide useful insight into performance, to have any lasting benefit proficiency testing must be performed on a continual basis at least every 3 months, as is the case with commercial schemes such as FAPAS.

The European Union has an established network of expert laboratories responsible for milk and milk products testing which is coordinated through a Community Reference Laboratory. Proficiency testing of these 19 laboratories was carried out in 1996 and 1998[106] to assess their performance in determining aflatoxin M_1 in milk samples. As might be expected, the performance of these expert laboratories was better than that of the greater number of other laboratories undertaking aflatoxin M_1 analysis, with only one or two laboratories (5 to 10%) not achieving satisfactory z-scores. This compares with 26% of some 74 laboratories who were found to be unsatisfactory or questionable in a 2002 round of FAPAS for aflatoxin M_1 in powdered milk which is illustrated in Figure 12.1. In this round, the assigned value for aflatoxin M_1 was 0.26 ng/g and a target standard deviation of 0.06 was employed which was derived from a modified Horwitz equation.[102] No doubt continued participation in proficiency testing leads to improved performance with time,[100] and, as has been shown for a network of specialist aflatoxin M_1 field laboratories,[107] that feedback leads to training, seeking technical advice, improved quality assurance, and method standardization, all of which can contribute to improvements.

The large datasets generated from proficiency testing over a period of time provide some insight into the relative performance of different analytical methods.

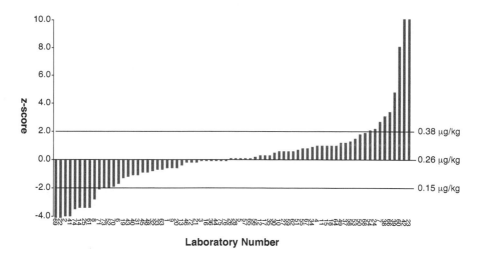

FIGURE 12.1 Z-scores for aflatoxin M_1 (0.26 μg/kg) in milk powder test material taken from 2002 FAPAS proficiency testing.

For the aflatoxin M_1 FAPAS round illustrated in Figure 12.1, of the 74 laboratories that took part, 66 participants (89%) used HPLC and 65 (87%) used affinity column clean-up, although two of these employing affinity column clean-up used TLC rather than HPLC. Although the number of fully validated methods for aflatoxin M_1 is quite limited, when asked to cite references for the methods employed some 23 sources were provided. Some of these cited methods are duplicates; for example, the AOAC *Official Methods of Analysis* is referenced separately to the 15th, 16th, and 17th editions, and some official methods may be the same as journal publications. This diversity of apparent sources does illustrate the extent to which laboratories tend not to standardize on methods. Many laboratories take pride in "customized" methods even if these mean deviating from the official method or that which was originally validated. Of the 5 participants who used ELISA to determine aflatoxin M_1 in the FAPAS round, none achieved satisfactory z-scores, although arguably 5 out of 74 may not be statistically significant to generalize. It is interesting, however, to note that of the 2 laboratories using TLC and the one using HPTLC, only the participant who cited the 1975 AOAC *Official Method of Analysis* obtained a satisfactory z-score. This illustrates well that, provided the methods being used are basically sound, the performance obtained has more to do with the infrastructure of the laboratory and skills of the individual analyst than employing modern clean-up techniques and sophisticated instrumental analysis.

12.11 CONCLUSIONS

This review has looked at the published literature on sampling and analysis of aflatoxins over a relatively small time interval. Despite being a mature area of science from an analytical standpoint, significant activity with regard to publications on aflatoxins took place. Sampling has moved up the agenda, driven by the need to have unified sampling plans for enforcement and trading purposes. Despite this obvious need, the area is still neglected. Although some progress was noted on developing a better theoretical understanding of sampling of peanuts, sampling for other commodities still seems to have been largely neglected. Progress was noted on the development of screening techniques for aflatoxins using sometimes quite innovative approaches. Although many of these techniques showed promise, it was seen that in many instances the work on development was not very well connected to the real problem areas, meaning that the sensitivity and areas of application were misjudged. Continued progress on the development of improved sample clean-up techniques has been observed, and it is encouraging to see these modern approaches being coupled to TLC as the chromatographic step. HPLC still remains the technique of choice for aflatoxin analysis, although a wide range of methods are applied and often customized by individual laboratories. Method validation is continuing but still many matrices have no validated methods available or validation has not been at the level of interest from a regulatory perspective.

REFERENCES

1. Commission Regulation (EC) No. 257/2002 of February 12, 2002, amending Regulation No. 194/97 setting maximum levels for certain contaminants in foodstuffs and Regulation (EC) No. 466/2001 setting maximum levels for certain contaminants in foodstuffs, *Off. J. Eur. Comm.*, L41/12, 2002.
2. Commission Regulation (EC) No. 472/2002 of March 12, 2002, amending Regulation No. 466/2001 setting maximum levels for certain contaminants in foodstuffs, *Off. J. Eur. Comm.*, L75/18, 2002.
3. Shepard, G.S., Analytical methodology for mycotoxins: recent advances and future challenges, in *Mycotoxins and Phycotoxins in Perspective at the Turn of the Millennium*, de Koe, W.J., Samson, R.A., van Egmond, H.P., Gilbert, J., and Sabino, M., Eds., Ponsen & Looyen, Wageningen, 2001, pp. 19–28.
4. Trucksess, M.W., Rapid analysis (thin layer chromatographic and immunological methods) for mycotoxins in foods and feeds, in *Mycotoxins and Phycotoxins in Perspective at the Turn of the Millennium*, de Koe, W.J., Samson, R.A., van Egmond, H.P., Gilbert, J., and Sabino, M., Eds., Ponsen & Looyen, Wageningen, 2001, pp. 29–40.
5. Lin, L., Zhang, J., Wang, P., Wang, Y., and Chen, J., Thin-layer chromatography of mycotoxins and comparison with other chromatographic methods, *J. Chromatogr. A.*, 815, 3–20, 1998.
6. Jaimez, J., Fente, C.A., Vazquez, B.I., Franco, C.M., Cepeda, A., Mahuzier, G., and Prognon, P., Review: application of the assay of aflatoxins by liquid chromatography with fluorescence detection in food analysis, *J. Chromatogr. A*, 882, 1–10, 2000.
7. Gilbert, J. and Anklam, E., Validation of analytical methods for determining mycotoxins in foodstuffs, *Trends Anal. Chem.*, 21, 468, 2002.
8. Whitaker, T.B., Sampling techniques, in M*ethods in Molecular Biology: Mycotoxin Protocols*, Vol. 157, Trucksess, M.W. and Pohland, A.E., Eds., Humana Press, Totowa, NJ, 2001, pp. 11–24.
9. Johansson, A.S., Whitaker, T.B., Hagler, W.M., Giesbrecht, F.G., Young, J.H., and Bowman, D.T., Testing shelled corn for aflatoxin. Part I. Estimation of variance components, *J. Assoc. Off. Anal. Chem. Int.*, 83, 1264, 2000.

10. Commission Directive 98/53/EEC of July 16, 1999, laying down the sampling methods and the methods of analysis for the official control of the levels for certain contaminants in foodstuffs, *Off. J. Eur. Comm.*, L201/93, 1999.

11. Whitaker, T.B., Giesbrecht, F.G., and Wu, J., Suitability of several statistical models to simulate observed distribution of sample test results in inspections of aflatoxin-contaminated peanut lots, *J. Assoc. Off. Anal. Chem. Int.*, 79, 981, 1996.

12. Johansson, A.S., Whitaker, T.B., Giesbrecht, F.G., Hagler, W.M., and Young, J.H., Testing shelled corn for aflatoxin. Part II. Modelling the observed distribution of aflatoxin test results, *J. Assoc. Off. Anal. Chem. Int.*, 83, 1270, 2000.

13. Whitaker, T.B., Springer, J., Defrize, P.R., de Koe, W.J., and Coker, R., Evaluation of sampling plans in the United States, United Kingdom, and the Netherlands to test raw shelled peanuts for aflatoxin, *J. Assoc. Off. Anal. Chem. Int.*, 78, 1010, 1995.

14. Johansson, A.S., Whitaker, T.B., Giesbrecht, F.G., Hagler, W.M., and Young, J.H., Testing shelled corn for aflatoxin. Part III. Evaluating the performance of aflatoxin sampling plans, *J. Assoc. Off. Anal. Chem. Int.*, 83, 1279, 2000.

15. Park, D.L., Whitaker, T.B., Giesbrecht, F.G., and Njapau, H., Performance of three pneumatic probe samplers and four analytical methods used to estimate aflatoxins in bulk cottonseed, *J. Assoc. Off. Anal. Chem. Int.*, 83, 1247, 2000.

16. Vandeven, M., Whitaker, T., and Slate, A., Statistical approach for risk assessment of aflatoxin sampling plan used by manufacturers for raw shelled peanuts, *J. Assoc. Off. Anal. Chem. Int.*, 85, 925, 2002.

17. Coker, R., Nagler, M.J., Defieze, P.R., Derksen, G.B., Buchholz, H., Putzka, H.A., Hoogland, H.P., Roos, A.H., and Boenke, A., Sampling plans for the determination of aflatoxin B_1 in large shipments of animal feedstuffs, *J. Assoc. Off. Anal. Chem. Int.*, 83, 1252, 2000.

18. Whitaker, T.B., Hagler, W.M, Giesbrecht, F.G., Dorner, J.W., Dowell, F.E., and Cole, R.J., Estimating aflatoxin in farmers' stock peanut lots by measuring aflatoxin in various peanut-grade components, *J. Assoc. Off. Anal. Chem. Int.*, 81, 61, 1998.

19. Whitaker, T.B., Hagler, W.M, and Giesbrecht, F.G., Performance of sampling plans to determine aflatoxin in farmers' stock peanut lots by measuring aflatoxin in high-risk-grade components, *J. Assoc. Off. Anal. Chem. Int.*, 82, 264, 1999.

20. Mascini, M., Affinity electrochemical biosensors for pollution control, *Pure Appl. Chem.*, 73, 23, 2001.

21. Mascini, M., Palchetti, I., and Marrazza, G., DNA electrochemical biosensors, *Fresenius J. Anal. Chem.*, 369, 15, 2001.

22. Dickens, J. and Sepaniak, M., Modular separation-based fiber-optic sensors for remote *in situ* monitoring, *J. Environ. Monit.*, 2, 11, 2000.

23. Andreou, V.G., Nikolelis, D.P., and Tarus, B., Electrochemical investigation of transduction of interactions of aflatoxin M_1 with bilayer lipid membranes (BLMs), *Anal. Chem. Acta*, 350, 121, 1997.

24. Andreou, V.G. and Nikolelis, D.P., Electrochemical transduction of interactions of aflatoxin M_1 with bilayer membranes (BLMs) for the construction of one-shot sensors, *Sensors Actuators*, B41, 213, 1997.

25. Andreou, V.G. and Nikolelis, D.P., Flow injection monitoring of aflatoxin M_1 in milk and milk preparations using filter-supported bilayer lipid membranes, *Anal. Chem.*, 70, 2366, 1998.

26. Siontorou, C.G., Andreou, V.G., Nikolelis, D.P., and Krull, U.J., Flow injection monitoring of aflatoxin M_1 in cheese using filter-supported bilayer lipid membranes with incorporated DNA, *Electroanalysis*, 12, 747, 2000.

27. Carlson, M.A., Bargeron, C.B., Benson, R.C., Fraser, A.B., Phillips, T.E., Velky, J.T., Groopman, J.D., Strickland, P.T., and Ko, H.W., An automated handheld biosensor for aflatoxin, *Biosens. Bioelectron.*, 14, 841, 2000.

28. Daly, S.J., Keating, G.J., Dillon, P.P., Manning, B.M., O'Kennedy, R., Lee, H.A., and Morgan, M.R.A., Development of surface plasmon resonance-based immunoassay for aflatoxin B$_1$, *J. Agric. Food Chem.*, 48, 5097, 2000.

29. Strachan, N.J.C., John, P.G., and Millar, I.G., Application of an automated particle-based immunosensor for the detection of aflatoxin B$_1$ in foods, *Food Agric. Immunol.*, 9, 177, 1997.

30. Carter, R.M., Jacobs, M.B., Lubrano, G.J., and Guilbault, G.G., Rapid detection of aflatoxin B$_1$ with immunochemical optrodes, *Anal. Letts.*, 30, 1465, 1997.

31. Aldao, M.A.J., Carpinella, M.C., Corelli, M., and Herrero, G.G., Competitive ELISA for quantifying small amounts of aflatoxin B$_1$, *Food Agric. Immunol.*, 7, 307, 1995.

32. Reddy, S.V., Mayi, D.K., Reddy, M.U., Thirumala-Devi, K., and Reddy, D.V.R., Aflatoxin B$_1$ in different grades of chillies (*Capsicum annum* L.) in India as determined by indirect competitive-ELISA, *Food Addit. Contam.*, 18, 553, 2001.

33. Pesavento, M., Domagala, S., Baldini, E., and Cucca, L., Characterization of an enzyme linked immunosorbent assay for aflatoxin B$_1$ based on commercial reagents, *Talanta*, 45, 91, 1997.

34. Bhattacharya, D., Bhattacharya, R., and Dhar, T.K., A novel signal amplification technology for ELISA based on catalysed reporter deposition: demonstration of its applicability for measuring aflatoxin B$_1$, *J. Immunol. Methods*, 230, 71, 1999.

35. Markaki, P. and Melissari, E., Occurrence of aflatoxin M$_1$ in commercial pasteurised milk determined with ELISA and HPLC, *Food Addit. Contam.*, 14, 451, 1997.

36. Kim, E.K., Shon, D.H., Ryu, D., Park, J.W., Hwang, H.J., and Kim, Y.B., Occurrence of aflatoxin M$_1$ in Korean dairy products determined by ELISA and HPLC, *Food Addit. Contam.*, 17, 59, 2000.

37. Malone, B.R., Humphrey, C.W., Romer, T.R., and Richard, J.L., Determination of aflatoxins in grains and raw peanuts by rapid procedure with fluorometric analysis, *J. Assoc. Off. Anal. Chem. Int.*, 83, 95, 2000.

38. Arim, R.H., Aguinaldo, A.R., Tanaka, T., and Yoshizawa, T., Optimization and validation of a minicolumn method for determining aflatoxins in copra meal, *J. Assoc. Off. Anal. Chem. Int.*, 82, 877, 1999.

39. AOAC, *Official Methods of Analysis of the AOAC International*, 16th ed., 4th ver., Association of Official Analytical Chemists, Gaithersburg, MD, 1998.

40. Yoshizawa, T., Yamashita, A., and Chokethaworn, N., Occurrence of fumonisins and aflatoxins in corn from Thailand, *Food Addit. Contam.*, 13, 163, 1996.

41. Ali, N., Sardjono, Yamashita, A., and Yoshizawa, T., Natural co-occurrence of aflatoxins and *Fusarium* mycotoxins (fumonisins, deoxynivalenol, nivalenol and zearalenone) in maize from Indonesia, *Food Addit. Contam.*, 15, 377, 1998.

42. Akiyama, H., Chen, D., Miyahara, M., Toyoda, M., and Saito, Y., Simple HPLC determination of aflatoxins B$_1$, B$_2$, G$_1$ and G$_2$ in nuts and corn, *J. Food Hygienic Soc. Jpn.*, 37, 195, 1996.

43. Ali, N., Hashim, N. H., and Yoshizawa, T., Evaluation and application of a simple and rapid method for the analysis of aflatoxins in commercial foods from Malaysia and the Philippines, *Food Addit. Contam.*, 16, 273, 1999.

44. Tanaka, T., Yoneda, A., Sugiura, Y., Inoue, S., Takino, M., Tanaka, A., Shinoda, A., Suzuki, H., Akiyama, H., and Toyoda, M., An application of liquid chromatography and mass spectrometry for determination of aflatoxins, *Mycotoxins*, 52, 107, 2002.

45. Stroka, J., Anklam, E., Joerissen, U., and Gilbert, J., Immunoaffinity column cleanup with liquid chromatography using post-column bromination for determination of aflatoxins in peanut butter, pistachio paste, and paprika powder: collaborative study, *J. Assoc. Off. Anal. Chem. Int.*, 83, 320, 2000.

46. Stroka, J., Anklam, E., Joerissen, U., and Gilbert, J., Determination of aflatoxin B_1 in baby food (infant formula) by immunoaffinity column cleanup liquid chromatography with postcolumn bromination: collaborative study, *J. Assoc. Off. Anal. Chem. Int.*, 84, 1116, 2001.

47. Nesheim, S., Trucksess, M.W., and Page, S.W., Molar absorptivities of aflatoxins B_1, B_2, G_1, and G_2 in acetronitrile, methanol, and toluene–acetonitrile (9+1) (modification of AOAC official method 971.22): collaborative study, *J. Assoc. Off. Anal. Chem. Int.*, 82, 251, 1999.

48. Delaunay, N., Pichon, V., and Hennion, M.-C., Immunoaffinity solid-phase extraction for the trace-analysis of low-molecular-mass analytes in complex sample matrices, *J. Chromatogr.*, B745, 15, 2000.

49. Dragacci, S. and Grosso, F., *Validation of an Analytical Method to Determine the Content of Aflatoxin M_1 in Milk and Milk Powder by Thin Layer Chromatography After Immunoaffinity Clean-Up*, report of IDF/IUPAC/IAEA joint project, June 2001.

50. Dragacci, S., Grosso, F., and Gilbert, J., Immunoaffinity column clean-up with liquid chromatography for determination of aflatoxin M_1 in liquid milk: collaborative study, *J. Assoc. Off. Anal. Chem. Int.*, 84, 437, 2001.

51. Govaris, A., Roussi, V., Koidis, P.A., and Botsoglou, N.A., Distribution and stability of aflatoxin M_1 during processing, ripening and storage of Telemes cheese, *Food Addit. Contam.*, 18, 437, 2001.

52. Kussak, A., Andersson, B., Andersson, K., and Nilsson, C.-A., Determination of aflatoxicol in human urine by immunoaffinity column clean-up and liquid chromatography, *Chemosphere*, 36, 1841, 1998.

53. Shantha, T., Critical evaluation of methods available for the estimation of aflatoxin B_1 in chili powder, *J. Food Sci. Technol.*, 36, 163, 1999.

54. Roch, O.G., Blinden, G., Coker, R.D., and Nawaz, S., The validation of a solid phase clean-up procedure for the analysis of aflatoxins in groundnut cake using HPLC, *Food Chem.*, 52, 93, 1995.

55. Bradburn, N., Coker R.D., and Blunden, G., A comparative study of solvent extraction efficiency and the performance of immunoaffinity and solid phase columns on the determination of aflatoxin B_1, *Food Chem.*, 52, 179, 1995.

56. Daradimos, E., Marcaki, P. and Koupparis, M., Evaluation and validation of two fluorometric HPLC methods for the determination of aflatoxin B_1 in olive oil, *Food Addit. Contam.*, 17, 65, 2000.

57. Simon, P., Delsaut, P., Lafontaine, M., Morele, Y., and Nicot, T., Automated column-switching high-performance liquid chromatography for the determination of aflatoxin M_1. *J. Chromatogr.*, B712, 95, 1998.

58. Nakajima, M., Mycotoxin analysis using immunoaffinity columns, in *Proc. Int. Symp. of Mycotoxicology 99, Mycotoxin Contamination: Health Risk and Prevention Project*, Chiba, Japan, September 9–10, 1999.

59. Sobolev, V.S. and Dorner, J.W., Clean-up procedure for determination of aflatoxins in major agricultural commodities by liquid chromatography, *J. Assoc. Off. Anal. Chem. Int.*, 85, 642, 2002.

60. Otta, K.H., Papp, E., and Bagócsi, B., Determination of aflatoxins in food by overpressured-layer chromatography, *J. Chromatogr. A*, 882, 11, 2000.

61. Stroka, J., Petz, M., Joerissen, U., and Anklam, E., Investigation of various extractants for the analysis of aflatoxin B_1 in different food and feed matrices, *Food Addit. Contam.*, 16, 331, 1999.

62. Kamimura, H., Nishijima, M., Yasuda, K., Ushiyama, H., Tabata, S., Matsumoto, S., and Nishima, T., Simple clean-up method for analysis of aflatoxins and comparison with various methods, *J. Assoc. Off. Anal. Chem. Int.*, 68, 458, 1985.

63. Castro, L. and Vargas, E.A., Determining aflatoxins B_1, B_2, G_1, G_2 in maize using florisil clean up with thin layer chromatography and visual and densitometric quantification, *Food Sci. Technol.*, 21, 115, 2001.

64. Vargas, E.A., Preis, R.A, Castro, L., and Silva, C.M.G, Co-occurrence of aflatoxins B_1, B_2, G_1, G_2, zearalenone and fumonisin B_1 in corn from Brazil, *Food Addit. Contam.*, 18, 981,2001.

65. Peng, Z., Yibing, Z., and Weidong, Z., Determination of aflatoxins B_1, B_2, G_1, G_2 in peanuts by high performance thin-layer chromatography with multifunction clean-up column, *Fenxi Ceshi Xuebao (J. Instrum. Anal.)*, 18, 62, 1999.

66. Goto, T., Marzuki, M.A., Daud, M.J., Oshibe, A., Nakamura, K., and Nagashima, H., Simple analytical method for aflatoxin contamination in dried oil palm frond (OPF) and OPF base feed, *Mycotoxins*, 52, 123, 2002.

67. Nawaz, S., Coker, R.D., and Haswell, S., HPTLC: a valuable chromatographic tool for the analysis of aflatoxins, *J. Planar Chromatogr.*, 8, 4, 1995.

68. de Koe, W.J., CEN approach to standardisation of methods for mycotoxin analysis, *Nat. Toxins*, 3, 318, 1995.

69. Stroka, J., van Otterdijk, R., and Anklam, E., Immunoaffinity column clean-up prior to thin-layer chromatography for the determination of aflatoxins in various food matrices, *J. Chromatogr. A*, 904, 251, 2000.

70. Skarkova, J. and Ostry V., An HPTLC method for confirmation of the presence of ultra-trace amounts of aflatoxin M_1 in human urine, *J. Planar Chromatogr.*, 13, 42, 2000.

71. Carman, A.S., Kuan, S.S., Ware G.M., and Umrigar, P., Robotic automated analysis foods for aflatoxin, *J. Assoc. Off. Anal. Chem. Int.*, 79, 456, 1996.

72. Li, F.-Q., Yoshizawa, T., Kawamura, O., Luo, X.Y., and Li, Y.-W., Aflatoxins and fumonisins in corn from the high-incidence area for human hepatocellular carcinoma in Guangxi, China, *J. Agric. Food. Chem.*, 49, 4122, 2001.

73. Whitaker, T., Horwitz, W., Albert, R., and Nesheim, S., Variability associated with analytical methods used to measure aflatoxin in agricultural commodities, *J. Assoc. Off. Anal. Chem. Int.*, 79, 476, 1996.

74. Papp, E., Bagócsi, B., H-Otta, K., Kovacsics-Ács, L., and Mincsovics, E., The role of over-pressured-layer chromatography among chromatographic methods for the determination of the aflatoxin content of fish, *J. Planar Chromatogr.*, 12, 383, 1999.

75. Otta, K.H., Papp, E., Mincsovics, E., and Záray G., Determination of aflatoxins in corn by use of the personal OPLC basic system, *J. Planar Chromatogr.*, 11, 370, 1998.

76. Papp, E., Farkas, A., Otta, H. K., and Mincsovics, E., Validation and robustness testing of an OPLC method for the determination of aflatoxins in wheat, *J. Planar Chromatogr.*, 13, 328, 2000.

77. Stroka, J. and Anklam, E., Development of a simplified densitometer for the determination of aflatoxins by thin layer chromatography, *J. Chromatogr. A*, 904, 263, 2000.

78. Liang, Y., Baker, M.E., Yeager, B.T., and Denton, M.B., Quantitative analysis of aflatoxins by high-performance thin-layer chromatography utilizing a scientifically operated charge-coupled device detector, *Analyt. Chem.*, 68, 3885, 1996.

79. Onji, Y., Okayama, A., Yasumura, K., and Tamaki, M., Two-dimensional liquid chromatographic separation of aflatoxins B_1, B_2, G_1, and G_2 in spices, *Mycotoxins*, 52, 115, 2002.

80. Scott, P.M. and Lawrence, G.A., Determination of aflatoxins in beer, *J. Assoc. Off. Anal. Chem. Int.*, 80, 1229, 1997.

81. Céspedes, A.E. and Diaz, G.J., Analysis of aflatoxins in poultry and pig feeds and feedstuffs used in Colombia, *J. Assoc. Off. Anal. Chem. Int.*, 80, 1215, 1997.

82. Scudamore, K.A. and Patel, S., Survey for aflatoxins, ochratoxin A, zearalenone and fumonisins in maize imported into the United Kingdom, *Food Addit. Contam.*, 17, 407, 2000.

83. Zhang, P., Zhang, Y., Zhao, W., and Li, Y., Determination of aflatoxins in peanut by high performance liquid chromatography using immunoaffinity column clean-up and on-line electrochemical derivatization, *Chin. J. Chromatogr.*, 18, 82, 2000.

84. MacDonald, S., Wilson, P., Barnes, K., Damant, A., Massey, R., Mortby, E., and Shepherd, M.J., Ochratoxin A in dried vine fruit: method development and survey, *Food Addit. Contam.*, 16, 253, 1999.

85. Kussak, A., Andersson, B., and Andersson, K., Immunoaffinity column clean-up for the high-performance liquid chromatographic determination of aflatoxins B_1, B_2, G_1, G_2, M_1 and Q_1 in urine, *J. Chromatogr. B*, 672, 253, 1995.

86. Papadopoulou-Bouari, A., Stroka, J., and Anklam, E., Comparison of two post-column derivatization systems, ultraviolet irradiation and electrochemical determination, for the liquid chromatography determination of aflatoxins in food, *J. Assoc. Off. Anal. Chem. Int.*, 85, 411–423, 2002.

87. Cepeda, A., Franco, C.M., Fente, C.A., Vázquez, B.I., Rodríguez, J.L., Prognon, P., and Mahuzier, G., Post-column exitation of aflatoxins using cyclodextrins in liquid chromatography for food analysis, *J. Chromatogr. A*, 721, 69, 1996.

88. Wei, J., Okerberg, E., Dunlap, J., Ly, C., and Shear, J.B., Determination of biological toxins using capillary electrokinetic chromatography with multiphoton-excited fluorescence, *Anal. Chem.*, 72, 1360, 2000.

89. Siméon, N., Myers, R., Bayle, C., Nertz, M., Stewart, J.K., and Couderc, F., Some applications of near-ultraviolet laser-induced fluorescence detection in nanomolar- and subnanomolar-range high-performanace liquid chromatography or micro-high-performance liquid chromatography, *J. Chromatogr.*, 913, 253, 2001.

90. Maragos, C.M. and Greer, J.I., Analysis of aflatoxin B_1 in corn using capillary electrophoresis with laser-induce fluorescence detection, *J. Agric. Food Chem.*, 45, 4337, 1997.

91. Holak, W., DiProssimo, V., and Malek, E.G., Reductive voltammetric HPLC detection of aflatoxins: determination of aflatoxin B_1 in foods, *J. Liq. Chrom. Rel. Technol.*, 20, 1057, 1997.

92. Elizalde-González, M.P., Mattusch, J., and Wennrich, R., Stability and determination of aflatoxins by high-performance liquid chromatography with amperometric detection, *J. Chromatogr. A*, 828, 439, 1998.

93. Janini, G.M., Muschik, G.M., and Issaq, H.J., Micellar electrokinetic chromatography in zero-eletroosmotic flow environment, *J. Chromatogr. B*, 683, 29, 1996.

94. Cappiello, A., Famiglini, G., and Tirillini, B., Determination of aflatoxins in peanut meal by LC/MS with a particle beam interface, *Chromatographia*, 40, 411, 1995

95. Kussak, A., Nilsson, C.-A., Andersson, B., and Langridge, J., Determination of aflatoxins in dust and urine by liquid chromatography/electrospray ionization tandem mass spectrometry, *Rapid Commun. Mass Spectrom.*, 9, 1234, 1995.

96. Trucksess, M.W, Dombrink-Kurtzman, M.A., Tournas, V.H., and White, K.D., Occurrence of aflatoxins and fumonisins in Incaparina from Guatemala, *Food Addit. Contam.*, 19, 671, 2002.

97. Pohland, A.E. and Trucksess, M.W., Mycotoxin method evaluation, in *Methods in Molecular Biology: Mycotoxin Protocols*, Vol. 157, Trucksess, M.W. and Pohland, A.E., Eds., Humana Press, Totowa, NJ, 2001, pp. 3–10.

98. International Union of Pure and Applied Chemistry, Guidelines for collaborative study procedure to validate characteristics of a method of analysis, *J. Assoc. Off. Anal. Chem. Int.*, 72, 694, 1989.

99. Gilbert, J., Quality assurance in mycotoxin analysis, *Food Nutr. Agric.*, 23, 33, 1999.

100. Key, P.E., Patey, A.L., Rowling, S., Wilbourne, A., and Worner, F., International proficiency testing of analytical laboratories for foods and feeds from 1990 to 1996: the experiences of the United Kingdom food analysis performance assessment scheme, *J. Assoc. Off. Anal. Chem. Int.*, 80, 895, 1997.

101. Horwitz, W., Kamps, R.K., and Boyer, K.W., Quality assurance in the analysis of foods for trace constituents, *J. Assoc. Off. Anal. Chem. Int.*, 63, 1344, 1980.

102. Thompson, M., Recent trends in inter-laboratory precision at ppb and sub-ppb concentrations in relation to fitness for purpose criteria in proficiency testing, *Analyst*, 125, 385, 2000.

103. Gilbert, J., Mathieson, K., and Owen, L., Results from an international mycotoxin proficiency testing scheme, in *Mycotoxins and Phycotoxins in Perspective at the Turn of the Millennium*, de Koe, W.J., Samson, R.A., van Egmond, H.P., Gilbert, J., and Sabino, M., Eds., Ponsen & Looyen, Wageningen, 2001, pp. 69–75.

104. Vongbuddhapitak, A., Trucksess, M.W., Atisook, K., Suprasert, D., and Horwitz, W., Laboratory proficiency testing of aflatoxins in corn and peanuts: a cooperative project between Thailand and the United States, *J. Assoc. Off. Anal. Chem. Int.*, 82, 259, 1999.

105. Weigert, P., Gilbert, J., Patey, A.L., Wood, R., and Barylko-Pikielna, N., Analytical quality assurance for the WHO GEMS/Food-EURO programme: results of 1993/94 laboratory proficiency testing, *Food Addit. Contam.*, 14, 399, 1997.

106. Dragacci, S., Grosso, F., Pfauwathel-Marchond, N., Fremy, J.M., Vernant, A., and Lombard, B., Proficiency testing for the evaluation of the ability of European Union National Reference laboratories to determine aflatoxin M_1 in milk at levels corresponding to the new European Union legislation, *Food Addit. Contam.*, 18, 405, 2001.

107. Dragacci, S. and Fremy, J.M., Proficiency testing for aflatoxin M_1 monitoring programme: a five-year experience in France, in *Mycotoxins and Phycotoxins: Developments in Chemistry, Toxicology and Food Safety*, Miraglia, M., van Egmond, H.P., Brera, C., and Gilbert, J., Eds., Alaken, Fort Collins, CO, 1998, pp. 151–157.

108. Reif, K. and Metzger, W., Determination of aflatoxins in medicinal herbs and plant extracts, *J. Chromatogr. A*, 692, 131, 1995.

109. Scott, P.M. and Trucksess, M.W., Application of immunoaffinity columns to mycotoxin analysis, *J. Assoc. Off. Anal. Chem. Int.*, 80, 941, 1997.

110. Ioannou-Haouri, E., Christodoulidou, M., Christou, E., and Constantinidou, E., Immunoaffinity column/HPLC determination of aflatoxin M_1 in milk, *Food Agric. Immunol.*, 7, 131, 1995.

111. Kussak, A., Andersson, B., and Andersson, K., Determination of aflatoxin in airborne dust from feed factories by automated immunoaffinity column clean-up and liquid chromatography, *J. Chromatogr. A*, 708, 55, 1995.

112. Sujatha, N., Suriakala, S., and Rao, B.S., Enzyme immunoassay for aflatoxin B_1–lysine adduct and its validation, *J. Assoc. Off. Anal. Chem. Int.*, 84, 1465, 2001.

113. Arim, R.H., Ferolin, C.A., and Dumada, L.M., Comparison of three methods for the determination of aflatoxin in copra meal, *Food Addit. Contam.*, 12, 415, 1995.

114. Dragacci, S., Gleizes, E., Fremy, J.M., and Candlish, A.A.G., Use of immunoaffinity chromatography as a purification step for the determination of aflatoxin M_1 in cheeses, *Food Addit. Contam.*, 12, 59, 1995.

115. DiProssimo, V.P. and Malek, E.G., Comparison of three methods for determining aflatoxins in melon seeds, *J. Assoc. Off. Anal. Chem. Int.*, 79, 1330, 1996.

116. Scholten, J.M. and Spanjer M.C., Determination of aflatoxin in pistachio and shells, *J. Assoc. Off. Anal. Chem. Int.*, 79, 1360, 1996.

117. Selim, M.I. and Popendorf, W., Aflatoxin B_1 in common egyptian foods, *J. Assoc. Off. Anal. Chem. Int.*, 79, 1124, 1996.

118. Lin, S.-S. and Fu, Y.-M., Determination of aflatoxins in liquor products by immunoaffinity column with fluorometry and HPLC, *J. Food Drug Analy.*, 5, 171, 1997.

119. Bhat, R.V., Vasanthi, S., Rao, B.S., Rao, R.N., Rao, V.S., Nagaraja, K.V., Bai, R.G., Prasad, C.A.K., Vanchinathan, S., Roy, R., Saha, S., Mukherjee, A., Ghosh., P.K., Toteja, G.S., and Saxena, B.N., Aflatoxin B_1 contamination in maize samples collected from different geographical regions of India: a multicentre study, *Food Addit. Contam.*, 14, 151, 1997.

120. El-Tahan, F.H., El-Tahan, M.H., and Shebl, M.A., Occurrence of aflatoxins in cereal grains from four Egyptian governorates, *Nahrung*, 44, 279, 2000.

121. Nakajima, M., Tsubouchi, H., Miyabe, M., and Ueno, Y., Survey of aflatoxin B_1 and ochratoxin A in commercial green coffee beans by high-performance liquid chromatography linked with immunoaffinity chromatography, *Food Agric. Immunol.*, 9, 77, 1997.

122. Vahl, M. and Jorgensen, K., Determination of aflatoxin in food using LC/MS/MS, *Lebensm Unters Forsch.*, 206, 243, 1998.

123. Arim, R.H., Aguinaldo, A.R., and Yoshizawa, T., Application of a modified minicolumn to detection of aflatoxins in corn, *Mycotoxins*, 48, 53, 1999.

124. Bilotti, L.G., Pinto, V.E.F., and Vaamonde, G., Aflatoxin production in three selected samples of triticale, wheat and rye grown in Argentina, *J. Sci. Food Agric.*, 80, 1981, 2000.

125. Medina-Martínez, M.S. and Martínez, A.J., Mold occurrence and aflatoxin B_1 and fumonisin B_1 determination in corn samples in Venezuela, *J. Agric. Food Chem.*, 48, 2833, 2000.

126. Horwitz, W., Evaluation of analytical methods used for regulation of foods and drugs, *Anal. Chem.*, 54, 67A, 1982

13 Recent Developments in Immunochemical Methods

Chris M. Maragos

CONTENTS

13.1. INTRODUCTION

The history of the development of analytical methods for detecting fungal toxins is rich and varied. Method development has followed a process somewhat akin to Darwinian evolution: Methods are selected based upon the characteristics most desirable to the analyst. Typically, this has led to the development of accurate and sensitive methods for their detection, with a recurring emphasis on improving the speed and lowering the costs of the assays. Like evolution, there have been radical developments, incremental developments, and techniques that have fallen from favor only to be rediscovered. This review focuses on recent developments in technologies for detection of mycotoxins, with a particular emphasis on the myriad forms of biosensors that have begun to appear. Specifically, recent developments in evanescent wave technologies (surface plasmon resonance, fiberoptic sensors), lateral flow and dipstick devices, fluorescence polarization and time-resolved fluorescence, microbead assays, and capillary electrophoretic immunoassays are described. The challenge for the emerging technologies is to demonstrate advantages over the more conventional, and better established, techniques in settings outside of the analytical laboratory.

Since the link was first made between chemical agents produced by fungi and disease in animals, technologies for detection of these mycotoxins have steadily advanced. As new analytical technologies have developed, they have been rapidly incorporated into mycotoxin testing strategies. The reasons for this rapid adaptation have been the desire to protect human health, economic incentives of protecting livestock from acute toxicity, gains in production obtained from reducing the chronic effects of exposure to mycotoxins, and testing requirements in order to meet contract specifications for minimum acceptable levels in foods and feeds. These forces have led to the continued experimentation and improvement in mycotoxin analytical testing. This review focuses on emerging technologies that may, in the future, find use in the monitoring of mycotoxins in agricultural commodities and foods.

Detection of mycotoxins themselves must be distinguished from the detection of mycotoxin-producing fungi. Historically, the fungi have been detected either visually (e.g., moldy grain) or indirectly by the effects they cause on foodstuffs as they grow. The growth of fungi within a foodstuff changes the physical and chemical composition of the food, and these changes can often be used advantageously to distinguish fungally infected material. Removing the bulk of fungal contamination can be expected to reduce the mycotoxin content of the material, provided the fungus is mycotoxigenic. Early studies used the bright greenish-yellow fluorescence (BGYF) of a kojic acid derivative as a marker for aflatoxin contamination. The effect was the basis for a fiberoptic device for detecting BGYF in corn kernels.[1] More recently, image analysis, machine vision systems, and infrared spectroscopy have all been used to detect the changes wrought by fungal infection.[2-8] The advantages of such techniques are that they may eventually allow the rapid sorting of commodities based on fungal content which, in turn, could be used as a tool to reduce exposure to the toxins. As such, the newer fungal detection technologies hold considerable promise. Nevertheless, the indirectness of the association of fungal content with mycotoxin content necessitates the detection of the fungal toxins themselves. The remainder of this review focuses on methods for the detection of mycotoxins.

Testing for mycotoxins is conducted under many different circumstances and for a variety of reasons, which has led to a proliferation in the number of test methods. Selecting the appropriate method depends on the intended use for the method. Factors such as the speed of the method, its accuracy, the skill level required to perform the assay, and the cost will all have an impact on method selection. The methods basically fall into two major categories: (1) those that can be conducted with minimal training in portable laboratories or the field (screening assays), and (2) those that must be conducted by more fully trained personnel in analytical laboratories. In all cases, obtaining a representative test sample of the overall lot is essential in order to ensure that the results of the test sample can be correctly ascribed to the lot. Sampling, subsampling, grinding, and extraction of commodities take considerable attention and time. In fact, these steps often require more time than some of the rapid assays for detecting the toxins; therefore, where possible, it is preferable to combine a rapid extraction technique with rapid assays in order to minimize the overall assay time.

Widely used methods include some of those that were developed when mycotoxins were first identified as chemical agents, such as thin-layer chromatography (TLC). The development of antibodies to the major mycotoxins in the 1970s and 1980s led to the increased use of enzyme-linked immunosorbent assays (ELISAs). The ELISAs are extensively used as screening methods, and over time commercial ELISA test kits have been developed, many of which have been validated through organizations such as AOAC International. The website of AOAC International (www.aoac.org) is a good resource for locating commercially available test kits. Refinements to ELISA technology continue, including the development of more sensitive amplification mechanisms.[9]

Chromatographic methods for mycotoxins have continuously been developed and improved. Commonly used liquid chromatographic methods include high-performance liquid chromatography (HPLC) with fluorescence detection for aflatoxins, zearalenone, ochratoxins, and (derivatized) fumonisins, as well as HPLC with ultraviolet detection for deoxynivalenol. Many of the trichothecene mycotoxins are commonly analyzed by gas chromatography (GC) with various detectors. This review cannot adequately address the nuances of the many chromatographic methods, and interested readers are directed to the excellent reviews by Sydenham and Shephard,[10] Shephard,[11] and Trucksess.[12] TLC, once a mainstay of mycotoxin analysis, has been supplanted by HPLC in many locations; however, given the significant advantages of the low cost of operation, the potential to test many samples simultaneously, and advances in instrumentation that allow quantification by image analysis or densitometry,[13,14] TLC remains a viable screening technique for mycotoxins.

Because of the advantages of specificity and selectivity, chromatographic separation combined with mass spectrometric (MS) detection has continued to expand as a laboratory-based method for detecting mycotoxins. HPLC–MS methods for all of the major and many of the minor mycotoxins have been published and continue to be developed and improved.[15-20] Clearly, the use of mass spectrometric methods can be expected to increase, particularly as they become easier to use and the costs of the instrumentation continues to fall.

Despite the considerable advantages of the chromatographic techniques, most remain laboratory-based assays because they require considerable skill and instrumentation to operate. On the other end of the analytical spectrum are the immunoassays: assays that use the inherent specificity of antibodies to bind target analytes. By far the majority of reported mycotoxins are low molecular weight (less than 1000 daltons), which restricts somewhat the formats of immunoassays that can be used for their detection. Most, but not all, mycotoxin immunoassays are competitive immunoassays of one of two types: (1) so-called "direct" assays, where the mycotoxin-specific antibody is attached to a surface, or (2) so-called "indirect" assays, where a mycotoxin or mycotoxin–protein conjugate is attached to a surface (Figure 13.1). The terminology is somewhat misleading, because both formats entail measurement of an enzymatic product, not direct detection of the mycotoxin itself. The distinction between whether antibody or antigen is attached to the surface is important and has implications for the formats of biosensors, as is discussed below.

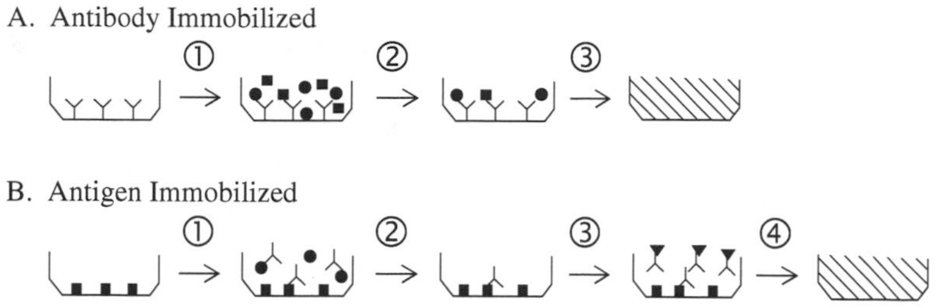

A. Antibody Immobilized

B. Antigen Immobilized

FIGURE 13.1 Two common immunoassay formats using either immobilized antibody or immobilized antigen. (A) With antibody (**Y**) immobilized, the steps are (1) addition of sample (toxin: ●) and toxin-enzyme conjugate (■) and incubation, (2) washing to remove unbound conjugate, and (3) addition of substrate, incubation, and measurement of colored product. (B) With antigen (■) immobilized, the steps are (1) addition of sample (toxin: ●) and antitoxin antibody (**Y**) and incubation, (2) washing to remove unbound antibody, (3) addition of secondary antibody–enzyme conjugate (**Y▼**) and incubation, and (4) washing to remove unbound conjugate, addition of substrate, incubation, and measurement of colored product.

13.2 SENSORS FOR DETECTING FUNGAL TOXINS

Many technologies exist for detecting low-molecular-weight materials. Those that have recently been applied to mycotoxin detection include evanescent wave technologies, lateral flow and dipstick test strips, fluorescence polarization, microbead assays, flow injection liposome immunoassays, capillary electrophoretic immunoassays, and flow injection lipid bilayer assays.

13.2.1 EVANESCENT WAVE TECHNOLOGIES

13.2.1.1 Fiberoptic Devices

When light is applied to some materials, such as optical fibers, it can, under the appropriate conditions, undergo a process known as *total internal reflection*. When this occurs, essentially all of the light that is applied (launched) to the surface is propagated through the fiber; however, a small portion of the applied light exits the fiber perpendicular to it in the form of an evanescent wave. The evanescent wave can also be formed when light is reflected off other surfaces, such as glass slides. The characteristics of the evanescent wave are influenced by the refractive index of the fiber, the refractive index of the surrounding material, and the incident light. A useful property of the evanescent wave is that its intensity decreases exponentially with distance from the interface between the fiber and the surrounding material.[21] This effect can be used in several ways. The first of these is with fiberoptic devices, where a binding event can be made to occur near the surface of the fiber. The second is with the induction of plasmons in a metal film, as in surface plasmon resonance.

With fiberoptic-based devices, the binding event can be monitored in several ways, analogous to the situation discussed above with ELISAs;[21] that is, either antibody or antigen can be attached to the surface of the fiber. Examples with mycotoxins include immunosensors for fumonisins and aflatoxins. In the former case, antibodies to fumonisin are attached to the surface of optical fibers. The fibers are then exposed to a sample mixed with fluorescently labeled fumonisin B_1 (FB_1-FL). The labeled and unlabeled FB_1 compete for binding to the surface of the fiber. After a washing step to remove unbound fluorophore, the amount of bound fluorophore is detected. This is possible because a small proportion of the fluorescence emission of the FB_1-FL is captured by the optical fiber, which transmits it to a sensitive detector. This device is capable of detecting fumonisin B_1 in maize samples within 8 minutes with moderate sensitivity, having a midpoint for the calibration curve (IC_{50}) of 70 ng FB_1 per mL.[22] The technique has been applied to corn samples extracted with methanol/water. Simple dilution of the methanolic extract, in order to reduce the methanol content, gave an assay with poor sensitivity, having an IC_{50} of 25,000 ng FB_1 per g maize. Concentrating the FB_1 with an immunoaffinity column improved the sensitivity of the assay but negated the primary advantage of the method — speed.[23]

A similar device was constructed for aflatoxin B_1 (AFB_1) using antiaflatoxin antibodies attached to the optical fiber.[23] Unlike fumonisins, the aflatoxins have a native fluorescence that can be monitored. The binding of aflatoxin to antibody increases the concentration of the fluorophore at the surface of the fiber, effectively resulting in a noncompetitive assay for aflatoxin (vs. the competitive format of the fumonisin assay). The major advantage of the noncompetitive format would be direct, rather than indirect, detection of the toxin. The fiberoptic device detected aflatoxin B_1, with a limit of determination of 2 ng AFB_1 per mL; however, small changes in the refractive index of the solution surrounding the fiber (i.e., sample) greatly affect the size of the evanescent wave and, therefore, the response.

A fluorescence-based immunosensor for AFB_1 not relying on the principle of evanescence has also been reported.[24] In this case, aflatoxin antibodies were immobilized to a membrane. The membrane was exposed to AFB_1 for 1 hour then washed and fitted onto the tip of an optical fiber connected to a fluorometer. The fluorescence of bound AFB_1 was then detected over the range of 0.05 to 20 ng/mL. Samples of corn and peanuts were tested after clean-up. Corn samples were extracted with methanol/water, treated with NaCl/zinc acetate, partitioned with benzene, dried, and reconstituted before testing. Peanut samples were extracted with acetonitrile/buffer overnight then centrifuged and the supernatant used directly. The limit of detection in buffer, peanut extract, and corn extract was 0.05 ng/mL. The same article also described two types of competitive assay where an aflatoxin–bovine serum albumin conjugate (AFB_1–BSA) was coated on the membranes. In both formats, free AFB_1 competed with bound AFB_1–BSA for aflatoxin antibody binding. In the first format, the aflatoxin antibody was unlabeled but was detected with a secondary antibody labeled with the enzyme alkaline phosphatase. An additional rinsing step was added to remove the excess secondary antibody before fitting the membrane onto the sensor. The amount of secondary antibody was then determined after the addition of a fluorogenic substrate. The limit of detection was 5 ng/mL in peanut extract. In the second format, the aflatoxin antibody was itself labeled with fluorescein, so the addition of substrate was not necessary. The limit of detection was 1 ng/mL in peanut extract.

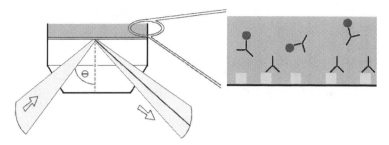

FIGURE 13.2 Schematic of a surface plasmon resonance biosensor for mycotoxins. The left panel depicts the incident light applied through a prism onto a glass slide, reflection of the light, and the formation of an evanescent wave. In the format shown, a mycotoxin or myc-otoxin–protein conjugate (antigen) is attached to the surface of the sensor chip, and antibody binding is detected. Competition between the immobilized antigen (□) and free toxin (●), from the sample, decreases the amount of antibody (Y) bound at the surface of the chip.

13.2.1.2 Surface Plasmon Resonance

The evanescent wave effect has also been applied using the phenomenon of surface plasmon resonance (SPR).[25] With SPR, light is used to excite plasmons (electron charge density waves) in a thin film of gold foil attached to the surface of a glass prism (Figure 13.2). The resonance is a coupling between the light energy and the surface plasmons in the gold film. When the resonance occurs, a resultant absorption of energy and a decrease in the intensity of the reflected light are observed. The angle of incident light at which this process occurs is known as the *resonance angle* (θ in Figure 13.2), and it is dependent upon the refractive indices of the prism and the sensor surface. If the incident light is applied in a fashion such that there are multiple incident angles (as shown in Figure 13.2, where the incident light is a wedge), then the characteristic drop at the resonance angle creates what amounts to a shadow within the reflected light.[26]

The evanescent wave extends outward from the surface of the gold foil into the surrounding solution. The intensity of the evanescent wave decays exponentially with distance from the surface. Materials that interact near the surface alter the refractive index of the surface, thereby changing the resonance angle. SPR sensors measure binding phenomena by detecting either the change in the resonance angle or the change in intensity of the reflected light. In either case, the magnitude of the response is affected by the amount (mass) of material that adheres to the sensor surface. The SPR sensors then, in a fashion, act as mass sensors. Devices using this technology are available commercially from several sources but can also be fabricated.

The formats for the SPR immunoassays mimic those of the ELISAs; namely, either antigen is attached to the surface or antibody is attached to the surface, analogous to the illustration in Figure 13.1. The schematic in Figure 13.2 illustrates the case where mycotoxin or a mycotoxin–protein conjugate (antigen) is attached to the surface of the chip, and the binding of mycotoxin-specific antibody is detected in a competitive assay. The alternative format is the attachment of the mycotoxin-specific antibody to the surface of the chip. In the latter case, the binding of toxin to the antibody can be measured in a noncompetitive assay.

Assays for mycotoxins using both formats have been described, although most have used antigen-modified surfaces to detect antibody binding. The first group to report assays of this form for mycotoxins was TNO in The Netherlands.[27] SPR assays have been described for AFB_1, deoxynivalenol (DON), zearalenone (ZEN), ochratoxin A (OA), and fumonisins. The majority of SPR applications for mycotoxins have used instrumentation commercially available from Pharmacia AB (Uppsala, Sweden). AFB_1 was detected by SPR using a format with AFB_1–BSA antigen attached to the sensor surface and competition between the bound antigen and AFB_1 in solution.[28] Two polyclonal antibody preparations were tested. AFB_1 standards were incubated with the aflatoxin antibodies for 10 minutes before being applied to the sensor. After an interval during which the antibody attached to the sensor surface the antibody/antigen interaction was disrupted with 1-M ethanolamine in 20% (v/v) acetonitrile in order to regenerate the surface of the sensor. The sensor had a linear range of detection between 3 and 98 ng AFB_1 per mL, which was slightly more sensitive than the same antibody preparation tested in an ELISA format (linear range, 12 to 25,000 ng/mL).

Because SPR measures antibody/antigen interaction, the technique can be used to select for high-affinity antibodies or antibody fragments. This approach was taken for the selection of single-chain antibody fragments for binding to AFB_1–BSA.[29] Two phage-display antibody libraries were panned against AFB_1–BSA, and the antibody fragments were screened for binding to AFB_1–BSA by SPR. The technique allowed the isolation of single-chain fragment variable (scFv) antibody domains with affinity for AFB_1. The scFv were then evaluated in a competitive SPR assay; although the limits of detection were not specified, the assay was shown to be able to detect a 50-nM solution of AFB_1 or AFG_1 (approximately 16 ng/mL). Antiaflatoxin scFv has also been used for the detection of AFB_1 in spiked extracts of grain.[30] The range of detection for the assay was between 3 and 195 ng AFB_1/mL in phosphate buffered saline and 0.75 to 48 ng/mL in spiked grain extracts. The type of grain used was not specified. The enhanced performance of the assay in the grain extracts may be due to the presence of 5% (v/v) methanol in the extracts, a situation also known to occur with some ELISAs for AFB_1.

Deoxynivalenol has also been detected using SPR.[31–33] DON was attached to the surface of the sensor using a DON–biotin conjugate and a streptavidin-coated sensor surface.[31] Wheat was extracted with aqueous methanol and centrifuged, and the extract was passed through a solid-phase extraction column (MycoSep®; Romer Labs) to remove impurities. The purified extract was combined with a rabbit polyclonal antibody before injection into the sensor. Greater response could also be attained by adding a secondary, anti-rabbit, antibody. Using the secondary antibody increased the signal fivefold but also shifted the working range toward higher concentrations. The assays were relatively rapid, with a 10-min sample preparation time and a 5-min analysis time. Recovery of DON from wheat spiked at 50 to 500 ng/g averaged $104 \pm 15\%$. The working range was between 130 and 10,000 ng DON per mL (equivalent to 390 to 3000 ng/g in samples), with an IC_{50} of 720 ng/mL.

Results by SPR were correlated with results from GC–MS and HPLC–UV of contaminated wheat.

Recently, Tüdos et al.[33] reported an assay for DON in wheat using SPR with a DON–casein conjugate immobilized on the sensor surface. After the antibody binding step, the sensor surface was regenerated with 6-M guanidine chloride, and the sensor could be used 500 times without significant loss of activity. The assay was used to detect DON in wheat extracted with acetonitrile/water. No sample clean-up was necessary; however, the samples had to be diluted before injection in order to reduce the solvent strength to minimize the affect on the DON antibodies. The assay had a working range of 2.5 to 30 ng DON per mL, and results correlated well between the sensor and HPLC–MS–MS for 8 wheat samples.

A technique for the detection of up to four mycotoxins simultaneously using SPR was recently reported.[32] The fluidics of the instrument, a BIACORE® 2000, were constructed such that the sensor surface contained four serially connected flow cells. As with the previously described SPR assays, sample was mixed with mycotoxin-specific antibodies before injection onto the sensor. Instead of immobilizing toxin–protein conjugates onto the sensor surface the toxins themselves were immobilized. The exception was for DON, which was immobilized as a DON–BSA conjugate. Samples were extracted with 90% (v/v) acetonitrile/water and a portion of the extract cleaned up with a solid-phase extraction column (MycoSep® 224 MFC), which bound impurities and allowed the toxins to pass through into the filtrate. The filtrate was diluted tenfold and mixed with the four antibodies (ZEN, DON, FB_1, AFB_1) before assay. Assays could be conducted within 25 minutes, including the sensor regeneration time.

The second SPR format — using antibody-modified surfaces to directly detect toxin binding noncompetitively — has been reported for the fumonisins.[34] It is possible with the fumonisins because of their larger molecular weight (721 daltons for FB_1) relative to other mycotoxins such as aflatoxin (312 daltons). Polyclonal antifumonisin antibodies were immobilized on the sensor surface. The latter assay had a limit of detection of standard solutions of FB_1 of 50 ng/mL and could be conducted in 10 minutes. Application of the assay to fumonisins in foods was not reported. The advantage of the immobilized antibody format is that it is noncompetitive; therefore, the response was directly proportional to the amount of toxin present. A second advantage is that a toxin–protein conjugate was not required.

13.2.2 Test Strips

A long-desired format for mycotoxin assays is one analogous to home pregnancy test kits, where the presence of the mycotoxin is directly detected in a rapid disposable device. Devices of this type are also known as *immunochromatographic tests*. A major impediment to the development of kits of this format for mycotoxins has been their low molecular weight. Unlike the detection of larger antigens, where multiple antibodies can be attached and used to make noncompetitive "sandwich" formats, the detection of low-molecular-weight toxins has relied upon competitive assays. A disposable device that uses a membrane-based, flow-through immunoassay has been available commercially for many years for detection of aflatoxin M_1 (AFM_1)

in milk (AflaCup®; International Diagnostic Systems Corp., St. Joseph, MI). With the AflaCup® format, the applied liquids flow through the membrane and are collected on an absorbent pad on the opposite side of the membrane. The label is enzymatic, which means that a substrate-incubation step must be included. This type of assay is also known as an enzyme-linked immunofiltration assay (ELIFA). A flow-through membrane immunossay for detection of ochratoxin A in wheat was also reported,[35] and a collaborative study of kits to detect OA and T-2 toxin has also been conducted.[36] The limits of detection were 4 ng/g and 50 ng/g for OA and T-2, respectively, in wheat, rye, maize, and barley.

Lateral flow devices differ from ELIFA in that the flow is directed laterally across the membrane rather than through it (parallel rather than perpendicular flow), analogous to thin-layer chromatography. Lateral flow devices can be made in several forms depending on which reagent is labeled (the toxin or the antibody) and the form of the label (enzymatic, labeled liposomes, or colloidal gold). A lateral flow device using an enzymatic marker, a lateral flow ELISA, was sold commercially for aflatoxins, OA, T-2 toxin, and ZEN by Editek (Burlington, NC).

A dipstick assay similar to a lateral flow device was developed for FB_1 in corn-based foods and was reported to have a visual limit of detection of 40 to 60 ng FB_1 per g sample.[37] In this format, the test strips have two lines: one line corresponding to antifumonisin antibody and the other to antihorseradish peroxidase antibody. Test strips are incubated in a tube containing the tracer (fumonisin–horseradish peroxidase) and the sample extract. After washing and the addition of substrate, the two lines are visualized. The anti-HRP line acts as a positive color control, while the presence of FB_1 is indicated by a reduction in the color at the fumonisin antibody line. Assay time is about 1 hour. A similar type of device was developed for T-2 toxin in wheat.[38]

An interesting adaptation of the aforementioned dipstick format was the application to the detection of multiple mycotoxins in wheat.[39] Using multiple mycotoxin-specific antibodies and multiple toxin–HRP conjugates, the technique was able to detect aflatoxin B_1, T-2 toxin, 3-acetyl-DON, roridin A, and ZEN. The response of the test (toxin-exposed) dipstick was compared to the response of a control dipstick (not exposed to toxin) for estimation of toxin presence.[39] The detection limits for spiked wheat samples were 30, 100, 600, 500, and 60 ng/g for AFB_1, T-2, 3-acetyl-DON, roridin A, and ZEN, respectively.

Commercial lateral flow devices for mycotoxins continue to be developed, with the goals of combining the negative control reaction on the same strip as the sample and shortening the required assay time. Interesting variations include the possibilities of using labeled liposomes or colloidal gold conjugates to avoid the enzymatic reaction step. A lateral flow device was constructed for aflatoxin B_1 using aflatoxin-modified liposomes.[40] The liposomes contained sulfo-rhodamine B, a visible (and fluorescent) dye. Aflatoxin-specific antibody was attached to the strip and the strip exposed to AFB_1. The labeled liposomes were then added and competed for binding to the antibody, with the color at the site of the antibody inversely proportional to the AFB_1 level. Assay times were 12 minutes. The device could detect as little as 20 ng AFB_1, although on a concentration basis the detection was relative poor, with the midpoint of the binding curve occurring at approximately 2000 ng/mL. Unfortunately, the liposomes also showed some instability to solvents. Notwithstanding this result, the assay demonstrates the possibility of shortening analysis times through the use of nonenzymatic labels.

Because of the ease of use of these devices, efforts to develop dipstick and lateral flow assays for mycotoxins are likely to continue, particularly with stable nonenzymatic labels. Recently, American Bionostica (Logan Township, NJ) in collaboration with R-Biopharm (Darmstadt, Germany) developed lateral flow devices for DON, fumonisins, and aflatoxins. Grain samples are extracted with buffer, and the extract is allowed to settle for 5 to 10 minutes. Several drops of the extract are then transferred to the test device (cassette). The test strips contain two lines, one of which is a negative control. Positive results are indicated by the decrease of intensity of red color at the test line. Further information on the devices can be obtained from R-Biopharm. Lateral flow test strips have also been developed by Charm Science, Inc. (Lawrence, MA). The strips measure AFM_1 in milk and use a portable hand-held instrument for quantitation. At the time this review was written, the test strips and reader were available commercially; however, no documentation on the performance characteristics of the assay was found. The assay is purported to detect AFM_1 at the European Union regulatory limit of 0.050 ng/mL in milk and requires 15 minutes to perform (www.charm.com).

13.2.3 FLUORESCENCE POLARIZATION AND TIME-RESOLVED FLUORESCENCE

Fluorescence polarization (FP) immunoassay has recently been described for a number of mycotoxins, including the aflatoxins, DON, fumonisins, and ZEN.[41–43] Unlike most of the other sensors described in this review, the FP immunoassays are solution-phase assays; that is, they can be conducted without the attachment of antibody or antigen to a solid surface.[44] The principle for FP immunoassay is illustrated in Figure 13.3. Fluorescence polarization detectors are indirectly measuring the rate of rotation of a fluorophore in solution. The rate of rotation is directly related to the size of molecules, with larger molecules rotating more slowly at a given temperature. With FP immunossay a mycotoxin–fluorophore conjugate (tracer) is used. The tracer has a low molecular weight and rotates rapidly in solution. The addition of antitoxin antibody results in the formation of an immune complex of the tracer with the antibody, effectively slowing the rate of rotation of the fluorophore and increasing the polarization. FP immunoassay therefore allows the detection of low-molecular-weight materials in solution without requiring a step to separate the "bound" and "unbound" label, a significant advantage over traditional ELISA techniques.

As with other immunoassays, the selection of appropriate antibody and tracer pairs is essential. While FP immunoassays can be conducted using either the rate of association (kinetic assays) or the endpoint of equilibrated mixture (batch or equilibration assays), in general the latter method may be preferable if untrained personnel will be performing the assays. The time it takes for the antibody/tracer/toxin combination to achieve equilibration is a critical aspect of FP immunoassays. This equilibration time can vary from 1 minute to over 15 minutes,

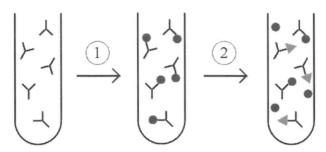

FIGURE 13.3 Fluorescence polarization (FP) immunoassay. Assays are performed by placing antimycotoxin antibody (**Y**) into a cuvette followed by: (1) addition of sample extract (toxin: ●) and blanking the instrument, then (2) addition of toxin–fluorophore (tracer: ▲) and incubation, during which the tracer and toxin compete for available antibody. Fluorescence polarization is measured without the need for separating the bound and unbound tracer (see text).

depending on the antibody/tracer combination selected. Rapid (30-second) and sensitive assays for deoxynivalenol were developed using a DON–fluorescein tracer; however, the assay did not come to equilibrium quickly, a potential problem if samples are tested by untrained personnel.[42] When a different antibody/tracer combination was used, though, a rapid (1-minute) and sensitive assay that quickly came to equilibrium was attained. The latter assay was used to quantitate DON in spiked or naturally contaminated wheat, but not maize, at levels greater than 500 ng/g; thus, when appropriate antibody/tracer combinations are used, rapid FP immunoassays can be developed.[42] This aspect is important in any competitive immunoassay but seems to be particularly important with FP immunoassays. The potential speed of FP assays combined with the portability of commercially available devices suggests this is a promising technology for mycotoxin detection.

Unlike fluorescence polarization immunoassays, time-resolved fluoroimmunoassays (TR-FIA) use the property of fluorescence lifetime. The rate of decay of fluorescence after a pulse of light at the excitation wavelength differs among different types of fluorophores. The fluorescence lifetime of some fluorophores, such as europium, are much longer than most fluorescent materials present in the matrix as background fluorescence; therefore, europium can be discriminated from background fluorescence without the need to blank the sample. This property is used to advantage in TR-FIAs. TR-FIAs were recently reported for α-zeralanol (zeranol) and α-zearalenol in bovine urine.[45] The principle of the assay was essentially that of a competitive ELISA as illustrated in Figure 13.1A. An anti-IgG was coated to the microtiter wells, followed by antizearalenol antibody and a zeranol–ovalbumin–europium conjugate. An advantage of the technique was that all the reagents could be adsorbed onto the surface of the wells, eliminating the need for a separate addition/mixing step during the assay. The bovine urine was cleaned up with an immunoaffinity column. The cleaned extract was added to the wells, and the plates were shaken and washed (to remove unbound conjugate). An enhancement solution was added, and the europium time-resolved fluorescence was measured. The technique was very sensitive, with limits of detection of 1.3 ng zeranol per mL and 5.6 ng α-zearalenol per mL in bovine urine. A TR-FIA was also developed several years ago for AFB_1 in soya seeds, dried figs, and raisins.[46] The limits of detection were 0.5 ng/g, indicating the method was sensitive enough to be used in these commodities.

13.2.4 CAPILLARY-BASED IMMUNOASSAYS

13.2.4.1 Microbead Assays

Immunoaffinity columns (IACs) have a long history of use in the clean-up of samples for mycotoxin analysis.[47] In the most common form, mycotoxin antibodies are coated on the surface of spherical beads and packed in a column. Diluted sample extract is applied to the column. The toxin adheres to the column, and most of the potentially interfering material is removed with a wash step. The toxin is then eluted by disrupting the immune complex, generally by increasing the solvent strength. In many cases, the eluted toxin can be derivatized and detected with a portable fluorometer (Vicam LP, Watertown, MA). Alternatively, the eluted toxin can be applied to an instrumental technique for further separation before quantitation. Assays using this concept are available commercially. Microbead assays are miniaturized versions of the IAC assays, often with the clean-up and detection steps performed in a single instrument. Although attaching antibodies to microbeads is the more direct approach, assays can also be conducted with antigen attached to the microbeads in competitive assays similar conceptually to ELISAs (Figure 13.4).

Recently, a handheld microbead sensor was developed for aflatoxins.[48] The sensor uses a small peristaltic pump to move fluids over a miniaturized affinity column containing aflatoxin antibodies. Samples in buffer solution are allowed to flow over the column, binding the aflatoxin. The column is then washed with buffer and eluted with methanol/water and the aflatoxin measured directly by fluorescence. The fluorescence detector uses a xenon arc lamp and a filter to select light at the excitation wavelength of 365 nm. Assays can be conducted within 2 minutes using a 1-mL sample volume. The fluorescence of aflatoxins is highly sensitive to the presence or absence of the C_{15}–C_{16} double bond. Aflatoxin B_2 (AFB_2) is more fluorescent than AFB_1. For many chromatographic methods for the aflatoxins, the C_{15}–C_{16} bond is reacted (e.g., with bromine, iodine, or trifluoroacetic acid) to yield more fluorescent derivatives, increasing the sensitivity of the assay. Commercial affinity columns also employ a developing (derivatization) solution to enhance fluorescence before detection in portable fluorometers, such as with the Vicam system. The aflatoxin microbead sensor has detected 1 mL of a 1.44-ng/mL solution of AFB_2. The range of detection for the device is reported to be 0.1 to 50 ng/mL for aflatoxin in buffer (the specific aflatoxin was not noted). The instrument is capable of holding about 500 mL of reagents, enough for approximately 100 assays before refilling. Given the history of the successful application of commercial IACs, when used in conjunction with a separate fluorometric detection step, the construction of a device combining both steps is a promising development, although the reuse of antibody-based affinity columns can be problematic. Issues such as fouling of the column, denaturation/renaturation of antibody, and leaching of antibody all impact the degree to which antibody-based affinity columns can be reused.

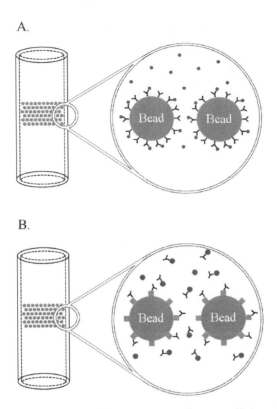

FIGURE 13.4 Formats of microbead immunoassays or immunoaffinity columns. (A) Immobilized antibody (**Y**), to which toxin binds. The beads are then washed and the toxin (●) eluted for detection. (B) Immobilized antigen (■), which competes with the toxin (●) for a limiting amount of antibody (**Y**) in solution. The beads are washed and a secondary, labeled antibody is added (not shown). After a second wash either the labeled antibody is detected directly (in the case of fluorescent labels) or substrate is added to yield a colored product (in the case of enzymatic labels).

Affinity columns utilizing bound antigen, rather than antibody, use a competitive rather than a noncompetitive format. A competitive format has a disadvantage in that the mycotoxin is indirectly detected, but it may offer the advantage of reusability if the antigen coating is stable. A commercial instrument, KinEXA®, available from Sapidyne Instruments (Idaho City, ID), performs many of the functions of an automated IAC assay using microbeads. This instrument was used by Strachan et al.[49] to develop an application for detection of aflatoxin B_1 in nut puree, peanut butter, and pistachio meal. The assay format is known as *sequential injection immunoassay* (SIIA), although it has also been called *flow-injection immunoassay* (FIIA). Beads were coated with an AFB_1–BSA conjugate. Assays were conducted by mixing sample with aflatoxin antibody (primary antibody) and pumping this mixture over the beads. A fluorescein-labeled secondary antibody was added, and the excess label was washed away. The fluorescence associated with the beads was then determined.

Assays were performed within 8 minutes; however, sample preparation/clean-up required an additional hour, which negated some of the potential advantages over ELISA. A similar assay, also using the KinEXA® apparatus, was used to detect ZEN standard solutions.[50] The beads were coated with ZEN–BSA antigen, and, as with the aflatoxin assay, a secondary antibody labeled with fluorescein was used. Assay time was described as less than 60 minutes. The assay was capable of detecting 5 ng ZEN per mL solution, but because food samples were not examined it is not possible to extrapolate a limit of detection in foods.

The SIIA format has also been applied to AFB$_1$ using an enzymatic rather than a fluorescent label.[51] The instrumentation is available commercially from FIALab Instruments (Bellevue, WA) and uses a small spectrometer rather than a fluorescence detector. As with the earlier work, the beads are coated with AFB$_1$–BSA. The secondary antibody is labeled with alkaline phosphatase (rather than fluorescein). A 15-min sample extraction/dilution was combined with a 10-min assay to detect AFB$_1$ in artificially contaminated pistachios over the range of 4 to 400 ng/g. The minimum concentration of AFB$_1$ detected was 0.2 ng/mL, equivalent to 4 ng AFB$_1$ per g sample, although matrix interferences were observed.

13.2.4.2. Flow Injection Liposome Immunoassay

A variant of FIIA involves the use of antigen-tagged liposomes instead of microbeads and is known as *flow-injection liposome immunoanalysis* (FILIA). The format has been applied to analysis of fumonisins in corn.[52] Fumonisin antibodies were coated onto protein A on the capillary walls. Extracts of samples were injected, followed by fumonisin-tagged liposomes. The liposomes were filled with a fluorescent marker (sulforhodamine B). After a wash to remove unbound liposomes, the liposomes were lysed with a detergent, and the fluorescence measured. As with an ELISA, the signal from the fluorophore was inversely proportional to the fumonisin concentration. The assays could be performed in 11 minutes, and the limit of detection was 0.1 ng (0.1 mL of a 1 ng FB$_1$ per mL solution) for the FILIA and 2.5 ng for the HPLC–fluorescence method. Recovery of FB$_1$ from spiked cornmeal ranged from 80 to 92% over the range of 1000 to 4000 ng FB$_1$ per g cornmeal, and the results for spiked samples compared favorably to HPLC. The assay also compared favorably to HPLC for detection of FB$_1$ in commercial corn products and corn-based feeds, suggesting this format has true potential for detecting mycotoxins in foods.

13.2.4.3 Capillary Electrophoretic Immunoassay

While the FIIA and SIIA involve immunoassays conducted in capillaries with micro-bead or antigen-tagged liposomes, the immunoassays can also be conducted without a supporting phase (e.g., in solution). Capillary electrophoresis (CE) is generally used as a chromatographic technique in which mycotoxins are separated from one another and from matrix components using electrical potential. When used as a chromatographic method, the toxins are isolated from food samples using clean-up methods analogous to HPLC, and the cleaned extracts are injected into the capillaries. After separation in an electrical field, the analytes are detected, typically using

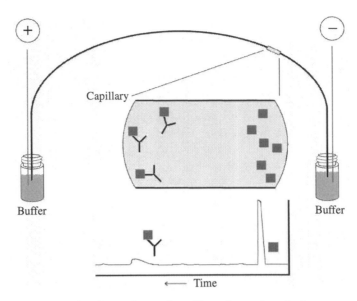

FIGURE 13.5 Schematic of one form of capillary electrophoretic immunoassay. In this format, antibody (**Y**) is combined with sample and a fluorescently labeled toxin (tracer: **■**). Bound and unbound tracer are separated in an electric field. In the presence of free toxin the amount of unbound tracer increases, and the amount of bound tracer decreases, changing the relative sizes of the two peaks.

fluorescence or ultraviolet absorbance. CE as a chromatographic method for mycotoxin analysis has been reviewed.[53]

Recent advances in mycotoxin detection with CE include the use of β-cyclodextrins combined with multiphoton excitation for aflatoxin detection[54] and the detection of patulin in apple juice by UV.[55] The former was a very sensitive method, having concentration detection limits for aflatoxins in the range of 0.2 to 0.4 nM (0.06 to 0.13 ng/mL). A method combining the detection of ochratoxins A and B with that of four aflatoxins has also been described.[56] Micellar electrokinetic capillary chromatography (MECC) is a variant of capillary zone electrophoresis that is particularly useful for detecting neutral compounds, such as the aflatoxins. An MECC-based method using an electronically controlled injection process (vs. the more generally used pressure or electrokinetic injection) for measurement of aflatoxin standard solutions was described.[57] The injection platform is interesting because it resembles those used in microchip formats. The reported limits of detection (S/N of 2) of aflatoxins in buffer ranged from 7.2 nM (2.3 ng/mL), for AFB$_2$ to 31 nM (10 ng/mL) for AFG$_1$.

The combination of CE with immunoassay (Figure 13.5) has also been used for analysis of fumonisins in maize.[58] After extraction of corn with water, a portion of the extract was mixed with antibody and a fluorescein-tagged fumonisin (tracer). Fumonisin in the sample competed with the tracer for binding to the antibody. Application of voltage resulted in a separation of the bound and unbound tracer. With increasing fumonisin in the sample, the level of bound tracer decreased, and the level of unbound tracer increased, signaling the presence of the toxin. The assays were relatively rapid, using a 4-min electrophoretic step and a 2-min wash of the capillary between samples. The sensitivity of the technique was highly dependent on the concentration of antibody used. At the optimum antibody concentration the midpoint for the calibration curves ranged from 500 to 1700 ng FB_1/mL. Unfortunately this level of sensitivity was only sufficient for analyzing maize samples containing substantial concentrations of FB_1 (greater than 10,000 ng/g). Sensitivity in this format is likely highly dependent on the relative affinity of the antibody for the fumonisin and the tracer under conditions of high electric field strength, which might be improved with a different fumonisin antibody.

Other, less well developed techniques also use capillaries to deliver reagents to multichannel devices, with the goal of multiple-analyte detection.[59] It is likely the improvements in microfluidics and miniaturization of sensor components will lead to the development of multichannel mycotoxin sensors, perhaps using sensor-on-a-chip technologies or array biosensors for mycotoxin detection.[60]

13.3   FUTURE CHALLENGES

Sensitive and reproducible quantitation of analytes present at low levels in complex matrices begets certain challenges in the development of the assays. Principally, these include ensuring that the sample being tested is representative of the larger lot and that the assays are sensitive enough and accurate enough for their intended use. The state of mycotoxin analysis is such that for most of the known mycotoxins current analytical techniques have overcome these obstacles. For the lesser known mycotoxins and for those mycotoxins that remain to be discovered, the challenges are to develop methods that can be used for routine analysis in laboratories. For most of the known mycotoxins, the remaining challenges are to render the analytical process more efficient through the application of new technologies that may be less labor intensive and therefore less expensive.

For laboratory-based assays an ongoing challenge has been the simultaneous detection of multiple toxins. Despite the efforts of researchers throughout the years to develop multiple mycotoxin assays, the need still exists for the detection of multiple families of mycotoxins from the same sample. For example, the potential co-occurrence of aflatoxins and fumonisins in corn suggests that screening for both groups of mycotoxins is warranted. Yet, the differences in the polarity of these toxins, the differences in their physical properties (fluorescence, UV absorbance, or lack thereof), and the concentration ranges of interest (ng/g vs. μg/g) have made simultaneous detection difficult. In this regard, the mass spectrometric methods hold considerable promise, as do those that use chromatography combined with multiple detectors.

Rapid detection of multiple toxins is also an area where emerging technologies for mycotoxin detection may find use. It is not difficult to envision antibody-based screening assays for multiple mycotoxins using array formats similar to those described for higher molecular weight toxins.[60] Recently, a biochip that uses surface-enhanced Raman scattering (SERS) microscopy was demonstrated to detect aflatoxins B_1 and G_1.[61] The chip uses aflatoxin antibodies or RNA polymerase to capture the aflatoxins. A Raman microscope was used to collect SERS spectra before and after exposure to the toxin, with a change in the spectra indicating the presence of the toxin. The concentration of aflatoxin that could be detected by this method was not described, but the potential to detect multiple toxins simultaneously using an array of antibodies is apparent.

The continued miniaturization of analytical instrumentation also opens up possibilities for handheld devices that perform the same duties as today's benchtop devices. This is particularly true for instruments measuring absorbance or fluorescence. The ongoing development of microfluidics and capillary-based assays (e.g., capillary electrophoresis, FIIA, SIIA) suggests that the development of assay-on-a-chip technology is in the near future.

Biosensors can also be constructed using binding events other than that of antibody/antigen. Examples include the flow injection assays developed for aflatoxin M_1 in milk based on lipid bilayer membranes.[62,63] In two formats, the AFM_1 was shown to interact directly with the bilayers and to inhibit the hybridization of single-stranded DNA oligomers. The pertubations in the bilayer were measured electrochemically. In the first format, the working range of AFM_1 standards was 1.9 to 20.9 nM (0.62 to 6.9 ng/mL); in the second format, the limit of detection was 0.5 nM (0.16 ng/mL), and the assays were very rapid — less than 1 minute.[63] In the non-DNA hybridization format, with the use of filter-supported bilayer membranes, AFM_1 was shown to alter the phase transition temperature of the membrane.[62] Detection using the electrochemical response was very rapid (10 seconds), and the assays had subnanomolar limits of detection. By adjusting the flow rate through the membranes, effects due to potential matrix interferences such as casein were minimized.[62] Milk and milk products spiked with AFM_1 showed a good agreement between the spiking level and the concentration detected in the range of 3.8 to 14.6 nM AFM_1 and at a rate of 4 samples per minute. A disposable electrochemical DNA-based biosensor has also been reported to detect aflatoxin B_1 at much higher levels (10,000 ng/mL).[64]

While the focus of this review has been on antibody-based technologies, the use of biologically derived binding elements is not inherently essential to the development of functional sensors (although, by definition, it *is* required for a biosensor). The improvement of antibodies and antibody fragments through recombinant techniques is one approach to improving immunoassay,[65,66] as is the development of novel mycotoxin binding peptides using combinatorial solid-phase synthesis.[67] Yet another alternative is the development of nonbiologically based binding and transduction elements. An example of the latter is molecularly imprinted polymers (MIPs). Usually, MIPs are synthesized using a template molecule similar in structure to the analyte. Functional monomers that interact with the template noncovalently are polymerized together using cross-linking monomers. The entrapped template is then removed and the polymer used to bind the analyte. Functional monomers that interact covalently with the template or analyte can also be used. High-affinity MIPs could essentially perform the same functions as antibodies in immunoassays and might benefit from greater solvent tolerance or tolerance to extremes of pH or ionic strength. Recently, MIPs have been reported for the ochratoxins,[68] DON, and ZEN.[69]

Although the affinities are not yet competitive with those of antibodies, the potential for further development is excellent.

As discussed at the beginning of this review, further progress can be expected on technologies that detect mycotoxigenic fungi as well. Detection of the fungi may involve detection of physical changes to the commodity (as with the previously mentioned color, fluorescence, and IR methods, and machine vision systems). The growth of fungi also cause chemical changes, some of which may be detectable by optical methods, or by alternative methods measuring changing volatile composition such as GC–MS or electronic noses.[70–72] Furthermore, the detection of DNA of mycotoxigenic fungi is possible, using a variety of polymerase chain reaction (PCR)-based methods such as random amplification of polymorphic DNA (RAPD), reverse transcription (RT)-PCR, competitive PCR, and real-time quantitative PCR. The latter techniques, with regard to detection of mycotoxigenic fungi, were recently reviewed.[73]

The aforementioned emerging technologies for mycotoxin detection are at various stages in the progression to useful analytical tools. Some have been tested and found, at least currently, to be poor candidates for further development. Some are advanced enough for field use. Many still face the challenge of making the transition from proof-of-concept assays using toxins in buffer solutions to analysis of food samples. Others have been demonstrated to work with food samples but still face the challenges of ease of use and validation by multiple laboratories. Despite these obstacles, detection technologies continue to advance, and the prospects for further improvements in mycotoxin detection methodology are excellent.

REFERENCES

1. McClure, W.F. and Farsaie, A., Dual-wavelength fiberoptic photometer measures fluorescence of aflatoxin contaminated pistachio nuts, *Trans. ASAE*, 204–207, 1980.
2. Pearson, T., Machine vision system for automated detection of stained pistachio nuts, *Lebensmitelw. U. Technol.*, 29, 203–209, 1996.
3. Hirano, S., Okawara, N., and Narazaki, S., Near-infrared detection of internally moldy nuts, *Biosci. Biotechnol. Biochem.*, 62, 102–107,1998.
4. Ruan, R., Ning, S., Song, A., Ning, A., Jones, R., and Chen, P., Estimation of *Fusarium* scab in wheat using machine vision and a neural network, *Cereal Chem.*, 75, 455–459, 1998.
5. Dowell, F.E., Ram, M.S., and Seitz, L.M., Predicting scab, vomitoxin, and ergosterol in single wheat kernels using near-infrared spectroscopy, *Cereal Chem.*, 76, 573–576, 1999.
6. Pearson, T., Wicklow, D.T., Maghirang, E.B., Xie, F., and Dowell, F.E., Detecting aflatoxin in single corn kernels by transmittance and reflectance spectroscopy, *Trans. ASAE*, 44, 1247–1254, 2001.
7. Dowell, F.E., Pearson, T.C., Maghirang, E.B., Xie, F., and Wicklow, D.T., Reflectance and transmittance spectroscopy applied to detecting fumonisin in single corn kernels infected with *Fusarium verticillioides*, *Cereal Chem.*, 79, 222–226, 2002.
8. Kos, G., Lohninger, H., and Krska, R., Fourier transform mid-infrared spectroscopy with attenuated total reflection (FT-IR/ATR) as a tool for the detection of *Fusarium* fungi on maize, *Vib. Spec.*, 29, 115–119, 2002.

9. Bhattacharya, D., Bhattacharya, R., and Dhar, T.K., A novel signal amplification technology for ELISA based on catalyzed reporter deposition: demonstration of its applicability for measuring aflatoxin B_1, *J. Immunol. Meth.*, 230, 71–86, 1999.

10. Sydenham, E.W. and Shephard, G.S., Chromatographic and allied methods of analysis for selected mycotoxins, in *Progress in Food Contaminant Analysis*, Gilbert, J., Ed., Chapman & Hall, New York, 1997, pp. 65–146.

11. Shephard, G.S., Analytical methodology for mycotoxins: recent advances and future challenges, in *Mycotoxins and Phycotoxins in Perspective at the Turn of the Millennium*, de Koe, W.J., Samson, R.A., van Egmond, H.P., Gilbert, J., and Sabino, M., Eds., Ponsen & Looyen, Wageningen, 2001, pp. 19–28.

12. Trucksess, M.W., Rapid analysis (thin layer chromatographic and immunochemical methods) for mycotoxins in foods and feeds, in *Mycotoxins and Phycotoxins in Perspective at the Turn of the Millennium*, de Koe, W.J., Samson, R.A., van Egmond, H.P., Gilbert, J., and Sabino, M., Eds., Ponsen & Looyen, Wageningen, 2001, pp. 29–40.

13. Karuna, R. and Sashidhar, R.B., Use of ion-exchange chromatography coupled with TLC-laser scanning densitometry for the quantitation of fumonisin B_1, *Talanta*, 50, 381–389, 1999.

14. Stroka, J. and Anklam, E., Development of a simplified densitometer for the determination of aflatoxins by thin-layer chromatography, *J. Chromatogr. A*, 904, 263–268, 2000.

15. Cappiello, A., Famiglini, G., and Tirillini, B., Determination of aflatoxins in peanut meal by LC/MS with a particle beam interface, *Chromatographia*, 40, 411–416, 1995.

16. Hartl, M. and Humpf, H.-U., Simultaneous determination of fumonisin B_1 and hydrolyzed fumonisin B_1 in corn products by liquid chromatography/electrospray ionization mass spectrometry, *J. Agric. Food Chem.*, 47, 5078–5083, 1999.

17. Zöllner, P., Jodlbauer, J., and Lindner, W., Determination of zearalenone in grains by high-performance liquid chromatography-tandem mass spectrometry after solid-phase extraction with RP-18 columns or immunoaffinity columns, *J. Chromatogr. A*, 858, 167–174, 1999.

18. Musser, S.M., Eppley, R.M., and Trucksess, M.W., Electrospray mass spectrometry for fumonisin detection and method validation, in *Mycotoxins and Food Safety*, DeVries, J.W., Trucksess, M.W., and Jackson, L., Eds., Kluwer Academic, New York, 2002, pp. 95–105.

19. Tanaka, T., Yoneda, A., Sugiura, Y., Inoue, S., Takino, M., Tanaka, A., Shinoda, A., Suzuki, H., Akiyama, H., and Toyoda, M., An application of liquid chromatography and mass spectrometry for determination of aflatoxins, *Mycotoxins*, 52, 107–113, 2002.

20. Plattner, R.D. and Maragos, C.M., Determination of deoxynivalenol and nivalenol in corn and wheat by liquid chromatography with electrospray mass spectrometry, *J. Assoc. Off. Anal. Chem. Int.*, 86, 61–65. 2003,

21. Thompson, R.B., Ligler, F.S. Chemistry and technology of evanescent wave biosensors, in *Biosensors with Fiberoptics*, Wise, D.L. and Wingard, L.B., Eds., Humana Press, Clifton, NJ, 1991, pp. 111–138.

22. Thompson, V.S. and Maragos, C.M., Fiberoptic immunosensor for the detection of fumonisin B_1, *J. Agric. Food Chem.*, 44, 1041–1046, 1996.

23. Maragos, C.M. and Thompson, V.S., Fiber-optic immunosensor for mycotoxins, *Nat. Toxins*, 7, 371–376, 1999.

24. Carter, R.M., Jacobs, M.B., Lubrano, G.J., and Guilbault, G.G., Rapid detection of aflatoxin B_1 with immunochemical optrodes, *Anal. Lett.*, 30, 1465–1482, 1997.

25. Liedberg, B., Nylander, C., and Lundström, I., Biosensing with surface plasmon resonance-how it all started, *Biosen. Bioelect.*, 10, i–ix, 1995.

26. Pharmacia Biosensor, *Surface Plasmon Resonance: A Description of the Detection Principle*, BIAtechnology Note 101, Pharmacia Biosensor AB, Uppsala, Sweden, 1995, pp. S-751–S782.

27. Van der Gaag, B., Burggraaf, R.A., and Wahlström, L., Application and development of a BIAcore for the detection of mycotoxins in food and feed, in *Abstracts of Papers*, 110th AOAC International Annual Meeting and Exposition, Orlando, FL, September 8–12, 1996, AOAC International, Gaithersburg, MD, 1996.

28. Daly, S.J., Keating, G.J., Dillon, P.P., Manning, B.M., O'Kennedy, R.O., Lee, H.A., and Morgan, M.R.A., Development of surface plasmon resonance-based immunoassay for aflatoxin B₁, *J. Agric. Food Chem.*, 48, 5097–5104, 2000.

29. Moghaddam, A., Løbersli, I., Gebhardt, K., Braunagel, M., and Marvik, O.J., Selection and characterization of recombinant single-chain antibodies to the hapten aflatoxin-B₁ from naive recombinant antibody libraries, *J. Immunol. Methods*, 254, 169–181, 2001.

30. Daly, S.J., Dillon, P.P., Manning, B.M., Dunne, L., Killard, A., and O'Kennedy, R.O., Production and characterization of murine single chain Fv antibodies to aflatoxin B₁ derived from a pre-immunized antibody phage display library system, *Food Agric. Immunol.*, 14, 255–274, 2002.

31. Schnerr, H., Vogel, R.F., and Niessen, L., A biosensor-based immunoassay for rapid screening of deoxynivalenol contamination in wheat, *Food Agric. Immunol.*, 14, 313–321, 2002.

32. Van der Gaag, B., Spath, S., Dietrich, H., Stigter, E., Boonzaaijer, G., van Osenbruggen, T., and Koopal, K., Biosensors and multiple mycotoxin analysis, *Food Control*, 14, 251–254, 2003.

33. Tüdos, A.J., Lucas-van den Bos, H.R., and Stigter, E.C.A., Rapid surface plasmon resonance-based assay of deoxynivalenol (DON), *J. Agric. Food Chem.*, 51, 5843–5848, 2003.

34. Mullett, W., Lai, E.P.C., and Yeung, J.M., Immunoassay of fumonisins by a surface plasmon resonance biosensor, *Anal. Biochem.*, 258, 161–167, 1998.

35. De Saeger, S. and Van Peteghem, C., Flow-through membrane-based enzyme immunoassay for rapid detection of ochratoxin A in wheat, *J. Food Prot.*, 62, 65–69, 1999.

36. De Saeger, S., Sibanda, L., Desmet, A., and Van Peteghem, C., A collaborative study to validate novel field immunoassay kits for rapid mycotoxin detection, *Int. J. Food Microbiol.*, 75, 135–142, 2002.

37. Schneider, E., Usleber, E., and Märtbauer, E., Rapid detection of fumonisin B₁ in corn-based food by competitive direct dipstick enzyme immunoassay/enzyme-linked immunofiltration assay with integrated negative control reaction, *J. Agric. Food Chem.*, 43, 2548–2552, 1995.

38. De Saeger, S. and Van Peteghem, C., Dipstick enzyme immunoassay to detect *Fusarium* T-2 toxin in wheat, *Appl. Environ. Microbiol.*, 62, 1880–1884, 1996.

39. Schneider, E., Usleber, E., Märtlbauer, E., Dietrich, R., and Terplan, G., Multimycotoxin dipstick enzyme immunoassay applied to wheat, *Food Addit. Contam.*, 12, 387–393, 1995.

40. Ho, J.A.A. and Wauchope, R.D., A strip liposome immunoassay for aflatoxin B₁, *Anal. Chem.*, 74, 1493–1496, 2002.

41. Maragos, C.M., Jolley, M.E., Plattner, R.D., and Nasir, M.S., Fluorescence polarization as a means for determination of fumonisins in maize, *J. Agric. Food Chem.*, 49, 596–602, 2001.

42. Maragos, C.M. and Plattner, R.D., Rapid fluorescence polarization immunoassay for the mycotoxin deoxynivalenol in wheat, *J. Agric. Food Chem.*, 50, 1827–1832, 2002.

43. Nasir, M.S. and Jolley, M.E., Fluorescence polarization (FP) assays for the determination of grain mycotoxins (fumonisins, DON vomitoxin and aflatoxins), *Comb. Chem. High Thr. Scr.*, 6, 267–273, 2003.

44. Checovich, W.J., Bolger, R.E., and Burke, T., Fluorescence polarization-a new tool for cell and molecular biology, *Nature*, 375, 254–256, 1995.

45. Cooper, K.M., Tuomola, M., Lahdenperä, S., Lövgren, T., Elliott, C.T., and Kennedy, D.G., Development and validation of dry reagent time-resolved fluoroimmunoassays for zeranol and α-zearalenol to assist in distinguishing zeranol abuse from *Fusarium* spp. toxin contamination in bovine urine, *Food Addit. Contam.*, 19, 1130–1137, 2002.

46. Bacigalupo, M.A., Ius, A., Meroni, G., Dovis, M., and Petruzzelli, E., Determination of aflatoxin B_1 in agricultural commodities by time-resolved fluoroimmunoassay and immunoenzymometric assay, *Analyst*, 119, 2813–2815, 1994.

47. Scott, P.M. and Trucksess, M.W., Application of immunoaffinity columns to mycotoxin analysis, *J. Assoc. Off. Anal. Chem. Int.*, 80, 941–949, 1997.

48. Carlson, M.A., Bargeron, C.B., Benson, R.C., Fraser, A.B., Phillips, T.E., Velky, J.T., Groopman, J.D., Strickland, P.T., and Ko, H.W., An automated, handheld biosensor for aflatoxin, *Biosen. Bioelect.*, 14, 841–848, 2000.

49. Strachan, N.J.C., John, P.G., and Miller, I.G., Application of an automated particle-based immunosensor for the detection of aflatoxin B_1 in foods, *Food Agric. Immunol.*, 9, 177–184, 1997.

50. Carter, R.M., Blake II, R.C., Mayer, H.P., Echevarria, A.A., Nguyen, T.D., and Bostanian, L.A., A fluorescent biosensor for detection of zearalenone, *Anal. Lett.*, 33, 405–412, 2000.

51. Garden, S.R. and Strachan, N.J.C., Novel colorimetric immunoassay for the detection of aflatoxin B_1, *Anal. Chim. Acta*, 444, 187–191, 2001.

52. Ho, J.A. and Durst, R.A., Detection of fumonisin B_1: comparison of flow-injection liposome immunoanalysis with high-performance liquid chromatography, *Anal. Biochem.*, 312, 7–13, 2003.

53. Maragos, C.M., Analysis of mycotoxins with capillary electrophoresis, *Sem. Food Anal.*, 3, 353–373, 1998.

54. Wei, J., Okerberg, E., Dunlap, J., Ly, C., and Shear, J.B., Determination of biological toxins using capillary electrophoretic chromatography with multiphoton-excited fluorescence, *Anal. Chem.*, 72, 1360–1363, 2000.

55. Tsao, R. and Zhou, T., Micellar electrokinetic capillary electrophoresis for rapid analysis of patulin in apple cider, *J. Agric. Food Chem.*, 48, 5231–5235, 2000.

56. Peña, R., Alcaraz, M.C., Arce, L., Ríos, A., and Valcárcel, M., Screening of aflatoxins in feed samples using a flow system coupled to capillary electrophoresis, *J. Chromatogr. A*, 967, 303–314, 2002.

57. Dickens, J. and Sepaniak, M., Modular separation-based fiber-optic sensors for remote *in situ* monitoring, *J. Environ. Monit.*, 2, 11–16, 2000.

58. Maragos, C.M., Detection of the mycotoxin fumonisin B_1 by a combination of immunofluorescence and capillary electrophoresis, *Food Agric. Immunol.*, 9, 147–157, 1997.

59. Narang, U., Gauger, P.R., Kusterbeck, A.W., and Ligler, F.S., Multianalyte detection using a capillary-based flow immunosensor, *Anal. Biochem.*, 255, 13–19, 1998.

60. Rowe-Taitt, C.A., Golden, J.P., Feldstein, M.J., Cras, J.J., Hoffman, K.E., and Ligler, F.S., Array biosensor for detection of biohazards, *Biosen. Bioelect.*, 14, 785–794, 2000.

61. Grow, A.E., Wood, L.L., Claycomb, J.L., and Thompson, P.A., New biochip technology for label-free detection of pathogens and their toxins, *J. Microbiol. Methods*, 53, 221–233, 2003.

62. Andreou, V. and Nikolelis, D., Flow injection monitoring of aflatoxin M_1 in milk and milk preparations using filter-supported bilayer lipid membranes, *Anal. Chem.*, 70, 2366–2371, 1998.

63. Siontorou, C.G., Nikolelis, D.P., Miernik, A., and Krull, U.J., Rapid methods for detection of aflatoxin M_1 based on electrochemical transduction by self-assembled metal-supported bilayer lipid membranes (s-BLMs) and on interferences with transduction of DNA hybridization, *Electrochim. Acta*, 43, 3611–3617, 1998.

64. Mascini, M., Palchetti, I., and Marrazza, G., DNA electrochemical biosensors, *Fresenius J. Anal. Chem.*, 369, 15–22, 2001.

65. Zhou, H-R., Pestka, J.J., and Hart, L.P., Molecular cloning and expression of recombinant phage antibody against fumonisin B_1, *J. Food Prot.*, 59, 1208–1212, 1996.

66. Yuan, Q., Hu, W., Pestka, J.J., He, S.Y., and Hart, L.P., Expression of a functional antizearalenone single-chain Fv antibody in transgenic *Arabidopsis* plants, *Appl. Environ. Microbiol.*, 66, 3499–3505, 2000.

67. Tozzi, C., Anfossi, L., Baggiani, C., Giovannoli, C., and Giraudi, G., A combinatorial approach to obtain affinity media with binding properties towards the aflatoxins, *Anal. Bioanal. Chem.*, 375, 994–999, 2003.

68. Jodlbauer, J., Maier, N.M., and Lindner, W., Towards ochratoxin A selective molecularly imprinted polymers for solid-phase extraction, *J. Chromatogr. A*, 945, 45–63, 2002.

69. Weiss, R., Freudenschuss, M., Krska, R., and Mizaikoff, B., Improving methods of analysis for mycotoxins: molecularly imprinted polymers for deoxynivalenol and zearalenone, *Food Addit. Contam.*, 20, 386–395, 2003.

70. Keshri, G. and Magan, N., Detection and differentiation between mycotoxigenic and non-mycotoxigenic strains of two *Fusarium* spp. using volatile production profiles and hydrolytic enzymes, *J. Appl. Microbiol.*, 89, 825–833, 2000.

71. Olsson, J., Börjesson, T., Lundstedt, T., and Schnürer, J., Volatiles for mycological quality grading of barley grains: determinations using gas chromatography-mass spectrometry and electronic nose, *Int. J. Food Microbiol.*, 59, 167–178, 2000.

72. Olsson, J., Börjesson, T., Lundstedt, T., and Schnürer, J., Detection and quantification of ochratoxin A and deoxynivalenol in barley grains by GC–MS and electronic nose, *Int. J. Food Microbiol.*, 72, 203–214, 2002.

73. Edwards, S.G., O'Callaghan, J., and Dobson, A.D.W., PCR-based detection and quantification of mycotoxigenic fungi, *Mycol. Res.*, 106, 1005–1025, 2002.

14 The Case for Monitoring *Aspergillus flavus* Aflatoxigenicity for Food Safety Assessment in Developing Countries

W. Thomas Shier, Hamed K. Abbas,
Mark A. Weaver, and Bruce W. Horn

CONTENTS

14.1 INTRODUCTION

Aflatoxins represent the most important single mycotoxin-related food safety problem in developed and developing countries, but the two types of countries are quite different with regard to how, when, and where aflatoxin production occurs and how the problem is addressed. In developed countries, aflatoxin levels are monitored postharvest by relatively expensive immunochemical or instrumental methods. It is assumed that the aflatoxin level measured will not change significantly during storage, and because storage conditions in developed countries are often nearly ideal this assumption is usually valid. In humid tropical developing countries, however, where crops intended for domestic consumption are often stored under far from ideal conditions, additional fungal proliferation and aflatoxin synthesis may occur. In developing countries with alternating dry and rainy seasons, most crop production occurs during the rainy season. Excellent storage conditions are usually present during the following dry season, but dangerous levels of aflatoxin may be produced during the subsequent rainy season before stored crops are consumed and the new crop is ready for harvest. Aflatoxigenic fungal contamination levels, readily assessed by cultural methods, may be the best predictors of susceptibility to aflatoxin production following harvest. Cultural tests have additional advantages in that they are relatively inexpensive and require less technical training to conduct. In developing countries, the most heavily contaminated crops could be scheduled for earliest consumption during the dry season before additional aflatoxin production can occur, whereas crops with low levels of aflatoxigenic fungal contamination could be more safely stored for consumption during the subsequent rainy season.

14.2 THE AFLATOXIN PROBLEM

Aflatoxins have been responsible for the most important contamination problems caused by known mycotoxins since they were first discovered in the early 1960s.[6] Aflatoxins are produced primarily by *Aspergillus flavus* Link: Fries, and *A. parasiticus* Speare, and they contaminate many commodities used for human food and animal feed.[20,41,64,86] Public health and food safety concerns have focused on aflatoxins because they are known to be mutagenic, teratogenic, carcinogenic, and immunosuppressive in animals and possibly in humans.[4,12–14,19,26,38,49,56,57,86]

TABLE 14.1
Comparison of Aflatoxin Problems in Developed and Developing Countries

Factor	Developed Countries	Developing Countries
Period of most aflatoxin production	Preharvest[61]	Postharvest[11]
Crops affected	Corn (maize, *Zea mays* L.),[54] peanuts (groundnuts, *Arachishypogaea* L.),[36] cottonseed (*Gossypium hirsutum* L.),[61] tree nuts[10]	Corn, peanuts, copra (*Cocos nucifera* L.), chickpeas (*Cicer arietinum* L.), millet (*Eleusine coracana* Gaertn), yam flour (*Dioscorea* spp.), cassava flour (*Manihot esculenta* Crantz)[11,59,66,69]
Number 1 concern	Regulatory costs for monitoring[61]	Chronic toxicity, including primary hepatocarcinoma, reduced immunity and rare acute toxicity[11,78]
Number 2 concern	Yield loss in animal feed[61]	Yield loss in animal feed[11,69]

14.3 COMPARISON OF AFLATOXIN IMPACTS IN DEVELOPED AND DEVELOPING COUNTRIES

Aflatoxins impact food safety in a variety of ways in developed and developing countries (Table 14.1). Some of the problems caused by aflatoxins are similar in both developed and developing countries, but the problems of greatest concern are different. One similarity is that the most important crops affected by aflatoxins are corn (maize, *Zea mays* L.)[54,83] and peanuts (groundnuts, *Arachis hypogaea* L.)[36] in both developed[59,61] and developing[11,59,69] countries. Other crops are affected in developed countries (e.g., cottonseed meal from *Gossypium hirsutum* L., tree nuts)[10] and in developing countries (e.g., copra, or coconut meal, *Cocos nucifera* L.; millet, *Eleusine coracana* Gaertn; chickpeas, *Cicer arietinum* L.; yams, *Dioscorea* spp.; cassava, *Manihot esculenta* Crantz),[11] but the quantities of corn and peanuts produced and their susceptibility to *A. flavus* and *A. parasiticus* contamination make these two crops central to the aflatoxin problem worldwide. A second worldwide similarity is the important association between yield loss and aflatoxin-contaminated animal feed, particularly in the case of corn, which is a major component of domesticated animal feeds in most parts of the world.

The impacts of differences in food safety on developed and developing countries are more numerous and more important. One difference that has far-reaching consequences is the time in the crop production cycle at which most aflatoxin production occurs. In developed countries, aflatoxin production occurs almost exclusively preharvest, whereas in developing countries aflatoxin production occurs both preharvest and postharvest.[11,69] In developed countries, the primary aflatoxin concerns for producers are the various regulatory costs,[61] whereas in developing countries the most important aflatoxin concerns are the health impacts.[11]

14.3.1 The Primary Aflatoxin Concern in Developed Countries: Regulatory Costs

Aflatoxin levels are carefully monitored and tolerance levels are set sufficiently low such that neither people nor domesticated animals are exposed to enough aflatoxins to cause detectable health effects;[62] however, these regulatory processes come at considerable cost.[61] The following is a discussion of six major cost areas for U.S. agriculture.

14.3.1.1 Crop Management Costs

A variety of crop management techniques can be used to minimize production of aflatoxins.[9] Preharvest techniques include many that reduce stress in the plants, notably irrigation and fertilization (which reduce drought and nutrient stresses, respectively), cultivation and herbicide application (which reduce crop-density stress), insecticide application (which reduces insect injury, an important infection route for *Aspergillus flavus* and *A. parasiticus*), and scheduling planting time to minimize drought and heat stress. Postharvest techniques for preventing additional aflatoxin production primarily involve drying crops immediately after harvest to <15% moisture content (e.g., with propane-fueled driers) and maintaining dry storage conditions until the crop has been used. All of these techniques require capital costs, material costs, and time expenditure. Costs of some aflatoxin-reducing crop management techniques, such as irrigation, fertilization, cultivation, and pesticide application, are offset by increased yield, but others are not. The total costs of crop management techniques carried out solely to reduce aflatoxin, as well as other aflatoxin reduction costs above those compensated for by increased yield, are not known and are difficult to estimate.[61]

14.3.1.2 Sampling Costs

With *Aspergillus flavus* contamination, infestation levels are far from uniform, making proper sampling critical for aflatoxin management.[27] Contaminated crops typically consist of a few extensively contaminated kernels, while the remaining kernels are largely uncontaminated. For example, one or two infested peanuts can contaminate a multiple-ton lot of peanut butter. Because of the coarseness of harvested crops, large sample sizes must be taken, finely ground, and thoroughly mixed to obtain a reliable sample for aflatoxin analysis. The remainder of the ground sample cannot be returned to the lot that was sampled and often is wasted. Corn sampling costs have been estimated at $20 to $30 per test and $2 to $3 per acre in the United States.[61]

14.3.1.3 Analytical Costs

Routine analysis for aflatoxins in industry typically uses commercially available immunochemical assays marketed for the purpose.[61] The assay kits are sensitive,

TABLE 14.2
Maximum Levels of Combined Aflatoxins Allowed in Various Use Categories of U.S. Corn (Maize, *Zea mays* L.)

Use Category	Level of Aflatoxins (ppm)
Alcohol fermentation	No limit
Feed for finishing cattle	300
Feed for finishing swine	200
Feed for poultry and breeding livestock	100
Feed for immature livestock	20
Feed for dairy animals	20
Food for direct human consumption	20
Maize for export to Europe	5

Source: Adapted from FDA, *Action Levels for Poisonous or Deleterious Substances in Human Food and Animal Feed*, U.S. Food and Drug Administration, Rockville, MD, 2000 (http://www.cfsan.fda.gov/~lrd/fdaact.html#afla).

quantitative, reliable, and relatively easy to use, but they are expensive, resulting in a substantial assay costs. Research applications typically use high-performance liquid chromatography (HPLC) with fluorescence detection, which has greater precision and distinguishes aflatoxins B_1, B_2, G_1, and G_2, which are not distinguished by immunochemical assays.[27] Instrumental assays are associated with high capital costs and require a highly trained operator. Neither type of assay can use a solid substrate, so the ground sample must be extracted with an organic solvent, adding significant effort and solvent disposal problems to the assay process.

14.3.1.4 Crop Value Shift/Crop Remediation Costs

In the United States and many other developed countries, aflatoxin levels determine crop quality and hence how crops can be used (Table 14.2). Thus, aflatoxin levels are a major determinant of crop value, with crop value being inversely related to aflatoxin level. When corn becomes aflatoxin-contaminated despite the best efforts of the grower (e.g., after hot, dry growing conditions), it may be possible to increase the value of aflatoxin-contaminated corn by suitable remediation techniques, such as diluting with more expensive low-aflatoxin material or screening.[65,79] Because aflatoxin levels are not uniform among kernels, with the highest aflatoxin levels being found in broken kernels, it is usually possible to substantially lower aflatoxin levels by screening to remove the damaged kernels, which are then discarded; however, costs are associated with any type of processing, and they may be greater than the added value of the crop.

14.3.1.5   Research

Research on methods to reduce aflatoxin contamination are an important and readily quantified component of the overall agricultural research program in the United States. Health benefits are expected to accrue from reductions in aflatoxin consumption, but they are difficult to quantify.

14.3.1.6   Insurance

Crop insurance protects growers from financial disasters of various types, including aflatoxin-caused losses, but it does so at a cost. An additional cost associated with insurance is the increased testing required to comply with insurance company requirements.[61]

14.3.2   THE PRIMARY AFLATOXIN CONCERN IN DEVELOPING COUNTRIES: HEALTH IMPACTS

The primary concern about aflatoxins in developing countries is centered on the toxic effects of direct human consumption of aflatoxin-contaminated agricultural products.[11] Of particular concern is chronic toxicity, although acute toxicity has been reported.[69] Concerns about chronic toxicity of aflatoxins have focused on the possibility that aflatoxins may act synergistically with industrial pollutants and other natural toxins in the environment, particularly environmental tumor promoters such as microcystins in drinking water and fumonisins that co-contaminate corn.[78] Both of these environmental tumor promoters meet the repeated exposure requirement for an effective tumor promoter. Concern that aflatoxins may cause cancer in the United States is not great, because the tumor type most often associated with aflatoxin exposure, primary hepatocellular carcinoma, is very rare. Most liver cancer in the United States is actually metastatic colon cancer, and the bulk of the primary hepatocellular carcinoma that does occur is associated with alcoholism, not aflatoxin consumption.

Direct toxicity of aflatoxins is a concern in developing countries at times when people are faced with starvation and must consume moldy food.[69] Most of the research on the role of aflatoxins in causing primary hepatocellular carcinoma has been carried out in East Asia or Africa where the disease has been endemic. A long-running controversy exists over whether primary hepatocellular carcinoma is caused by aflatoxins, hepatitis B virus, or both, but a consensus appears to have developed that both are causes and that they strongly synergize each other.[78] Some of the earliest studies, conducted when aflatoxin levels were presumably higher than now, have found that aflatoxin was the primary cause, whereas more recent studies have found hepatitis B virus to be the primary cause. The availability of an effective vaccine against hepatitis B virus is expected to change the relative importance of the two causes of primary hepatocellular carcinoma in Asia, where the vaccine represents a less expensive option for preventing the disease than aflatoxin reduction;[11] however, in many parts of Africa both options are too expensive.

Another major concern for chronic toxicity to aflatoxin is its possible effects on immunity. Aflatoxins have been reported to reduce immunity in chickens,[52] and they may reduce immunity in humans.[11,51] Reduced immunity contributes to death by communicable diseases, particularly in children and the elderly. Loss of life caused by aflatoxins by this mechanism is difficult to quantify but may exceed all other causes combined. Although cases of death by acute toxicity of aflatoxins (nonviral hepatitis) have been documented,[69] they are very rare.

14.4 AFLATOXIN MONITORING IN DEVELOPED COUNTRIES

Maintaining food safety is viewed as an important government responsibility in developed countries.[61,62] Mycotoxin management is carried out aggressively for a limited number of generally recognized problem mycotoxins, notably aflatoxins, ochratoxins, fumonisins, deoxynivalenol, patulin, and zearalenones. Little attention is given to (1) mycotoxins that are not officially recognized by the government (e.g., cyclopiazonic acid, *Stachybotrys* toxins), (2) interactions between official mycotoxins (e.g., aflatoxins plus fumonisins co-contaminating corn), (3) interactions between official mycotoxins and nutrients, or (4) derivatives of official mycotoxins formed by metabolic action or by thermal or chemical action during food processing with a few exceptions (e.g., aflatoxin M_1). Governments of developed countries pass laws and government agencies promulgate regulations based on the law and available data on the toxicity of the mycotoxin, the frequency of occurrence and range of concentrations observed, the range of commodities affected, and the availability of useable assays. The passing of the regulatory laws that initiate this process is influenced by regulatory climates in other countries and a trade-off between domestic political factors related to the food producing and processing industries and to the public. Government agencies formulate regulations mandated by these laws on the basis of animal toxicity data, epidemiological data (if available), exposure assessments based on measured toxin concentrations in foods, and the need for an adequate food supply. Frequently the action level selected for regulation is that which is achievable with reasonably good manufacturing practices. For example, low levels of aflatoxin are permitted in peanut butter in the United States even though laws are in place that block addition of carcinogenic additives. In practice, this does not affect food safety, because risk assessments that underlie mycotoxin regulations in developed countries incorporate large margins of safety.

Regulatory agencies in developed countries usually stipulate the sampling techniques to be used for each mycotoxin in each commodity. This is particularly important for aflatoxins, because the percentage of infected, contaminated kernels is relatively low. These regulations include the number, size, and distribution of samples taken per ton for each regulated commodity.

Government regulations define how agricultural products can be used (Table 14.2) and hence affect their value, based on mycotoxin levels measured postharvest with approved analytical techniques. A wide variety of analytical methods for the detection and quantification of aflatoxins in agricultural commodities has been published,[27,45,48,81] including: (1) thin-layer chromatography (TLC),[72] (2) high-performance liquid chromatography (HPLC),[68,70,73] (3) liquid chromatography/mass spectroscopy (LC/MS),[3] (4) enzyme-linked immunosorbent assay (ELISA),[53,74] and (5) immunoaffinity columns with fluorescence measurement (Vicam).[46,47] Some of the published methods are only suitable for research applications. To be suitable for regulatory applications, an analytical method must be reliable, preferably simple, and sensitive down to the lowest level selected for regulatory action. Acceptable methods must be approved by recognized expert bodies such as the Association of Official Analytical Chemists (AOAC) International or the European Standardization Committee (CEN). The latest edition of the *Official Methods of the AOAC International* lists about 40 methods for mycotoxins, including many aflatoxin methods suited for specific commodities, all of which have been extensively validated. Expert agencies also provide standards, calibration samples with known mycotoxin levels, and reference samples of commodities certified to be free of the mycotoxin. These agencies have also developed analytical training programs and certification programs for technicians and laboratories. Among the many methods developed and validated for aflatoxins, the two most common strategies appear to be (1) immunoaffinity column clean-up followed by HPLC with fluorescence detection, often with post-column electrochemical bromination to enhance fluorescence, and (2) silica or C_{18} minicolumn clean-up followed by ELISA with one of about a dozen commercially available antibody-based test kits.[27] All methods require a sampling procedure, with its associated labor and sample loss costs, and extraction with organic solvents, with associated disposal problems. Immunoaffinity columns and commercial ELISA kits have high unit costs, and instrumental methods such as HPLC have high capital costs for instrumentation; however, to growers the major cost is perceived to be the loss in crop value from segregation of their crops into a lower value category due to the aflatoxin level. A grower may choose to use a remediation technique such as screening to increase the value of the crop, but the cost of the remediation procedure plus reassay may exceed the added value.[61] Because regulations are based on no-effect levels, farmers are unlikely to ever observe overt toxicity of a regulated mycotoxin such as aflatoxin. They do, however, occasionally see feed refusal and even overt toxicity from unregulated toxins, particularly when crops have been grown in environments that favor mycotoxin production. Thus, mycotoxin management is government driven in both domestic and export markets, and the costs are borne primarily by producers, who derive no benefit from them, while the intended beneficiaries, the consumers, never notice them. In general, cost–benefit analysis does not appear to play an important role in shaping developed country mycotoxin regulation practices, particularly in Europe, where the 2-ppb action level is maintained at enormous cost per life saved.

14.5 PROBLEMS ASSOCIATED WITH AFLATOXIN MONITORING IN DEVELOPING COUNTRIES

Exports of agricultural products to developed countries are often an important source of foreign exchange for developing countries, and exports may continue even when poor people in the exporting country are starving. Food products destined for the export market must necessarily be handled according to practices prescribed by the destination country, including measurement of aflatoxin levels by instrumental or immunochemical methods.[8,61,62] These agricultural products are generally of the highest quality the developing country has to offer, and the postharvest handling conditions are comparable to those in developed countries. Under these conditions, the assumption that aflatoxin levels will not change during storage and handling is valid, and the additional costs of aflatoxin testing and high-quality storage are borne by the higher value of the agricultural product. At issue here are the food safety monitoring practices of developing countries for agricultural products intended for the domestic market.[11] The following are some of the problems encountered in attempting to introduce developed country food safety monitoring practices into developing countries without modification:

1. Assay materials are too expensive to be absorbed into the price received for agricultural products in the developing country domestic market.
2. Although a sufficient number of well-trained personnel may be available to staff testing centers for those agricultural products destined for the export market, they are not enough to test the much larger volume in the domestic market product stream.
3. Marketing and distribution networks in developing countries are much more limited than in developed countries, so the producer does not have a similar range of options for using agricultural products with different levels of aflatoxin contamination. Most of the agricultural products grown in developing countries already have their use predetermined before harvest (e.g., direct consumption by a subsistence farmer), so the aflatoxin level in the crop is not useful knowledge. When starvation is the only alternative to consuming aflatoxin-contaminated crops, contaminated commodities will be consumed regardless of the measured aflatoxin level, so nothing is to be gained by measuring it. To make matters worse, corn is the crop most commonly cultivated by subsistence farmers worldwide, because it produces a crop when soil quality is too poor to support other crops such as rice.[28] Unfortunately, corn is very susceptible to contamination by mycotoxins, including aflatoxin.[55,83]
4. The assumption that aflatoxin levels determined postharvest will remain constant throughout the storage life of an agricultural product is often not valid in a developing country setting. If additional aflatoxin production is likely to occur during the next rainy season, then the value measured postharvest is meaningless and an unnecessary expense.

Occasionally, governments of developing countries have been forced to implement developed country management practices as a condition for receiving development loans, even when they know those practices will be ineffective or counterproductive in the developing country setting.[32] Developed countries' practice of using only postharvest aflatoxin level measurements to manage food safety programs should not be imposed on domestic markets of developing countries until it has been rigorously established that the potential for postharvest aflatoxin production does not exist.

14.6 THE RATIONALE FOR MONITORING AFLATOXIGENIC FUNGAL CONTAMINATION LEVELS IN DEVELOPING COUNTRIES

Aflatoxin levels are used in developed countries and in international commerce as a major measure of crop quality, in that levels of the toxin are used to classify crop products into various use categories, which then determine value. In this system, the highest quality food commodities are directed toward human consumption and other sensitive applications, while the lowest quality crops are used as animal feed or in extreme cases for ethanol fermentation or fuel.[75] Many developing countries with serious aflatoxin contamination problems cannot provide funding or the personnel necessary to maintain the type of analytical laboratory required to monitor aflatoxin levels in all lots of foods and feeds produced in the country.[11] Furthermore, the system used in developed countries is based on the underlying assumption that aflatoxin content can be determined by immunochemical or instrumental methods in an agricultural product at postharvest and that aflatoxin content will remain constant throughout the storage lifetime of the crop. This assumption is probably valid as long as crops are stored under near ideal storage conditions at 15% or less moisture to inhibit fungal metabolism. These conditions are generally met in developed countries and for high-quality crops slated for export to them; however, in developing countries, particularly in the tropics where storage conditions are often less than ideal, this assumption often breaks down and postharvest production of aflatoxin by contaminating *Aspergillus flavus* is a clear danger. This assumption also may break down in the case of U.S. foreign aid grains that are exposed to poor storage conditions during ocean shipping and subsequent handling in the recipient country. Postharvest mycotoxin production is the most probable explanation for reports[71] of U.S. foreign aid corn being contaminated with mycotoxins at levels far higher than normally encountered in U.S. commerce. The possibility of postharvest mycotoxin production is one of the factors that support managing food safety by monitoring incidence and severity of contamination of foods by aflatoxigenic fungi, rather than only measuring aflatoxin levels. This approach is particularly attractive in tropical countries where wet and dry seasons alternate, with the majority of corn production occurring in the rainy season. Corn is then stored for consumption during the subsequent dry season and the following rainy season until the new crop is harvested. The dry season provides near ideal storage conditions, so corn consumed during that period is as safe as when harvested; however, when the next rainy season begins, storage conditions usually deteriorate, and the possibility of additional aflatoxin production becomes a concern. If extensive postharvest production of aflatoxin occurs in stored crops, the amount of additional aflatoxins produced would be expected to correlate better under any given set of conditions with the level of infestation by viable aflatoxigenic fungi than with the previously determined postharvest level of aflatoxins. In principle, knowing the level of contamination with aflatoxigenic fungi in agricultural products would allow minimization of aflatoxin ingestion by those consuming the products. That is, crops contaminated with the highest levels of viable fungal spores could be consumed during the dry season, when aflatoxin production would be minimal and the food would still be relatively safe. The crops that should be reserved for consumption during the rainy season are those with the lowest levels of *A. flavus* and *A. parasiticus* contamination which are less likely to have additional aflatoxin synthesis. This strategy is designed to minimize total production of aflatoxins and thus the total exposure to aflatoxin in people who must consume the crops. It will also spread the aflatoxin exposure which cannot be avoided over the maximum period in the hope that the rate of DNA damage will never exceed the person's repair capacity. In this type of analysis, it is important to differentiate between aflatoxigenic and non-aflatoxigenic fungi. Contamination with substantial levels of non-aflatoxigenic fungi may actually render agricultural products partially resistant to the formation of additional aflatoxins, because non-aflatoxigenic fungi may compete with aflatoxigenic fungi for available substrate.[21]

14.7   CULTURAL METHODS FOR AFLATOXIGENICITY ASSESSMENT

Many developing countries with serious aflatoxin contamination problems cannot provide either the funds or the personnel for monitoring aflatoxin levels in all lots of foods and feeds. Furthermore, the high-quality storage conditions necessary to make aflatoxin measurements a valid tool for managing food safety are often lacking. This situation has created much interest in developing and using cultural methods for aflatoxigenicity assessment.[1,2] This type of method could be used at least as a prescreen to identify those lots of agricultural products that are the best candidates for the export market and to identify those lots with poor storage potential that should be used immediately.

14.7.1   Sample Preparation

Species of *Aspergillus* that produce aflatoxins are ubiquitous and easily isolated from nature. Samples from various parts of a uniform lot of the agricultural commodity are usually ground to a powder or are homogenized in water in a blender, then diluted with known volumes of sterile water. Suspensions are plated on an agar medium (dilution plated) to obtain quantitative estimates of the population density expressed as colony-forming units (CFU)/g.[20,34,36,40]

14.7.2   Selective Culture Conditions

Aspergillus flavus and *A. parasiticus* are not fastidious in their nutritional requirements and will grow on nearly all commonly prepared media for fungi. Isolation of these fungi on agar media instead relies on their sensitivity to certain antibiotics relative to other fungi, their ability to grow at relatively high temperatures (37°C), and their tolerance of low moisture content in the growth medium. The most commonly used media for dilution plating contain the antibiotics dichloran or rose bengal for restricting fungal colony diameter.[17,25,39,58] Antibiotics against bacteria are also added, and incubation at 37°C inhibits the growth of many soil fungi that would interfere with the detection of aflatoxigenic species. Various formulations of dichloran–rose bengal medium permit the accurate identification of many aspergilli, including *A. flavus* and *A. parasiticus*, directly on the dilution plate.[36,58] Other media rely on low water activity for selection of aflatoxigenic *Aspergillus* species. Sodium chloride is often used to adjust the water activity;[30,31] however, identification of *A. flavus*, *A. parasiticus*, and related species is not possible in the presence of NaCl, so isolates must be subcultured to another medium such as Czapek agar for final identification.[37] What is needed, but is not yet available (see below), is a widely accepted, single-step culture method that allows for both the identification of aflatoxigenic fungi and an assessment of their aflatoxigenicity.

14.7.3 IDENTIFICATION OF AFLATOXIGENICITY

Aflatoxins B_1 and B_2 produce an intense blue fluorescence visible at approximately 450 nm when exposed to long-wavelength (365 nm) ultraviolet (UV) light. This property is the basis of a variety of qualitative and quantitative analytical methods for the measurement of aflatoxins in extracts,[27,45,60] and it also is the basis of some of the cultural methods for identifying aflatoxigenicity in fungal isolates. These methods are based on identifying the fluorescence of the aflatoxins produced by a colony growing on agar medium. Other cultural methods for identifying aflatoxigenicity are empirically based and detect the visible color of pigments the colonies produce.

14.7.3.1 Blue Fluorescence

Blue fluorescence of aflatoxins has been used to develop qualitative cultural methods for detecting aflatoxin production by colonies of *Aspergillus* species grown on suitable media, such as potato dextrose agar and coconut agar.[18,33,42–44,63,80] Cotty[16] developed a simple technique in which aflatoxins produced by colonies on solid medium in culture tubes were quantified by measuring fluorescence with a scanning densitometer. Yabe et al.[85] used UV photography as a rapid method to screen for aflatoxin-producing species on GY-agar medium; even small colonies only 36 hours old produced aflatoxins, and many colonies could be examined on a single plate. Aflatoxin-producing isolates appeared as gray or black colonies in the UV photographs, whereas nonproducing isolates appeared as white colonies. Aflatoxins B_1 and G_1 were primarily responsible for absorbing UV light in this study, but the possibility of different blue fluorescent materials, such as oxidized kojic acid, being produced by other strains remains a concern.

14.7.3.2 Cyclodextrin-Enhanced Blue Fluorescence

The blue fluorescence of aflatoxin B_1 under UV light is significantly enhanced in both liquid and solid media by treatment with various fluorescence enhancers such as iodine and cyclodextrins. Lemke et al.[43] developed a simple mini-assay for detecting aflatoxin-producing isolates after 3 to 10 days in coconut extract broth using iodine derivatization, which enabled about a 100-fold increase in sensitivity compared to aflatoxin B_1 without derivatization. Fluorescence emission of aflatoxins B_1 and G_1 is substantially enhanced when complexed with cyclodextrins (CDs), which have been used to improve a variety of mycotoxin analytical methods,[24,35,67,76,77] including liquid chromatography.[15] β-CD has been adapted for qualitative cultural methods by adding it to a suitable agar medium. β-CD enhances detection of aflatoxin production by *Aspergillus flavus* and *A. parasiticus* through blue fluorescence under 365-nm light.[23,50]

14.7.3.3   Yellow Pigment

Production of yellow to orange pigments by aflatoxigenic *Aspergillus flavus* was first described by Wiseman et al.[84] Arseculeratne et al.[5] observed pigment production by the second day in *A. flavus* colonies on coconut agar medium; however, Lin and Dianese[44] were the first to associate the bright yellow pigment production in the medium with aflatoxigenicity in *A. flavus* as detected by blue fluorescence of aflatoxins. The yellow pigmentation was produced earlier than the blue fluorescence, and it was not observed in colonies that did not produce aflatoxins. Yellow pigment was secreted into the medium, but it was most easily visualized on the reverse side of colonies grown on semitransparent agar media such as potato dextrose agar. Lin and Dianese[44] reported that the degree of yellow pigmentation was proportional to blue fluorescence, but Davis et al.[18] and Gupta and Gopal[33] identified some media in which semiquantitiative differences occurred.

14.7.3.4   Ammonium Hydroxide Vapor-Induced Color Change

Saito and Machida[63] introduced a rapid, sensitive method for identification of aflatoxin-producing and -nonproducing strains of *Aspergillus flavus* and *A. parasiticus*. The method was developed empirically but validated using a collection of 120 strains of *A. flavus*, *A. parasiticus*, *A. oryzae*, and *A. sojae* that were characterized with respect to aflatoxin production by HPLC and UV fluorescence methods. With this method *A. flavus* colonies are grown on a suitable agar medium (e.g., potato dextrose agar). The dish is first inverted, then one or two drops of concentrated ammonium hydroxide solution are placed on the inside of the lid, and the bottom of the Petri dish is inverted over it. The undersides of aflatoxin-producing colonies quickly turn plum-red, but essentially no color change occurs on the undersides of non-aflatoxigenic colonies. We have shown (Shier et al., in preparation) that the color change is due to yellow pigments, identified as aflatoxin biosynthetic intermediates, that undergo reversible pH-dependent color changes like pH indicator dyes. The yellow pigments are presumably the same ones that form the basis of the aflatoxigenicity test of Lin and Dianese.[44] Identification of the pigments as aflatoxin biosynthetic intermediates provides both a rationale for the effectiveness of these two empirical tests and a basis for predicting some conditions under which false positives and false negatives might be expected to occur.

14.7.3.5   Combined Aflatoxigenicity Test

Abbas et al.[1,2] demonstrated that three of the culture-based aflatoxigenicity tests described above can be carried out in the same Petri dish and still allow sampling by two analytical methods. Colonies of *Aspergillus* spp. grown on potato dextrose agar containing 0.3% wt/vol β-cyclodextrin are examined on the undersides under natural light for bright-yellow pigmentation,[33,44] then under long-wavelength (365 nm) UV light to visualize aflatoxin as blue fluorescent zones. The same Petri dishes are inverted over 0.5 mL of 25 to 27% ammonium hydroxide on the lid of the dish to identify aflatoxigenic colonies by the color change from yellow to plum-red. Aflatoxins can be quantified in small plugs cut from the agar medium by TLC, ELISA, or HPLC after extraction with 70% methanol.

14.8 ADVANTAGES AND DISADVANTAGES OF MONITORING AFLATOXIGENIC FUNGAL LEVELS IN DEVELOPING COUNTRIES

A major incentive for developing a practical cultural test for aflatoxigenic fungal levels is to provide a tool for managing food safety in developing countries, where measuring aflatoxin levels may not be possible because of cost or availability of testing materials. A practical cultural test for aflatoxigenic fungal levels may also be useful in developed countries as an adjunct to measuring aflatoxin levels when there are reasons to suspect that the grain will be subjected to poor storage conditions before use; however, currently available cultural methods have both advantages and disadvantages. One of the most important advantages of cultural methods in a developing country setting is that they are less expensive to conduct than even thin-layer chromatography,[1,2] which is often not an option due to limited availability of silica gel. Cultural methods use simple equipment that is readily available in developing countries, and maintenance of the equipment is manageable. Pressure-cookers are readily available for media sterilization, and ambient temperature is generally satisfactory for incubation of cultures. Cultural methods use supplies that are readily recycled in a developing country, where wages are low enough that it is less expensive to use glassware that can be washed and resterilized than to use the disposable plasticware that is popular in developed countries. Required materials, including media components, are relatively inexpensive and are generally stable enough not to deteriorate before use. Because cultural methods involve relatively low technology, personnel are available in developing countries who can be readily trained to conduct the assays. Sampling for cultural assays is done with sterile water. Because no organic solvents are needed, costs are low and no environmental problems are associated with solvent disposal.

The simplicity and low cost of cultural methods means that they become practical in certain social and economic niches for which aflatoxin level measurements are not practical. Cultural methods can be conducted on smaller lot sizes and at more widely dispersed testing centers. Cultural methods can be made available to farmers who cannot afford the expense of having aflatoxin level determinations done. Positive measurements of aflatoxigenic fungal levels are probably better predictors of storage potential than are aflatoxin levels, even if they are not better predictors of food safety.

The major disadvantage of cultural methods for measuring aflatoxigenic fungi is that they do not directly measure the toxicity of the food or feed product. Analytical methods for determining aflatoxin levels are easier to translate into toxicity, particularly if the method used is specific with respect to aflatoxin B_1, the most toxic of the aflatoxins. Another disadvantage is that cultural methods are slow, typically taking 3 to 5 days. They are certainly not rapid enough to be used dockside before unloading a ship. Faster ways to measure the aflatoxigenic potential of fungi contaminating crops are available, such as DNA probe-based assays,[29,45] but they lack the advantages of simplicity and low cost.

Cultural methods are widely regarded as being less sensitive than analytical methods. Because the two types of tests measure different things, this is an inappropriate comparison, but even inappropriate comparisons are barriers to implementation of novel methodology. Because many analytical methods are sensitive to well below the limits of toxicity, the practical advantage of sensitivity is dubious. Many unanswered scientific questions remain (see below) that need to be addressed before cultural methods can be useful as regulatory tools. Cultural methods have not been standardized, with the result that they vary in limit of detection, sensitivity, accuracy and precision, and limitations and areas of application. Until standardized, well-characterized methods have been developed, validated, and widely accepted, government officials will not consider cultural methods as either alternate or additional tools for managing food safety.

14.9 ADDITIONAL STUDIES NEEDED

The great majority of research on aflatoxin contamination of agricultural products has been conducted in developed countries. Because aflatoxin production in developed countries occurs almost exclusively preharvest, research has focused almost exclusively on prevention of preharvest production of aflatoxins. Less research has been done on factors that affect postharvest production of aflatoxins, although studies have been conducted on optimal storage conditions and on remediation methods that are applicable to developing country needs.[65,79] The following are a few examples of the many unmet aflatoxin research needs in developing countries:

1. A simplified, inexpensive, readily-used method for selectively culturing and quantifying levels of aflatoxigenic fungi in major agricultural products is needed. For it to be used in developing countries, such a method would have to allow quantitation of the levels of aflatoxigenic fungi in a sample on a minimum number of plates (two to three dilutions) without subculturing. Species identification is not of primary importance for this application, but aflatoxigenicity of fungal isolates is. Most studies have found that the majority of aflatoxigenic field isolates are *Aspergillus flavus* in the United States[1] and in other countries.[7,63] While progress has been made in combining aflatoxigenicity tests,[2] they have yet to be combined with selective media that facilitate quantitation. Any such test would have to be extensively validated before it could be introduced. A cultural test for aflatoxigenic fungi might also be useful in developed countries as an alternative to more expensive analytical tests for aflatoxin levels in northern tier regions, such as Canada and the bordering U.S. states, where aflatoxins are infrequently detected. A cultural test for aflatoxigenicity

might also be useful in addition to measuring aflatoxin levels in export grains, if the test could be shown to be a good predictor of stability in storage and shipping.

2. A validated, quantitative cultural test for aflatoxigenicity would be more readily accepted if we had a better understanding of how good a predictor of food quality and storage stability postharvest aflatoxigenic fungal levels are. Also needed is a better understanding of the factors that affect the kinetics of postharvest aflatoxin production in each major agricultural product. That is, studies are needed to determine effects of (1) storage humidity, (2) storage temperature, (3) storage duration, (4) crop type, and (5) crop maturation level on aflatoxin production in stored agricultural products at high, medium, and low *A. flavus* contamination levels. Because aflatoxigenic fungi are not the only factors affecting food safety and storage stability, it will be necessary to study how aflatoxigenic fungi interact with those other factors. Also, little research has been done on aflatoxin production at levels high enough to cause acute toxicity.

3. The effectiveness of biocontrol methods in which soil or crops are inoculated with nontoxigenic *A. flavus* or with bacteria has been extensively studied in the United States for preharvest prevention of aflatoxin production;[21] however, only a limited number of studies have been conducted on the application of this strategy to the prevention of postharvest aflatoxin production.[22] It would be a particularly attractive strategy for prevention of aflatoxin production in crops such as copra (coconut) for which preharvest infection by aflatoxigenic fungi is not a significant concern. Biocontrol methods using non-aflatoxigenic strains of *A. flavus* would not complicate food safety management using cultural methods, because cultural methods selectively monitor the aflatoxigenic fungi.

4. Relatively little research has been conducted on postharvest remediation of aflatoxin contamination.[65] Remediation by ammoniation has not been endorsed by developed country regulatory agencies, which may be the reason why it is not widely practiced in developed or developing countries. Similarly, relatively little research has been done on postharvest remediation of contamination by aflatoxigenic fungi. Most remediation studies have focused on removing aflatoxin, not on removing aflatoxigenic fungi. Harvest time and conditions are usually selected to maximize yield. If the factors affecting postharvest aflatoxin production in typical developing country storage conditions were better known, it might be possible to reduce aflatoxin production by making appropriate choices before harvest. It would be useful to know the source and location within or on the stored agricultural product of the fungi that ultimately produce aflatoxins during postharvest storage.[55] This will clearly vary with crop type. For example, in corn, is dust on the kernels the most important source of aflatoxigenic *A. flavus* inoculum for postharvest aflatoxin production, or is the inoculum source primarily preharvest infestation of the kernels or cobs? If dust on the kernels is a source of inoculum, washing the kernels would be a remediation strategy; if the cob were the source, shelling as soon as dry

would be a remediation strategy. Does the cob retain moisture that favors postharvest aflatoxin production in the kernels, or does it help prevent aflatoxin production by reducing compaction in storage, permitting better aeration and faster redrying if the crop inadvertently gets wet during storage?

5. Is there a role for extension outreach education in reducing postharvest production of aflatoxins in developing countries? That is, would it help to teach subsistence farmers the importance of keeping their agricultural products dry during postharvest storage, or do they already know, but just don't have the means to protect their stored crops properly?

14.10 CONCLUSION

We have ample reason to believe that cultural assays for assessing contamination of crops with aflatoxigenic fungi have a potential role along with analyzing aflatoxin levels in predicting possible postharvest production of aflatoxins in crops stored under less than ideal conditions. Suboptimal storage conditions are encountered in developing countries in regions with rainy seasons or in ocean shipping of foreign aid grains. Cultural methods have the additional advantages of being less expensive and less technically demanding than immunochemical or instrumental methods used for postharvest mycotoxin monitoring in industrialized countries.

REFERENCES

1. Abbas, H.K., Zablotowicz, R.M., Weaver, M.A., Horn, B.W., Xie, W., and Shier, W.T., Comparison of cultural and analytical methods for determination of aflatoxin production by Mississippi Delta *Aspergillus* isolates, *Can. J. Microbiol.*, 50, 193–199, 2004.
2. Abbas, H.K., Shier, W.T., Horn, B.W., and Weaver, M.A., Cultural methods for aflatoxin detection. *J. Toxicol. Toxin Rev.*, 23, 295–315, 2004.
3. Abbas, H.K., Williams, W.P., Windham, G.L., Pringle, III, H.C., Xie, W., and Shier, W.T., Aflatoxin and fumonisin contamination of commercial corn (*Zea mays*) hybrids in Mississippi, *J. Agric. Food Chem.*, 50, 5246–5254, 2002.
4. Alpert, M.E., Hutt, M.S. R., Wogan, G.N., and Davidson, C.S., Association between aflatoxin cancer of food and hepatoma frequency in Uganda, *Cancer*, 28, 253–260, 1971.
5. Arseculeratne, S.N., de Silva, L.M., Wijesundera, S., and Bandunatha, C.H.S.R., Coconut as a medium for the experimental production of aflatoxin, *Appl. Microbiol.*, 18, 88–94, 1969.
6. Aspilin, F.D. and Carnghan, R.B.A., The toxicity of certain groundnut meal for poultry with special reference to their effect on ducklings, *Vet. Res.*, 73, 1215–1219, 1961.
7. Bilgrami, K.S. and Choudhary, A.K., Impact of habitats on toxigenic potential of *Aspergillus flavus*, *J. Stored Prod. Res.*, 29, 351–355, 1993.
8. Boutrif, E. and Canet, C., Mycotoxin prevention and control FAO programmes, *Rev. Méd. Vét.*, 149, 681–694, 1998.
9. Bruns, H.A., Controlling aflatoxin and fumonisin in maize by crop management, *J. Toxicol. Toxin Rev.*, 22, 153–173, 2003.

10. Campbell, B.C., Molyneux, R.J., and Schatzki, T.F., Current research on reducing pre- and postharvest aflatoxin contamination of U.S. almond, pistachio and walnut, *J. Toxicol. Toxin Rev.*, 22, 225–266, 2003.

11. Cardwell, K.F. and Henry, S.H., Risk of exposure to and mitigation of effect of aflatoxin on human health: a West African example, *J. Toxicol. Toxin Rev.*, 23, 217–247, 2004.

12. CAST, *Aflatoxin and Other Mycotoxins: An Agricultural Perspective*, Report No. 80, Council for Agricultural Science and Technology, Ames, IA, 1979.

13. CAST, *Mycotoxins: Economic and Health Risks*, Report No. 116, Council for Agricultural Science and Technology, Ames, IA, 1989.

14. CAST, *Mycotoxins: Risks in Plant, Animal and Human Systems*, Report No. 139, Council for Agricultural Science and Technology, Ames, IA, 2003.

15. Chiavaro, E., Asta, C.D., Galaverna, G., Biancardi, A., Gambarelli, E., Dossena, A., and Marchelli, R., New reversed-phase liquid chromatographic method to detect aflatoxins in food and feed with cyclodextrins as fluorescence enhancers added to the eluent, *J. Chromatogr. A*, 937, 31–40, 2001.

16. Cotty, P.J., Simple fluorescence method for rapid estimation of aflatoxin levels in a solid culture medium, *Appl. Environ. Microbiol.*, 54, 274–276, 1988.

17. Cotty, P.J., Comparison of four media for the isolation of *Aspergillus flavus* group fungi, *Mycopathologia*, 125, 157–162, 1994.

18. Davis, N.D., Iyer, S.K., and Diener, U.L., Improved method of screening for aflatoxin with a coconut agar medium, *Appl. Environ. Microbiol.*, 53, 1593–1595, 1987.

19. DiPaolo, J.A., Elis, J., and Erwin, H., Teratogenic response by hamsters, rats and mice to aflatoxin B, *Nature*, 215, 638–639, 1967.

20. Dorner, J.W., Simultaneous quantitation of *Aspergillus flavus*, *A. parasiticus* and aflatoxin in peanuts, *J. Assoc. Off. Anal. Chem. Int.*, 85, 911–916, 2002.

21. Dorner, J.W., Biological control of aflatoxin contamination of crops, *J. Toxicol. Toxin Rev.*, 23, 425–450, 2004.

22. Dorner, J.W. and Cole, R.J., Effect of application of non-toxigenic strains of *Aspergillus flavus* and *A. parasiticus* on subsequent aflatoxin contamination of peanuts in storage, *J. Stored Prod. Res.*, 38, 329–339, 2002.

23. Fente, C.A., Ordaz, J.J., Vazquez, B.I., Franco, C.M., and Cepeda, A., New additive for cultural media for rapid identification of aflatoxin-producing *Aspergillus* strains, *Appl. Environ. Microbiol.*, 67, 4858–4862, 2001.

24. Franco, C.M., Fente, C.A., Vazquez, B.I., Cepeda, A., Mabuzier, G., and Prognon, P., Interaction between cyclodextrins and aflatoxins Q_1, M_1, and P_1 fluorescence and chromatographic studies, *J. Chromatogr. A*, 815, 21–29, 1998.

25. Frisvad, J.C., Filtenborg, O., Lund, F., and Thrane, U., New selective media for the detection of toxigenic fungi in cereal products, meat and cheese, in *Modern Methods in Food Mycology*, Samson, R.A., Hocking, A.D., Pitt, J.I., and King, A.D., Eds., Elsevier, Amsterdam, 1992, 275–284.

26. Georggiett, O.C., Muino, J.C., Montrull, H., Brizuela, N., Avalos, S., and Gomez, R.M., Relationship between lung cancer and aflatoxin B_1, *Rev. Fac. Cien. Med. Univ. Nac. Cordoba*, 57, 95–107, 2000.

27. Gilbert, J. and Vargas, E.A., Advances in sampling and analysis for aflatoxins in food and animal feed, *J. Toxicol. Toxin Rev.*, 22, 381–422, 2003.

28. Ginsburg, N., The Philippines, in *The Pattern of Asia*, Ginsburg, N., Ed., Prentice-Hall, Englewood Cliffs, NJ, 1958, pp. 321–343.

29. Guo, B.Z., Yu, J., Holbrook, C.C., Lee, R.D., and Lynch, R.E., Application of differential display RT-PRC and EST/microarray technologies to the analysis of gene expression in response to drought stress and elimination of aflatoxin contamination in corn and peanut, *J. Toxicol. Toxin Rev.*, 22, 287–312, 2003.

30. Griffin, G.J., Ford, R.H., and Garren, K.H., Relation of *Aspergillus flavus* colony growth on three selective media to recovery from naturally infested soil, *Phytopathology*, 65, 704–707, 1975.

31. Griffin, G.J., Smith, E.P., and Robinson, T.J., Population patterns of *Aspergillus flavus* group and *A. niger* group in field soils, *Soil Biol. Biochem.*, 33, 253–257, 2001.

32. Grundy, J., Healy, V., Gorgolon, L., and Sandig, E., Overview of devolution of health services in the Philippines, *Rural Remote Health*, 3, 220 2003 (http://rrh.deakin.edu.au).

33. Gupta, A. and Gopal, M., Aflatoxin production by *Aspergillus flavus* isolates pathogenic to coconut insect pests, *World J. Microbiol. Biotechnol.*, 18, 325–331, 2002.

34. Hartog, B.J. and Notermans, S., The detection and quantification of fungi in food, in *Introduction to Food-Borne Fungi*, Samson, R.A. and van Reenen-Hoekstra, E.S., Eds., Centraalbureau voor Schimmelcultures, Baarn, Netherlands, 1988, pp. 222–230.

35. Hongyo, K., Itoh, Y., Hifumi, E., Takeyasu, A. and Uda, T., Comparison of monoclonal antibody based enzyme-linked immunosorbent assay with thin layer chromatography and liquid chromatography for aflatoxin B_1 determination in naturally contaminated corn and mixed feed, *J. Assoc. Off. Anal. Chem. Int.*, 75, 307–312, 1992.

36. Horn, B.W. and Dorner, J.W., Soil populations of *Aspergillus* species from section *Flavi* along a transect through peanut-growing regions of the United States, *Mycologia*, 90, 767–776, 1998.

37. Horn, B.W., Greene, R.L., and Dorner, J.W., Effect of corn and peanut cultivation on populations of *Aspergillus flavus* and *A. parasiticus* in southwestern Georgia, *Appl. Environ. Microbiol.*, 61, 2472–2475, 1995.

38. Hussein, H.S. and Brasel, J.M., Toxicity, metabolism, and impact of mycotoxins on humans and animals, *Toxicology*, 167, 101–134, 2001.

39. King, Jr., A.D., Hocking, A.D., and Pitt, J.I., Dichloran-rose bengal medium for enumeration and isolation of molds from foods, *Appl. Environ. Microbiol.*, 37, 959–964, 1979.

40. Klich, M.A., Tiffany, L.H., and Knaphus, G., Ecology of the aspergilli of soils and litter, in Aspergillus: *Biology and Industrial Applications*, Bennett, J.W. and Klich, M.A., Eds., Butterworth-Heinemann, Boston, 1992, pp. 329–353.

41. Leitao, J., de Saint Blanquat, G., Bailly, J.R., and Paillas, C., Quantitation of aflatoxins from various strains of *Aspergillus* in foodstuffs, *J. Chromatogr.*, 435, 229–234, 1988.

42. Lemke, P.A., Davis, N.D., and Creech, G.W., Direct visual detection of aflatoxin synthesis by minicolonies of *Aspergillus* species, *Appl. Environ. Microbiol.*, 55, 1808–1810, 1989.

43. Lemke, P.A., Davis, N.D., Lyer, S.K., Creech, G.W., and Diener, U.L., Fluorometric analysis of iodinated aflatoxin in minicultures of *Aspergillus flavus* and *Aspergillus parasiticus*, *J. Industr. Microbiol.*, 3, 119–125, 1988.

44. Lin, M.T. and Dianese, J.C., A coconut-agar medium for rapid detection of aflatoxin production by *Aspergillus* spp., *Phytopathology*, 66, 1466–1499, 1976.

45. Maragos, C.M., Emerging technologies for mycotoxins detection, *J. Toxicol. Toxin Rev.*, 23, 317–344, 2004.

46. Maragos, C.M. and Thompson, V.S., Fiber-optic immunosensor for mycotoxins, *Nat. Toxins*, 7, 371–376, 1999.

47. Nasir, M.S. and Jolley, M.E., Development of a fluorescence polarization assay for the determination of aflatoxins in grains, *J. Agric. Food Chem.*, 50, 3116–3121, 2002.
48. Nilufer, D. and Boyacioglu, D., Comparative study of three different methods for the determination of aflatoxins in tahini, *J. Agric. Food Chem.*, 50, 3375–3379, 2002.
49. Ong, T., Aflatoxin mutagenesis, *Mutation Res.*, 32, 35–58, 1975.
50. Ordaz, J.J., Fente, C.A., Vazquez, B.I., Franco, C.M., and Cepeda, A., Development of a method for direct visual determination of aflatoxin production by colonies of the *Aspergillus flavus* group, *Int. J. Food Microbiol.*, 83, 219–225, 2003.
51. Oswald, I.P. and Comera, C., Immunotoxicity of mycotoxins, *Rev. Méd. Vét.*, 149, 585–590, 1998.
52. Padmanaban, V.D., Role of aflatoxins as immunomodulators, *J. Toxicol. Toxin Rev.*, 8, 239–245, 1989.
53. Patey, A.L., Sharman, M., Wood, R., and Gilbert, J., Determination of aflatoxin concentrations in peanut butter by enzyme-linked immunosorbent assay (ELISA): study of three commercial ELISA kits, *J. Assoc. Off. Anal. Chem. Int.*, 72, 965–969, 1989.
54. Payne, G.A., Aflatoxins in maize, *CRC Crit. Rev. Plant Sci.*, 10, 423–440, 1992.
55. Payne, G.A., Process of contamination by aflatoxin-producing fungi and their impact on crops, in *Mycotoxins in Agriculture and Food Safety*, Sinha, K.K. and Bhatnagar, D., Eds., Marcel Dekker, New York, 1998, pp. 279–306.
56. Peraica, M., Radiae, B., Luciae, A., and Pavloviae, M., Toxic effects of mycotoxins in humans, *Bull. World Health Org.*, 77, 754–766, 1999.
57. Pier, A.C., Effects of aflatoxin on immunity, *J. Am. Vet. Med. Assoc.*, 163, 1268–1269, 1973.
58. Pitt, J.I., Collaborative study on media for detection and differentiation of *Aspergillus flavus* and *A. parasiticus*, and the detection of aflatoxin production, in *Modern Methods in Food Mycology*, Samson, R.A., Hocking, A.D., Pitt, J.I., and King, A.D., Eds., Elsevier, Amsterdam, 1992, pp. 303–308.
59. Pittet, A., Natural occurrence of mycotoxins in foods and feeds: an updated review, *Revue Méd. Vét.*, 149, 479–492, 1998.
60. Pons, Jr., W.A. and Goldblatt, L.A., Physicochemical assay of aflatoxin, in *Aflatoxin*, Goldblatt, L.A., Ed., Academic Press, New York, 1969, pp. 77–105.
61. Robens, J. and Cardwell, K., The costs of mycotoxin management to the USA: management of aflatoxins in the United States, *J. Toxicol. Toxin Rev.*, 22, 139–152, 2003.
62. Rosner, H., Mycotoxin regulations: an update, *Rev. Méd. Vét.*, 149, 679–680, 1998.
63. Saito, M. and Machida, S., A rapid identification method for aflatoxin-producing strains of *A. flavus* and *A. parasiticus* by ammonia vapor, *Mycoscience*, 40, 205–211, 1999.
64. Scott, P.M., Mycotoxins: review, *J. Assoc. Off. Anal. Chem. Int.*, 70, 276–281, 1987.
65. Scott, P.M., Industrial and farm detoxification processes for mycotoxins, *Rev. Méd. Vét.*, 149, 543–548, 1998.
66. Scussel, V.M., Aflatoxin and food safety: recent South American perspectives, *J. Toxicol. Toxin Rev.*, 23, 179–216, 2004.
67. Seidel, V., Poglits, E., Schiller, K., and Lindner, W., Simultaneous determination of ochratoxin A and zearalenone in maize by reversed-phase high-performance liquid chromatography with fluorescence detection and beta-cyclodextrin as mobile phase additive, *J. Chromatogr.*, 635, 227–235, 1993.
68. Seitz, L.M., Comparison of methods of aflatoxin analysis by high-pressure liquid chromatography, *J. Chromatogr.*, 104, 81–91, 1975.
69. Shephard, G.S., Aflatoxin and food safety: recent African perspectives, *J. Toxicol. Toxin Rev.*, 22, 267–286, 2003.

70. Sobolev, V.S. and Dorner, J.W., Cleanup procedure for determination of aflatoxins in major agricultural commodities by liquid chromatography, *Food Chem. Contam.*, 85, 642–645, 2002.

71. Stockenstrom, S., Sydenham, E.W., and Shephard, G.S., Fumonisin B_1, B_2, and B_3 content of commercial unprocessed maize imported into South Africa from Argentina and the USA during 1992, *Food Addit. Contam.*, 15, 676–680, 1998.

72. Stroka, J. and Anklam, E., Development of a simplified densitometer for the determination of aflatoxins by thin-layer chromatography, *J. Chromatogr. A*, 904, 263–268, 2000.

73. Trucksess, M.W., Stack, M.E., Nesheim, S., Albert, R.H., and Romer, T.R., Multifunctional column coupled with liquid chromatography for determination of aflatoxins B_1, B_2, G_1 and G_2 in corn, almonds, Brazil nuts, peanuts and pistachio nuts: collaborative study, *J. Assoc. Off. Anal. Chem. Int.*, 77, 1512–1521, 1994.

74. Trucksess, M.W., Young, K., Donahue, K.F., Morris, and D.K., Comparison of two immunochemical methods with thin layer chromatographic methods for determination of aflatoxins, *J. Assoc. Off. Anal. Chem. Int.*, 73, 425–428, 1990.

75. FDA, *Action Levels for Poisonous or Deleterious Substances in Human Food and Animal Feed*, U.S. Food and Drug Administration, Rockville, MD, 2000 (http://www.cfsan.fda.gov/~lrd/fdaact.html#afla).

76. Vazquez, M.L., Cepeda, A., Prognon, P., Mabuzier, G., and Blais, J., Cyclodextrins as modifiers of the luminescence characteristics of aflatoxins, *Anal. Chim. Acta*, 255, 343–350, 1991.

77. Vazquez, M.L., Franco, C.M., Cepeda, A., Prognon, P., and Mabuzier, G., Liquid-chromatographic study of the interaction between aflatoxins and beta-cyclodextrin, *Anal. Chim. Acta*, 269, 239–247, 1992.

78. Wang, J.-S. and Tang, L., Epidemiology of aflatoxin exposure and human liver cancer, *J. Toxicol. Toxin Rev.*, 23, 249–271, 2004.

79. Watts, C.M., Chen, Y.C., Ledoux, D.R., Bermudez, A.J., and Rottinghaus, G.E., Effects of multiple mycotoxins and a hydrated sodium calcium aluminosilicate in poultry, *Int. J. Poultry Sci.*, 2, 372–378, 2003.

80. Wei, D.-L., Chen, W.-L., Wei, R.-D., and Jong, S.-C., Identity and aflatoxins producing ability of *Aspergillus* reference cultures, in *Toxigenic Fungi: Their Toxins and Health Hazards*, Kurata, H. and Ueno, Y., Eds., Elsevier, Amsterdam, 1984, pp. 87–97.

81. Whitaker, T., Horwitz, W., Albert, R., and Nesheim, S., Variability associated with analytical methods used to measure aflatoxin in agricultural commodities, *J. Assoc. Off. Anal. Chem. Int.*, 79, 476–485, 1996.

82. Wicklow, D.T., Shotwell, O.L., and Adams, G.L., Use of aflatoxin-producing ability medium to distinguish aflatoxin-producing strains of *Aspergillus flavus*, *Appl. Environ. Microbiol.*, 41, 697–699, 1981.

83. Widstrom, N.W., The aflatoxin problem with corn grain, *Adv. Agron.*, 56, 219–280, 1996.

84. Wiseman, H.G., Jacobson, W.C., and Harmeyer, W.C., Note on removal of pigments from chloroform extracts of aflatoxin cultures with copper carbonate, *J. Assoc. Off. Anal. Chem. Int.*, 50, 982–983, 1967.

85. Yabe, K., Ando, Y., Ito, M., and Terakado, N., Simple method for screening aflatoxin-producing molds by UV photography, *Appl. Environ. Microbiol.*, 53, 230–234, 1987.

86. Yiannikouris, A. and Jouany, J.P., Mycotoxins in feeds and their fate in animals: a review, *Animal Res.*, 51, 81–99, 2002.

15 Application of Technology of Gene Expression in Response to Drought Stress and Elimination of Preharvest Aflatoxin Contamination

Baozhu Z. Guo, C. Corley Holbrook, Jiujiang Yu, Dewey R. Lee, and Robert E. Lynch

CONTENTS

15.1 INTRODUCTION

A major milestone in biological science was the sequencing of the human genome which provided fundamentally new ways of studying the human body.[1-3] Likewise, with regard to the complexity of factors involved in preharvest aflatoxin contamination of corn and peanut crops, genomics could tremendously impact our understanding of host resistance mechanisms, genetic improvement of resistance to insects, invasion by *Aspergillus* spp., and improvement in drought tolerance. The complete decoding of the 3-billion-letter human genetic codes marked an important milestone in biomedical research, suggesting that the human genome may contain fewer than the expected 50,000 to 100,000 genes. No matter how many genes are encoded in the human genome, only a fraction of them is expressed at any given time in any given cell within the human body. This is also true in the plant genome. To better understand plant response to stress, more information is needed on the dynamics of gene expression in plants and how their expression is controlled in the context of a cell as a function of time and space.

Corn and peanut become contaminated with aflatoxins when subjected to prolonged periods of heat and drought stress. To meet the challenge of preventing preharvest aflatoxin contamination, more detailed understanding of the expression and function of the genetic material of corn and peanut in response to biotic/abiotic stresses will be needed. Moreover, the genes that control functions leading to plant reactions to environmental stress and fungal infection must be identified. In this paper, we will discuss drought stress, aflatoxin contamination, molecular tools used to study the genetic response to drought stress, and genetic engineering approaches to control aflatoxin contamination. Research objectives include "prospecting" for useful plant genes that can be characterized and transferred into plants. Genomic research will help identify and understand the function and control of genes to improve the desired traits. Identifying and characterizing those genes that control significant biological processes and agronomic performance are crucial in the development of genetic approaches for control of preharvest aflatoxin contamination.

15.2 AFLATOXIN CONTAMINATION AND ENVIRONMENTAL FACTORS

Aspergillus flavus and *A. parasiticus* can colonize seed of several agricultural crops including corn and peanut. This can result in the contamination of the seed with aflatoxins, which are toxic fungal metabolites. These fungi are ubiquitous, being found virtually everywhere in the world. They are soil borne, but prefer to grow on high nutrient media (e.g., seeds). *A. flavus* appears to be the primary aflatoxin-producing fungus on these commodities, although *A. parasiticus* also occurs frequently on peanut. Both fungi produce a family of related aflatoxins; the ones most commonly produced by *A. flavus* are B_1 and B_2, while *A. parasiticus* produces two additional aflatoxins, G_1 and G_2. Damage due to insects or environmental stress (drought) can enable the fungi to invade seeds where they thrive at high temperatures and extremely dry conditions, such as those frequently experienced in the southern

United States during the summer. The development of crop lines with reduced aflatoxin contamination would be a valuable development in alleviating this world-wide problem for human and animal health.

Plant stresses, depending on the type of stress and the type of plant, may include factors affecting plant survival, growth, and development of seed for harvest. Tremendous efforts have been made by scientists worldwide to study the mechanisms of the environmental factors that affect crop yield.[4-9] Aflatoxin contamination in preharvest corn is affected by many factors, including drought, temperature, humidity, planting date, irrigation, tillage, insect damage, resistance, or susceptibility.[10] Among these factors, resistance to insects, fungal infection and aflatoxin formation, and drought are genetic properties of the crop variety. We have spent years trying to decipher the genetic mechanisms of resistance or susceptibility to insect damage, fungal invasion, and tolerance to adverse environmental conditions in relation to the level of aflatoxin contamination in preharvest corn.[11-16] Likewise, the action of aflatoxin biosynthesis has also been investigated extensively.[17,18] Our goal is to reduce or eliminate aflatoxin contamination by screening for genetic traits that contribute to a greater resistance to insect damage and to A. flavus infection as well as tolerance to environmental stresses, such as drought. Although significant progress has been made,[19-21] the problem is far from solved.

15.3 DROUGHT STRESS/TOLERANCE AND AFLATOXIN CONTAMINATION

Several agronomic practices can reduce preharvest aflatoxin contamination. These include the use of pesticides, altered cultural practices (such as irrigation), and the use of resistant varieties. Although resistant varieties are not currently available, long-term research projects are ongoing to develop varieties that resist preharvest aflatoxin contamination. Holbrook et al.[22] developed a large-scale field screening technique to directly measure field resistance to preharvest aflatoxin contamination in peanut. This technique uses subsurface irrigation in a desert environment to allow an extended period of drought stress in the pod zone while keeping the plant alive. In initial field tests conducted in the desert environment without subsurface irrigation, peanut plants died and their seeds rapidly dehydrated in the soil before contamination could occur. The use of a small amount of subsurface irrigation, to prolong plant viability during the drought stress, resulted in higher and more consistent contamination. Sanders et al.[23] also observed high levels of aflatoxin contamination when peanuts in the pod zone were artificially stressed with heat and drought while keeping plants nonstressed by providing root zone irrigation.

Drought tolerance is a characteristic that has the potential to serve as an indirect selection tool for resistance to preharvest aflatoxin contamination. Holbrook et al.[24] evaluated the resistance to preharvest aflatoxin contamination in a set of genotypes that had been documented as having varying levels of drought tolerance[25] and determined the correlation of drought tolerance characteristics with aflatoxin contamination. Drought tolerance was very effective in reducing aflatoxin contamination in Tifton, GA, and significant positive correlations were observed between aflatoxin contamination and leaf temperature, and between aflatoxin contamination and visual stress ratings. A significant negative correlation was also observed between aflatoxin contamination and yield under drought stressed conditions. Leaf temperature, visual stress ratings, and yield are all less variable and expensive to measure than aflatoxin contamination. These characteristics may be useful as indirect selection tools for reduced aflatoxin contamination.

A similar relationship between drought tolerance and reduced aflatoxin contamination has been observed in a drought-tolerant peanut cultivar in Australia.[26] The cultivar, "Streeton," has up to 40% lower aflatoxin contamination during years of high aflatoxin incidence in comparison to other commercial cultivars. Physiological studies have shown that the lower aflatoxin incident is associated with better root water uptake, resulting in better maintenance of plant water status during severe end-of-season drought.

In corn, research has been conducted to evaluate drought tolerance of corn germplasm in rain-out shelters for 3 years. In rain-out shelter screening for drought-tolerant germplasm, we identified and selected several corn lines with excellent drought tolerance based on a "stay-green" character.[19] We also evaluated lines selected from the GT-MAS:gk population that have drought tolerance.[13,14] Multiple-location field evaluation of commercial hybrids for drought tolerance and aflatoxin production demonstrated that drought-tolerant commercial lines, in general, had lower aflatoxin contamination under drought conditions.[18] This positive association of drought tolerance with lower aflatoxin production is encouraging, and hybrids made from drought-tolerant lines will be tested further to evaluate drought tolerance, yield, and aflatoxin contamination.

15.4 GENETIC ENGINEERING AND PREVENTION OF AFLATOXIN FORMATION

Genetic engineering approaches to control aflatoxin contamination in corn and peanut have focused on three main areas: resistance to the fungus, inhibition of aflatoxin production, and resistance to insects. The focus on resistance to insects is a result of the intimate relation between insect damage and aflatoxin contamination.[27–30] *Aspergillus flavus* and *A. parasiticus* are able to survive and out-compete other fungi under hot, dry conditions. These conditions are also conducive to the development of outbreak populations of certain insects, such as the lesser cornstalk borer, *Elasmopalpus lignosellus* (Zeller), in the United States, and termites (*Odontotermes* spp. and *Microtermes* spp.) in Africa that feed on peanut pods/kernels. Other insects such as the corn earworm, *Helicoverpa zea* (Boddie), and the fall armyworm, *Spodoptera frugiperda* (Smith), damage kernels as they feed in an ear of corn, which provides a direct avenue for infection by *A. flavus* and *A. parasiticus*, exacerbating the infection and contamination of ears with *A. flavus* and aflatoxin.[31] The highest levels of aflatoxin contamination in both corn and peanut are usually associated with insect damage.[29,31] Indeed, aflatoxin contamination in peanuts from insect-damaged pods is 30 to 60 times greater than that in undamaged pods. Thus, one approach to reduce aflatoxin contamination is to reduce insect damage.

15.4.1 INSECT RESISTANCE IN TRANSGENIC CROPS

The bacterium *Bacillus thuringiensis* (Bt) is ubiquitous and unique in that it produces a protein (termed Cry proteins because of their crystalline nature) that is toxic to certain insects. Over 240 insecticidal Cry proteins have been identified and sequenced.[32] Each of these proteins is encoded by a single gene. Corn, cotton, potato, and other crops have been genetically engineered to express one of these proteins for insect control. Transgenic Bt crops have been commercially available since the mid-1990s. In 2001, genetically engineered crops were grown on 130 million acres worldwide, up 19%, or almost 20 million acres, from 2000. Of this total, 88.2 million acres were planted in transgenic crops in the United States in 2001 and included soybean, cotton, corn, and potato. Herbicide resistance accounted for 77% of the total acreage planted to transgenic crops, Bt crops accounted for 15%, and stacked genes for herbicide and insect resistance accounted for 8%. Registration of Bt crop varieties was recently renewed for another 7 years.[33]

The primary target of Bt transgenic corn is the European corn borer, *Ostrinia nubilalis* (Hübner). This insect not only reduces the yield of corn grown in the Midwest by an estimated $1 billion annually[34] but is also associated with ear infections with *Fusarium* spp. and *A. flavus*.[35] Field studies in the Midwest with transgenic corn have consistently shown that hybrids that express the BT11 and MON810 events have a significantly lower incidence and severity of *Fusarium* ear rot and significantly lower concentrations of fumonisins than isogenic corn lines without the Bt gene.[36–38] These events produce the Cry1Ab toxin in all parts of the corn plant including silks and kernels. Events that do not express the Bt toxin in the kernels are less effective in reducing European corn borer damage and *Fusarium* ear rot.[37,39]

Although present, the European corn borer is not the major pest of corn in the South and Southeast, and the relationships between reduced insect damage in transgenic corn and aflatoxin in southern grown corn is not as clear as that for fumonisins in midwestern grown corn. There are two reasons for this difference. First, the corn earworm and fall armyworm are the major pests of corn in the South, and commercially available Bt corn hybrids are not as effective against these insects as they are against the European corn borer. Second, the environmental conditions conducive to the infection of corn with *Aspergillus flavus* and formation of aflatoxin are also much more severe, on average, in the South and Southeast than they are in the Midwest. In the South and Southeast, the corn earworm, fall armyworm, and southwestern corn borer (*Diatraea grandiosella* Dyar) are the major lepidopterous pests of corn. Ear damage by the corn earworm and fall armyworm can be quite extensive and lead to increased levels of aflatoxin contamination under appropriate environmental conditions. In the Midwest, Bt corn reduced kernel infection by *A. flavus* and lowered aflatoxin concentrations in BT11 and MOB810 hybrids;[37] however, in the Southeast, no such relationship between insect resistance in Bt corn (YieldGard, BT11, MON810) and aflatoxin concentration could be established.[40] Although Yield-Gard corn did reduce the percentage of infested ears and the number of larvae in the ears, slower larval development did occur in ears of the resistant plants. Under heavy fall armyworm infestations, YieldGard corn did not reduce the percentage of infested ears but did reduce the rate of larval development and the amount of kernel damage. Sims et al.[41] reported reduced corn earworm feeding damage and reduced larval development on 8 of 12 independently transformed lines of corn containing a Cry1Ab gene. Williams et al.[42] reported significantly less fall armyworm leaf feeding damage, reduced survival, and slower larval growth on Bt corn (BT11 event) and near immunity to feeding by the southwestern corn borer. These differences in the effect of Bt transgenic plants on corn insects is directly related to the susceptibility of the insects to the Cry1Ab protein; LC_{50} values ranged from 2.22 to 7.89 ng/cm^2 for the European corn borer,[43] considerably lower than the 70.3 to 221.3 ng/cm^2 for the corn earworm[44] and lower than the 0.36 to 10.22 µg/cm^2 for the fall armyworm.[44] Windham et al.[46] reported that corn hybrid N6800Bt had a lower southwestern corn borer damage rating and about a 50% reduction in aflatoxin concentration than N6800 when they were artificially infested with *A. flavus* spores and southwestern corn borer larvae. Research conducted in South Texas with Cry2Ab, Cry1Ab, and non-Bt isolines showed a positive correlation between the number of fall armyworm larvae per ear with ear insect injury rating at harvest and with aflatoxin content.

Peanut has also been genetically engineered to contain the Cry1Ac gene, which confers resistance to feeding by the lesser cornstalk borer (LCB).[47] This gene also confers resistance to the corn earworm and velvebean caterpillar but not to the fall armyworm (Lynch, unpublished data). The transgenic peanut is primarily aimed at control of the LCB because this insect is intimately associated with aflatoxin contamination. Only external scarification of peanut pods by LCB is needed to enhance infection of peanut kernels with *Aspergillus flavus*.[29] Field tests have been conducted to evaluate the efficacy of the Bt peanut in reducing lesser damage and aflatoxin contamination under drought stress.[48] In 2000, no difference was observed in the percentage of pods showing scarification due to LCB feeding on transgenic vs. nontransgenic peanut pods. The aflatoxin concentration in scarified, transgenic peanut pods was significantly lower than in scarified, nontransgenic pods. The experiment was repeated in 2001, but aflatoxin analyses have not yet been reported.

15.4.2 Fungal Resistance and Inhibition of Toxin Production in Transgenic Crops

Progress has been made in the development of crop resistance to aflatoxin through genetic engineering. Research in Peggy Ozias-Akins' lab in Tifton, GA, on aflatoxin reduction is using a three-tiered approach: (1) resistance to insect damage using a Bt gene, (2) resistance to fungal growth using the tomato anionic peroxidase gene (*tap1*) or an antifungal peptide D4E1, and (3) inhibition of the aflatoxin biosynthetic pathway using the lipoxygenase gene *lox1*.[48]

Art Weissinger, at North Carolina State University, is testing transgenic peanut containing synthetic Peptidyl Membrane Interactive Molecules (Peptidyl MIMs™) developed by Demegen, Inc.[49] His group developed transgenic peanut encoding D5C, an α-helical peptide that is highly active against *Aspergillus flavus*. In a test of 15 lines that carried the D5C transgene, none contained D5C mRNA, and the peptide was not detectable using western blots. Furthermore, D5C transgenic peanut plants produced significantly fewer pods than control plants. Subsequent tests indicated that D5C was phytotoxic to peanut at levels required to kill *A. flavus*. Demegen, Inc., has also developed other antimicrobial peptides that may warrant testing for *A. flavus* inhibition in transgenic plants.[50] D4E1 has emerged as one of the most active peptides against several species of bacteria and fungi. Activity against *A. flavus* is also present but at a lower level than that for other pathogens. Research is either planned or underway to integrate this gene in several crop species.

Charles Woloshuk and colleagues[51] at Purdue University are investigating the possibility that transgenic corn containing an α-amylase inhibitor will inhibit *Aspergillus flavus* infection. Their previous research had indicated that α-amylase produced by *A. flavus* may facilitate colonization and aflatoxin production in corn kernels. They also found that the α-amylase inhibitor from *Lablab purpureus* inhibits α-amylase production in several fungi but not those from animals or plants. It also inhibits conidia germination and hypha growth of *A. flavus*.

15.5 MOLECULAR TOOLS TO STUDY GENE EXPRESSION

Plants tolerate environmental stress because of numerous physiological adaptations, which have been attributed to the function of various genes.[52] For example, in *Arabidopsis thaliana*, transcription of *RD* (responsive to dehydration)[53] and *COR* (cold responsive)[54] genes are activated by hyperosmotic or cold stress. The plant hormone abscisic acid (ABA) activates transcription of some *RD* and *COR* genes, while *PLD* (phospholipase D) gene transcription is activated by drought stress.[55–58] The genetic control of these traits for tolerance to abiotic stresses is complex. Drought tolerance, for example, may be determined by many genetic factors. Quite a number of plant features contribute to drought tolerance and include both physiological and biological elements such as waxy skin layer on plant surfaces, size and number of stomata, extensiveness of root system, respiration rate, and nutritional status. These factors are genetically controlled. The isolation of one of these genes for a specific function is not easy, and the determination of all of these genes is almost impossible using traditional genetics and cloning techniques. The "one-gene-at-a-time" approach for analyzing gene expression is wholly inadequate. The development of differential-display, reverse-transcription PCR (DD-RT-PRC) and expressed sequence tag (EST) methods provided new tools for isolating more genes. It is now possible to locate multiple genes that enable plants to withstand biotic and abiotic stresses. Several major tools are used for gene expression analysis, four of which are discussed briefly here: DD-RT-PCR, EST/microarray, proteomics, and transgenes/genetic transformation.

15.5.1 EXPRESSED GENE DIFFERENTIAL DISPLAY

Liang and Pardee[59] first described DD-RT-PCR, which is a powerful and cost-effective method to detect variations in mRNA expression. DD-RT-PCR technology was developed to identify and isolate selectively those genes that are expressed in a temporally and spatially regulated manner in different tissues and organs. The technique uses a limited number of short arbitrary primers in combination with the

anchored oligo-dT primers to systematically amplify and visualize a certain proportion of the expressed genes (mRNA) in an organism or tissue. In cowpea,
sunflower, and tomato, cDNA libraries constructed from drought-induced mRNA
have been used to characterize genes associated with drought response. Differential
display fragments can then be used as probes to screen the cDNA library to get the
full-length drought-inducible genes. Using DD-RT-PCR, we have identify mRNA
transcripts that are up- or downregulated due to drought stress. In addition, differences in the composition of selected metabolite levels between the drought-tolerant
and -susceptible genotypes following drought stress may be determined.

To investigate gene expression patterns in response to induced drought stress in
plants we have used DD-RT-PCR to differentiate gene expression in drought-susceptible and drought-tolerant corn and peanut.[60,61] Polymorphic mRNA transcripts
have been identified. Some cDNA fragments that were up- or downregulated by
induced drought stress have been cloned and sequenced. Using this method, we
identified a novel *PLD* gene,[57,58] which encodes a putative phospholipase D, a
primary enzyme responsible for the drought-induced degradation of membrane phos-
pholipids in plants. The *PLD* gene expression under drought stress has been studied
in the greenhouse using two peanut lines, Tifton 8 (drought tolerant) and Georgia
Green (drought sensitive). Northern analyses showed that the *PLD* gene expression
was induced sooner by drought stress in Georgia Green than in Tifton 8.[57] After the
PLD gene in peanut is completely characterized, we will attempt gene silencing
using genetic transformation to suppress *PLD* gene expression and induce drought
tolerance. The limitation of DD-RT-PCR is that it can be used to identify only those
genes that are amplified by a few arbitrary primers within hundreds and perhaps
thousands of expressed genes. In order to identify and isolate all of the expressed
genes, expressed sequence tag (EST) offers the best solution.

15.5.2 EXPRESSED SEQUENCE TAG AND MACRO/MICROARRAY

Expressed sequence tag (EST) is used to sequence cDNA (DNA copies of RNAs)
clones in an expressed cDNA library and identify all of the unique sequences (genes)
to study their functions. Generating sequences from cDNA fragments can be used
to discover new genes and to assess their expression levels in the representative
tissue.[62,63] The level of an mRNA species in a tissue is reflected by the frequency
of occurrence of its corresponding EST in a cDNA library. EST technologies are
attractive because they do not rely on established sequence data from the organism
under study, and they also fit well with labs already equipped to carry out high-
throughput DNA sequencing.[64] Auxiliary techniques to reduce the amount of
sequencing include subtraction hybridization,[64] representational difference analysis
(RDA),[66] and suppression subtractive hybridization (SSH).[67] The identified cDNA
sequences, either fragments or homologous oligoes, can be used to fabricate a DNA
microarray for functional study.

DNA microarrays or a gene chip typically consist of thousands of immobilized
DNA sequences present on a miniaturized surface the size of a microscope slide.
Arrays are used to analyze a sample for the presence of gene variations or mutations

(genotyping) or for patterns of gene expression.[68] Microarrays are distinguished from macroarrays in that the DNA spot size is smaller, allowing for the presence of thousands of DNA sequences instead of the hundreds present on macroarrays. The samples of cDNAs are then prepared for expression analysis. The DNA samples are tagged with a radioactive or fluorescent label and applied to the array. Single-strand DNA will bind to a complementary strand of DNA. At positions on the array where the immobilized DNA recognizes a complementary DNA in the sample, binding or hybridization occurs. The labeled sample DNA marks the exact positions on the array where binding occurs, allowing automatic detection. The output consists of a list of hybridization events reflecting the presence or relative abundance of specific DNA sequences that are present in the sample, thus indicating how much a gene is turned on or off.

The mode of action, metabolism, and biosynthesis of aflatoxins have been extensively studied in the last decade.[17,69–75] For a better understanding of the genetic control and regulation of toxin production by *Aspergillus flavus* and the mechanism of toxin production in response to environmental conditions such as drought stress and temperature, fungal EST and macro-/microarray programs are being carried out at the USDA–ARS Southern Regional Research Center in New Orleans, LA,[75,76] and USDA–ARS Labs at Tifton, GA. Currently, about 8000 expressed unique genes have been identified from the *A. flavus* EST programs. A microarray containing these identified *A. flavus* genes will be produced to study gene expression and regulation and to identify factors involved in the plant–microbe interaction. The *A. flavus* EST program will help to identify genes that could be used to inhibit fungal growth or aflatoxin formation by the fungi. The EST and macro-/microarray projects in corn and peanut have been initiated in Tifton, GA, to study the gene expression profile of drought response based on suppression subtractive hybridization.[77] The preliminary ESTs show that some plant defense genes have been identified, such as a small cysteine-rich antifungal protein, Ca^{2+}/H^+-exchanging protein, peroxidase, 14-3-3-like protein, glutathione *S*-transferase, and trypsin inhibitor. The first batch of 1345 ESTs has been released to GenBank. Four hundred unigenes have been selected from these ESTs and arrayed on glass slides for gene expression analysis, and 44 EST-derived SSR markers have been characterized for cultivated peanut, in which over 20% SSR produced polymorphic markers among 24 cultivated peanut genotypes.[78,79]

15.5.3 PROTEOMICS

Proteomics is the identification and examination of the proteins produced by a cell type and an organism.[80] The term *proteome* refers to all the proteins expressed by a genome, thus proteomics involves the identification of proteins in the organism and the determination of their role in physiological and biochemical functions. To study the proteins directly and to identify their genes is another effective method for gene expression analysis. Identifying drug receptors and inhibitory factors has tremendous potential and practical applications for the pharmaceutical industry. The approximately 30,000 genes defined by the Human Genome Project translate into 300,000 to 1 million proteins when alternate splicing and posttranslation modifications are considered. Although a genome remains unchanged to a large extent, the proteins in any particular tissue change dramatically as genes are turned on and off in response to its environment. As sequencing of the entire genomes of many prokaryotes and eukaryotes has been completed, the technology of proteomics is necessary to separate proteins from each other and to study proteins. The main way this has been achieved is through one- or two-dimensional polyacrylamide gel electrophoresis (2-D PAGE).[81–83] Using 2-D PAGE, the separation of several thousands of different proteins can be achieved in one gel.

As a reflection of the dynamic nature of the proteome, some researchers prefer to use the term *functional proteome* to describe all the proteins produced by a specific cell in a single time frame.[84] Riccardi et al.[82] reported that protein profiles change in response to water deficits in corn. The induced changes of protein profile in leaf tissue of 3-week-old plants in response to drought or water deficit were studied by 2-D electrophoresis. Out of a total of 413 plants, 78 showed a significant quantitative variation (increase or decrease), and 38 of those exhibited a different expression in different genotypes. Eleven proteins increased by a factor of 1.3 to 5 in stressed plants, and 8 proteins were detected only in stressed plants. Some proteins are already known to be involved in the response to water stress (responsive to ABA). Most cellular processes are carried out by multiprotein complexes. Through proteomics, new plant resistance genes could be identified and DNA markers could be derived from these proteins that could be used as markers for breeding selection or genetic transformation, such as antifungal proteins identified from corn kernels.[85–87]

15.5.4 TRANSGENES/GENETIC TRANSFORMATION

Molecular techniques allowed the identification, isolation, and characterization of genes that encode specific protein products controlling plant development (see above discussion on molecular tools). Genetic engineering is the next step to modify the genome of plants to contain and express foreign genes or modify native or endogenous genes to alter/enhance/suppress the traits of a plant in a specific manner (see earlier discussion on genetic engineering). Such foreign and modified genes are referred to as *transgenes*.

15.5.4.1 Expression Vector

Plant transformation involves the construction of an expression vector that will function in plant cells. Such a vector is comprised of DNA, including a gene under the control of or linked to a regulatory element, such as a promoter. Expression vectors include at least one genetic marker linked to a regulatory element (a promoter) that allows transformed cells containing the marker to be either recovered by negative selection, such as inhibiting growth of cells that do not contain the selectable marker gene, or by positive selection by screening for the product encoded by the genetic marker. One commonly used selectable marker gene for plant transformation is the neomycin phosphotransferase II (*nptII*) gene, which when placed under the control of plant regulatory signals confers resistance to kanamycin.[88]

Another commonly used selectable marker gene is the hygromycin phosphotrans-ferase gene, which confers resistance to the antibiotic hygromycin.[89] Other selectable marker genes that confer resistance to antibiotics include gentamycin acetyl trans-ferase,[90] streptomycin phosphotransferase, aminoglycoside-3′-adenyl transferase,[91] and bleomycin resistance.[92] Selectable marker genes may also confer resistance to herbicides such as glyphosate, glufosinate, or broxynil.[93] GUS (β-glucuronidase) and luciferase represent another class of marker genes for plant transformation and require screening of presumptively transformed plant cells rather than direct genetic selection of transformed cells for resistance to an antibiotic.[94,95] More recently, a gene encoding green fluorescent protein (GFP) has been utilized as a marker for gene expression.[96]

15.5.4.2 Promoter

Genes included in expression vectors must be driven by a nucleotide sequence containing a regulatory element, a promoter. Several types of promoters are now well known in plant transformation. A plant promoter is capable of initiating tran-scription in plant cells. Promoters under developmental control include promoters that preferentially initiate transcription in certain tissues, such as leaves, roots, or seeds. Such promoters are referred to as being tissue preferred or tissue specific, such as the phaseolin gene[97] and light-induced promoter.[98] An inducible promoter is one that is under environmental control. Tissue-specific, tissue-preferred, and inducible promoters comprise the class of nonconstitutive promoters. A constitutive promoter is one that is active under most environmental conditions, such as the 35S promoter from CaMV,[99] rice actin,[100] or corn ubiquitin promoter.[101,102] With an inducible promoter, the rate of transcription increases in response to an inducing agent. A constitutive promoter is linked to a gene for expression or to a nucleotide sequence encoding a signal sequence that is linked to a gene for expression.

15.5.4.3 Methods for Transformation

Numerous methods for plant transformation have been developed, including biolog-ical and physical. One method for introducing an expression vector into plants is based on the natural transformation system of *Agrobacterium*.[103] *A. tumefaciens* and *A. rhizogenes* are plant pathogenic soil bacteria that can genetically transform plant cells. The Ti and Ri plasmids of *A. tumefaciens* and *A. rhizogenes*, respectively, carry genes responsible for genetic transformation of the plant.[104] Another method is referred to as direct gene transfer, microprojectile-mediated transformation wherein DNA is carried on the surface of microprojectiles. The expression vector is introduced into plant tissues with a biolistic device (gene gun) that accelerates the microprojectiles to penetrate plant cell walls and membranes.[105,106] In maize, several target tissues can be bombarded with DNA-coated microprojectiles in order to produce transgenic plants, including callus, immature embryos, and meristematic tissue. In peanut, the most reliable method for the introduction of foreign DNA is microprojectile bombardment of embryogenic tissue cultures.[107]

15.6   SUMMARY AND PROSPECTS

In traditional genetics, a trait of interest is targeted and then research to identify the gene that caused, or coded, for that trait is conducted for several years. In the new paradigm of genomics, however, we take the opposite approach in that we map out all of the genes of an organism first, and then work to determine their functions. The first step is known as structural genomics, and the second step is functional genomics.[108–110] The information obtained from genomics can be applied to the development of commercial crops for high yield with no or low aflatoxin contamination through genetic engineering.[111] Practical examples of genetic engineering are the genetically improved (Bt) corn that protects against insects and the genetically engineered cotton that protects against the bollworm.[112] These innovative products not only increase crop yields but also dramatically reduce the cost for insecticides and the chance for environmental contamination.

Genes are key components in manipulating plants and animals for more desirable and economic and agronomic traits. To reduce yield losses and to study genetic factors involved with plant stresses, the National Science Foundation granted $8.4 million to the "Functional Genomics of Plant Stress Tolerance Project," which is being conducted by scientists at Purdue University, the University of Arizona, and Oklahoma State University. The corn genomics project is expected to define and discover the full suite of genes in corn as a route to new fundamental discoveries in plant biology and to find immediate application in basic research for use in the commercial arena. Corn genomics promises development of new commercial corn varieties that are able to withstand environmental stresses such as drought and heat, as well as resistance to insects and plant pathogens. A peanut genomics project will be launched soon.

Expressed sequence tag/microarray technology can be used to detect an entire set of genes transcribed under specific conditions and to study the biological functions of genes of interest. EST and microarray technology provides a tool for rapid identification of genes of interest expressed by plants under fungal challenged or environmental stress conditions. They can help in our understanding of the biological functions, coordination of gene expression in response to internal and external factors, mechanisms of plant–fungal interaction, plant–environmental interaction, fungal pathogenicity antifungal properties, and the mechanism of genetic regulation in relation to plant tolerance to biotic and abiotic stresses. This technology allows us to study a complete set of genes simultaneously for screening and identifying the most important host-resistance and stress-tolerance genes among hundreds or even thousands of relevant genes that could be used in genetic engineering for developing commercial crops. Our *Aspergillus flavus*/corn/peanut EST/microarray programs are expected to provide valuable information on the prevention and elimination of aflatoxin contamination in these crops.

In the effort to prevent preharvest aflatoxin contamination in corn and peanut, knowledge obtained from the *Aspergillus flavus* EST/microarray program can be integrated into the corn and peanut genomics programs for identifying host-resistance and stress-tolerance genes, and, at the same time, identifying biological targets for antifungal growth or inhibition of toxin formation by fungi. Corn and peanut genomics combined with the *A. flavus* EST/microarray project will give us more specific genetic information to target critical regulatory components and genes involved in aflatoxin biosynthesis. These genes can then be engineered into commercial crops to alleviate the problems of preharvest aflatoxin contamination of food and feed.

REFERENCES

1. Lander, E.S., et al., Initial sequencing and analysis of the human genome, *Nature*, 409, 860–921, 2001.
2. Subramanian, G., Adams, M.D., Venter, J.C., and Broder, S., Implications of the human genome for understanding human biology and medicine, *J. Am. Med. Assoc.*, 286, 2296–2307, 2001.
3. Venter, J.C. et al., The sequence of the human genome, *Science*, 291, 1304–1351, 2001.
4. Cochard, H., Xylem embolism and drought-induced stomatal closure in maize, *Planta*, 215, 466–471, 2002.
5. Norton, S.B., Cormier, S.M., Smith, M., Jones, R.C., and Schubauer-Berigan, M., Predicting levels of stress from biological assessment data: empirical models from the eastern corn belt plains, Ohio, USA, *Environ Toxicol Chem.*, 21, 1168–1175, 2002.
6. Kolesnichenko, A.V., Pobezhimova, T.P., Grabelnych, O.I., and Voinikov, V.K., Stress-induced protein CSP 310: a third uncoupling system in plants, *Planta*, 215, 279–286, 2002.
7. Polidoros, A.N., Mylona, P.V., and Scandalios, J.G., Transgenic tobacco plants expressing the maize cat2 gene have altered catalase levels that affect plant-pathogen interactions and resistance to oxidative stress, *Transgenic Res.*, 10, 555–569, 2001.
8. Sauter, A. and Hartung, W., The contribution of internode and mesocotyl tissues to root-to-shoot signalling of abscisic acid, *J. Exp. Bot.*, 53, 297–302, 2002.
9. Horn, B.W., Greene, R.L, and Dorner, J.W., Effect of corn and peanut cultivation on soil populations of *Aspergillus flavus* and *A. parasiticus* in southwestern Georgia, *Appl. Environ. Microbiol.*, 61, 2472–2475, 1995.
10. Widstrom, N.W., Guo, B.Z., and Wilson, D.M., Integration of crop management and genetics for control of preharvest aflatoxin contamination of corn, *J. Toxicol. Toxin Rev.*, 22,199–227, 2003.
11. Guo, B.Z., Chen, Z.-Y., Brown, R.L., Lax, A.R., Cleveland, T.E., Russin, J.S., Mehta, A.D., Selitrennikoff, C.P., and Widstrom, N.W., Germination induces accumulation of specific proteins and antifungal activities in corn kernels, *Phytopathology*, 87, 1174–1178, 1997.
12. Guo, B.Z., Widstrom, N.W., Cleveland, T.E., and Lynch, R.E., Control of preharvest aflatoxin contamination in corn: fungus–plant–insect interactions and control strategies, *Recent Res. Devel. Agric. Food Chem.*, 4, 165–176, 2000.
13. Guo, B.Z., Li, R., Widstrom, N.W., Lynch, R.E., and Cleveland, T.E., Genetic variation in the maize population GT-MAS:gk and the relationship with resistance to *Aspergillus flavus*, *Theo. Appl. Genet.*, 103, 533–539, 2001.
14. Guo, B.Z., Butron, A., Li, H., Widstrom, N.W., and Lynch, R.E., Restriction fragment length polymorphism assessment of the heterogeneous nature of maize population GT-MAS:gk and field evaluation of resistance to aflatoxin production by *Aspergillus flavus*, *J. Food Product.*, 65, 167–171, 2002.

15. Butrón, A., Li, R.G., Guo, B.Z., Widstrom, N.W., Snook, M.E., Cleveland, T.E., and Lynch, R.E., Molecular markers to increase corn earworm resistance in a maize population, *Maydica*, 46, 117–124, 2001.

16. Lynch, R.E., Guo, B.Z., Timper, P., and Wilson, J.P., United States Department of Agriculture–Agricultural Research Service: research on improving host-plant resistance to pests, *Pest Manage. Sci.*, 59, 718–727, 2003.

17. Bhatnagar, D., Cotty, P.J., and Cleveland, T.E., Genetic and biological control of aflatoxigenic fungi, in *Microbial Food Contamination*, Wilson, C.L. and Droby, S., Eds, CRC Press, Boca Raton, FL, 2001, pp. 207–240.

18. Yu, J., Genetics and biochemistry of mycotoxin synthesis, in *Handbook of Fungal Biotechnology*, 2nd ed., Arora, D.K., Ed., Marcel Dekker, New York, 2002.

19. Li, H., Butrón, A., Jiang, T., Guo, B.Z., Coy, A.E., Lee, R.D., Widstrom, N.W., and Lynch, R.E., Evaluation of corn germplasm tolerance to drought stress and effects on aflatoxin production, in *Proc. Aflatoxin/Fumonisin Elimination Workshop*, Yosemite, CA, October 25–27, 2000.

20. Guo, B.Z., Widstrom, N.W., Holbrook, C.C., Lee, R.D., Coy, A.E., and Lynch, R.E., Molecular genetic analysis of resistance mechanisms to aflatoxin formation in corn and peanut, *Mycopathologia*, 155, 78, 2002.

21. Guo, B.Z., Cao, Y., Coy, A.E., Lee, R.D., Holbrook, C.C., and Lynch, R.E., Evaluation of drought tolerance and relationship with aflatoxin contamination, *Phytopathology*, 92, S33, 2002.

22. Holbrook, C.C., Matheron, M.E., Wilson, D.M., Anderson, W.F., Will, M.E., and Norden, A.J., Development of a large-scale field system for screening peanut for resistance to preharvest aflatoxin contamination, *Peanut Sci.*, 21, 20–22, 1994.

23. Sanders, T.H., Cole, R.J., Blankenship, P.D., and Dorner, J.W., Aflatoxin contamination of peanut from plants drought stressed in pod or root zones, *Peanut Sci.*, 20, 5–8, 1993.

24. Holbrook, C.C., Kvien, C.K., Ruckers, K.S., Wilson, D.M., and Hook, J.E., Preharvest aflatoxin contamination in drought tolerant and intolerant peanut genotypes, *Peanut Sci.*, 27, 45–48, 2000.

25. Rucker, K.S., Kvien, C.K., Holbrook, C.C., and Hook, J.E., Identification of peanut genotypes with improved drought avoidance traits, *Peanut Sci.*, 21, 14–18, 1995.

26. Cruickshank, A.L., Wright, G.C., Rachaputi, N.R., "Streeton": an aflatoxin tolerant peanut cultivar for the Australian peanut industry, *Proc. Amer. Peanut Res. Educ. Soc.*, 32, 27, 2000.

27. Widstrom, N.W., The aflatoxin problem with corn grain, *Adv. Agron.*, 56, 219–280, 1996.

28. Cole, R.J., Dorner, J.W., and Holbrook, C.C., Advances in mycotoxin elimination and resistance, in *Advances in Peanut Science*, Pattee, H.E. and Stalker, H.T., Eds., American Peanut Research and Education Society, Stillwater, OK, 1995, pp. 456–474.

29. Lynch, R.E. and Wilson, D.M., Enhanced infection of peanut, *Arachis hypogaea* L., seeds with *Aspergillus flavus* group fungi due to external scarification of peanut pods by the lesser cornstalk borer, *Elasmopalpus lignosellus* (Zeller), *Peanut Sci.*, 18, 110–116, 1991.

30. Bowen, K.L. and Mack, T.P., Relationship of damage from the lesser cornstalk borer to *aspergillus flavus* contamination in peanuts, *J. Entomol. Sci.*, 28, 29–42, 1993.

31. McMillian, W.W., Wilson, D.M., and Widstrom, N.W., Aflatoxin contamination of preharvest corn of Georgia: a six-year study of insect damage and visible *Aspergillus flavus*, *J. Environ. Qual.*, 14, 200–202, 1985.

32. Crickmore, N., Zeigler, D.R., Schnepf, E., Van Rie, J., Lereclus, D., Baum, J, Bravo, A., and Dean, D.H., Bacillus thuringiensis *Toxin Nomenclature*, 2002 (http://www.biols.susx.ac.uk/Home/Neil_Crickmore/Bt/index.html).

33. EPA, Bacillus thuringiensis *Plant-Incorporated Protectants*, Biopesticide registration action document, U.S. Environmental Protection Agency, Washington, D.C., 2001 (http://www.epa.gov/pesticides/biopesticides/reds/brad_bt_pip2.htm).

34. Ostlie, K.R., Hutchison, W.D., and Hellmich, R.L., *Bt Corn and European Corn Borer*, NCR publication 602, University of Minnesota, St. Paul, 1997, 18 pp.

35. Dowd, P.F., Involvement of arthropods in the establishment of mycotoxigenic fungi under field conditions, in *Mycotoxins in Agriculture and Food Safety*, Sinha, K.K. and Bhatagnar, D., Eds., Marcel Dekker, New York, 1998, pp. 307–350.

36. Munkvold, G.P., Hellmich, R.L., and Showers, W.B., Reduced Fusarium ear rot and symptomless infections in kernels of maize genetically engineered for European corn borer resistance, *Phytopathology*, 87, 1071–1077, 1997.

37. Munkvold, G.P. and Hellmich, R.L., Comparison of fumonisin concentration in kernels of transgenic maize hybrids and nontransgenic hybrids, *Plant Dis.*, 83, 130–138, 1999.

38. Dowd, P.F. and Munkvold, G.P., Association between insect damage and fumonison derived from field-based insect control strategies, in *Proc. 40th Annual Corn Dry Milling Conf.*, Peoria, IL, June 3–4, 1999.

39. Munkvold, G.P. and Hellmich R.L., *Genetically Modified, Insect Resistant Corn: Implications for Disease Management*, APSnet feature, 1999 (http://www.aps-net.org/online/feature/BtCorn/Top.html).

40. Buntin, G.D., Lee, R.D., Wilson, D.M., and McPherson, R.M., Evaluation of YieldGard transgenic resistance for control of fall armyworm and corn earworm (Lepidoptera: Noctuidae) on corn, *Florida Entomol.*, 84, 37–42, 2001.

41. Sims, S.R., Pershing, J.C., and Reich, B.J., Field evaluation of transgenic corn containing a *Bacillus thuringiensis* Berliner insecticidal protein gene against *Helicoverpa zea* (Lepidoptera: Noctuidae), *J. Entomol. Sci.*, 31, 340–346, 1996.

42. Williams, W.P., Sagers, J.B., Hanten, J.A., Davis, F.M., and Buckley, P.M., Transgenic corn evaluated for resistance to fall armyworm and southwestern corn borer, *Crop Sci.*, 37, 957–962, 1997.

43. Marçon, P.C., Young, L.J., Steffey, K.L., and Siegfried, B.D., Baseline susceptibility of European corn borer (Lepidoptera: Crambidae) to *Bacillus thuringiensis* toxins, *J. Econ. Entomol.*, 92, 279–285, 1999.

44. Siegfried, B.D., Spencer, T., and Nearman, J., Baseline susceptibility of the corn earworm (Lepidoptera: Noctuidae) to the Cry1Ab toxin from *Bacillus thuringiensis*, *J. Econ. Entomol.*, 93, 1265–1268, 2000.

45. Lynch, R.E., Hamm, J.J., Myers, R.E., Guyer, D., and Stein, J., Baseline susceptibility of the fall armyworm (Lepidoptera: Noctuidae) to Cry1Ab toxin: 1998–2000, *J. Entomol Sci.*, 38(3), 377–385, 2003.

46. Windham, G.L., Williams, W.P., and Davis, F.M., Effects of the southwestern corn borer on *Aspergillus flavus* kernel infection and aflatoxin accumulation in maize hybrids, *Plant Dis.*, 83, 535–540, 1999.

47. Singsit, C., Adang, M.J., Lynch, R.E., Anderson, W.F., Wang, A., Cardineau, G., and Ozias-Akins, P., Expression of a *Bacillus thuringiensis* CryIAb gene in transgenic peanut plants and its efficacy against lesser cornstalk borer, *Transgenic Res.*, 5, 1–8, 1996.

48. Ozias-Akins, P., Yang, H., Perry, E., Akasaka, Y., Niu, C., Holbrook, C., and Lynch, R.E., Transgenic peanut for preharvest aflatoxin reduction, *Mycopathologia*, 155, 98, 2002.

49. Weissinger, A., Wu, M., Liu, Y.S., Ingram, K., Rajasekaran, K., and Cleveland, T.E., Development of transgenic peanut with enhanced resistance against preharvest aflatoxin contamination, *Mycopathologia*, 155, 97, 2002.

50. Zorner, P.S., Antimicrobial peptide technology to prevent fungal and bacterial diseases of crops, *Mycopathologia*, 155, 99, 2002.

51. Woloshuk, C.P., Huh, G.H., and Fakhoury, A., Progress toward determining if alpha-amylase inhibitors can reduce aflatoxin contamination in maize, *Mycopathologia*, 155, 102, 2002.

52. Hasegawa, P.M., Bressan, R.A., Zhu, J.K., and Bohnert, H.J., Plant cuticular and molecular responses to high salinity, *Annu. Rev. Plant Physiol. Plant Mol. Biol.*, 51, 463–499, 2000.

53. Yamaguchi-Shinozaki, K., Koizumi, M., Urao, S., and Shinozaki, K., Molecular cloning and characterization of 9 cDNAs for genes that are responsive to desiccation to *Arabidopsis thaliana*: sequence analysis of one cDNA clone that encodes a putative transmembrane channel protein, *Plant Cell Physiol.*, 33, 217–224, 1992.

54. Hajela, R.K., Horvath, D.P., Gilmour, S.J., and Thomashow, M.F., Molecular cloning and expression of COR (cold-regulated) genes in *Arabidopsis thaliana*, *Plant Physiol.*, 93, 1246–1252, 1990.

55. Maarouf, E.I.H., Zuily-Fodil, Y., Gareil, M., d'Arcy-Lameta, and Pham-Thi, A.T., Enzymatic activity and gene expression under water stress of phopholipase D in two cultivars of *Vigna unguiculata* L. Walp. differing in drought tolerance, *Plant Mol. Biol.*, 39, 1257–1265, 1999.

56. Sang, Y., Zheng, S., Li. W., Huang, B., and Wang, X., Regulation of plant water loss by manipulating the expression of phospholipase Dalpha, *Plant J.*, 28, 135–144, 2001.

57. Guo, B.Z., Cao, Y., Xu, G., Holbrook, C.C., and Lynch, R.E., Characterization of phospholipase D (PLD) in peanut and *PLD* expression associated with drought stress, in *Proc. 34th American Peanut Research and Education Society Conf.*, Research Triangle, NC, July 16–19, 2002.

58. Xu, G., Guo, B.Z., Holbrook, C.C., and Lynch, R.E., Identification and partial sequence of a *PLD*-like gene encoding for phospholipase D in peanut, *J. Peanut Sci.*, 30, 1–10, 2001.

59. Liang, P. and Pardee, A.B., Differential display of eucaryotic messenger RNA by means of the polymerase chain reaction, *Science*, 257, 967–971, 1992.

60. Cao, Y.G., Guo, B.Z., Lee, R.D., and Lynch, R.E., Identification of putative genes relating to drought stress in maize by differential display of mRNA, *Mycopathologia*, 155, 90, 2002.

61. Xu, G., Guo, B.Z., and Lynch, R.E., Identification of the drought-inducible genes in peanut by mRNA differential display, *Mycopathologia*, 155, 92, 2002.

62. Ewing, R.M., Kahla, A.B., Poirot, O., Lopez, F., Audic, S., and Claverie, J.M., Large-scale statistical analyses of rice ESTs reveal correlated patterns of gene expression, *Genome Res.*, 9, 950–959, 1999.

63. Mekhedov, S., Martínez de Ilárduya, O., and Ohlrogge, J., Toward a functional catalog of the plant genome: a survey of genes for lipid biosynthesis, *Plant Physiol.*, 122, 389–401, 2000.

64. Adams, M.D., Kelley, J.M., Gocayne, J.D., Dubnick, M., Polymeropoulos, M.H., Xiao, H., Merril, C.R., Wu, A., Olds, B., Moreno, R.F., Kerlavage, A.R., McCombie, W.R., and Venter, J.C., Complementary DNA sequencing: expressed sequence tags and human genome project, *Science*, 252, 1651–1656, 1991.

65. Sargent, T.D., Isolation of differentially expressed genes, *Methods Enzymol.*, 152, 423–432, 1987.

66. Hubank, M. and Schatz, D.G., Identifying differences in mRNA expression by representational difference analysis of cDNA, *Nucl. Acids. Res.*, 25, 5640–5648, 1994.

67. Diatchenko, L., Lau, Y.F., Campbell, A.P., Chenchik, A., Moqadam, F., Huang, B., Lukyanov, S., Lukyanov, K., Gurskaya, N., Sverdlov, E.D., and Siebert, P.D., Suppression subtractive hybridization: a method for generating differentially regulated or tissue-specific cDNA probes and libraries, *Proc. Natl. Acad. Sci. USA*, 12, 6025–6030, 1996.

68. Aharoni, A. and Vorst, O., DNA microarrays for functional plant genomics, *Plant Mol. Biol.*, 48, 99–118, 2002.

69. Cleveland, T.E. and Bhatnagar, D., Molecular regulation of aflatoxin biosynthesis, in *Mycotoxins, Cancer and Health*, Vol. 1, Bray, G.A. and Ryan, D.H., Eds, Pennington Center Nutrition Series, Pennington Biomedical Research Center, Baton Route, LA, 1991, pp. 270–287.

70. Cleveland, T.E., Cary, J.W., Brown, R.L., Bhatnagar, D., Yu, J., Chang, P.K., Chlan, C.A., and Rajasekaran, K., Use of biotechnology to eliminate aflatoxin in preharvest crops, *Bull. Inst. Compr. Agric. Sci. Kinki Univ.*, 5, 75–90, 1997.

71. Chang, P.-K., Cary, J.W., Bhatnagar, D., Cleveland, T.E., Bennett, J.W., Linz, J.E., Woloshuk, C.P., and Payne, G.A., Cloning of the *Aspergillus parasiticus apa-2* gene associated with the regulation of aflatoxin biosynthesis, *Appl. Environ. Microbiol.*, 59, 3273–3279, 1993.

72. Chang, P.-K., Ehrlich, K.C., Yu, J., Bhatnagar, D., and Cleveland, T.E., Increased expression of *Aspergillus parasiticus aflR*, encoding a sequence-specific DNA binding protein, relieves nitrate inhibition of aflatoxin biosynthesis, *Appl. Environ. Microbiol.*, 61, 2372–2377, 1995.

73. Payne, G.A. and Brown, M.P., Genetics and physiology of aflatoxin biosynthesis, *Annu. Rev. Phytopathol.*, 36, 329–362, 1998.

74. Yu, J., Chang, P.-K., Cary, J.W., Wright, M., Bhatnagar, D., Cleveland, T.E., Payne, G.A., and Linz, J.E., Comparative mapping of aflatoxin pathway gene clusters in *Aspergillus parasiticus* and *Aspergillus flavus*, *Appl. Environ. Microbiol.*, 61, 2365–2371, 1995.

75. Yu, J., Bhatnagar, D., Cleveland, T.E., and Nierman, W.C., *Aspergillus flavus* EST technology and its applications for eliminating aflatoxin contamination, *Mycopathologia*, 155, 6, 2002.

76. Yu, J., Proctor, R.H., Brown, D.W., Abe, K., Gomi, K., Machida, M., Hasegawa, F., Nierman, W.C., Bhatnagar, D., and Cleveland, T.E., Genomics of economically significant *Aspergillus* and *Fusarium* species, *Appl. Mycol. Biotechnol.*, 4, 1–35, 2004.

77. Luo, M., Guo, B.Z., Dang, P., Lee, R.D., Holbrook, C.C., Niedz, R.P., and Lynch, R.E., Gene expression profiling in kernel developing stages as influenced by drought stress in corn and peanut, in *Proc. Second Fungal Genomics, Third Fumonisin Elimination, and 15th Aflatoxin Elimination Workshop*, San Antonio, TX, October 23–25, 2002.

78. Luo, M., Dang, P., Guo, B.Z., He, G., Holbrook, C.C., Bausher, M.G., and Lee, R.D., Generation of expressed sequence tags (ESTs) for gene discovery and marker development in cultivated peanut, *Crop Sci.*, 45, 346–353, 2005.

79. He, G., Meng, R., Gao, H., Guo, B., Gao, G., Newman, M., Pittman, R., and Prakash, C.S., Simple sequence repeat markers for botanical varieties of cultivated peanut (*Arachis hypogaea* L.), *Euphytica*, 142, 131–136, 2005.

80. Wilkins, M.R., Sanchez, J.C., Gooley, A.A., Appel, R.D., Humphery-Smith, I., Hochstrasser, D.F., and Williams, K.L., Progress with proteome projects: why all proteins expressed by a genome should be identified and how to do it, *Biotech. Genet. Eng. Rev.*, 13, 19–50, 1996.

81. Chen, Z.-Y., Brown, R.L., Lax, A.R., Guo, B.Z., Cleveland, T.E., and Russin, J.S., Resistance to *Aspergillus flavus* in corn kernels is associated with a 14-kDa protein, *Phytopathology*, 88, 276–281, 1998.

82. Santoni, V., Bellini, C., and Caboche, M., Use of two-dimensional protein-pattern analysis for the characterization of *Arabidopsis thaliana* mutants, *Planta*, 192, 557–566, 1994.

83. Riccardi, F., Gazeau, P., Vienne, D.de., and Zivy, M., Protein changes in response to progressive water deficit in maize: quantitative variation and polypeptide identification, *Plant Physiol.*, 117, 1253–1263, 1998.

84. Gavin, A.C., Bosche, M., Krause, R., Grandi, P., Marzioch, M., Bauer, A., Schultz, J., Rick, J.M., Michon, A.M., and Cruciat, C.M., Functional organization of the yeast proteome by systematic analysis of protein complexes, *Nature*, 415, 141–147, 2002.

85. Chen, Z.Y., Brown, R.L., Russin, J.S., Lax, A.R., and Cleveland, T.E., A corn trypsin inhibitor with antifungal activity inhibits *Aspergillus flavus* alpha-amylase, *Phytopathology*, 89, 902–907, 1999.

86. Chen, Z.Y., Brown, R.L., Lax, A.R., Cleveland, T.E., and Russin, J.S., Inhibition of plant-pathogenic fungi by a corn trypsin inhibitor, *Appl. Environ. Microbiol.*, 65, 1320–1324, 1999.

87. Chen, Z., Brown, R.L., Cleveland, T.E., and Damann, K.E., The use of proteomics to elucidate factors regulating the corn–*Aspergillus flavus* interaction, *Mycopathologia*, 155, 14, 2002.

88. Fraley, R.T., Rogers, S.G., Horsch, R.B., Sanders, P.R., and Flick, J.S., Expression of bacterial genes in plant cells *Agrobacterium tumefaciens*, *Proc. Natl. Acad. Sci. USA*, 80, 4803–4807, 1983.

89. Elzen, P.van den, Lee, K.Y., Townsend, J., and Bedbrook, J., Simple binary vector for DNA transfer to plant cells, *Plant Mol. Biol.*, 5, 149–154, 1985.

90. Hayford, M.B., Medford, J.I., Hoffman, N.L., Rogers, S.G., and Klee, H.J., Development of a plant transformation selection system based on expression of genes encoding gentamicin acetyltransferases, *Plant Physiol.*, 86, 1216–1222, 1988.

91. Svab, Z., Harper, E.C., Jones, D.G., and Maliga, P., Aminoglycoside-3′-adenyltransferase confers resistance to spectinomycin and streptomycin in *Nicotiana tabacum*, *Plant Mol. Biol.*, 14, 197–205, 1990.

92. Hille, J., Verheggen, F., Roelvink, P., Franssen, H., Kammen, A., and van, Zabel, P., Bleomycin resistance: a new dominant selectable marker for plant cell, *Plant Mol. Biol.*, 7, 171–176, 1986.

93. Stalker, D.M., McBride, K.E., and Malyj, L.D., Herbicide resistance in transgenic plants expressing a bacterial detoxification gene, *Science*, 242, 419–423, 1988.

94. Jefferson, R.A., The GUS reporter gene system, *Nature*, 342, 837–838, 1989.

95. Koncz, C., Olsson, O., Langridge, W.H.R., Schell, J., and Szalay, A.A., Expression and assembly, of functional bacterial luciferase in plants, *Proc. Natl. Acad. Sci. USA*, 84, 131–135, 1987.

96. Sheen, J., Hwang, S., Niwa, Y., Kobayashi, H., and Galbraith, D.M., Green-fluorescent protein as a new vital marker in plant cells, *Plant J.*, 8, 777–784, 1995.

97. Murai, N., Sutton, D.W., Murray, M.G., Slighton, J.L., and Merlo, D.J., Phaseolin gene from bean is expressed after transfer to sunflower via tumor-inducing plasmid vectors genetic engineering, Ti plasmid, *Agrobacterium tumifaciens*, *Science*, 222, 476–482, 1983.

98. Timko, M.P., Kausch, A.P., Castresana, C., Fassler, J., Herrera-Estrella, L., Broeck, G., van den, Montagu, M., van, Schell, J., and Cashmore, A.R., Light regulation of plant gene expression by an upstream enhancer-like element, *Nature*, 318, 579–582, 1985.

99. Odell, J.T., Knowlton, S., Lin, W., and Mauvais, C.J., Properties of an isolated transcription stimulating sequence derived from the cauliflower mosaic virus 35S promoter, *Plant Mol. Biol.*, 10, 263–272, 1988.

100. McElroy, D., Zhang, W., Cao, J., and Wu, R., Isolation of an efficient actin promoter for use in rice transformation, *Plant Cell*, 2, 163–171, 1990.
101. Christensen, A.H. and Quail, P.H., Sequence analysis and transcriptional regulation by heat shock of polyubiquitin transcripts from maize, *Plant Mol. Biol.*, 12, 619–632, 1989.
102. Christensen, A.H., Sharrock, R.A., and Quail, P.H., Maize polyubiquitin genes: structure, thermal perturbation of expression and transcript splicing, and promoter activity following transfer to protoplasts by electroporation, *Plant Mol. Biol.*, 18, 675–689, 1992.
103. Horsch, R., Fraley, R., Rogers, S., Fry, J., Klee, H., Shah, D., McCormick, S., Niedermeyer, J., and Hoffmann, N., *Agrobacterium*-mediated transformation of plants, *Plant Biol.*, 3, 317–329, 1986.
104. Kado, C.I., Molecular mechanisms of crown gall tumorigenesis, *CRC Crit. Rev. Plant Sci.*, 10, 1–32, 1991.
105. Klein, T.M., Wolf, E.D., Wu, R., and Sanford, J.C., High-velocity microprojectiles for delivering nucleic acids into living cells, *Nature*, 327, 70–73, 1987.
106. Ye, G.N., Daniell, H., and Sanford, J.C., Optimization of delivery of foreign DNA into higher-plant chloroplast, *Plant Mol. Biol.*, 15, 809–819, 1990.
107. Ozias-Akins, P. and Gill, R., Progress in the development of tissue culture and transformation methods applicable to the production of transgenic peanut, *Peanut Sci.*, 28, 123–131, 2001.
108. Kantety, R.V., La Rota, M., Matthews, D.E., and Sorrells, M.E., Data mining for simple sequence repeats in expressed sequence tags from barley, maize, rice, sorghum and wheat, *Plant. Mol. Biol.*, 48, 501–510, 2002.
109. Fernandes, J., Brendel, V., Gai, X., Lal, S., Chandler, V.L., Elumalai, R.P., Galbraith, D.W., Pierson, E.A., and Walbot, V., Comparison of RNA expression profiles based on maize expressed sequence tag frequency analysis and micro-array hybridization, *Plant Physiol.*, 128, 896–910, 2002.
110. Woo, Y.M., Hu, D.W., Larkins, B.A., and Jung, R., Genomics analysis of genes expressed in maize endosperm identifies novel seed proteins and clarifies patterns of zein gene expression, *Plant Cell*, 13, 2297–2317, 2001.
111. Estruch, J.J., Carozzi ,N.B., Desai, N., Duck, N.B., Warren, G.W., and Koziel, M.G., Transgenic plants: an emerging approach to pest control, *Nat. Biotechnol.*, 15, 137–141, 1997.
112. Dowd, P.F., Biotic and abiotic factors limiting efficacy of Bt corn in indirectly reducing mycotoxin levels in commercial fields, *J. Econ. Entomol.*, 94, 1067–1074, 2001.

16 Biological Control of Aflatoxin Crop Contamination

Joe W. Dorner

CONTENTS

16.1 INTRODUCTION

Aflatoxin contamination of crops is a worldwide problem that compromises the safety of food and feed and is devastating to the agricultural economies of specific commodity industries and regions where it occurs. Aflatoxin refers to a group of four mycotoxins (B_1, B_2, G_1, and G_2) produced in crops primarily by the closely related fungi, *Aspergillus flavus* and *A. parasiticus*.[1] Aflatoxins are potent hepatotoxins and carcinogens,[2,3] and their quantity in food and feed is closely monitored and regulated in most countries.[4] For example, the U.S. Food and Drug Administration (FDA) action level for total aflatoxins in food is 20 ppb (ng/g), while the European Union has a maximum level of 2 ppb for B_1 and 4 ppb for total aflatoxins.[5,6] Strains of *A. flavus* vary greatly in their ability to produce aflatoxins; for example, toxigenic strains typically produce only B_1 and B_2, but most strains of *A. parasiticus* typically produce all four toxins.[1] In addition to aflatoxins, many strains of *A. flavus* produce the mycotoxin cyclopiazonic acid, which is also a natural contaminant of a variety of crops .[7,8] Many strategies, including biological control, are being investigated to manage, reduce, and ultimately eliminate aflatoxin contamination of crops.[9] Different organisms have been investigated as potential biocontrol agents, including bacteria, yeasts, and fungi. The purpose of this article is to review progress to date in developing technology for biological control of aflatoxin contamination in a variety of crops.

16.2 BACTERIA AND YEASTS

Kimura and Hirano[10] isolated a strain of *Bacillus subtilis* (NK-330) that inhibited growth and aflatoxin production by *Aspergillus flavus* and *A. parasiticus* in the laboratory. Autoclaved peanuts and corn were coinoculated with fungal conidia and bacterial cells, and aflatoxin production by the toxigenic fungi was almost completely inhibited. *B. subtilis* prevented aflatoxin contamination in corn in field tests when ears were inoculated with the bacterium 48 hours before inoculation with *A. flavus*;[11] however, no reduction in aflatoxin occurred when bacteria were inoculated 48 hours after inoculation with *A. flavus*. *Bacillus subtilis* (NK-330) did not inhibit aflatoxin contamination of farmers' stock peanuts when it was applied to pods prior to warehouse storage for 56 days.[12] Because the proliferation of *A. flavus* that occurs in peanut kernels during storage is predominately a result of infection that occurred in the field,[13] the bacteria were unable to prevent proliferation by *A. flavus* that had already infected kernels. This same strain of *B. subtilis* (NK-330) was tested in peanut plots for control of preharvest aflatoxin contamination (unpublished data). An aqueous suspension of bacterial cells was applied to soil at the time peanuts were planted and also was sprayed over plants mid-season before peanuts were subjected to late season drought stress. No reduction in aflatoxin contamination of peanuts resulted from these treatments. The tests demonstrated that, even though *B. subtilis* NK-330 can be highly inhibitory to aflatoxin production under laboratory conditions, it was very difficult to place the bacterial cells at the necessary site, which is the point of kernel infection by *A. flavus*, under field conditions. Studies were discontinued because the bacterium could not be delivered in such a way that it could prevent or inhibit *A. flavus* infection and growth in peanut kernels in the field.

Several bacterial species were evaluated in greenhouse and field experiments for biological control of *Aspergillus flavus* infection and aflatoxin contamination of peanuts.[14] Peanut seeds were treated with the bacteria prior to planting, and bacterial suspensions were applied as a soil drench (greenhouse) or sprayed over the row (field) at the mid-peg stage (80 to 90 days after planting). Only one bacterial strain (*Xanthomonas maltophila*) produced a significant reduction ($p = 0.05$) in *A. flavus* infection of pods at harvest in both the greenhouse and field studies. One strain of *Pseudomonas putida* reduced the incidence of *A. flavus* on harvested seed. Lack of late-season drought resulted in very low levels of aflatoxin contamination with no significant differences among treatments. Further development of biological control of aflatoxin in peanuts using bacteria has not been reported.

Six of 892 bacterial isolates indigenous to cotton inhibited *Aspergillus flavus* growth in an *in vitro* assay using inoculated cottonseed.[15] One of those isolates, *Pseudomonas cepacia* (D1), significantly reduced *A. flavus* damage to cotton locules by 41 to 100% when the bacterium was inoculated simultaneously with *A. flavus* in field studies. Further work showed a reduction in the level of *A. flavus*-infected cottonseed when plants were spray-inoculated with a suspension of D1;[16] however, no reports have shown that treatment with D1 or other bacteria under field conditions produced significant reductions in aflatoxin contamination of cottonseed.

Saprophytic yeasts isolated from fruits of almond, pistachio, and walnut trees inhibited aflatoxin production by *Aspergillus flavus in vitro*.[17] A strain of *Candida krusei* and a strain of *Pichia anomala* reduced aflatoxin production by 96 and 99%, respectively, in a Petri dish assay. Efforts are underway to apply these yeasts to almond and pistachio orchards to determine their potential for aflatoxin reduction under crop production conditions.[18]

16.3 COMPETITIVE FUNGI

The greatest success to date regarding biological control of aflatoxin contamination in the field has been achieved through competitive exclusion by applying non-aflatoxigenic strains of *Aspergillus flavus* and *A. parasiticus* to the soil of developing crops. These strains are typically referred to as atoxigenic or nontoxigenic, but those designations are often used with reference to production of aflatoxins only. Strains of *Aspergillus* species used for biological control may or may not produce other toxins or toxic biosynthetic precursors to aflatoxin. The applied strains occupy the same niche as the naturally occurring toxigenic strains and compete for crop substrates. Preharvest aflatoxin contamination of most crops is associated with drought or high temperature stresses or insect damage that occur during the crop maturation period.[19–21] For competitive exclusion to be effective, the competing strains must be present at highly competitive levels when conditions make the crop susceptible to infection. In theory, the strain that has been applied to the soil then displaces naturally present wild-type strains when infections of the crop occur. Two primary factors, therefore, determine the effectiveness of this strategy. First, the applied strains must be truly competitive and dominant relative to the toxigenic strains that are already present. Second, the formulation used to apply the competing strains must be effective in delivering the necessary quantity of conidia to achieve a competitive advantage. In addition, the timing of that application is crucial for ensuring that the necessary competitive level is present when the threat of crop infection is greatest.

Fungi used for competitive exclusion should be both nontoxigenic and competitive. Species of *Aspergillus* are capable of producing not only aflatoxins but also a variety of other toxins and toxic precursors to aflatoxin, including cyclopiazonic acid, sterigmatocystin and related compounds, and the versicolorins.[22] If a strain that is applied to soil predominantly infects a crop, the metabolites produced by that strain will likely contaminate that crop. While reducing aflatoxin contamination is a primary goal of this strategy, it should not be accomplished with the replacement of aflatoxin with another toxin even though that toxin may be perceived to be less harmful than aflatoxin.

Cotty[23] investigated the ability of seven non-aflatoxigenic strains of *Aspergillus flavus* to reduce aflatoxin contamination of cottonseed when they were coinoculated with toxigenic strains in greenhouse experiments. Six of the non-aflatoxigenic strains significantly reduced the amount of aflatoxin produced in cottonseed by the toxigenic strain. Strain 36 (AF36) produced the largest reduction in aflatoxin under these conditions, and it was subsequently shown to reduce aflatoxin contamination of cottonseed in the field when applied on colonized wheat seed.[24] This strain has become the basis of an aflatoxin control program for cottonseed in Arizona that has been extensively tested under an Environmental Protection Agency (EPA) experimental use permit.[25]

Brown et al.[26] conducted inoculation experiments with corn in field plots. When ears were either coinoculated with AF36 and a toxigenic strain of *Aspergillus flavus* or inoculated with AF36 24 hours prior to inoculation with the toxigenic strain, subsequent aflatoxin concentrations were significantly reduced compared to inoculation with the toxigenic strain alone.

Dorner et al.[27] showed that application of different non-aflatoxigenic strains of *Aspergillus parasiticus* to soil reduced preharvest aflatoxin contamination when peanuts were exposed to late-season drought and temperature stress; however, one of those strains (NRRL 18991), which was originally isolated from soil, was subsequently shown to produce *O*-methylsterigmatocystin (OMST), the immediate biosynthetic precursor to aflatoxin B_1.[28] Analysis of peanuts from soil treated with that strain showed that not only was aflatoxin reduced but also the concentrations of OMST in peanuts were increased.[27] An ultraviolet-induced mutant of that strain (NRRL 18786) was also tested and shown to reduce aflatoxin contamination,[27] but it was subsequently found to produce versicolorin A. Although these strains proved to be competitive in the infection of peanuts and produced reductions in aflatoxin, they were not deemed appropriate biocontrol agents because of the metabolites they produced.

Several naturally occurring, nontoxigenic strains of *Aspergillus flavus* were tested as potential biocontrol agents in greenhouse experiments with peanuts by coinoculating the root zone with a toxigenic strain.[29] Six of the nontoxigenic strains produced significant reductions in aflatoxin contamination of kernels when compared with inoculation with the toxigenic strain alone. One strain (AU 32) prevented aflatoxin contamination of peanuts when root regions were inoculated 1 day before inoculation with the toxigenic strain.

Other strains of *Aspergillus flavus* and *A. parasiticus* have been shown to be effective in reducing aflatoxin contamination of crops. *A. flavus* NRRL 21882, a naturally occurring strain isolated from a peanut in Georgia in 1991, has been used in several studies that have demonstrated its efficacy for reducing contamination in the field. This strain is the active ingredient in an EPA-registered biopesticide called Afla-Guard®. A color mutant of this strain, NRRL 21368, was used in several early studies and also found to be effective when used in conjunction with a color mutant of *A. parasiticus* (NRRL 21369).[30,31]

Other species that have shown promise include *Aspergillus oryzae* and *A. sojae*, domesticated strains of *A. flavus* and *A. parasiticus*, respectively, which are commonly referred to as koji molds. They are used in the food industry in fermentations that lead to the production of soy sauce and other products. Only limited testing was done with these species, and they did not appear to be as competitive as *A. flavus* and *A. parasiticus*.[32] A one-year study was conducted at the National Peanut Research Laboratory in which *A. niger* was applied to peanut soils; however, results clearly showed no reduction in aflatoxin as a result of the *A. niger* application (unpublished data).

16.4 FORMULATIONS

The formulation is the combination of competitive strain and carrier/substrate used to establish the competitive strain in the field. In this type of biological control (biocompetitive exclusion), the goal is to have a dominant population of the competitive strain established at the time the crop is susceptible to infection by *Aspergillus flavus*. Although this method of biological control is different from the more classical form in which the applied organism causes disease or death of the target pest, any formulation used to apply a nontoxigenic strain of *A. flavus* to soil is considered to be a biopesticide by the EPA. As such, the formulation must be registered before it can be used commercially. Many of the various methods used to formulate microbial pesticides for control of plant diseases and weed and insect pests have recently been reviewed.[33,34] This chapter focuses only on formulations used for the application of nontoxigenic strains of *Aspergillus* species to reduce aflatoxin contamination.

In initial studies with peanuts, suspensions of homogenized cultures of *Aspergillus parasiticus* (primarily conidia) were applied to emerged plants or directly to the soil surface prior to planting.[27] Whereas this direct application of conidia resulted in significant reductions in aflatoxin contamination, it was not deemed cost effective for large-scale field applications. Cotty applied *A. flavus* to cotton plots by spraying a conidial suspension over plants prior to first bloom and by applying wheat seeds that were colonized with the fungus.[24] The spray treatment did not reduce aflatoxin in cottonseed compared with controls, but the wheat seed application produced significant reductions in 2 consecutive years. The technique of using solid-state fermentation to colonize a small grain, such as wheat[24,35] and rice,[30,31] has been used in several studies to produce the biocontrol formulation. In this process, the grain is sterilized, inoculated with a conidial suspension of the competitive strain, and cultured with agitation to prevent or limit fungal sporulation. After the desired culture period, the colonized grain is dried at temperatures not exceeding 60°C so as not to kill the fungus. The goal is to colonize the grain with the fungus to the extent that when it is applied to the field the competitive strain will resume growth and produce an abundance of conidia on the surface of the grain. Those conidia are then disseminated in the soil, where they can compete with naturally occurring aflatoxigenic strains already present; thus, the grain serves both as a carrier for delivery of the competitive strain to the field and as a substrate for growth and sporulation after application. This method is more cost effective than producing the massive amounts of conidia in the laboratory that would be required to achieve the same population density of the competitive fungus in the field. Bock and Cotty[35] investigated this methodology for producing colonized wheat seed and suggested that the most cost-effective use of the technique would require an inoculation of 10^6 conidia per kg of seed at 25% moisture and an incubation period of 18 hours at 31°C.

Other formulations have been produced in which conidia or mycelia of the desired strain are encapsulated in a matrix of suitable substrate. Daigle and Cotty[36] encapsulated mycelia of *A. flavus* in pellets composed of sodium alginate, corn cob grits, and wheat gluten. Spore yield in the laboratory on a per gram basis was greater with the pellets (4.0×10^9/g) than with the colonized wheat seed (1.0×10^9/g) after

7 days of incubation, but Bock and Cotty[35] concluded that the additional spore yield was not advantageous enough to justify the additional cost of the alginate formulation. Estimated costs of the raw materials to produce the alginate formulation ranged from \$2.53 to \$5.76 per kg, whereas the cost of wheat was \$0.18 to 0.26 per kg.

A process for making pasta has been applied to the production of a mycoherbicide formulation in which fungal propagules are incorporated in a wheat gluten matrix. Dough prepared from wheat flour, filler, fungus, and water is rolled into thin sheets, air dried, and ground into granules called "Pesta."[37] Large quantities of Pesta can be produced by twin-screw extrusion in which the shape and size of the granules is determined by the diameter or shape of the holes in the die of the extruder.[38] The extrusion process was used successfully to produce Pesta containing a variety of biocontrol fungi, including nontoxigenic strains of *Aspergillus flavus* and *A. parasiticus*. Pesta was prepared by incorporating pure conidia of the fungi[38] or by first culturing the fungi on rice flour and incorporating the fungus-infested flour.[39] After extrusion, Pesta granules were dried in a fluid bed dryer at 50°C for 1.0 to 1.5 hours. Drying resulted in about a 14% loss in *A. flavus* propagules but no loss in propagules of *A. parasiticus*.[38]

Dorner et al.[40] conducted an evaluation of three formulations of nontoxigenic color mutant strains of *Aspergillus flavus* and *A. parasiticus* for control of preharvest aflatoxin contamination of peanuts. Formulations included solid-state fermented rice, Pesta, and corn-flour-based granules. Formulations were applied to peanut test plots for 2 years, and peanuts were exposed to late-season drought conditions conducive for aflatoxin contamination. All formulations were effective in delivering competitive levels of the nontoxigenic strains to soil, with the solid-state fermented rice producing the highest population of those fungi in soil. Aflatoxin contamination in total kernels appeared to be reduced by all formulations in the first year, but differences were not statistically significant (Table 16.1). In the second year of the study, all formulations produced statistically significant reductions in aflatoxin compared with controls, but no significant differences were observed among the three formulation treatments. The average reduction in aflatoxin in total kernels was 92% compared with peanuts from untreated control plots.[40]

Although these various formulation techniques have proven to be effective for delivering biocontrol agents to the field, many will have little or no practical use because of the costs associated with their production. The cost of raw materials may be considered too high, such as with alginate pellets.[35] Steps in processing also may introduce excessive costs, such as the relatively low-temperature drying associated with production of Pesta.[38] Even solid-state fermentation of the fungi on wheat or rice, which has low raw material costs, has limited production capacity because of batch processing that may take 2 to 3 days per batch. Solid-state fermentation also requires low-temperature drying that will not greatly reduce the number of viable fungal propagules in the formulation. When considering aflatoxin contamination from an economic standpoint, the costs associated with reducing contamination must be justified based upon the economic benefits to be gained from that reduction. The cost of aflatoxin contamination varies among commodities and even among segments of a commodity industry, such as the peanut industry.[41] Profit margins associated with production of specific crops are extremely tight, and additional costs to reduce

TABLE 16.1
Mean Aflatoxin Concentrations in Peanuts from Soil Treated with Different Formulations of Nontoxigenic Strains of A. flavus (NRRL 21368) and A. parasiticus (NRRL 21369) for 2 Consecutive Years

Formulation	1996[a] (ng/g)	1997[a] (ng/g)
Control	119.8 a	405.5 a
Rice	5.0 a	43.9 b
Pesta	30.6 a	20.4 b
Corn flour	13.8 a	29.9 b

[a] Means followed by a different letter are significantly different (Student–Newman–Keuls method, $p < 0.05$).

Source: Dorner, J.W. et al., *Biol. Control*, 26, 318–324, 2003. With permission.

aflatoxin may not be economically justifiable; therefore, a biological control formulation not only must be effective but must also be relatively inexpensive to produce and apply.

A simple, fast, and economical formulation technique was developed in which conidia of nontoxigenic *Aspergillus* species are coated and trapped onto the surface of a small grain, such as hulled barley.[42] This is accomplished by suspending conidia in vegetable oil, spraying the conidial suspension onto the hulled barley at 1.5% by weight, and then adding 2.5% by weight of diatomaceous earth. Conidia can be purchased inexpensively from companies in Japan that produce *Aspergillus* conidia for use in the koji fermentation industry. Because of the lipophilic nature of the conidia, they can be suspended easily in any of various vegetable oils. Common seed coating equipment can be used to apply an even coating of the conidial suspension to the hulled barley, which was found to be an ideal substrate for rapid growth and sporulation of *A. flavus* on its surface. The diatomaceous earth adheres to the oil-coated barley, absorbs the oil, and entraps the conidia so that they do not escape during handling. The coated formulation is free flowing and can be applied with common on-farm granular application equipment. Several advantages are associated with this formulation: It can be produced in a flow-through seed coater enabling a production capacity of several tons per hour. Raw ingredient costs are very low, with approximately 90% of the cost associated with the substrate (hulled barley) itself. Sterilization of the substrate is not necessary as with formulations produced by solid-state fermentation because, with the quantity (10^6 CFU/g) of conidia applied, rapid growth and sporulation by *A. flavus* results. Additionally, costs associated with drying the formulation are eliminated because water is not used in any phase of the process.

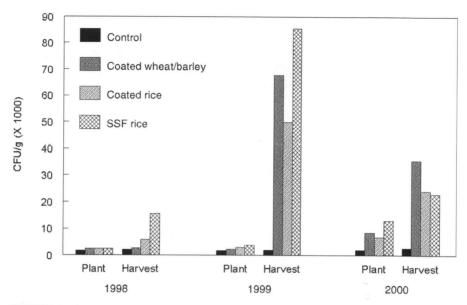

FIGURE 16.1 Population densities of all strains (wild-type and applied) of *Aspergillus flavus* and *A. parasiticus* in soils inoculated with different formulations of nontoxigenic strains. Soils were sampled immediately after planting and immediately prior to harvest from 1998 to 2000. The coated wheat formulation was applied only in 1998 and was replaced by coated barley in 1999/2000.

Coated formulations of nontoxigenic strains of *Aspergillus flavus* (NRRL 21882) and *A. parasiticus* (NRRL 21369) were compared with formulations produced by solid-state fermentation of rice in a 3-year field study.[43] In the first year (1998), substrates included spore-coated wheat, spore-coated rice, and solid-state fermented (SSF) rice. Spore-coated wheat was not as effective in establishing a competitive population of the nontoxigenic strains in soil as spore-coated rice and SSF rice, probably because the hull of the wheat prevented rapid fungal growth and sporulation (Figure 16.1). In 1999, the spore-coated wheat formulations were replaced by spore-coated hulled barley. Hulled barley had proven in the laboratory to be an excellent substrate for rapid growth by the applied fungi. At harvest in 1999, each of the three formulations had produced high soil populations of competitive strains, with the SSF rice formulation producing the highest population. By planting time of the third year, soil populations in the treated plots had declined significantly from the levels at the preceding harvest. Soil populations at harvest of the third year did not differ significantly among the three formulation treatments, which were all significantly higher than the control. Only in 1999 were field conditions conducive for preharvest aflatoxin contamination. Results (Table 16.2) showed that spore-coated formulations using hulled barley and rice were as effective as SSF rice in significantly reducing aflatoxin contamination by an average of 81.4%. Although significant aflatoxin contamination did not occur in year 3, peanuts were colonized by *A. flavus* and *A. parasiticus*. Even though soil populations of *A. flavus* and *A. parasiticus* were significantly higher in treated plots (Figure 16.1), the overall quantity of *A. flavus*

TABLE 16.2
Mean Aflatoxin Concentrations in 1999 Crop-Year Peanuts Grown in Soil Treated with Three Different Biocontrol Formulations

Formulation	Aflatoxin (ng/g)[a]	Percent Reduction (%)
Control	671.3 a	—
Solid-state fermented rice	90.1 b	86.6
Spore-coated rice	154.5 b	77.0
Spore-coated hulled barley	130.6 b	80.5

[a] Values are the means of 16 replications. Means followed by a different letter are significantly different ($p < 0.05$).

TABLE 16.3
Density of *Aspergillus flavus* and *A. parasiticus* and the Incidence of Toxigenic Strains in Peanuts Grown in Soil Treated with Three Different Biocontrol Formulations

Formulation	CFU/g[a]	Percent Toxigenic (%)
Control	8466 a	60.0 a
Solid-state fermented rice	4288 a	11.2 b
Spore-coated rice	6350 a	19.1 b
Spore-coated hulled barley	4680 a	15.4 b

[a] Values are the means of 16 replications. Means followed by a different letter are significantly different ($p < 0.05$).

and *A. parasiticus* in peanuts was no higher in treated peanuts than in controls (Table 16.3). However, the composition of *A. flavus* and *A. parasiticus* in peanuts from treated soils consisted of predominately nontoxigenic strains (Table 16.3). The coated hulled-barley formulation recently received EPA registration as a biopesticide for use on peanuts (http://www.epa.gov/oppbppd1/biopesticides/ingredients/tech_docs/brad_006500.pdf). A private company, Circle One Global, Inc., is marketing the product under the trade name Afla-Guard®.

16.5 FUNGAL DISPERSAL

A study conducted to monitor movement of conidia following application of non-toxigenic strain inoculum to peanut soil indicated that conidia remained near the soil surface.[44] Even after repeated rainfall events or application of water through irrigation, conidia were retained in the upper layers of the soil; however, dispersal of conidia was observed down peanut furrows where the land was sloped. Little movement perpendicular to peanut rows occurred. Retention of conidia near the soil surface is important for biological control in peanuts because peanuts are developing in the upper 5 cm of soil. It is also important for biological control in aerial crops such as corn and cotton so primary inoculum can be easily dispersed by wind and insects.[44] In applications of nontoxigenic *A. flavus* to cotton fields in Arizona, dispersal of conidia to fields that were not treated has been observed, with adjacent untreated fields sometimes showing large increases in the incidence of the applied strain.[45] It was noted that the incidence of applied strains in adjacent fields was variable, possibly indicating the importance of wind direction in dispersal.

16.6 CROPS

16.6.1 PEANUTS

Initial studies with this biocontrol strategy in peanuts began in 1987 using a naturally occurring strain of *A. parasiticus* (NRRL 18991).[27] Homogenized liquid cultures of the fungus were applied over the peanut row at 32 and 100 days after planting. Although these were the only applications of the fungus, peanuts from inoculated soil were analyzed for aflatoxin for 3 consecutive years. Reduced aflatoxin concentrations in peanuts from treated soil were found in each of the years compared with peanuts from untreated soil. Aflatoxin reductions in peanuts from soil treated only in 1987 were greatest in 1988, with aflatoxin in edible-category peanuts averaging 1 ppb compared with 96 ppb in edible peanuts from untreated soil. An ultraviolet-induced mutant of NRRL 18991 (NRRL 18786) was tested in 1989 using two different inoculum levels of homogenized fungal cultures. In this experiment, soil was inoculated 57 days before peanuts were planted. Aflatoxin was reduced by 88 and 93% in the low and high inoculum treatments, respectively, further demonstrating the potential for reduction of aflatoxin contamination of peanuts under field conditions.

Additional evidence for the efficacy of this strategy in reducing aflatoxin in peanuts was obtained in a 2-year study on the effect of inoculum rates.[30] Inoculum consisted of rice colonized by nontoxigenic color mutants of *Aspergillus flavus* (NRRL 21368) and *A. parasiticus* (NRRL 21369) applied at rates of 0, 20, 100, and 500 pounds per acre. Reductions in aflatoxin contamination ranged from 74.3% in 1995 for the low inoculum rate to 99.9% that same year with the high rate (Table 16.4). Regression analysis showed a significant ($p < 0.05$) trend toward decreasing aflatoxin concentrations in peanuts with increasing amounts of inoculum applied (year 1, $R^2 = 0.40$; year 2, $R^2 = 0.66$). The lowest inoculum rate of 20 pounds per acre produced reductions in aflatoxin contamination of 78.2 and 74.3% in years 1 and 2, respectively, while the 500-pound-per-acre rate resulted in a 99.9% reduction in year 2. Although the high rate is impractical from an economic standpoint, it demonstrates the degree of control of aflatoxin contamination that potentially can be achieved. It may be indicative of the kind of control that may be achieved if multiyear applications of practical amounts produce an ever-increasing displacement of toxigenic strains by nontoxigenic strains.

TABLE 16.4
Aflatoxin Concentrations in Peanuts from Soils Inoculated with
Varying Rates of Fungal-Colonized Rice in 1994 and 1995

	1994		1995	
Inoculum Rate (lb/ac)	Aflatoxin (ng/g)	Percent Reduction (%)	Aflatoxin (ng/g)	Percent Reduction (%)
Control	337.6	—	718.3	—
20	73.7	78.2	184.4	74.3
100	34.8	89.7	35.9	95.0
500	33.3	90.1	0.4	99.9

Source: Dorner, J.W. and Cole, R.J., *Biol. Control*, 12, 171–176, 1998. With permission.

An 8-year field study (1995 to 2002) in southwestern Georgia was conducted to measure the long-term effects of applying nontoxigenic strains of *Aspergillus flavus* and *A. parasiticus* to soil. Six distinct 0.25-acre plots were treated with various nontoxigenic strains using different formulations and application rates during those years (Table 16.5). Six equivalent untreated control plots were separated from treated plots by approximately 220 m to limit the influence nontoxigenic strains on control plots while still growing peanuts under the same environmental conditions. Peanuts

TABLE 16.5
Nontoxigenic Strains, Type of Formulation, and Application Rates Used in a Long-Term Field Study of Biological Control of Aflatoxin Contamination of Peanuts

Year	Nontoxigenic Strain(s)	Formulation	Rate (lbs/acre)[a]
1995	*A. flavus* (NRRL 21368) and *A. parasiticus* (NRRL 21369)	Colonized rye	275
1996	*A. flavus* (NRRL 21368) and *A. parasiticus* (NRRL 21369)	Pesta	200
1997	*A. flavus* (NRRL 21368) and *A. parasiticus* (NRRL 21369)	Colonized rice	25
1998	*A. flavus* (NRRL 21368) and *A. parasiticus* (NRRL 21369)	Colonized rice	20
1999	*A. flavus* (NRRL 21368) and *A. parasiticus* (NRRL 21369)	Colonized rice	20
2000[b]	None	None	None
2001[c]	None	None	None
2002	*A. flavus* (NRRL 21882)	Coated barley	20

[a] When two strains were applied, the rate was an equal mixture of separately produced formulations of each strain.

[b] Plots were planted to rye and no inoculation was done.

[c] Plots were neither planted nor inoculated, but a substantial stand of volunteer rye was present.

TABLE 16.6

Mean Aflatoxin Concentrations in Peanuts at Harvest from Plots Treated and Not Treated (Control) with Biocompetitive Fungi in Drought Years of 1997, 1999, and 2002

Treatment	1997[a]	1999[b]	2002[c] Harvest 1	Harvest 2
Control	603.5 ng/g	516.8 ng/g	39.7 ng/g	88.7 ng/g
Treated	50.8 ng/g	54.1 ng/g	0.7 ng/g	1.4 ng/g
Reduction	91.6%	89.5%	98.2%	98.4%

[a] Values are the means of eight determinations with an average sample size of 3 kg.

[b] Values are the means of six determinations with an average sample size of 9 kg.

[c] Samples were harvested two times at one week apart. Values are the means of six determinations with an average sample size of 33.6 kg.

were subjected to natural late-season drought stress only during 1997, 1999, and 2002; thus, preharvest aflatoxin contamination did not occur in the other years. Significant ($p < 0.05$) reductions in aflatoxin in peanuts from treated soil were seen in each of those 3 years (Table 16.6). From 1995 to 1999, soil was inoculated with color mutants of *A. flavus* and *A. parasiticus* (Table 16.5); however, in 2002 only the naturally occurring nontoxigenic strain of *A. flavus* (NRRL 21882) was applied. Prior studies had indicated that this strain was more competitive than the color mutant (NRRL 21368) derived from it.[31] Nevertheless, the color mutants produced significant reductions in aflatoxin in 1997 and 1999, and the long-term effect coupled with the application of NRRL 21882 in 2002 produced dramatic reductions (>98%) in peanuts from two separate harvests (Table 16.6). Analysis of peanuts from the 2002 test for the quantity and toxigenicity of *A. flavus* and *A. parasiticus* showed a significantly (P < 0.01) higher quantity of total *A. flavus* and *A. parasiticus* in control peanuts (166,000 CFU/g) than in treated peanuts (7300 CFU/g). The quantity of toxigenic strains of *A. flavus* and *A. parasiticus* was also much higher in control peanuts (165,000 CFU/g) than in treated peanuts (500 CFU/g). The incidence of toxigenic strains of *A. flavus* and *A. parasiticus* in control peanuts was >99% compared with an incidence of only 7% in treated peanuts. It may be surprising that peanuts from untreated soil contained significantly more *A. flavus* and *A. parasiticus* than did peanuts from soil to which nontoxigenic strains were applied. Evidently, the nontoxigenic strains (predominately *A. flavus* NRRL 21882) were very effective in displacing toxigenic strains but possibly were not as aggressive in colonizing the peanut substrate. Soil populations of toxigenic and nontoxigenic strains of *A. flavus* and *A. parasiticus* were measured in the spring and fall of each year beginning in 1996 (a year after initial inoculations) and are shown in Figure 16.2. Total populations of *A. flavus* and *A. parasiticus* fluctuated considerably over time, but in treated plots the population was consistently dominated by nontoxigenic strains, whereas in control plots the population was predominately toxigenic at all times. Inoculation

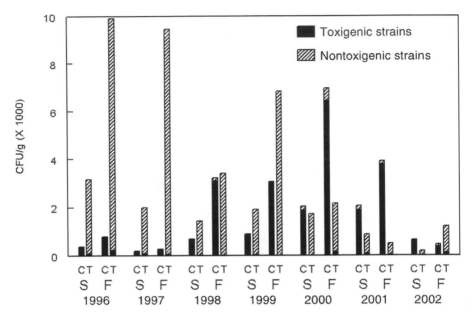

FIGURE 16.2 Population densities of toxigenic and nontoxigenic strains of *Aspergillus flavus* and *A. parasiticus* in soil of control (C) and treated (T) plots sampled in the spring (S) and fall (F) over the course of 7 years. See Table 16.5 for details concerning specific strains, formulations, and rates applied in each year.

rates for the first 2 years (1995 and 1996) were quite high (Table 16.5), but after 1997 the total population in treated plots was often no higher and sometimes less than that in control plots. In the final year, when the percent aflatoxin reduction was greatest in treated peanuts, the total population in treated plots was less than 2000 CFU/g at harvest. This demonstrates that long-term inoculations of approximately 20 lb/ac can produce good control of aflatoxin contamination without greatly altering the total population of *A. flavus* and *A. parasiticus* in soil.

Not only does application of nontoxigenic strains of *Aspergillus* to soil reduce levels of preharvest aflatoxin contamination in peanuts, but it also has a carryover effect, reducing contamination that may occur during long-term bulk storage.[13] Treated and control peanuts from the 1998 and 1999 field studies described above were stored separately in a miniature warehouse and subjected to storage conditions that would be conducive to aflatoxin contamination. Peanuts entering the warehouse in 1998 were not contaminated, but peanuts in 1999 were contaminated in the field (Table 16.7). In 1998, peanuts from soil not treated with nontoxigenic strains (control) experienced a large increase in aflatoxin during storage (from 0.0 to 78.0 ppb) while peanuts from treated soil contained only 1.4 ppb after storage, a 98% reduction in contamination. Peanuts from both treated and nontreated soil were contaminated at harvest in 1999, although peanuts from treated soil contained 89.5% less aflatoxin than control peanuts. Although aflatoxin increased in both groups during storage, peanuts from treated soil contained 96.7% less aflatoxin than control peanuts after storage. Aflatoxin increased during storage by 22-fold in control peanuts compared

TABLE 16.7

Mean Aflatoxin Concentrations in Peanuts Prior to and After Storage in 1998 and 1999

Treatment	1998		1999	
	Prior to Storage (ng/g)	After Storage (ng/g)	Prior to Storage (ng/g)	After Storage (ng/g)
Control	0.0	78.0	516.8	11,579.3
Treated	0.0	1.4	54.1	380.0

Source: Dorner, J.W. and Cole, R.J., *J. Stored Prod. Res.*, 38, 329-339, 2002. With permission.

with a 7-fold increase in treated peanuts. Half of the peanuts from control and treated plots were sprayed with a conidial suspension of the nontoxigenic strains (NRRL 21368 and 21369) prior to storage, but that treatment had only a slight effect in reducing storage contamination. The greatest effect in reducing storage contamination was seen in peanuts from soil that had been treated. Data from this study strongly indicate that the proliferation of fungi that occurs in peanuts during storage is a result of infection that occurred in the field. Because aflatoxin contamination of peanuts that occurs during storage is still a major problem for the peanut industry, treatment of soil with appropriate nontoxigenic strains of *A. flavus* and *A. parasiticus* offers a legitimate added benefit.

16.6.2 COTTON

In initial experiments involving biological control of aflatoxin contamination of cottonseed, cotton bolls were coinoculated with a toxigenic strain of *Aspergillus flavus* and various atoxigenic strains.[23] Significant reductions in aflatoxin contamination were noted with six of the atoxigenic strains, and one strain (AF36) was chosen for further experiments. In coinoculation experiments between AF36 and a toxigenic strain (AF13), AF36 reduced aflatoxin contamination in cottonseed by 82 to 100%.[46] It was suggested that the reduction was partly due to the ability of AF36 to competitively exclude the toxigenic strain during the infection process and also to competition between the strains for available nutrients. Even when bolls were coinoculated with only half as many conidia of AF36 as with the toxigenic strain, an equivalent reduction in aflatoxin contamination occurred compared with coinoculation of equal amounts.

A 2-year field study was conducted to determine the effectiveness of field applications of AF36 in excluding toxigenic strains during cotton boll infection and in reducing aflatoxin contamination of cottonseed.[24] When AF36 was applied to soil with the colonized wheat seed formulation, a significant reduction in the quantity of aflatoxin in harvested seed exhibiting bright greenish-yellow fluorescence (BGYF) was found in both years. In year 2, seeds not exhibiting BGYF were not analyzed, but in year 1 aflatoxin concentrations in non-BGYF seeds were not reduced. Overall soil populations of *Aspergillus flavus* were significantly higher in treated plots at harvest in year 1 but not significantly different in year 2. The incidence of the applied strain in soil was not significantly different between control and treated plots in either year, indicating the probable spread of AF36 from the area to which it was applied to control plots. The overall quantity of *A. flavus* on the harvested crop was not different between control and treated plots, but the incidence of AF36 was significantly higher on cottonseed from treated plots.

An experimental use permit (EUP) was granted by the EPA for large-scale testing of AF36-colonized wheat seed beginning in 1996.[25] About 120 acres (three fields) were treated at 10 lb/ac with the colonized-wheat-seed formulation by growers using modified Gandy boxes. Fungal and aflatoxin analyses indicated that AF36 displaced toxigenic strains and reduced aflatoxin contamination of cottonseed.[47] Prior to application of AF36-colonized wheat, the incidence of AF36 in soils ranged from 1.2 to 8.6% of the total *Aspergillus flavus* population; however, at harvest AF36 was the dominant strain found on cottonseed, comprising 74.2 to 98.6% of total *A. flavus* on seed surfaces. The incidence of AF36 in soil of treated fields averaged 85.3% a year after application, indicating a strong survival rate for the strain. In 1997, the EPA approved aerial application in addition to ground application, and the treated acreage was increased to 463 acres.[47] Treatments were applied between May 30 and June 18, and it was determined that displacement of toxigenic strains by AF36 was highly dependent on the time of application, with earlier applications (before June 3) being more effective than applications made after June 10.[48] The project continued in 1998 with 499 acres treated with AF36 between April 24 and July 9. The growing season in 1998 was characterized by abnormally cold weather early in the season, and this prevented the necessary growth and sporulation by the fungus in fields receiving earliest applications.[48]

In 1998, the Arizona Cotton Research and Protection Council (ACRPC) assumed responsibility for the development of a grower-owned facility for the production of commercial-scale quantities of the AF36 wheat seed formulation and establishment of protocols for area-wide implementation.[49] Initial efforts to scale up production of the formulation resulted in a product that did not compare well with laboratory-produced material;[50] therefore, significant design changes in equipment and the manufacturing process were undertaken, with an anticipated production capacity of 6000 lb per day by the end of 2002.[51] The EUP was expanded in 1999 to allow treatment of up to 20,000 acres,[52] and steady increases in treated acreage occurred with 19,975 acres being treated in 2001.[51] During the time of the expanded EUP (1999 to 2001), variable results were seen in different areas, with incidences of AF36 associated with the crop ranging from 30% to >90% in treated areas.[51,53] The poorer results were attributed to poor-quality inoculum and poor cotton canopy development, which resulted in inadequate conditions for growth and spread of the applied fungus.[53] In general, results of the program have been promising, and in 2001, 82% of treated field cottonseed tested at <20 ppb of aflatoxin while all control seed lots were >100 ppb.[51] In 2003, the EPA issued a registration for AF36 for treatment of cotton in Arizona and Texas (http://www.epa.gov/oppbppd1/biopesticides/ingredients/ tech_docs/brad_006456.pdf).

16.6.3 CORN

A modest amount of work has been done in the area of biological control of aflatoxin contamination of corn even though it is a major commodity that is subject to frequent outbreaks of contamination, particularly during hot, dry growing seasons. Initial experiments showing a potential for biocontrol of aflatoxin contamination of corn through application of nontoxigenic strains of *Aspergillus flavus* were reported in 1991.[26] Ears wounded with a cork borer were coinoculated with a toxigenic and a nontoxigenic (AF36) strain of *A. flavus*. A reduction in preharvest aflatoxin contamination of 79% resulted when ears were coinoculated with both strains compared with inoculation by the toxigenic strain alone. When ears were inoculated with AF36 24 hours prior to inoculation with the toxigenic strain, an average reduction of 95% was achieved. Postharvest experiments were also conducted in which harvested kernels were first inoculated with the nontoxigenic strain, incubated for 24 hours, dried and stored for 8 days, and then inoculated with the toxigenic strain and incubated for 12 days. Results showed that prior inoculation with the nontoxigenic strain produced significant reductions in aflatoxin of 67 to 83% compared with inoculation by the toxigenic strain alone.

Field studies were conducted over 4 years in which nontoxigenic color mutants of *Aspergillus flavus* (NRRL 21368) and *A. parasiticus* (NRRL 21369) were applied to soil in eight corn plots using a formulation of colonized rice.[31] In the fourth year of the study, NRRL 21368 was replaced with a naturally occurring nontoxigenic strain of *A. flavus* (NRRL 21882). Equivalent untreated control plots were separated from treated plots by about 1 km. After initial inoculation, soil populations of *A. flavus* and *A. parasiticus* remained significantly higher in treated soil. Over the course of the experiment, the applied strain of *A. parasiticus* was the dominant strain in soil, comprising 67 to 95% of the total *A. flavus* and *A. parasiticus* population; however, corn kernels were rarely infected with *A. parasiticus*. When the *A. flavus* color mutant (NRRL 21368) was part of the inoculum (first 3 years), the percentage of kernels infected by wild-type *A. flavus* was significantly reduced in treated plots without increasing the overall infection of kernels by *A. flavus* and *A. parasiticus*; however, upon changing inoculum to include the naturally occurring nontoxigenic strain of *A. flavus* (NRRL 21882), a significantly higher infection rate of kernels was seen with that strain. Environmental conditions conducive to preharvest aflatoxin contamination occurred only in the last 2 years of the study. During those 2 years, significant reductions of 87 and 66% in aflatoxin contamination of corn were achieved. Further studies to refine and optimize a biological control strategy for aflatoxin contamination of corn have not been pursued.

16.7 CONCLUSIONS

Many organisms have been investigated as potential biological control agents for aflatoxin contamination of crops. Whereas organisms such as bacteria and yeasts have shown promise in laboratory assays by inhibiting *Aspergillus flavus* growth or aflatoxin production, they have not been successful in preventing contamination of crops in the field. The probable reason is the difficulty associated with applying the organism so it can be effective under the hot, dry conditions associated with aflatoxin contamination and at the sites where infection and growth by *A. flavus* occur. The most successful biological control approach to date has been with the application of nontoxigenic strains of *A. flavus* and *A. parasiticus* to soil where they competitively exclude toxigenic strains. The nontoxigenic strains have been formulated in a variety of ways for delivery to the field, but the most effective method has been to combine the fungi with small grain, either through brief fermentation or coating conidia on the surface. The grain serves as a carrier for delivery to the field and as a substrate for growth and sporulation after application. Soil populations of nontoxigenic strains increase dramatically after application, thus providing a competitive advantage when crops are susceptible to *A. flavus* invasion. After the growing season, the overall soil population of *A. flavus* and *A. parasiticus* declines to a level that can be supported by that particular soil, but the toxigenic to nontoxigenic strain composition has been dramatically changed. Although total soil populations of *A. flavus* are increased after application of the nontoxigenic strain, data have consistently shown that total colonization of crops by *A. flavus* is not increased; however, the incidence of toxigenic *A. flavus* in the crop is greatly reduced. The result has been consistent reduction in aflatoxin contamination of crops, often averaging as much as 90%. This technology has advanced to the point that one product (AF36) has been registered by the EPA for treatment of cotton in Arizona and Texas and another (Afla-Guard®) has been approved for use on peanuts.

REFERENCES

1. Diener, U.L., Cole, R.J., Sanders, T.H., Payne, G.A., Lee, L.S., and Klich, M.A., Epidemiology of aflatoxin formation by *Aspergillus flavus*, *Annu. Rev. Phytopathol.*, 25, 249–270, 1987.
2. Cullen, J.M. and Newberne, P.M., Acute hepatoxicity of aflatoxins, in *The Toxicology of Aflatoxins*, Eaton, D.L. and Groopman, J.D., Eds., Academic Press, San Diego, 1994, pp. 3–26.
3. Roebuck, B.D. and Maxuitenko, Y.Y., Biochemical mechanisms and biological implications of the toxicity of aflatoxins as related to aflatoxin carcinogenesis, in *The Toxicology of Aflatoxins*, Eaton, D.L. and Groopman, J.D., Eds., Academic Press, San Diego, 1994, pp. 27–43.
4. van Egmond, H.P., Mycotoxins: regulations, quality assurance and reference materials, *Food Addit. Contam.*, 12, 321–330, 1995.
5. Wood, G.E. and Trucksess, M.W., Regulatory control programs for mycotoxin-contaminated food, in *Mycotoxins in Agriculture and Food Safety*, Sinha, K.K. and Bhatnagar, D., Eds., Marcel Dekker, New York, 1998, pp. 459–481.
6. Commission Regulation (EC) No 1525/98, *Off. J. Eur. Comm.*, L201, 43–46, 1998.
7. Horn, B.W. and Dorner, J.W., Regional differences in production of aflatoxin B_1 and cyclopiazonic acid by soil isolates of *Aspergillus flavus* along a transect within the United States, *Appl. Environ. Microbiol.*, 65, 1444–1449, 1999.
8. Dorner, J.W., Recent advances in analytical methodology for cyclopiazonic acid, in *Mycotoxins and Food Safety*, DeVries, J.W., Trucksess, M.W., and Jackson, L.S., Eds., Kluwer Academic/Plenum Press, New York, 2002, pp. 107–116.

9. Robens, J.F. and Riley, R.T., Eds., Special Issue: Aflatoxin/Fumonisin Elimination and Fungal Genomics Workshops, Phoenix Arizona, October 23–26 2001, *Mycopathologia*, 155, 2002.

10. Kimura, N. and Hirano, S., Inhibitory strains of *Bacillus subtilis* for growth and aflatoxin-production of aflatoxigenic fungi, *Agric. Biol. Chem.*, 52, 1173–1179, 1988.

11. Cuero, R.G., Duffus, E., Osuji, G., and Pettit, R., Aflatoxin control in preharvest maize: effects of chitosan and two microbial agents, *J. Agr. Sci.*, 117, 165–169, 1991.

12. Smith, Jr., J.S., Dorner, J.W., and Cole, R.J., Testing *Bacillus subtilis* as a possible aflatoxin inhibitor in stored farmers stock peanuts, *Proc. Am. Peanut Res. Educ. Soc.*, 22, 35, 1990.

13. Dorner, J.W. and Cole, R.J., Effect of application of nontoxigenic strains of *Aspergillus flavus* and *A. parasiticus* on subsequent aflatoxin contamination of peanuts in storage, *J. Stored Prod. Res.*, 38, 329–339, 2002.

14. Mickler, C.J., Bowen, K.L., and Kloepper, J.W., Evaluation of selected geocarposphere bacteria for biological control of *Aspergillus flavus* in peanut, *Plant Soil*, 175, 291–299, 1995.

15. Misaghi, I.J., Cotty, P.J., and Decianne, D.M., Bacterial antagonists of *Aspergillus flavus*, *Biocontr. Sci. Technol.*, 5, 387–392, 1995.

16. Misaghi, I.J., Management of aflatoxin contamination of cottonseed in Arizona, in *Proc. Aflatoxin Elimination Workshop*, St. Louis, MO, October 24–25, 1994, Robens, J.F., Ed., Agricultural Research Service, U.S. Department of Agriculture, Beltsville, MD, 1994, p. 56.

17. Hua, S.-S.T., Baker, J.L., and Flores-Espiritu, M., Interactions of saprophytic yeasts with a *nor* mutant of *Aspergillus flavus*, *Appl. Environ. Microbiol.*, 65, 2738–2740, 1999.

18. Hua, S.-S.T., Biological control of aflatoxin in almond and pistachio by preharvest yeast application in orchards, in Special Issue: Aflatoxin/Fumonisin Elimination and Fungal Genomics Workshops, Phoenix, AZ, October 23–26 2001, *Mycopathologia*, 155, 65, 2002.

19. Cole, R.J., Sanders, T.H., Dorner, J.W., and Blankenship, P.D., Environmental conditions required to induce preharvest aflatoxin contamination of groundnuts: summary of six years' research, in *Aflatoxin Contamination of Groundnut: Proceedings of the International Workshop*, ICRISAT Center, October 6–9, 1987, Patancheru, India, Hall, S.D., Ed., 1989, pp. 279–287.

20. Cotty, P.J. and Lee, L.S., Aflatoxin contamination of cottonseed: comparison of pink bollworm damaged and undamaged bolls, *Trop. Sci.*, 29, 273–277, 1989.

21. Payne, G.A., Aflatoxin in maize, *CRC Crit. Rev. Plant Sci.*, 10, 423–440, 1992.

22. Cole, R.J. and Cox, R.H., *Handbook of Toxic Fungal Metabolites*, Academic Press, New York, 1981, 937 pp.

23. Cotty, P.J., Effect of atoxigenic strains of *Aspergillus flavus* on aflatoxin contamination of developing cottonseed, *Plant Dis.*, 74, 233–235, 1990.

24. Cotty, P.J., Influence of field application of an atoxigenic strain of *Aspergillus flavus* on the populations of *A. flavus* infecting cotton bolls and on the aflatoxin content of cottonseed, *Phytopathology*, 84, 1270–1277, 1994.

25. Cotty, P.J., Howell, D.R., and Sobek, E.A., The EPA approved experimental use program for *Aspergillus flavus* AF 36, in *Proc. Aflatoxin Elimination Workshop*, Fresno, CA, Oct 28–29, 1996, Robens, J.F. and Cleveland, T.E., Eds., Agricultural Research Service, Beltsville, MD, U.S. Department of Agriculture, 1996, p. 3.

26. Brown, R.L., Cotty, P.J., and Cleveland, T.E., Reduction in aflatoxin content of maize by atoxigenic strains of *Aspergillus flavus*, *J. Food Prot.*, 54, 623–626, 1991.

27. Dorner, J.W., Cole, R.J., and Blankenship, P.D., Use of a biocompetitive agent to control preharvest aflatoxin in drought stressed peanuts, *J. Food Prot.*, 55, 888–892, 1992.
28. Brown, M.P., Brown-Jenco, C.S., and Payne, G.A., Genetic and molecular analysis of aflatoxin biosynthesis, *Fungal Genet. Biol.*, 26, 81–98, 1999.
29. Chourasia, H.K. and Sinha, R.K., Potential of the biological control of aflatoxin contamination in developing peanut (*Arachis hypogaea* L.) by atoxigenic strains of *Aspergillus flavus*, *J. Food Sci. Technol.*, 31, 362–366, 1994.
30. Dorner, J.W., Cole, R.J., and Blankenship, P.D., Effect of inoculum rate of biological control agents on preharvest aflatoxin contamination of peanuts, *Biol. Control*, 12, 171–176, 1998.
31. Dorner, J.W., Cole, R.J., and Wicklow, D.T., Aflatoxin reduction in corn through field application of competitive fungi, *J. Food Prot.*, 62, 650–656, 1999.
32. Dorner, J.W., Cole, R.J., Horn, B.W., and Blankenship, P.D., Evaluation of *Aspergillus oryzae* and *A. sojae* as potential biological control agents for preharvest aflatoxin contamination of peanuts, *Proc. Am. Peanut Res. Educ. Soc.*, 31, 58, 1999.
33. Fravel, D.R., Connick, Jr., W.J., and Lewis, J.A., Formulation of microorganisms to control plant diseases, in *Formulation of Microbial Biopesticides, Beneficial Microorganisms, Nematodes, and Seed Treatments*, Burges, H.D., Ed., Kluwer Academic, Dordrecht, 1998, pp. 187–202.
34. McGuire, M.R., Connick, W.J., and Quimby, P.C., Formulation of microbial pesticides, in *Controlled-Release Delivery Systems for Pesticides*, Sher, H.B., Ed., Marcel Dekker, New York, 1999, pp. 173–193.
35. Bock, C. and Cotty, P.J., Wheat seed colonized with atoxigenic *Aspergillus flavus*: characterization and production of a biopesticide for aflatoxin control, *Biocontr. Sci. Technol.*, 9, 529–543, 1999.
36. Daigle, D.J. and Cotty, P.J., Formulating atoxigenic *Aspergillus flavus* for field release, *Biocontr. Sci. Technol.*, 5, 175–184, 1995.
37. Connick, Jr., W.J., Boyette, C.D., and McAlpine, J.R., Formulation of mycoherbicides using a pasta-like process, *Biol. Control*, 1, 281–287, 1991.
38. Daigle, D.J., Connick, Jr., W.J., Boyette, C.D., Lovisa, M.P., Williams, K.S., and Watson, M., Twin-screw extrusion of 'Pesta'-encapsulated biocontrol agents, *World J. Microbiol. Biotechnol.*, 13, 671–676, 1997.
39. Daigle, D.J., Connick, W.J., Boyette, C.D., Jackson, M.A., and Dorner, J.W., Solid-state fermentation plus extrusion to make biopesticide granules, *Biotechnol. Tech.*, 12, 715–719, 1998.
40. Dorner, J.W., Cole, R.J., Connick, W.J., Daigle, D.J., McGuire, M.R., and Shasha, B.S. Evaluation of biological control formulations to reduce aflatoxin contamination in peanuts, *Biol. Control*, 26, 318–324, 2003.
41. Lamb, M.C. and Sternitzke, D.A., Cost of aflatoxin to the farmer, buying point, and sheller segments of the southeast United States peanut industry, *Peanut Sci.*, 28, 59–63, 2001.
42. Cole, R.J. and Dorner, J.W., Biological Control Formulations Containing Spores of Nontoxigenic Strains of Fungi for Toxin Control of Food Crops, U.S. Patent 6,306,3860, October 23, 2001.
43. Dorner, J.W., Combined effects of biological control formulations, cultivars, and fungicides on preharvest aflatoxin contamination of peanuts, *Proc. Am. Peanut Res. Educ. Soc.*, 34, 62, 2002.

44. Horn, B.W., Greene, R.L., Sorensen, R.B., Blankenship, P.D., and Dorner, J.W., Conidial movement of nontoxigenic *Aspergillus flavus* and *A. parasiticus* in peanut fields following application to soil, *Mycopathologia*, 151, 81–92, 2001.

45. Cotty, P.J., Long-term influences of atoxigenic strain applications on *Aspergillus flavus* communities in commercial agriculture, in *Proc. Aflatoxin Elimination Workshop*, Atlanta, GA, October 20–22, 1999, Robens, J. and Cary, J.W., Eds., Agricultural Research Service, U.S. Department of Agriculture, Beltsville, MD, 1999, p. 82.

46. Cotty, P.J. and Bayman, P., Competitive exclusion of a toxigenic strain of *Aspergillus flavus* by an atoxigenic strain, *Phytopathology*, 83, 1283–1287, 1993.

47. Cotty, P.J. and Sobek, E.A., The use of *Aspergillus flavus* to prevent aflatoxin contamination in commercial agriculture, in *Proc. Aflatoxin Elimination Workshop*, Memphis, TN, October 26–28, 1997, Robens, J. and Dorner, J., Eds., Agricultural Research Service, U.S. Department of Agriculture, Beltsville, MD, 1997, p. 76.

48. Cotty, P.J., Improving aflatoxin management with atoxigenic strains: requirements and obstacles, in *Proc. Aflatoxin Elimination Workshop*, St. Louis, MO, October 25–27, 1998, Robens, J. and Wicklow, D., Eds., Agricultural Research Service, U.S. Department of Agriculture, Beltsville, MD, 1998, p. 78.

49. Antilla, L. and Cotty, P.J., Development and construction of a facility to manufacture commercially useful quantities of atoxigenic strain inoculum, in *Proc. Aflatoxin Elimination Workshop*, St. Louis, MO, October 25–27, 1998, Robens, J. and Wicklow, D., Eds., Agricultural Research Service, U.S. Department of Agriculture, Beltsville, MD, 1998, p. 79.

50. Cotty, P.J., Antilla, L., Ploski, J., Kobbeman, K., and Bock, C.H. Utilizing atoxigenic strains of *A. flavus* to manage aflatoxins in commercial cotton. Part I. Commercial scale manufacture of inoculum, in *Proc. Aflatoxin Elimination Workshop*, Fish Camp, CA, October 25–27, 2000, Robens, J.F., Cary, J.W., and Campbell, B.W., Eds., Agricultural Research Service, U.S. Department of Agriculture, Beltsville, MD, 2000, pp. 130–131.

51. Antilla, L. and Cotty, P.J., The ARS–ACRPC partnership to control aflatoxin in Arizona cotton: current status, in Special Issue: Aflatoxin/Fumonisin Elimination and Fungal Genomics Workshops, Phoenix, AZ, October 23–26, 2001, *Mycopathologia*, 155, 64, 2002.

52. Antilla, L. and Cotty, P.J., Production of commercially useful quantities of atoxigenic strain inoculum, in *Proc. Aflatoxin Elimination Workshop*, Atlanta, GA, October 20–22, 1999, Robens, J. and Cary, J.W., Eds., Agricultural Research Service, U.S. Department of Agriculture, Beltsville, MD, 1999, pp. 83–84.

53. Antilla L. and Cotty, P.J., Utilizing atoxigenic strains of *A. flavus* to manage aflatoxins in commercial cotton. Part II. Field aspects, in *Proc. Aflatoxin Elimination Workshop*, Fish Camp, CA, October 25–27, 2000, Robens, J.F., Cary, J.W., and Campbell, B.W., Eds., Agricultural Research Service, U.S. Department of Agriculture, Beltsville, MD, 2000, pp. 132–133.

17 Breeding Corn to Reduce Preharvest Aflatoxin Contamination

Javier Betrán, Tom Isakeit, Gary Odvody, and Kerry Mayfield

CONTENTS

17.1 INTRODUCTION

Aflatoxin is a mycotoxin produced by *Aspergillus flavus* Link:Fr. that causes aflatoxicosis in livestock and hepatic cancer in humans.[1] Preharvest aflatoxin contamination in corn (*Zea mays* L.) is a chronic problem in the southern United States that
limits maize marketability and causes economic losses.[2-4] Approaches to reduce
aflatoxin include: cultural practices and crop management, host plant resistance
through breeding or genetic engineering, and biocontrol (e.g., atoxigenic strains).[5,6]
Genetic variation for response to aflatoxin has been found in corn,[7-10] and sources
of resistance such as inbreds Mp420, Mp313E, Mp715, Tex6, and population GT-
MAS:gk have been identified;[11-14] however, the majority of these sources of resistance lack agronomic performance, which precludes their direct use in commercial
hybrids. In addition, no competitive commercial hybrids are available that are resistant to aflatoxin; therefore, the objectives of several research groups are the transfer
of resistance from these sources of resistance to elite inbreds and hybrids and the
search for resistance in elite commercial material. In this chapter, we describe our
efforts at the Texas Agricultural Experiment Station (Texas A&M University) in
screening and developing maize inbreds and hybrids that reduce aflatoxin contamination and have good agronomic performance.

17.2 EXPERIMENTAL APPROACHES TO
EVALUATING CORN GERMPLASM
FOR RESPONSE TO AFLATOXIN

17.2.1 INOCULATION AND AFLATOXIN QUANTIFICATION

We use two methods of inoculation: (1) the nonwounding silk channel inoculation
technique,[15] where ears are inoculated 6 to 10 days after silking with 3 mL of the
conidial suspension (~10^7/mL) with a syringe, and (2) the colonized kernel technique, where colonized autoclaved corn kernels are placed on the soil surface
between treatment rows when the first hybrids reach mid-silk stage. Both methods
have been effective to discriminate genotypes and detect significant differences.
Aflatoxin levels are higher in ears inoculated with the silk channel technique as
compared with ears from the same plots that were not inoculated and relied upon
colonization by indigenous *Aspergillus flavus* in the environment (Figure 17.1);
however, the silk channel technique may not evaluate all possible host resistance
factors. The silk channel technique bypasses potential morphological barriers, such
as husk coverage or tightness, or chemical inhibitors that prevent silk colonization,[16]
but these mechanisms of resistance can come into play when using the colonized
kernel technique. The limitation of the colonized kernel technique is the susceptibility to environmental factors extraneous to the study, such as heavy rains, which

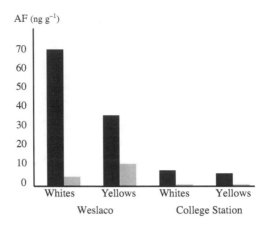

FIGURE 17.1 Aflatoxin content (ng/g) for inoculated ears with the silk channel inoculation technique (left bars) and noninoculated ears (right bars) in white and yellow hybrids in two environments.

may interfere with sporulation of the fungus on kernels and movement of conidia into the ears. With either inoculation technique, ears are hand harvested after kernel moisture in all hybrids is below 15%. Ears are then husked, rated for insect injury and visible fungal colonization, dried, shelled, and bulked. The whole kernel samples are ground using a Romer mill (Union, MO). Aflatoxin is quantified using 50-g subsamples from each plot with monoclonal antibody affinity columns and fluorescence determination using the Vicam Aflatest system (Watertown, MA). Aflatoxin content is expressed in ng/g (ppb).

17.2.2 Field Experimental Designs and Data Analysis

Aflatoxin accumulation shows high spatial and environmental variation; therefore, the use of optimal experimental designs and field layout can reduce the error, increase the precision of mean estimates, and, consequently, improve selection. Several field experimental designs are used in the evaluation for response to aflatoxin of inbred and hybrids. The most common are randomized complete-block design (RCBD), incomplete lattices,[17] and, more recently, row-and-column designs among replicated designs.[18] The application of restricted maximum likelihood (REML) methods to estimate variance components in mixed linear models is becoming a useful tool to deal with in-trial spatial variability *a posteriori* in field aflatoxin trials.[19] The spatial variation requires inoculation and a high number of replications, commonly three or greater. We have occasionally used up to nine replications, pooling them by groups of three to quantify aflatoxin. SAS® procedures and REML tools are applied to analyze the data. Logarithmic transformation of aflatoxin contents in parts per billion (log ng/g) is commonly used in the analysis to equalize variance and normalize the data. Antilogarithmic values of best-adjusted means are used to report the results. The use of resistant and susceptible checks is helpful to determine the efficiency of the inoculation, the reference aflatoxin levels for genotypes under evaluation, the detection of spatial variation in single trials, and the comparison of results across locations. The checks should have maturities and levels of inbreeding similar to the tested germplasm. We use inbreds such as CML176, CML269, CML288, and Tx772 as resistant checks and Tx114, Tx811, CML285, and Tx714 as susceptible checks. Among hybrids we have used Pioneer Brand P31B13, Tx110 × Tx114, and floury *opaque 2* hybrids (e.g., SR660) as susceptible checks and CML176 × CML269, FR2128 × NC300, and CML288 × Tx772 as resistant checks.

17.2.3 ENVIRONMENTS FOR AFLATOXIN EVALUATION

We have used three locations located in south and central Texas where aflatoxin contamination is a frequent problem: Weslaco (latitude 26°09′, elevation 22.5 m), Corpus Christi (latitude 27°46′, elevation 12.9 m), and College Station (latitude 30°37′, elevation 96 m). Plots at College Station and Weslaco are 6.40 m long and 0.75 m apart and are 7.90 m long and 0.96 m apart at Corpus Christi. No insecticides are applied after planting. Trials are planted at normal times in Weslaco (middle of February) and College Station (early March). Drought and heat stress is induced by late planting at Corpus Christi (4 weeks later than usual planting time) and by limited irrigation at Weslaco and College Station. A certain degree of drought stress increases the predisposition to aflatoxin contamination and permits the screening for drought tolerance at the same time. In most recent trials with the silk channel inoculation technique, we have used two row plots. After harvesting the inoculated ears by hand, we record combine grain yield, grain moisture, and test weight. This dual evaluation for aflatoxin and agronomic performance allows the selection of most resistant genotypes having the desired agronomic characteristics.

17.3 GENETIC PARAMETERS FOR AFLATOXIN RESPONSE

17.3.1 REPEATABILITIES FOR SINGLE ENVIRONMENT TRIALS

Response to aflatoxin accumulation has been assumed to be a low-heritable trait that is strongly influenced by environmental conditions. In field trials from 2001 to 2003, we have estimated how much of the observed variation in aflatoxin content of hybrids and inbreds is associated with genetic effects of test genotypes. Repeatabilities (i.e., genetic variation/total variation) for logarithmic transformation of aflatoxin at individual trials were higher than expected (Figure 17.2).[20] Inbred line trials were more consistently repeatable than hybrid trials, with average repeatability estimates for yellow inbreds the highest, at 0.88. Trials at Corpus Christi of both white and yellow hybrids for all years showed the highest repeatability estimates per location (average = 0.85), followed by Weslaco (average = 0.69) and College Station (average = 0.46). Hence, some locations, such as Corpus Christi, exhibit greater genetic variation than those that are less conducive for aflatoxin accumulation such as College Station. High aflatoxin accumulation averages were associated with high repeatabilty estimates. The identification of locations with better screening capacity that improves repeatability could facilitate genetic progress toward aflatoxin resistance in corn. Proper field experimental design and analysis, inoculation with *Aspergillus flavus*,

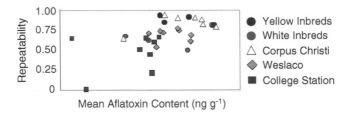

FIGURE 17.2 Repeatability estimates for logarithmic transformation of aflatoxin content (ng/g) in individual trials of inbreds and hybrids at three Texas locations.

an adequate number of replications and plants measured, the application of drought stress, and uniform soils and treatments, as well as reliable data collection, have reduced error and subsequently improved repeatability (or heritability) and the potential for genetic progress.

17.3.2 GENOTYPE AND ENVIRONMENTAL INTERACTION

Although experimental approaches at single locations generated useful information, the results across locations were more variable. Repeatability estimates across locations were intermediate and lower than at individual locations due to the proportion of environmental and genotype by environment interaction components in relation to the genetic component. Genotypes performed differently relative to each other in different environments. The relative performance of genotypes across environments can change the rank of genotypes among environments, creating crossover interactions and low genetic correlations among environments. This type of interaction has strong consequences in the magnitude of response to selection. The correlation of aflatoxin accumulation for the same genotypes across locations was variable. In experiments with yellow and white hybrids, the phenotypic correlation between our three testing Texas locations were either nonsignificant or significant and positive but below 0.5. These results indicate the necessity for multilocation testing in several environments in order to identify the most consistent stable sources of resistance across environments. For this reason, the South East Regional Aflatoxin Test (SERAT) was established. SERAT is a collaborative project involving several breeding programs that provides a testing network of environments across major growing areas affected by aflatoxin contamination. With this collaborative regional testing, we expect to identify the most stable sources of aflatoxin resistance and to assess the magnitude and nature of genotype–environment interactions for aflatoxin. A major factor that can vary by location beyond the physical environment and stress are biological factors or biological stresses, especially insects. Insects include stalk borers of various species, corn earworm, fall armyworm, spider mites that may increase susceptibility to drought stress, and corn rootworm.

17.3.3 INBRED–HYBRID CORRELATION FOR AFLATOXIN

The relationship between the response of inbred lines and their hybrids to aflatoxin accumulation and the degree of transmission of resistance to aflatoxin accumulation

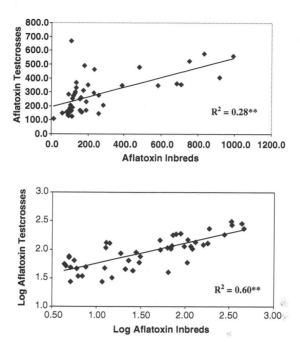

FIGURE 17.3 Regression of aflatoxin and its logarithmic transformation across locations in testcrosses on means for inbreds at Weslaco, TX, in 2002.

to hybrids are important issues in developing resistant hybrids. Aflatoxin accumulation in inbreds has been greater than in their corresponding hybrids. The possibility of using inbred line information as prediction of hybrid performance is desirable to reduce the number of evaluations of hybrids. For aflatoxin accumulation the correlation between line and testcross performance has been variable among testers. The amount of genetic variation among the inbreds tested and the type of tester may influence the correlation between line and testcross performance.[21] A resistant tester can reduce the correlation due to favorable alleles masking effects of alleles present in lines while susceptible tester can improve both the correlation and the genetic variation among testcrosses. In the evaluation of 48 inbreds and their testcrosses with a susceptible tester, Tx804, the correlation between inbreds and testcrosses was 0.53 for aflatoxin (Figure 17.3), suggesting that for this set of genotypes aflatoxin accumulation in inbreds had some predictive value for its expression in testcrosses; however, we have found different results in other studies where the correlation between inbred and hybrids have been of low predictive value.[22] In general, the relation between inbreds and their hybrids for aflatoxin has been variable depending on the germplasm and experimental approaches. Although the predictive value of inbred line performance as indicative of hybrid performance can be variable depending on the environment, degree of inbreeding, and lines and tester used, aflatoxin accumulation in inbreds does not appear to be fully predictive of hybrid performance. Hence, hybrid testing is required to identify the inbreds with the best breeding values for aflatoxin reduction as well as the most resistant hybrid combinations.

17.4 PLANT TRAITS ASSOCIATED WITH RESPONSE TO AFLATOXIN

The identification of heritable traits correlated with aflatoxin contamination and their subsequent use in the selection process can increase the rate of progress in developing less susceptible corn hybrids. Aflatoxin has been associated with several plant traits, including husk coverage and tightness,[23,24] physical and chemical characteristics of the seed pericarp,[25,26] drought and heat tolerance,[27] resistance to insects (e.g., corn earworm),[28,29] kernel integrity,[23] maturity and adaptation to the local environments,[24] endosperm texture,[22] and resistance factors in kernels that reduce fungal development or aflatoxin formation.[30]

17.4.1 HUSK COVERAGE AND MATURITY

The relationship between aflatoxin and husk coverage and maturity was assessed in a study with 25 commercial field and food maize hybrids with different maturities: full-season (>115 days to relative maturity [DRM]), intermediate (95 to 115 DRM), and early (DRM < 95).[24] Maturity was measured as days from planting to date at which 50% of the plants in the plot exhibited emerged silks, and husk coverage was visually rated on a scale of 1 (good) to 5 (poor) (1 = husk leaves extended more than 2.54 cm from the tip of the ear, 2 = husk leaves covering the tip of the ear between 0 and 2.54 cm, 3 = husk leaves of the same length than the ear and no grain exposed, 4 = husk leaves shorter than the ear and tip kernels exposed, and 5 = few husk leaves with more than a few kernels exposed). The correlation between silking date and aflatoxin accumulation was significant and negative (−0.59**), and the correlation between husk cover and aflatoxin content was significant and positive (0.77**) (Figure 17.4). Early-maturing hybrids with loose, poorly covered husks had more aflatoxin than full-season hybrids that had better husk coverage. This trait is selected in opposing directions between the midwestern and southeastern United States. In the Midwest, loose husks are preferred to allow faster drying in the field before harvest, while in the southeastern states tight and long husks are preferred to reduce or prevent insect and fungal damage. Maturity and husk coverage are closely correlated and their effects are difficult to separate, as later hybrids have more plant and husk leaves than early hybrids. The results in this particular study have been similar to the relationship of maturity and husk coverage in other hybrid trials suggesting that these two traits can be use in selection to reduce aflatoxin.[22,23]

17.4.2 ENDOSPERM TYPE

Endosperm hardness is defined as the proportion of hard to soft endosperm. There are genetic differences for horny/floury ratios, pericarp thickness, and cell structure among corn lines and hybrids. Hardness can be estimated visually in the field or with a light box. We have measured endosperm texture as visual rating from 1 (flint = round crown kernel and vitreous appearance) to 5 (dent = kernels with pronounced dentation and high proportion of floury endosperm) in most of the aflatoxin trials. With both inbreds and hybrids, aflatoxin was positively correlated with endosperm texture. Aflatoxin in white hybrids was positively correlated with texture ratings at

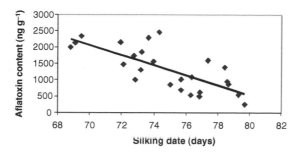

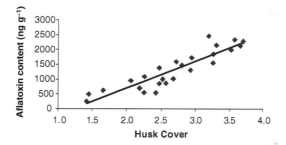

FIGURE 17.4 Relationship between aflatoxin concentration (ng/g) and maturity and husk coverage of full, intemediate, and early season commercial hybrids inoculated with *Aspergillus flavus* across Weslaco and College Station, TX.

College Station (0.53**) and Corpus Christi (0.62**) in a diallel among white food inbreds.[31] The correlation between endosperm texture and aflatoxin for 48 inbreds evaluated in Weslaco, TX, was 0.49** and for their testcrosses, 0.61**, across three locations[32]. Furthermore, the expression of this trait in parental inbreds was associated with aflatoxin in the testcrosses (Figure 17.5). This apparent association between endosperm texture and aflatoxin could be the result of a direct effect of the endosperm on the pathogen or an indirect effect, as a hard endosperm can help to maintain kernel integrity.

17.4.3 Kernel Integrity

The capability of grain kernels to maintain physical integrity is an important trait in reducing aflatoxin accumulation and maintaining grain quality. Kernel injuries in the pericarp and endosperm caused by insects, such as corn earworm, *Helicoverpa zea* (Boddie), and environmental stresses (stress cracks) predispose them to fungal infection. Kernel integrity is associated with good husk coverage, endosperm hardness, and insect resistance.[23] We have measured kernel integrity with a visual rating scale (1 = all ears without split kernels or damaged by insects to 5 = most of the ears with splits and/or insect damage). Also, at Corpus Christi we rate insect injury by the length of the insect galleries on the ear.[33] Aflatoxin in yellow hybrids has been positively correlated with insect damage ratings (0.66**) and ear injury (0.55**).[21] In another experiment, the correlation between kernel integrity ratings

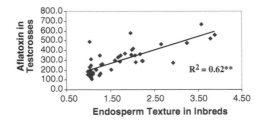

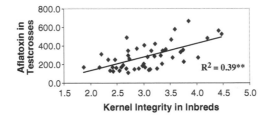

FIGURE 17.5 Regression of aflatoxin content across locations in test crosses on means for endosperm texture (rated visually from 1 = flint to 5 = dent) and kernel integrity (rated visually from 1 = all ears without splits kernels or damaged by insects to 5 = most of the ears with splits and/or insect damage) in inbreds at Weslaco, TX (2002).

and aflatoxin was 0.53** for inbreds and 0.75** for their testcrosses.[32] In the same experiment, and as in the case of endosperm texture, kernel integrity in parental inbreds was associated with aflatoxin in their testcrosses (Figure 17.5).

17.4.4 Drought and Heat Tolerance and Adaptation

Drought is one of the main environmental limitations on yield in rainfed areas in the southern United States. Drought and high temperatures during flowering and grain filling periods are common in Texas. Corn hybrids that tolerate drought and heat stress and have adaptation to southern U.S. growing areas can reduce aflatoxin risk and provide enhanced grain yield. Drought-susceptible, poorly adapted hybrids are more vulnerable to aflatoxin accumulation than well-adapted, drought-tolerant hybrids. Significant improvements have been observed in both temperate and tropical maize for drought tolerance at flowering.[34,35] Drought-tolerant germplasm in the form of populations (e.g., TS6, La Posta Sequia), synthetics (ZM521), inbreds (CML339, CML343, CML444), and hybrids have been developed in exotic subtropical and tropical corn. In addition, significant QTL consistent across genetic backgrounds and environments have been identified for different yield components, morphological traits, and physiological parameters associated with drought tolerance.[36] This germplasm and genomic information from these exotic sources can be used to introduce new alleles for drought tolerance in temperate germplasm. In our program, we are using drought-tolerant exotic inbreds in combination with temperate lines to enhance drought tolerance and adaptation and aflatoxin resistance. We emphasize traits associated with drought tolerance such as anthesis–silking interval, delayed senescence (i.e., stay-green), and grain yield in line selection.[37,38]

TABLE 17.1
Aflatoxin Accumulations and Rank of White Food Corn Inbreds at Weslaco in 2001 and 2002 and at College Station in 2002

	Weslaco 2001			College Station 2002		Weslaco 2002	
Inbred	ng/g	Rank	Inbred	ng/g	Rank	ng/g	Rank
Tx114	897.5	5	Tx114	8.50	11	321.3	14
Tx130	810.0	3	Tx130	0.75	2	49.3	10
Tx110	1300.0	7	Tx110	376.50	14	1125.0	15
CML78	422.5	2	CML78	1.25	4	7.5	3
CML322	2675.0	15	CML322	5.00	7	67.3	11
CML311	1612.5	11	CML311	300.70	13	140.8	12
CML373	1550.0	10	CML373	3.50(5)	5	0.7	2
CML384	1327.5	8	CML384	5.50	9	37.0	6
CML385	2150.0	14	CML269	0.00	1	15.8	4
CML343	862.5	4	CML343	16.70	12	31.3	5
T39	2070.0	13	T35	5.25	8	41.0	8
T35	897.5	6	Y21	462.70	15	0.0	1
Y9121	1360.0	9	Tx811	4.75	6	44.8	9
Tx8007	2067.5	12	Tx807	0.75	3	38.3	7
CML176	115.3	1	CML176	5.50	10	175.5	13
Average	1341.2		Average	79.80		157.1	
LSD (0.05)	1203.0		LSD (0.05)	461.10		411.9	

17.5 EVALUATION OF INBRED LINES

17.5.1 WHITE INBREDS

White subtropical, tropical, and temperate inbreds have been evaluated in our program for aflatoxin during recent years. Significant differences among inbreds were detected in all locations. At Weslaco during the 2001 season, the average aflatoxin was 1341.2 ng/g (range, 115.3 to 2675.0 ng/g) (Table 17.1).[31] The inbreds with the lowest aflatoxin contamination were CML176, CML78, and Tx130. At College Station in 2002, the average aflatoxin accumulation was 79.8 ng/g (range, 0.0 to 462.7 ng/g); the inbreds with the lowest aflatoxin were CML269, Tx130, and Tx807. At Weslaco in 2002, the average aflatoxin was 157.1 ng/g (range, 0.0 to 1125.0 ng/g); the inbreds with the lowest aflatoxin were Y21, CML373, and CML78. At Weslaco in 2003, the average aflatoxin was 178.1 ng/g (range, 0.0 to 649.1 ng/g); the inbreds with the lowest aflatoxin were CML78, CML176 and CML269. The inbreds with the most consistent lowest aflatoxin levels across evaluations have been CML176, CML269, CML78, Tx807, and Tx130. Most of the less susceptible lines have subtropical or tropical origin while the most susceptible inbreds have temperate origin (Figure 17.6).

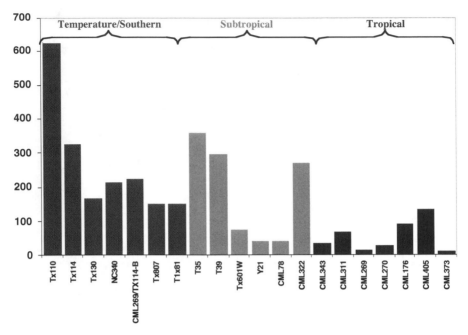

FIGURE 17.6 Aflatoxin content for temperate, subtropical, and tropical inbreds in Weslaco, TX, in 2003 season.

17.5.2 YELLOW INBREDS

Yellow inbreds have been evaluated in Weslaco, TX, from 2001 to 2003. Response to aflatoxin of yellow inbreds has been variable among years (i.e., high genotype by environmental interaction). Significant differences among inbreds were detected in all three seasons. In 2001, the average aflatoxin was 1343.17 ng/g, with a range of 452.5 to 2750.0 ng/g (Table 17.2).[39] The inbreds showing less susceptibility were CML289, Tx601Y, and Tx732. In the 2002 season in Weslaco, the average aflatoxin was 532.76 ng/g, with a range of 26.75 to 1905.9 ng/g. The inbreds showing less susceptibility were Tx772, NC300, and CML338. In the 2003 season, the average aflatoxin was 491.03 ng/g, with a range of 10.5 to 2575 ng/g. The inbreds showing less susceptibility were TxXQ69-B4, TxXQ69-B2, and Tx772. Overall, yellow inbreds CML323, Tx772, CML288, NC300, FR2128, CML338, and CML161 and experimental lines TxX69s have shown reduced levels of aflatoxin.

17.5.3 SPECIALTY CORN INBREDS

Fatty acid composition in the seed can affect the degree of fungi sporulation and aflatoxin production. We evaluated the response to aflatoxin contamination of corn lines with different fatty acid content derived from germplasm enhancement of maize (GEM) breeding crosses. GEM-derived lines with high linoleic/low oleic and low linoleic/high oleic were evaluated for aflatoxin accumulation at Weslaco and College Station, TX, during 2002, and at Weslaco during 2003. On average,

TABLE 17.2
Aflatoxin Content for Yellow Inbred Lines Evaluated in Weslaco, TX, in the 2001 to 2003 Seasons Under Inoculation

2003			2002			2001		
	Aflatoxin			Aflatoxin			Aflatoxin	
Inbred	ng/g	Rank	Inbred	ng/g	Rank	Inbred	ng/g	Rank
B104	610.5	14	B104	166.7	6	B104	1450.0	9
B97	2575.0	19	B97	1495.0	13	B97	2087.5	13
CML285	32.3	5	CML285	1577.5	14	CML285	2750.0	15
CML288	497.5	13	CML288	436.3	11	CML288	995.0	7
CML323	877.5	16	CML323	365.5	10	CML289	452.5	1
CML325	1332.5	18	CML325	157.0	5	CML294	777.5	5
CML338	267.5	11	CML338	46.0	3	CML323	952.5	6
FR2128	465.0	12	FR2128	780.0	12	CML338	1725.0	10
NC300	58.3	7	NC300	27.0	2	FR2128	1877.5	12
Tx601y	—	—	Tx601y	125.1	4	NC300	1280.0	8
Tx714	1322.5	17	Tx714	230.0	8	Tx601y	457.5	2
Tx732	622.5	15	Tx732	343.8	9	Tx714	1875.0	11
Tx770	210.3	10	Tx760	1905.0	15	Tx732	460.0	3
Tx772	19.0	2	Tx770	168.5	7	Tx770	682.5	4
TxXQB2	23.0	3	TX772	26.8	1	TX772	2325.0	14
TxXQB35	145.8	9	Average	532.8		Average	1343.2	
TxXQB36	25.8	4	LSD (0.05)	1156.3		LSD (0.05)	864.0	
TxXQB47	10.5	1						
TxXQB411	63.3	8						
TxXQB5	56.3	6						
Average	491.0							
LSD (0.05)	805.8							

high oleic/low linoleic lines had less aflatoxin content than low oleic/high linoleic lines at each location and across locations (Table 17.3); however, the range for aflatoxin among the low oleic/high linoleic lines was much greater than among the high oleic/low linoleic lines. Furthermore, the GEM lines with the lowest aflatoxin across locations were the low oleic/high linoleic lines DKXL380:S08A12-24-B and BR52060:S0212-25-B. Therefore, with this reduced sample of inbreds nonconclusive differences were observed between high oleic/low linoleic and low oleic/high linoleic GEM lines. QPM hybrids were less susceptible to aflatoxin than commercial hybrids in our experiments (Table 17.4).[32,40] Because the development of QPM germplasm involved selection of genotypes resistant to ear rot, insect resistance, kernel integrity, and modified kernel texture while simultaneously improving agronomic characteristics, QPM germplasm represents a potential source of resistance to aflatoxin.[41] White and yellow QPM hybrids had better husk cover, less ear rot, and less aflatoxin compared to non-QPM commercial checks.[40] Genotypes *opaque 2* with floury soft endosperm have been consistently more susceptible than quality

TABLE 17.3
Aflatoxin Content of GEM-Derived Lines with Different Composition of Oleic and Linoleic Fatty Acids and Resistant and Susceptible Checks at College Station and Weslaco, TX, and Across Locations in 2002 and 2003

	Aflatoxin Content (ng/g)			
GEM Line	College Station 2002	Weslaco 2002	Weslaco 2003	Average Across Locations
High oleic/low linoleic (HO–LL)				
CUBA164:S1511b-15-B	19.8	207.5	623.4	283.6
DKXL380:S08a12-12-B	23.5	790.0	641.0	484.8
DKB844:N11b17-21-B	47.2	354.3	189.1	196.9
AR16026:S1704-32-B	180.1	557.5	508.2	415.3
Average HO–LL	67.7	477.3	490.4	345.1
Low oleic/high linoleic (LO–HL)				
DKB830:S11a17-35-B	35.9	1925.0	2709.9	1557.0
DKXL380:S08A12-24-B	132.4	26.3	369.7	176.1
BR52060:S0212-25-B	179.5	95.5	260.1	178.4
FS8B(T):N1802-35-1-B	259.5	1417.3	1635.9	1104.2
Average LO–HL	151.8	866.0	1243.9	753.9
Resistant checks				
CML176	0.0	1.3	26.4	9.2
Tx601	7.1	28.0	76.9	37.3
Susceptible checks				
Tx110	11.5	1475.0	823.4	770.0
Tx732	167.6	692.5	146.9	335.6
Overall average	90.3	630.8	706.7	474.8
LSD (0.05)	237.2	746.4	604.9	320.3

protein maize (QPM), its high lysine counterpart, also homozygous o_2o_2 but with vitreous endosperm.[32,42]

17.6 EVALUATION OF INBREDS IN HYBRIDS

The breeding value of inbreds is estimated in hybrid combinations across locations. We emphasize the evaluation and selection of inbreds based on their combining abilities and their performance in hybrids. To reduce aflatoxin in corn, in addition to selecting germplasm that is consistently resistant across environments, it is also important to select inbreds with good expression of resistance across hybrid combinations; that is, inbreds that transmit resistant factors to the hybrids in a stable manner across genetic backgrounds should be selected. In the same way that multiyear and multilocation evaluation permits the identification of lines with the most consistent resistance, the evaluation of inbreds in multiple hybrid combinations facilitates the

TABLE 17.4

Aflatoxin Content of Quality Protein Maize (QPM) Hybrids and Commercial Checks at Three Texas Locations and Across Locations in 2002 Season Under Inoculation

| Maize | Aflatoxin Content (ng/g) | | | |
	Weslaco	College Station	Corpus Christi	Average Across Locations
QPM hybrids				
TxXQ69-B5-4 × Tx804	66.1	0.0	116.7	50.8
TxXQ69-B4-11 × Tx804	11.2	10.7	130.0	58.2
TxXQ69-B5-7 × Tx804	88.1	42.2	110.0	74.9
TxXQ69-B6-8 × Tx804	82.8	6.3	163.3	76.8
CML161 × CML170	43.4	0.6	193.3	77.3
Commercial checks				
P31B13	551.9	65.6	376.7	324.1
P32R25	108.8	43.9	500.0	212.7
RX897	307.5	156.3	286.7	247.8
DK668	692.0	7.4	346.7	352.0
Average (60 entries)	326.6	105.7	596.9	343.1
LSD (0.05)	410.6	158.6	782.4	356.7

selection of least susceptible inbreds across hybrid combinations. Following are brief summaries of our efforts in the evaluation of hybrids for aflatoxin.

17.6.1 WHITE HYBRIDS

Significant differences among the hybrids were detected in all locations. The average aflatoxin in 2001 was 126.9 ng/g at College Station, 872.7 ng/g at Corpus Christi, and 487.9 ng/g at Weslaco (Table 17.5).[31] Hybrid CML269 × CML176 was the least susceptible and most consistent hybrid across locations. Commercial checks and hybrids with Tx114 and Tx110 were among the most susceptible hybrids. The average aflatoxin in 2002 was 192.2 ng/g at Weslaco and 9.8 ng/g at College Station. At College Station, the colonized kernels inoculation technique was used, but in this environment the levels of aflatoxin were too low to differentiate among the hybrids. Tx114 hybrids were still susceptible under these conditions. At Weslaco, the hybrids with the lowest aflatoxin were CML269 × CML176 and CML78 × CML269.

17.6.2 YELLOW HYBRIDS

Significant differences among the hybrids were detected in all locations, except in College Station in 2002, where we used the colonized kernels inoculation technique. The average aflatoxin in 2001 for yellow hybrids involving subtropical and temperate

TABLE 17.5
Aflatoxin Content and Rank for White Hybrids Evaluated at College Station, Corpus Christi, and Weslaco, TX, in the 2001 to 2002 Seasons Under Inoculation

Hybrid	College Station 2001		Corpus Christi 2001		Weslaco 2001	
	ng/g	Rank	ng/g	Rank	ng/g	Rank
CML269 × CML176	35.0	6	133.3	1	73.0	1
CML269 × Tx807	73.5	10	333.3	7	320.5	10
CML269 × CML384	45.3	3	156.7	3	399.5	17
CML384 × CML176	156.3	25	210.0	4	205.0	3
Tx807 × Mp313E	106.5	15	136.7	2	750.0	26
CML322 × Tex6	23.0	1	1326.7	25	290.0	9
Commercial Checks						
P32H39 Pioneer	74.5	12	440.0	12	380.0	14
RX901W Asgrow	82.3	11	363.3	8	580.0	25
RX921W Asgrow	117.3	20	4800.0	30	383.5	15
Average (30 entries)	126.9		872.7		487.9	
LSD (0.05)	157.5		378.9		569.0	

Hybrid	Weslaco 2002		Corpus Christi 2002	
	ng/g	Rank	ng/g	Rank
CML269 × CML176	0.0	1	25.6	2
CML78 × CML269	10.9	2	72.2	7
CML311 × CML176	39.4	7	47.3	3
CML78 × CML176	19.9	4	93.2	6
Tx114 × CML176	104.9	14	78.6	5
Tx807 × CML176	22.1	5	130.3	11
Commercial Checks				
P30G54 Pioneer	817.2	30	422.0	21
1851W Wilson	163.2	19	225.0	17
RX949W Asgrow	81.6	10	611.2	26
RX951W Asgrow	16.5	3	438.1	22
1910W	165.2	20	93.4	9
Average (30 entries)	192.2		319.6	
LSD (0.05)	429.6		356.2	

lines was 131.5 ng/g at College Station, 530.7 ng/g at Weslaco, and 1682.2 ng/g at Corpus Christi.[39] The responses of hybrids at Weslaco and Corpus Christi in 2001 were different, as illustrated by the different rankings. The least susceptible hybrids at Weslaco were Tx601Y × NC300 and CML161 × CML170; at Corpus Christi, the commercial checks DK668 and RX889. The average aflatoxin in 2002 was 20.4

TABLE 17.6

Aflatoxin Content for Less Susceptible Yellow Hybrids Evaluated in Two Texas Locations in the 2002 and 2003 Seasons Under Inoculation

Weslaco 2002		Corpus Christi 2002	
Hybrid	Aflatoxin (ng/g)	Hybrid	Aflatoxin (ng/g)
CML323 × NC300	9.8	FR2128 × NC300	112.3
CML323 × CML288	11.5	NC300 × CML288	181.8
FR2128 × NC300	16.5	CML288 × CML285	212.7
(LH235 × 236) × CML288	33.4	Tx770 × CML288	255.9
(LH235 × 236) × CML285	34.3	(235×236) × CML288	332.7
Commercial Checks			
P31B13	1200.0	P31B13	2570.0
P32R25	413.7	P32R25	724.7
RX897	100.7	RX897	628.3
DK687	634.4	DK687	212.8
Average (30 entries)	220.1		925.0
Maximum	1200.0		2852.6
LSD (0.05)	335.2		1363.3

Weslaco 2003		Corpus Christi 2003	
Hybrid	Aflatoxin (ng/g)	Hybrid	Aflatoxin (ng/g)
FR2128 × NC300	4.7	CML338 × Tx772	9.5
CML338 × NC300	33.7	B104 × Tx772	11.9
FR2128 × CML288	37.6	LH195 × Tx772	17.6
Tx770 × Tx745	41.9	Tx772 × CML288	20.5
CML323 × CML288	43.3	NC300 × Tx745	23.6
Commercial Checks			
P31B13	338.0	P31B13	506.7
P32R25	168.0	P32R25	576.7
RX897	50.6	RX897	156.9
DK668	90.6	DK668	154.0
Average (45 entries)	217.5		186.8
Maximum	1373.3		896.7
LSD (0.05)	384.7		318.2

ng/g at College Station, 220.13 ng/g at Weslaco, and 925.0 ng/g at Corpus Christi (Table 17.6). The hybrids with the lowest aflatoxin across locations were FR2128 × NC300, TX770 × CML288, and NC300 × CML288. Average aflatoxin in 2003 was 186.8 ng/g at College Station, 217.49 ng/g at Weslaco, and 40.73 ng/g at Corpus Christi. The least susceptible hybrids were CML338 × Tx772 and B104 × Tx772 at

College Station and FR2128 × NC300 and CML338 × NC300 at Weslaco. Both inoculation techniques were effective to induce aflatoxin, but the levels and ranges were higher with the silk channel inoculation technique than with the colonized kernels inoculation technique. The relative aflatoxin accumulation in hybrids changed substantially with the location and was not consistent. Nevertheless, yellow inbreds such as CML288, NC300, FR2128, CML338, Tx772, and CML161 had less aflatoxin in several hybrids and locations. The less susceptible hybrids to aflatoxin involved subtropical or exotic adapted inbreds with hard endosperm. In general, their hybrids were more resistant to aflatoxin than current commercial hybrids.

17.6.3 TESTCROSSES

As the numbers of lines to be tested at various stages of inbreeding increase over time, their evaluation in all possible hybrid combinations is not feasible; therefore, testcrossing with appropriate testers has been adopted extensively to evaluate the relative combining ability of experimental inbred lines. For example, in 2002, we evaluated 48 inbreds developed in our program in testcrosses with Tx804, a susceptible inbred.[32] The levels of aflatoxin contamination for testcrosses averaged 596.78 ng/g at Corpus Christi, ranging from 268.5 to 2063.2 ng/g; 325.12 ng/g at Weslaco, ranging from 85.2 ng/g to 948.2 ng/g; and 105.72 ng/g at College Station, ranging from 75.4 to 229.5 ng/g. The group of inbreds consistently with the lowest aflatoxin accumulation both in inbreds and testcrosses at all locations originated from CIMMYT Population 69 when compared with other groups and commercials checks. These Population 69 inbreds have flinty endosperm, orange grain color, intermediate maturities, and dark green leaves. The most susceptible hybrids were testcrosses from inbreds developed from CIMMYT Temperate × Tropical High-Oil population and opaque commercial hybrids SR470, SL53, and SR660. Aflatoxin accumulation for standard nonopaque commercial hybrids (293.5 ng/g for P31B13, 223.0 ng/g for P32R25, 250.9 ng/g for Rx897, and 330.4 ng/g for DK668) was higher on average (310.5 ng/g) than for Population 69 (199.4 ng/g) and QPM hybrids (230.6 ng/g).

17.6.4 DIALLELS

Diallel is a mating design commonly used to estimate the general (GCA) and specific combining ability (SCA) effects of inbreds and the relative importance of general and specific combining ability in hybrid performance.[43] Two diallels among six local and exotic white and six yellow maize inbreds were evaluated at three locations in Texas in 2000.[10] White hybrids with low aflatoxin were CML269 × TxX24 and CML269 × CML176. CML269, CML176, and CML322 were the white inbreds with the lowest most consistent aflatoxin in hybrids and had the best GCA for aflatoxin resistance. Yellow hybrids with low aflatoxin were FR2128 × Mp715, Tx772 × Mp715, and Tx772 × CML326. Tx772 and FR2128 had the best GCA for reduced aflatoxin across locations or at specific locations. Tx772 is an Argentine inbred with flinty endosperm and good husk coverage.[44] The most prevalent type of gene action was variable and inconsistent across environments. The relative importance of additive vs. nonadditive effects has been variable depending on the testing environment,

TABLE 17.7

General Combining Ability (GCA) Effect Estimates for Aflatoxin Content of White Food Inbreds at Specific Locations and Across Locations

| | Aflatoxin Content (ng/g) | | | | |
| | College Station | | Weslaco | | Across |
Inbreds	2001	2002	2001	2002	Locations
Tx114	3.5	−93.6	−195.2	149.5	−33.9
Tx130	46.5	164.6	−85.0	48.4	43.6
Tx110	−0.8	−79.4	−511.9	175.4	−104.2
CML78	−48.2	−22.7	−553.9	−139.3	−191.0
CML311	20.4	−31.4	143.4	−90.6	10.4
CML322	−14.5	−126.2	791.8	−68.1	145.7
CML269	−6.8	188.6	410.9	−75.1	129.4
LSD (0.05)	64.7	235.3	225.6	107.6	157.6

method of inoculation, and sampling procedure. In another diallel among elite subtropical (CML311, CML78, CML322) and temperate (Tx114, Tx110, Tx130) white food inbreds, the average aflatoxin was 101.2 ng/g at College Station in 2001, 659.2 ng/g at Weslaco in 2001, and 170.9 ng/g at Weslaco in 2002.[45] The hybrids with the lowest AF across evaluations were Tx110 × CML78, CML269 × Tx110, and CML78 × CML311. Inbreds CML78 and TX110 had the best GCA for reduced aflatoxin (Table 17.7).

17.6.5 FACTORIAL DESIGNS

Factorial designs such as North Carolina II (NCII) permit the evaluation of general and specific combining ability between heterotic groups. Thirteen exotic inbred lines of tropical and subtropical (CML343, CML311, CML269, CML270, CML176, CML322, CML405, T35, T39, Y21, Tx601W) and temperate (NC340, Tx130) origins were crossed following a NCII design with three testers (Tx114, CML78, Tx110) and their single cross combinations (Tx114 × CML78, Tx114 × Tx110, Tx110 × CML78) to generate single crosses (SCs) and three-way crosses (TWCs).[46] The resulting 78 SCs and TWCs and commercial checks (Pioneer Brand P30G54, P32H39, Wilson 1851W, Asgrow hybrids Rx949W and Rx953W) were evaluated in 2003 at College Station and Weslaco under inoculation. Significant differences were found among hybrids for aflatoxin accumulation at single locations and across locations. Hybrid CML176 × CML78 was the least susceptible across locations (35.17 ng/g) and at WE (27.74 ng/g) (Table 17.8). Tropical line CML270 was the least susceptible (102.91 ng/g) in hybrid combinations, followed by CML269 and T35. Among the testers, subtropical line CML78 was the most resistant in SC and TWC hybrids. No differences were observed between SC and TWC for aflatoxin accumulation.

TABLE 17.8

Aflatoxin Content for White Food Single Crosses and Three-Way Crosses Evaluated Under Inoculation Across Texas Locations in 2003

		Aflatoxin Content (ng/g)					
		Single-Cross Hybrids			Three-Way-Cross Hybrids		
Lines	Average Lines	Tx114	CML78	Tx110	CML78 × Tx110	Tx114 × CML78	Tx114 × Tx110
CML343	208.8	293.7	110.2	313.2	198.9	159.3	177.5
CML311	129.1	96.3	95.7	148.8	96.2	121.7	216.2
CML269	106.2	194.4	49.9	67.7	84.8	141.2	99.2
CML270	102.9	60.7	77.6	69.9	112.5	226.3	70.5
CML176	117.4	224.7	35.2	82.8	97.7	69.3	195.0
CML322	203.2	249.5	100.5	375.3	241.9	114.8	137.3
CML405	224.7	227.0	114.9	506.3	63.0	134.3	302.8
NC340	234.8	148.3	134.0	247.5	526.1	269.2	83.8
T35	135.5	79.5	76.2	235.5	131.6	49.0	241.5
T39	144.1	187.8	173.3	48.8	53.3	201.7	199.5
Tx130	243.3	430.0	101.7	93.2	161.7	317.7	355.8
Y21	288.6	148.4	76.3	826.3	91.3	219.2	370.0
Tx601W	202.8	71.5	45.7	153.2	319.9	319.9	307.3
Average testers		185.5	91.6	243.7	167.6	180.3	212.0
LSD (0.05)	96.3						

17.6.6 Generation Mean Analysis

In generation mean analysis (GMA), means of different generations (e.g., P1, P2, F1, F2, BC1P1, BC1P2) are used to estimate genetic effects in a cross between two inbreds. Some of these generations are genetically homogeneous (P1, P2, F1), which helps to determine environmental and error variation, and the remainder are segregating (F2, BC1P1, BC1P2). We have used GMA to characterize and validate the presence of resistant factors in inbreds such as CML176, CML161, and CML269. The average aflatoxin content at Weslaco, TX, in 2003 was 7.7 ng/g for CML176, 303.3 ng/g for Tx114, 28.9 ng/g for F1 hybrid, 64.2 ng/g for the F2 generation, 29.7 ng/g for the BC to CML176, and 100.7 ng/g for the BC to Tx114. The average aflatoxin content was 8.0 ng/g for CML269, 425.0 ng/g for Tx114, 230.7 ng/g for F1 hybrid, 417.7 ng/g for the F2 generation, 293.1 ng/g for the BC to CML269, and 355.6 ng/g for the BC to Tx114. The average aflatoxin content was 40.0 ng/g for CML161, 646.7 ng/g for Tx804, 40.1 ng/g for F1 hybrid, 149.4 ng/g for the F2 generation, 150.3 ng/g for the BC to CML161, and 254.9 ng/g for the BC to Tx804. In all three cases, backcrosses to the most resistant parent were less susceptible than backcrosses to the susceptible parent, which is further evidence of the presence of resistant genetic factors in these lines.

17.6.7 COMMERCIAL HYBRIDS

Field screening of commercial hybrids for aflatoxin vulnerability has been conducted in South Texas under dryland conditions since 1990. Screening was conducted primarily at two Corpus Christi locations differing in potential for drought stress. Experiments were planted late to increase the probability of drought stress, especially from silking to maturity. Inoculation with a high-aflatoxin-producing *Aspergillus flavus* (NRRL3357) was conducted using either the nonwounding silk channel technique or the colonized kernel technique (after 1999). Commercial hybrids varied greatly in their vulnerability to aflatoxin accumulation, especially in years of greater drought stress. Despite year-to-year variability in relative levels of aflatoxin accumulation the hybrids most susceptible and resistant to aflatoxin were among the most consistent in their relative rank among hybrids being evaluated. Hybrids with moderate or conditional vulnerability were more difficult to rank and differentiate because they had similar intermediate aflatoxin accumulation or had variable response across locations and years. Open-husked hybrids, including Mo17 × B73, were more vulnerable to aflatoxin accumulation than tighter husked hybrids, regardless of maturity. The most aflatoxin-susceptible, open-husked hybrids also generally had the highest loss of kernel integrity, including highly visible silk cut. On vulnerable hybrids, silk cut was most common on a normal or higher yield crop exposed to rapidly increasing drought and heat stress after silking. Silk cut was less apparent or mostly absent when early season or season long drought stress affected yield potential and kernel size; however, the same hybrids were still among the most vulnerable to aflatoxin accumulation and had poor kernel quality or other loss of kernel integrity.

Forty mostly commercial, hybrids (110–125 RM) were tested for aflatoxin response in 1994 and 1995 at Corpus Christi and Temple, TX, to determine their relative risk for aflatoxin accumulation at both Texas locations. In 1994, the lowest and highest average aflatoxin values for individual hybrids were 607/3667, 287/2033, 330/3100, and 380/7233 ng/g at the Corpus Christi moderate- and high-drought-stress-potential sites and Temple first and second dates of planting, respectively. In 1995, these aflatoxin values were 550/3700, 727/8067, and 283/3333 ng/g at the Corpus Christi moderate- and high-drought-stress-potential sites and Temple (single planting date), respectively. QPM hybrid Tx807 × Tx811 had the lowest average rank for aflatoxin accumulation across all locations and years. This hybrid also had no detectable silk cut at Corpus Christi in 1995. The most aflatoxin-susceptible hybrid at all locations and years had incidences of silk cut ranging from 17 to 56% of total kernels at Corpus Christi in 1995. The initiation of any loss of kernel integrity in response to drought stress may vary between hybrids and could be an important factor in aflatoxin and other mycotoxin accumulation by harvest. As an example, one of most aflatoxin-resistant hybrids at all sites and years had a surprisingly high incidence of silk cut; however, silk cut was apparently initiated at kernel moistures low enough to preclude visible fungal colonization, and size of the splits was very small. Conversely, the most aflatoxin susceptible hybrid in this test had silk cut initiation at kernel moistures as high as 50% in subsequent years at Corpus Christi. After the mid-1990s, most hybrids highly vulnerable to silk cut were removed from

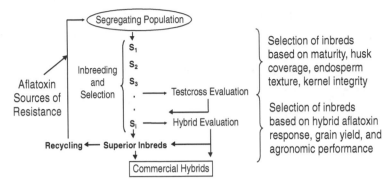

FIGURE 17.7 General scheme for the development of corn inbreds and hybrids resistant or tolerant to aflatoxin with agronomic performance.

the South Texas market; however, some current hybrids develop significant loss of kernel quality and integrity including generally low levels of silk cut under some drought stress environments. No hybrid currently marketed in South Texas is resistant to aflatoxin, and these hybrids vary considerably in their relative vulnerability to aflatoxin accumulation. That aflatoxin variability is not associated with the presence or absence of any transgenic trait although these traits may influence aflatoxin accumulation under some environments.

17.7 OVERVIEW OF DEVELOPMENT OF INBREDS AND HYBRIDS THAT REDUCE THE RISK OF AFLATOXIN

The general process to develop maize hybrids begins with the creation of a source segregating breeding population that is used to develop inbred lines through inbreeding and selection (Figure 17.7). Selected inbreds are then evaluated in hybrid combinations across locations to select superior hybrids and to estimate their combining abilities. This process presents opportunities to select inbreds that reduce aflatoxin and have good yield potential and agronomic performance. Source populations can be created by hybridization of inbreds that carry resistant factors to aflatoxin with elite lines that have adaptation and agronomic performance. We use multiparent crosses among temperate-adapted inbreds and exotic subtropical and tropical resistant inbreds. During the first generation of inbreeding (S_1 to S_4), traits associated with aflatoxin resistance that show high heritabilities and are easy to measure are used to select a reduced number of inbreds for testcross performance. Some of these traits are husk coverage, maturity, synchrony between silking and pollen shed, kernel integrity, endosperm hardness, and visual incidence of ear rot. Additional attention is devoted to agronomic traits, such as standability, plant morphology (low ear placement, erect leaves), stay-green, and plant vigor. The selected fraction of S_4 inbreds possessing the desirable traits are evaluated in testcrosses with representative testers for the heterotic groups commonly used in the United States, stiff stalk synthetic (SSS) and non-stiff stalk synthetic (NSSS). These testers are elite lines commonly used in commercial hybrid production susceptible to aflatoxin (e.g., currently we are using LH195 and LH210 as the SSS and NSSS testers, respectively). Testcrosses are evaluated in few representative locations for grain yield and agronomic performance. The best testcrosses are reevaluated for aflatoxin response under inoculation and drought stress. The parental inbreds of less susceptible testcrosses are then crossed with more testers from the opposite heterotic group, and the resulting hybrids are evaluated in multiple locations, including evaluations for aflatoxin response. This extensive wide area evaluation permits hybrid selection for adaptation, yield potential, stability, and reduced aflatoxin risk. Environments are representative of the most common farmer field conditions. The most resistant SS and NSS lines with desirable agronomic performance are advanced for further evaluation and characterization (e.g., mating designs and QTL mapping). By transferring complementary aflatoxin resistance mechanisms to different heterotic groups, we can pyramid them in SS × NSS hybrid combinations.

17.8 CONCLUSIONS AND CURRENT DIRECTIONS

Experimental screening techniques and inoculation have facilitated the display of genetic differences and increased heritability in aflatoxin evaluations. The response of inbreds to aflatoxin accumulation varies, depending upon the environment and the genetic background; therefore, their evaluation in several hybrid combinations and multiple environments under inoculation is necessary to identify the most consistent resistant germplasm. It seems plausible to select for associated traits having high heritabilities and strong correlation with low aflatoxin, in addition to low aflatoxin accumulation in inbreds and hybrids to reduce the risk of aflatoxin contamination. Low aflatoxin accumulation was associated with good husk coverage, flinty endosperm texture, good kernel integrity, high grain yield, and late maturities. The less susceptible inbreds in hybrids across evaluations in Texas have been CML176, CML269, and Tx807 among the whites and CML288, Tx772, CML161, Tx69Q's, FR2128, and NC300 among the yellows.

Exotic inbreds constitute a reservoir of alleles and allele combinations for aflatoxin resistance that, once identified, can be used in plant breeding in the United States; therefore, we are continuing our effort to introduce exotic germplasm and evaluate and select it for response to aflatoxin under the environmental conditions of Texas (Figure 17.8). After field confirmation of resistance, we characterize the resistance factors present in these sources through mating designs and genetic mapping. Currently, we have an ongoing research project to identify QTL for genetic resistance factors present in inbreds CML176, CML161, CML269, and Tx772. Marker-assisted selection can be used to introgress specific genomic regions containing genes for resistance and to recover progenies carrying the desired genomic regions in elite backgrounds. Molecular markers can also help to increase the probability of recovering transgressive segregants in crosses between inbreds carrying different resistant factors and to reduce number of seasons by selecting in off seasons nurseries. Our ultimate goal is to combine aflatoxin resistant factors with yield potential and agronomic performance.

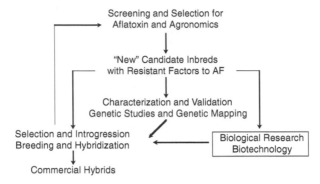

FIGURE 17.8 General flow of activities at the aflatoxin research program at Texas A&M University.

ACKNOWLEDGMENTS

We thank the personnel at the Research Station in Weslaco and Corpus Christi for their assistance conducting the aflatoxin trials. This research has been funded by the Texas Corn Producers Board and USDA–ARS competitive grants.

REFERENCES

1. Castegnaro, M. and McGregor, D., Carcinogenic risk assessment of mycotoxins, *Rev. Med. Vet.*, 149, 671–678, 1998.
2. Widstrom, N.W., The aflatoxin problem with corn grain, *Adv. Agron.*, 56, 219–280, 1996.
3. Cardwell, K., Scientists weigh costs of mycotoxin-contaminated crops, *CSANews*, 46(10), 2001.
4. CAST, *Mycotoxins: Risks in Plant, Animal and Human Systems*, Technology Report No. 139, Council on Agricultural Science and Technology, Ames, IA, 2003.
5. Brown, R., Bhatnagar, D., Cleveland, T.E., and Cary J.W., Recent advances in preharvest prevention of mycotoxin contamination, in *Mycotoxins in Agriculture and Food Safety*, Sinha, K.K. and Bhatnagar, D., Eds., Marcel Dekker, New York, 1998, pp. 351–379.
6. Widstrom, N.W., Breeding strategies to control aflatoxin contamination of maize through host plant resistance. in *Aflatoxin in Maize: Proceedings of the Workshop*, Zuber, M.S., Lillehoj, E.B., and Renfro, B.L., Ed., CIMMYT, Mexico, 1987, pp. 212–220.
7. Widstrom, N.W., McMillian W.W., and Wilson, D.M., Segregation for resistance to aflatoxin contamination among seeds on an ear of hybrid maize, *Crop Sci.*, 27, 961–963, 1987.
8. Scott, G.E. and Zummo, N., Sources of resistance in maize to kernel infection by *Aspergillus flavus* in the field, *Crop Sci.*, 28, 504–507, 1988.
9. Campbell K.W. and White D.G., Evaluation of corn genotypes for resistance to *Aspergillus* ear rot, kernel infection, and aflatoxin production, *Plant Dis.*, 79, 1039–1042, 1995.
10. Betrán, F.J., Isakeit, T., and Odvody, G., Aflatoxin accumulation of white and yellow maize inbreds in diallel crosses, *Crop Sci.*, 42, 1894–1901, 2002.
11. Scott, G.E. and Zummo, N., Registration of Mp313E germplasm line of maize, *Crop Sci.*, 30, 1378, 1990.

12. Scott, G.E. and Zummo, N., Registration of Mp420 germplasm line of maize, *Crop Sci.*, 32, 1296, 1992.

13. Williams, W.P. and Windham, G.L., Registration of Mp715 maize germplasm line, *Crop Sci.*, 41, 1374, 2002.

14. McMillian, W.W., Widstrom, N.W., and Wilson, D.M., Registration of GT-MAS:gk maize germplasm, *Crop Sci.*, 33, 882, 1993.

15. Zummo, N. and Scott, G.E., Evaluation of field inoculation techniques for screening maize genotypes against kernel infection by *Aspergillus flavus* in Mississippi, *Plant Dis.*, 73, 313–316, 1989.

16. Zeringue, Jr., H.J., Identification and effects of maize silk volatiles on cultures of *Aspergillus flavus*, *J. Agric. Food Chem.*, 48, 921–925, 2000.

17. Patterson, H.D. and Williams, E.R., A new class of resolvable incomplete block designs, *Biometrika*, 63, 83–89, 1976.

18. Cullis, B.R. and Gleeson, A.C., Spatial analysis of field experiments: an extension to two dimensions, *Biometrics*, 47, 1449–1460, 1991.

19. Gilmour, A.R., Cullis, B.R., and Verbyla, A.P., Accounting for natural and extraneous variation in the analysis of field experiments, *J. Agric. Biol. Env. Stat.*, 2, 269–293, 1997.

20. Edwards, M.L., Mayfield, K., Isakeit, T., Odvody, G., and Betrán, F.J., Repeatability of aflatoxin trials in white and yellow maize, in *Annual Meetings Abstracts* (CD-ROM), American Society of Agronomy, Madison, WI, 2003.

21. Betrán, F.J., Bänziger, M., and Menz, M., Corn breeding, in *Corn: Origin, History, Technology, and Production*, Smith, W., Betrán, F.J., and Runge, E., Eds., John Wiley & Sons, New York, 2004.

22. Betrán, F.J., Isakeit, T., Odvody, G., and Mayfield, K., Maize germplasm evaluation for aflatoxin resistance in Texas, *Mycopathologia*, 155, 81, 2002.

23. Odvody, G.N., Spencer, N., and Remmers, J., A description of silk cut, a stress-related loss of kernel integrity in preharvest maize, *Plant Dis.*, 81, 439–444, 1997.

24. Betrán, F.J. and Isakeit, T., Aflatoxin contamination in maize hybrids with different maturities, *Agron. J.*, 96, 565–570, 2004.

25. Guo, B.Z., Russin, J.S., Cleveland, T.E., Brown, R.L., and Widstrom, N.W., Wax and cutin layers in maize kernels associated with resistance to aflatoxin production by *Aspergillus flavus*, *J. Food Prot.*, 58, 296–300, 1995.

26. Guo, B.Z., Widstrom, N.W., Holbrook, C.C., Lee, R.D., and Lynch, R.E., Molecular genetic analysis of resistance mechanisms to aflatoxin formation in corn and peanut, *Mycopathologia*, 155, 78, 2001.

27. Payne, G.A., Aflatoxin in maize, *CRC Crit. Rev. Plant Sci.*, 10, 423–440, 1992.

28. McMilliam, W.W., Wilson, D.M., and Widstrom, N.W., Aflatoxin contamination of preharvest corn in Georgia: a six-year study of insect damage and visible *Aspergillus flavus*, *J. Environ. Qual.*, 14, 200–202, 1985.

29. Windham, G.L., Williams, W.P., and Davis, F.M., Effects of the southwestern corn borer on *Aspergillus flavus* kernel infection and aflatoxin accumulation in maize hybrids, *Plant. Dis.*, 83, 535–540, 1999.

30. Brown, R.L., Cleveland, T.E., Chen, Z., Gembeh, S.V., Menkir, A., Moore, S., Jeffers, D., Damann, K.E., and Bhatnagar, D., The identification of maize kernel resistance traits through comparative evaluation of aflatoxin-resistant with susceptible germplasm, *Mypathologia*, 155, 77, 2001.

31. Betrán, F.J., Isakeit, T., Transue, D., Mayfield, K., Bhatnagar, S., Makumbi, D., Ganunga, R., and Pietsch, D., Response of white food corn to aflatoxin contamination, *Mycopathologia*, 157, 495, 2004.

32. Betrán, F.J., Isakeit, T., Odvody, G., Bhatnagar, S., and Mayfield, K., Aflatoxin accumulation and associated traits in maize inbreds and their testcrosses, in *Proc. Aflatoxin/Fumonisin Workshop*, Savannah, GA, October 13–15, 2003.

33. Widstrom, N.W. An evaluation of methods for measuring corn earworm injury, *J. Econ. Entomol.*, 60, 791–794, 1967.

34. Beck, D., Betrán, F.J., Bänziger, M. et al., Progress in developing drought and low soil nitrogen tolerance in maize, in *Proc. 51st Annual Corn and Sorghum Seed Research Conference*, American Seed Trade Association, Washington, D.C., 1997.

35. Edmeades, G.O., Bolaños, J., Chapman, S.C., Lafitte, H.R., and Bänziger, M., Selection improves drought tolerance in tropical maize populations. I. Gains in biomass, grain yield, and harvest index, *Crop Sci.*, 39, 1306–1315, 1999.

36. Ribaut J.-M., Bänziger, M., Betrán, F.J., Jiang, C., Edmeades, G.O., Dreher, K., and Hoisington, H., Use of molecular markers in plant breeding: drought tolerance improvement in tropical maize, in *Quantitative Genetics, Genomics, and Plant Breeding*, Manjit, S.K., Ed., CABI, Wallingford, 2002.

37. Bolaños, J. and Edmeades, G.O., The importance of the anthesis-silking interval in breeding for drought tolerance in tropical maize, *Field Crops Res.*, 48, 65–80, 1996.

38. Betrán, F.J., Beck, D., Edmeades, G.O., and Bänziger, M., Secondary traits in parental inbreds and hybrids under stress and non-stress environments in tropical maize, *Field Crops Res.*, 83, 51–65, 2003.

39. Mayfield, K., Jones, B., Lutz, L., Blackwelder, A., Isakeit, T., Odvody, G., and Betrán, F.J., Aflatoxin accumulation in maize inbreds and hybrids, in *Proc. Aflatoxin and Fumonisin Workshop*, Savannah, GA, October 13–15, 2003.

40. Bhatnagar, S., Betrán, F.J., and Transue, D., Agronomic performance, aflatoxin accumulation and protein quality of subtropical and tropical QPM hybrids in southern USA, *Maydica*, 48, 113–124, 2003.

41. Vasal S.K., High quality protein corn, in *Specialty Corns*, Hallauer, A.R., Ed., CRC Press, Boca Raton, FL, 2001, pp. 85–129.

42. Nielsen, K., Kirst, M., Payne, G., and Boston, R., Protection of kernels from infection by *A. flavus* is reduced in Opaque 2 maize, in *Proc. of the Aflatoxin and Fumonisin Workshop*, San Antonio, TX, October 23–25, 2002.

43. Baker R.J. Issues in diallel analysis, *Crop Sci.*, 18, 533–536 1978.

44. Llorente, C.F., Betrán, F.J., Bockholt, A., and Fojt III, F., Registration of Tx772, *Crop Sci.*, 44, 1036, 2003.

45. Transue, D.K., Bhatnagar, S., Mayfield, K., and Betrán, F.J., Diallel analysis among temperate and subtropical white inbred testers: agronomic performance, heterotic response, and aflatoxin accumulation, in *Annual Meetings Abstracts* (CD-ROM), American Society of Agronomy, Madison, WI, 2003.

46. Maideni, F., Magorokosho, C., Ganunga, R., Makumbi, D., Mayfield, K., and Betrán, F.J., Comparative performance of single and three-way white maize hybrids, in *Annual Meetings Abstracts* (CD-ROM), American Society of Agronomy, Madison, WI, 2003.

18 Enhancing Maize with Resistance to *Aspergillus flavus* Infection and Aflatoxin Accumulation

W. Paul Williams, Gary L. Windham, and Paul M. Buckley

CONTENTS

18.1 INTRODUCTION

Preharvest kernel infection by *Aspergillus flavus* Link:Fries and the subsequent accumulation of aflatoxin in maize, *Zea mays* L., grain were first recognized as a major problem in the southeastern United States during the 1970s.[1–6] Aflatoxin contamination reached high levels in 1977. A field survey conducted in Georgia indicated that aflatoxin levels exceeded 20 ng/g in 90% of the samples evaluated.[7] Maize grain with aflatoxin levels exceeding 20 ng/g is banned from interstate commerce, and over 90% of the maize grown in the Southeast in 1977 was contaminated with aflatoxin.[8] Aflatoxin levels in many samples exceeded 1000 ng/g. Although aflatoxin has remained a chronic problem in the Southeast, it has tended to be more localized in most years.[9,10] Not until 1998 did aflatoxin contamination reach levels comparable to those attained in 1977.[11,12] Losses to aflatoxin-contaminated maize in Arkansas, Louisiana, Mississippi, and Texas were estimated at $85,000,000. Differences in aflatoxin contamination from year to year and among locations have frequently been attributed to variations in weather-related factors and differences in insect feeding.[13-17] High temperatures and drought stress have shown the most consistent associations with high levels of aflatoxin contamination.[9,11-13] Differences among hybrids have also contributed to variations in aflatoxin levels.[3,11,14]

18.2 ESTABLISHING A BREEDING PROGRAM AT MISSISSIPPI STATE

The heightened awareness in the 1970s of preharvest aflatoxin contamination in maize led to the initiation of several research programs that addressed the problem. One such program was initiated by USDA–ARS at Mississippi State, MS, under the leadership of Gene E. Scott. The primary objective of this research program was to identify, develop, and release maize germplasm with resistance to aflatoxin contamination. Growing aflatoxin-resistant hybrids was generally considered to be the most practical method for reducing or eliminating contamination of maize grain.

18.2.1 DEVELOPING GERMPLASM EVALUATION TECHNIQUES

One of the first challenges confronting Scott and his coworkers was determining how to quantify resistance to *Aspergillus flavus* infection and aflatoxin accumulation. King and Scott[18] evaluated two kernel wounding techniques and two nonwounding techniques to inoculate developing ears 20 days after midsilk with an *A. flavus* conidia suspension. Ears were harvested 40 days later, and kernels that did not exhibit physical damage were assayed for *A. flavus* infection. Inoculations made with a pinbar, a single 100-mm-long row of 35 sewing pins mounted in a plastic bar, resulted in higher levels of infection and better differentiation among hybrids than the other techniques. The pinbar was adopted as the standard inoculation technique for germplasm screening; however, comparisons between the pinbar and other techniques continued.[19,20] During the 1980s, susceptibility to *A. flavus* was measured as the percentage of infected kernels because analyzing grain samples for aflatoxin content was too expensive using methods available at that time. The availability of the Vicam AflaTest® (Watertown, MA) permitted aflatoxin analysis on a scale necessary for germplasm screening. With the transition from quantifying resistance by determining kernel infection to analyzing grain samples for aflatoxin content, the side-needle technique replaced the pinbar technique for inoculating ears.[20] With this technique, a spore suspension is injected underneath the husk with a tree-marking gun fitted with a 14-gauge hypodermic needle. Unlike with the pinbar technique, few kernels, if any, are damaged with the side-needle technique.

18.2.2 IDENTIFYING AFLATOXIN-RESISTANT GERMPLASM

Using the pinbar and other inoculation techniques, numerous maize genotypes were screened for resistance to *Aspergillus flavus* kernel infection during the 1980s.[21,22] The release in 1988 of Mp313E, a line developed from "Tuxpan," marked the first release of a maize germplasm line as a source of resistance to *A. flavus*.[23] A second germplasm line, Mp420, derived from "Yellow Mosby" and "Hill Yellow Dent," was released in 1991.[24]

18.3 CURRENT EFFORTS TO IDENTIFY NEW SOURCES OF RESISTANCE

New sources of resistance are essential for a breeding program with the objective of developing and releasing aflatoxin resistant germplasm. The search for maize germplasm with resistance to aflatoxin contamination continues at Mississippi State. Germplasm accessions that had not previously been evaluated for aflatoxin contamination were obtained through the germplasm enhancement of maize (GEM) project and the International Maize and Wheat Improvement Center (CIMMYT) in 2001. These accessions were evaluated to identify potentially useful sources of resistance.

18.3.1 MATERIALS AND METHODS

Sixty-two germplasm accessions obtained through the GEM project together with aflatoxin-resistant and susceptible genotypes were grown in a randomized complete block design with three replications. Nineteen accessions obtained through CIM-MYT were grown in a randomized complete block design with two replications. Both experiments were planted April 20, 2001, at the Plant Science Research Center at Mississippi State University. Each plot consisted of a single row with 20 plants. Rows were 4 m long and spaced 1 m apart. Blocks were bordered on each side with two rows of a commercial maize hybrid. Beginning when silks had emerged from 50% of the ears of the earliest maturing plots, all plants were inoculated with a spore suspension containing 9×10^7 *Aspergillus flavus* conidia per milliliter and a spreader sticker (Hi-Yield Chemical Co.; Bonham, TX). The suspension was applied to the silks and husks of the top ear of each plant weekly for 5 weeks using a backpack sprayer (Solo; Newport News, VA). *A. flavus* isolate NRRL3357, which is known to produce aflatoxin in corn, was used in preparing the inoculum.[25,26] The top ear from each plant in a plot was hand harvested approximately 60 days after the initial *A. flavus* inoculation. Ears were dried at 38°C for 7 days before shelling. The grain was mixed by pouring through a sample splitter twice and then ground using a Romer mill (Union, MO). Aflatoxin contamination was determined in a 50-g subsample from each plot by the Vicam AflaTest®. Plot means for aflatoxin contamination were used in an analysis of variance. To equalize variances, data were transformed by adding 1 and taking the logarithm of each number (log[y+1]) prior to statistical analysis. Means were compared by Fisher's protected least significant difference (LSD) test ($p = 0.05$).

18.3.2 RESULTS AND DISCUSSION

Aflatoxin levels ranged from a low of 4 ng/g for a resistant single cross, Mp716 × Mp92:673, to 4236 ng/g for B73, a susceptible inbred line (Table 18.1). Aflatoxin level for Mp92:673, a line selected for resistance to aflatoxin contamination, was 53 ng/g. Aflatoxin contamination is generally higher for inbred lines than for the more vigorous single crosses. This is illustrated by B73 × Mo17 and its parental inbreds. Aflatoxin levels were 4236, 1218, and 605 ng/g for B73, Mo17, and B73 × Mo17, respectively. Although aflatoxin contamination was high for most of the GEM accessions, 8 accessions did not differ significantly from the resistant check, Mp92:673. These will be evaluated further. Those that continue to exhibit resistance to aflatoxin contamination will be incorporated into the breeding program. The results of the evaluations of the 19 genotypes obtained from the CIMMYT breeding program are given in Table 18.2. Some of these genotypes had shown some indication of resistance to ear molds in CIMMYT trials although they had not been evaluated for resistance to aflatoxin contamination. The level of resistance in this group of genotypes was quite high. Four genotypes exhibited aflatoxin levels less than 20 ng/g. On the other hand, the genotypes MBR-ET White F2-202-2-3-X-B-B-#-# and MBR-ET White F2-113-2-1-X-B-B-# exhibited high levels of contamination. The genotypes that exhibited the lowest levels of contamination will be further evaluated. Locating and identifying germplasm that will provide new sources of resistance are critical to our breeding program. Unfortunately, most of the germplasm that we evaluate has little resistance to aflatoxin contamination. During our initial evaluations, our intent was to eliminate many of the susceptible genotypes as efficiently as possible; therefore, we generally plant only two or three replications for our initial evaluations. In the successive evaluations, we generally plant at least five replications. It is in these evaluations that we differentiate between susceptible escapes and genotypes that are resistant to aflatoxin contamination.

18.4 EVALUATION OF INBRED LINES AND ADVANCED BREEDING LINES

A primary objective of our research program is to develop and release germplasm lines with resistance to aflatoxin contamination. It seems expedient, then, to evaluate germplasm lines that were selected for attributes other than resistance to aflatoxin contamination as well. These lines have generally been developed as a result of considerable time and expense. Because the lines are already highly inbred, any lines that exhibit resistance to aflatoxin contamination would be quite valuable.

18.4.1 MATERIALS AND METHODS

A group of inbred lines that were developed in Mississippi during the 1940s and 1950s were evaluated for aflatoxin contamination at Mississippi State in 2000. A group of advanced breeding lines that were developed primarily for resistance to

TABLE 18.1
Aflatoxin Accumulation in Germplasm Accessions from the GEM Project Grown at Mississippi State in 2001 and Inoculated by Spraying an *Aspergillus flavus* Spore Suspension on Developing Ears

Genotype	Aflatoxin (ng/g)	Genotype	Aflatoxin (ng/g)
B73	4236a	CHO5015:N15-44-1-B-B	680d–o
FS8B(T):N1802-32-1-B-B	3768ab	CHO5015:N15-169-1-B-B	672d–o
CHO5015:N12-50-1-B-B	3474a–c	CHO5015:N15-182-1-B-B	672d–o
CHO5015:N12-92-1-B-B	2951a–d	CUBA164:S2008a-23-1-B-B	637e–o
CHO5015:N15-166-1-B-B	2156a–e	CHO5015:N12-183-1-B-B-S1B	611e–o
CHO5015:N15-87-1-B-B	2134a–e	B73 × Mo17	605e–o
DREP150:N2011d-13-1-B-B	1780a–e	CHO5015:N12-36-1-B-B	583e–o
FS8B(T):N1802-45-1-1S1B-B-B	1722a–f	CHO5015:N12-140-1-B-B	571e–o
CHO5015:N15-183-1-B-B	1650a–g	CHO5015:N12-102-1-B-B	553e–o
CHO5015:N12-84-1-B-B	1588a–g	CHO5015:N12-99-1-B-B	550e–p
CHO5015:N15-8-1-B-B	1560a–g	UR13085:NO215-21-1-B-B	528e–p
CHO5015:N12-20-1-B-B	1400a–h	DKXL370:N11a20-2-1-B-B	509e–p
CHO5015:N12-49-1-B-B	1316a–i	CHO5015:N12-13-1-B-B	501e–p
CHIS775:S1911b-16-1-1-B	1231a–i	CHO5015:N15-162-1-B-B	424f–p
Mo17	1218a–i	CHO5015:N12-18-1-B-B	418f–p
CHO5015:N12-145-1-B-B	1109a–j	CHO5015:N15-143-1-B-B	405f–p
CHO5015:N12-26-1-B-B	1108a–j	CHO5015:N15-98-1-B-B	393f–p
UR13085:N0215-14-1-B-B	1096a–j	CHO5015:N12-38-1-B-B	383g–p
CHO5015:N15-149-1-B-B	1045a–k	CUBA164:S2008a-6-1-B-B	377g–p
CHO5015:N12-33-1-B-B	1039a–k	CHO5015:N15-3-1-B-B	338h–q
UR13085:N0215-3-1-B-B	1023a–k	CHO5015:N12-12-1-B-B	333h–q
CHO5015:N12-61-1-B-B	1003a–l	CHO5015:N12-130-1-B-B	324h–q
CHO5015:N12-79-1-B-B	986a–l	CHO5015:N12-37-1-B-B	310i–q
CHO5015:N12-94-1-B-B	972a–m	GA209 × SC212m	258j–q
CHO5015:N15-82-1-B-B	946b–n	FS8B(T):N1802-36-1-B-B	240k–r
DKXL370:N11a20-31-1-B-B	900b–n	UR13085:N0215-2-1-B-B	225l–r
CHO5015:N15-101-1-B-B	868b–n	CHO5015:N12-131-1-B-B	218m–r
FS8B(T):N1802-35-1-B-B	855b–o	CHO5015:N12-147-1-B-B	216n–r
DK212T:S0610-14-1-B-B	804c–o	CHO5015:N12-32-1-B-B-S1B	214n–r
CHO5015:N12-126-1-B-B	796c–o	CHO5015:N12-7-1-B-B	191o–r
CHO5015:N15-184-1-B-B	772d–o	UR13085:N0215-11-1-B-B	117p–r
CHO5015:N12-21-1-B-B	738d–o	CHO5015:N12-43-1-B-B	79qr
CHO5015:N12-123-1-B-B	722d–o	Mp92:673	53r

Note: Means followed by the same letter do not differ at $p = 0.05$. Tests of significance were performed on transformed [$\log(y+1)$] means using Fisher's protected LSD before converting values back to the original scale.

TABLE 18.2

Aflatoxin Accumulation in Germplasm Accessions Obtained from CIMMYT, Grown at Mississippi State in 2001, and Inoculated by Spraying an *Aspergillus flavus* Spore Suspension on Developing Ears

Genotype	Aflatoxin (ng/g)
MBR-ETWhiteF2-202-2-3-X-B-B-#-#	1566a
MBR-ETWhiteF2-113-2-1-X-B-B-#	900ab
MBR-ETWhiteF2-147-2-3-X-B-B-#-B-#	388a–c
DERRC215-3-1-#2-1##-##	379a–c
SAMTSR-76-1-1-B-1-B-B-B-B-5-##-B10	259a–c
MBR-ETWhiteF2-96-1-2-X-B-B-#-B-#	236a–c
MBR-ETWhiteF2-263-1-1-X-B-B-#-#	166a–d
MBR-ETWhiteF2-176-4-2-X-B-B-#-B-#	147a–d
(P36STE-28*36STE-38)BBB-###-B8	125b–d
CML175-B-BP68Qc1HC77-2-3-7-B-2-3-1-B-1-B*6	113b–d
MBR-ETWhiteF2-261-1-2-X-B-B-#B-#	84b–e
(6304Q/6303Q)-xb-6-1-3-3-B-B-B	57c–e
6206Q-10-xb-3-2-B-B-B	56c–e
P22STEC2-11-B14	46c–f
CML155P62c3HC163-2-1-3#-1-1-1-1-B-1-B-B-#-B-B	40c–f
(CAFS113-2F1)x(CAFS82-1-4)-2-#2-3-2-1-#-#-#	17d–g
MBR-ETWhiteF2-112-1-1-X-B-B-#-B-#	9e–g
P25C5HC246-3-1-BB-2-#-B10	4fg
DERRC215-7-1-#2-1##-##	1g

Note: Means followed by the same letter do not differ at $p = 0.05$. Tests of significance were performed on transformed means [$\log(y+1)$] using Fisher's protected LSD before converting values back to the original scale.

southwestern corn borer and fall armyworm were evaluated for resistance to aflatoxin contamination in 2001. Each year lines were grown in single row plots of 20 plants that were planted in a randomized complete block design with five replications. In 2000, the experiment was planted on April 21. In 2001, the experiment was planted April 20. The side-needle inoculation technique was used for both experiments.[20] The top ear of each plant in a plot was inoculated approximately 14 days after silks had emerged from 50% of the plants in the plot. *Aspergillus flavus* isolate NRRL3357 was used as inoculum both years. Inoculum was prepared as described by Windham and Williams.[11] The top ears from each plant in a plot were harvested 60 days after midsilk. Aflatoxin and data analyses were performed as previously described.

TABLE 18.3
Aflatoxin Accumulation in Mississippi Inbred Lines
Inoculated with an *Aspergillus flavus* Spore Suspension Using
the Side-Needle Technique at Mississippi State in 2000

Inbred Line	Aflatoxin (ng/g)	Inbred Line	Aflatoxin (ng/g)
Mp319	2565a	Mp305	554c–e
Mp331	2468a	Mp496	517c–e
Mp460	2192a	Mp1	490c–e
Mp448	1899a	Mp307	480c–e
Mp416	1841a	Mp440	479c–e
Mp412	1776a	Mp424	415de
Mp351	1755a	Mp337	376de
Mp428	1623ab	Mp408	357de
Mp339	1384a–c	Mp492	271e
Mp420	1021a–d	Mp462	258e
Mp333	995a–d	Mp410	247e
Mp488	586b–e	Mp482	209e

Note: Means followed by the same letter do not differ at $p = 0.05$. Tests of significance were performed on transformed mean [log(y+1)] using Fisher's protected LSD.

18.4.2 RESULTS AND DISCUSSION

The results of the evaluation of the older Mississippi inbred lines are presented in Table 18.3. Aflatoxin levels were relatively high for all lines and ranged from a low of 209 ng/g for Mp482 to 2565 ng/g for Mp319. Mp420, which was released by Scott and Zummo[24] as a source of resistance to aflatoxin contamination, was highly contaminated (1021 ng/g). Although none of the lines exhibited high levels of resistance, some lines such as Mp410, Mp462, Mp482, and Mp492 could prove useful in breeding for aflatoxin resistance.

The results of the evaluations of inbred lines and advanced breeding lines performed in 2001 are presented in Table 18.4. Mp715, which was released in 1999, had the lowest level of aflatoxin contamination at 14 ng/g.[27] At 9289 ng/g, SC212m was most highly contaminated. Mp494 and Mp92:673 were selected for resistance to aflatoxin contamination and did not differ significantly from the released germplasm lines Mp313E and Mp420.[23,24] Other lines that did not differ significantly from Mp313E or Mp420 were Mp97:161, Mp95:513, Mp97:160, Mp95:512, Mp97:155, and Mp716. These six lines were selected for resistance to leaf-feeding resistance by southwestern corn borer and fall armyworm; however, only Mp716 has been released.[28] Although these lines were selected for resistance to leaf feeding, less insect damage to ears has also been observed. It is likely that the lower level

TABLE 18.4

Aflatoxin Accumulation in Inbred and Advanced Breeding Lines Inoculated with an *Aspergillus flavus* Spore Suspension Using the Side-Needle Technique at Mississippi State in 2001

Genotype	Aflatoxin (ng/g)	Genotype	Aflatoxin (ng/g)
SC212m	9289a	Ab24E	757fg
Tx114	6093a	SC229	621gh
GA209	4667ab	Mp95:519	573g–i
GT-MAS:gk-3-4-1-1-1-1-B	4184a–c	(Mp305 × T202)-2-10-1-1-1-B	463g–j
Mp713	2284b–d	Mp716	290h–k
Tx5885	2060cd	Mp97:155	262i–k
Mp97:154	1829de	Mp95:512	251jk
Mp714	1760de	Mp97:160	231jk
Mp339	1665d–f	Mp95:513	226j–l
Va35	1606d–f	Mp97:161	182k–m
Tex6	1560d–f	Mp420	180k–m
Mp95:535	864e–g	Mp313E	100lm
(Mp305 × T202)-2-9-2-1-1-B	830e–g	Mp92:673	97m
GT-MAS:gk-5-3-1-1-1-1-B	826e–g	Mp494	83m
(Mp305 × T202)-1-6-2-1-1-B	819e–g	Mp715	14n

Note: Means followed by the same letter do not differ at $p = 0.05$. Tests of significance were performed on transformed means $[\log(y+1)]$ using Fisher's protected LSD before converting values back to the original scale.

of aflatoxin contamination may have been due at least in part to reduced insect damage. Other lines with resistance to southwestern corn borer (*Diatraea grandiosella* Dyar) and fall armyworm (*Spodoptera frugiperda* [J.E. Smith]), including Mp713 and Mp714, exhibited high levels of aflatoxin contamination.[29]

Inbred lines that have been used frequently as susceptible checks in our research program, including Mp339, GA209, and SC212m, exhibited high levels of aflatoxin contamination. Two lines selected from the population GT-MAS:gk differed significantly for aflatoxin contamination. GT-MAS:gk-3-4-1-1-1-1-B showed an extremely high aflatoxin level of 4184 ng/g. GT-MAS:gk was developed and released by USDA–ARS at Tifton, GA.[30] As a population, it has exhibited good resistance to aflatoxin contamination.

Test crosses have been made with lines that exhibited resistance to aflatoxin contamination. These crosses will be evaluated not only for aflatoxin contamination but also for yield and other agronomic qualities.

18.5 PERFORMANCE OF AFLATOXIN-RESISTANT LINES IN CROSSES

The performance of an inbred line in crosses with other inbred lines provides additional information on its potential usefulness in a breeding program. Single crosses among inbred lines were evaluated for aflatoxin accumulation in 2000 and 2001.

18.5.1 MATERIALS AND METHODS

18.5.1.1 Diallel Cross

Ten inbred lines were chosen as parents of a diallel cross. Two of the lines, Mp313E and Mp420, had been released as sources of resistance to aflatoxin accumulation.[23,24] A third line, Mp80:04, has also exhibited resistance to aflatoxin accumulation; however, it has not been released. The other seven parental lines are susceptible to aflatoxin contamination. The 10 inbred lines were crossed in all possible combinations, and the resulting 45 single-cross hybrids were planted in a randomized complete block design with four replications on April 27, 2000. The experiment was conducted as previously described. Inoculations were made 14 days after midsilk using the side-needle technique. Grain was harvested and analyzed for aflatoxin contamination, and data were analyzed as in the other experiments. Variation among single crosses was partitioned into general and specific combining ability components using Griffin's Method 4, Model I.[31] Estimates of general combining ability (GCA) effects were also calculated.

18.5.1.2 Single-Cross Evaluation

A second experiment was grown in 2001. Twelve single crosses were planted on April 22, 2001 in a randomized complete block design with 10 replications. This group included crosses among most of the aflatoxin-resistant lines that had been identified and developed at Mississippi State. Another group of lines from the breeding program were evaluated in testcrosses for aflatoxin accumulation in 2003. Two experiments were planted on April 21: One included testcrosses with T173, and the other included testcrosses with NC300. Each experiment consisted of 30 testcrosses and hybrid checks planted in a randomized complete block design with three replications. The experimental protocol and data analyses were as previously described. The testcrosses evaluated for resistance to aflatoxin accumulation in 2003 were evaluated for yield in experiments planted at Mississippi State on April 19, 2002. Each experiment consisted of 26 testcrosses and commercial hybrid checks planted in a randomized complete block design with four replications. The single-row plots were approximately 4 m long and spaced approximately 1 m apart. Plots were thinned to 25 plants after seedling. Grain was harvested with an Almaco HP harvester (Nevada, IA), dried, and weighed. Yields were converted to kg/ha at 15.5% moisture.

18.5.2 Results and Discussion

18.5.2.1 Diallel Cross

The results of the evaluation of the 45 single crosses constituting the diallel set of crosses are given in Table 18.5. The two crosses with the lowest levels of aflatoxin contamination were Mp80:04 × T165 (50 ng/g) and Mp339 × Mp80:04 (93 ng/g). The four crosses with the highest levels of aflatoxin contamination each had SC212m as one parent: Mp488 × SC212m (2356 ng/g), Mp305 × SC212m (1427 ng/g), SC212m × SC213 (1218 ng/g), and Ab24E × SC212m (1078 ng/g). Aflatoxin levels for the three classes of crosses were 603 ng/g for susceptible × susceptible (S×S), 298 ng/g, for susceptible × resistant (S×R), and 160 ng/g for resistant × resistant (R×R). Aflatoxin levels for the S×R crosses were approximately 50% of those of the S×S crosses, and aflatoxin levels of the R×R crosses were approximately 25% of the S×S crosses. These results indicate that one resistant parent can substantially reduce aflatoxin levels. In crosses with other inbred lines, Mp80:04 exhibited significantly lower levels of aflatoxin accumulation and SC212m significantly higher levels than the other parental inbreds (Table 18.6). General combining ability was a significant source of variation, but specific combining ability was not. Estimates of specific combining ability (SCA) effects indicated that Mp313E and Mp80:04 contributed significantly to aflatoxin-resistant single crosses (Table 18.6). SC212m and SC213 contributed toward single crosses that were significantly more susceptible. These results indicate that Mp313E and Mp80:04 should be useful sources of resistance to aflatoxin contamination in hybrid development.

18.5.2.2 Single-Cross Evaluation

The results of the evaluation of 12 single crosses for resistance to aflatoxin contamination in 2001 are presented in Table 18.7. Crosses with two resistant parents exhibited the lowest levels of aflatoxin contamination. The two crosses between two susceptible inbred lines, GA209 × SC212m and Mp339 × SC212m, exhibited significantly higher levels of aflatoxin accumulation than all other crosses. As indicated earlier, Mp716 was developed and released as a source of resistance to southwestern corn borer and fall armyworm, but it exhibited some resistance to aflatoxin contamination when evaluated with other inbred and advanced breeding lines (Table 18.4). Its performance in the cross Mp714 × Mp716 was consistent with that of an aflatoxin-resistant line (Table 18.7). Yields of testcrosses with T173 were generally higher than the yields of testcrosses with NC300 (Table 18.8 and Table 18.9). The testcross yields, however, were not as high as the commercial hybrid checks, DK687 and 3223. This indicates that additional selection for higher yields and improved combining ability may be necessary if these lines are to be used in marketable hybrids. Aflatoxin levels were higher for the T173 testcrosses than the NC300 testcrosses (Table 18.8 and Table 18.9). The three commercially available hybrids exhibited high levels of aflatoxin contamination in both experiments. Several of the testcrosses exhibited low levels of aflatoxin contamination. Advanced breeding lines that performed well with both testers included Mp95:512 and Mp97:161, which had been selected for resistance to southwestern corn borer

TABLE 18.5

Aflatoxin Accumulation in Single Crosses Grown at Mississippi State in 2000 and Inoculated with an *Aspergillus flavus* Spore Suspension Using the Side-Needle Technique

Single Cross	Classification[a]	Aflatoxin (ng/g)	Single Cross	Classification[a]	Aflatoxin (ng/g)
Ab24E × Mp305	S×S	331e–k	Mp313E × SC213	R×S	134j–m
Ab24E × Mp313E	S×R	285f–l	Mp313E × T165	R×S	209h–l
Ab24E × Mp339	S×S	329e–k	Mp339 × Mp420	S×R	470b–i
Ab24E × Mp420	S×R	199h–l	Mp339 × Mp488	S×S	151i–m
Ab24E × Mp488	S×S	392c–j	Mp339 × Mp80:04	S×R	93lm
Ab24E × Mp80:04	S×R	252g–l	Mp339 × SC212m	S×S	354d–k
Ab24E × SC212m	S×S	1078a–d	Mp339 × SC213	S×S	495b–h
Ab24E × SC213	S×S	762a–g	Mp339 × T165	S×S	281f–l
Ab24E × T165	S×S	559d–k	Mp420 × Mp488	R×S	195h–l
Mp305 × Mp313E	S×R	301f–k	Mp420 × Mp80:04	R×R	115k–m
Mp305 × Mp339	S×S	381d–j	Mp420 × SC212m	R×S	248h–l
Mp305 × Mp420	S×R	443c–i	Mp420 × SC213	R×S	412c–j
Mp305 × Mp488	S×S	296f–l	Mp420 × T165	R×S	416c–j
Mp305 × Mp80:04	S×R	288f–l	Mp488 × Mp80:04	S×R	303f–k
Mp305 × SC212m	S×S	1427ab	Mp488 × SC212m	S×S	2356a
Mp305 × SC213	S×S	279f–l	Mp488 × SC213	S×S	814a–f
Mp305 × T165	S×S	284f–l	Mp488 × T165	S×S	299f–k
Mp313E × Mp339	R×S	258f–l	Mp80:04 × SC212m	R×S	279f–l
Mp313E × Mp420	R×R	195h–l	Mp80:04 × T165	R×S	50m
Mp313E × Mp488	R×S	229h–l	SC212m × SC213	S×S	1218a–c
Mp313E × Mp80:04	R×R	169h–l	SC212m × T165	S×S	475b–i
Mp313E × SC212m	R×S	969a–e	SC213 × T165	S×S	297f–k

[a] S indicates a line that is susceptible to aflatoxin contamination; R indicates a line selected for resistance to aflatoxin contamination.

Note: Means followed by the same letter do not differ at $p = 0.05$. Tests of significance were performed on transformed [$\log(y+1)$] means using Fisher's protected LSD before converting values back to the original scale.

and fall armyworm, showed promising levels of resistance to aflatoxin. Another line, (Mp313E × Va35)-1-2-1-1, also exhibited resistance to aflatoxin.

18.6 CONCLUSIONS AND FUTURE DIRECTIONS

The performance of Mp313E and Mp715 as lines and in crosses indicates that they possess adequate levels of resistance to aflatoxin accumulation to be useful in hybrid development. Other lines such as Mp494, Mp80:04, and Mp92:673, which have not been released, are also promising sources of resistance. Several lines including Mp95:512, Mp97:155, and Mp97:161 developed as sources of resistance to leaf

TABLE 18.6
Means for Each Inbred Line in Crosses and Estimates of General Combining Ability Effects for Aflatoxin Accumulation for Diallel Cross Evaluated at Mississippi State in 2000

Inbred Line	Mean in Crosses (ng/g)[a]	GCA Effect (log[ng/g+1])[b]
SC212m	720a	0.88**
SC213	429b	0.27*
Ab24E	383b	0.18
Mp305	379b	0.17
Mp488	371b	0.15
Mp339	280c	−0.17
Mp420	269c	−0.21
T165	259c	−0.26
Mp313E	256c	−0.28*
Mp80:04	170d	−0.73**

[a] Means followed by the same letter do not differ at $p = 0.05$ (Fisher's protected LSD).
[b] * and ** indicate significant differences from 0 at $p = 0.05$ and $p = 0.01$, respectively.

TABLE 18.7
Aflatoxin Accumulation in Single Crosses Grown at Mississippi State in 2001 and Inoculated with an *Aspergillus flavus* Conidial Suspension Using the Side-Needle Technique

Single Cross	Aflatoxin (ng/g)
GA209 × SC212m	834a
Mp339 × SC212m	765a
Mp92:673 × Tx114	269ab
Mp714 × Mp716	223bc
Mp313E × Mp420	74c–e
Mo18W × Mp313E	47d–f
Mp494 × Mp715	46d–f
Mp715 × Mp92:673	42d–f
Mp313E × Mp715	28e–f
Mp313E × Mp494	23f

Note: Means in a column followed by the same letter do not differ at $p = 0.05$. Tests of significance were performed on transformed means [$\log(y+1)$] using Fisher's protected LSD before converting back to the original scale.

TABLE 18.8
Mean Values for Yield and Aflatoxin Accumulation in Maize Testcrosses with T173 Evaluated at Mississippi State in 2002 and 2003

Genotype	Yield (kg/ha)[a]	Aflatoxin (ng/g)[b]
Mp95:512 × T173	5887b–e	35e–h
Mp95:535 × T173	6571bc	415ab
Mp97:154 × T173	7157a–c	256a–d
Mp97:155 × T173	5880b–e	83b–g
Mp97:161 × T173	6162b–d	46d–g
Mp92:673 × T173	6911bc	234a–d
Mp313E × T173	7031a–c	79b–g
Mp420 × T173	6722bc	116a–g
Mp715 × T173	6159b–d	126a–g
Va35 × T173	4795de	220a–d
GTmas:gk-3-4-1-1-1-1-1-1 × T173	6789bc	130a–g
(Mp715 × Va35)-1-3-1-1- × T173	7161ab	294a–c
(Mp715 × Va35)-1-4-1-1- × T173	6068be	174a–f
(Mp313E × Va35)-1-1-2-1 × T173	3769c–e	83b–g
(Mp313E × Va35)-1-1-4-1 × T173	5607b–e	331ab
(Mp313E × Va35)-1-1-7-1 × T173	6048b–e	129a–g
(Mp313E × Va35)-1-1-8-1- × T173	4459e	34f–h
(Mp313E × Va35)-1-1-10-1 × T173	7087a–c	187a–f
(Mp313E × Va35) -1-2-1-1 × T173	5850b–e	27gh
(Mp313E × Va35)-1-2-3-1 × T173	6412b–d	58c–g
(Mp313E × Va35)-1-3-4-1 × T173	7164ab	113a–g
(Mp313E × Va35)-1-3-5-1 × T173	6869bc	205a–d
NC300 × T173	7035a–c	117a–g
Mp313E × Mp420	109a–g	—
Mp313E × Mp715	7h	—
Mp339 × SC212m	194a–e	—
GA209 × SC212m	254a–d	—
DK687	7203ab	319a–c
3223	8580a	262a–c
TV2100	5663b–e	566a

[a] Mean yields are expressed in kg/ha at 15.5% moisture and were obtained in 2002.

[b] Tests of significance were performed on transformed means [log(y+1)] before converting means back to the original scale. Means for aflatoxin accumulation were obtained in 2003.

Note: Means in a column followed by the same letter do not differ at $p = 0.05$ (Fisher's protected LSD).

TABLE 18.9

Mean Values for Yield and Aflatoxin Accumulation in Maize Testcrosses with NC300 Evaluated at Mississippi State in 2002 and 2003

Genotype	Yield (kg/ha)[a]	Aflatoxin (ng/g)[b]
Mp95:512 × NC300	4431hi	9e–h
Mp95:535 × NC300	6065c–g	32d–h
Mp97:154 × NC300	6441c–e	47c–f
Mp97:155 × NC300	4813f–i	30d–h
Mp97:161 × NC300	5799d–h	13e–h
Mp92:673 × NC300	13e–h	—
Mp313E × NC300	7083b–d	68e–h
Mp420 × NC300	4167i	12c–e
Mp715 × NC300	6121c–f	13e–h
Va35 × NC300	4705f–i	45e–h
GTmas:gk-3-4-1-1-1-1-1-1 × NC300	6936c–e	77c–e
(Mp715 × Va35)-1-3-1-1- × NC300	7081b–d	4gh
(Mp715 × Va35)-1-4-1-1- × NC300	6509c–e	21e–h
(Mp313E × Va35)-1-1-2-1 × NC300	4571g–1	11e–h
(Mp313E × Va35)-1-1-4-1 × NC300	6468c–e	11e–h
(Mp313E × Va35)-1-1-7-1 × NC300	7022cd	23d–h
(Mp313E × Va35)-1-1-8-1- × NC300	5446e–i	29d–h
(Mp313E × Va35)-1-1-10-1 × NC300	6189c–f	11e–h
(Mp313E × Va35) -1-2-1-1 × NC300	6580c–e	3h
(Mp313E × Va35)-1-2-3-1 × NC300	5856d–h	28d–h
(Mp313E × Va35)-1-3-4-1 × NC300	6136c–f	5f–h
(Mp313E × Va35)-1-3-5-1 × NC300	7156b–d	14e–h
NC300 × T173	6865c–e	210a–d
Mp313E × Mp420	40c–g	—
Mp313E × Mp715	27d–h	—
Mp339 × SC212m	207a–d	—
GA209 × SC212m	347a–c	—
DK687	8616ab	645ab
3223	9896a	805a
TV2100	7582bc	325a–c

[a] Mean yields are expressed in kg/ha at 15.5% moisture and were obtained in 2002.

[b] Tests of significance were performed on transformed means $[\log(y+1)]$ before converting means back to the original scale. Means for aflatoxin accumulation were obtained in 2003.

Note: Means in a column followed by the same letter do not differ at $p = 0.05$ (Fisher's protected LSD).

feeding by southwestern corn borer and fall armyworm exhibited resistance to aflatoxin contamination, both as lines per se and in testcrosses. Unfortunately, these lines did not show good combining ability for yield in testcrosses. Further evaluation will be necessary to determine their potential value in developing aflatoxin-resistant maize hybrids. Most of the aflatoxin-resistant lines that have been identified lack desirable agronomic qualities. For them to be truly useful, the aflatoxin resistance must be combined with good agronomic characteristics. Efforts are underway to identify quantitative trait loci (QTL) associated with aflatoxin resistance. Both marker-assisted selection and conventional breeding methods are being used to transfer aflatoxin resistance into lines with good agronomic qualities. Research to identify and isolate proteins and genes associated with aflatoxin resistance in these lines has been initiated. As genes are identified, their roles in expression of aflatoxin resistance will be determined. Because aflatoxin contamination is highly sensitive to environmental stresses that are not well defined, research will be conducted to determine how gene expression is affected by physiological stress. Progress has been made toward the goal of developing and deploying aflatoxin resistant hybrids; however, much remains to be done. Both conventional and novel approaches will be essential to eliminate aflatoxin contamination in maize.

ACKNOWLEDGMENTS

This manuscript is a joint contribution of USDA–ARS and the Mississippi Agricultural and Forestry Experiment Station. It is published as Journal No. J10497 of the Mississippi Agricultural and Forestry Experiment Station.

REFERENCES

1. Anderson, H.W., Nehring, E.W., Wechser, W.R., Aflatoxin contamination of corn in the field, *J. Agric. Food Chem.*, 23(4), 775–782, 1975.
2. Lillehoj, E.B., Kwolek, W.F., Shannon, G.M., Shotwell, O.L, and Hesseltini, C.W., Aflatoxin occurrence in 1973 corn at harvest. I. A limited survey in the southeastern U.S., *Cereal Chem.*, 52(5), 603–611, 1974.
3. Lillehoj, E.B., Kwolek, W.F. Manwiller, A., Durant, J.A., and LaPrade, J.C., Horner, E.S., Reid, J, Zuber, M.S. Aflatoxin production in several corn hybrids grown in South Carolina and Florida, *Crop Sci.*, 16(4), 483–485, 1976.
4. Shotwell, O.L., Aflatoxin in corn, *J. AOCS*, 54(93), 216A–224A, 1977.
5. Zuber, M.S., Calvert, O.H., Lillehoj, E.B., and Kwolek, W.F., Preharvest development of aflatoxin B_1 in corn in the United States, *Phytopathology*, 66(9), 1120–1121, 1976.
6. Wilson, D.M., McMillian, W.W., and Widstrom, N.W., Field aflatoxin contamination in south Georgia, *J. AOCS*, 56(9), 798–799, 1979.
7. McMillian, W.W., Wilson, D.M., and Widstrom, N.W., Insect damage, *Aspergillus flavus* ear mold and aflatoxin contamination in south Georgia corn fields in 1977, *J. Environ. Qual.*, 7(4), 564–566, 1978.
8. Zuber, M.S. and Lillehoj, E.B., Status of the aflatoxin problem in corn, *J. Environ. Qual.*, 8(1), 1–5, 1979.
9. Payne, G.A., Aflatoxin in maize, *CRC Crit. Rev. Plant Sci.*, 10(5), 423–440, 1992.
10. Widstrom, N.W., The aflatoxin problem in corn grain, *Adv. Agron.*, 56, 219–280, 1996.
11. Windham, G.L. and Williams, W.P., *Aflatoxin Accumulation in Commercial Corn Hybrids in 1998*, Mississippi Agricultural and Forest Experiment Station Research Report No. 22(8), Mississippi State University, Mississippi State, 1999, pp. 1–4.

12. Windham, G.L. and Williams, W.P., Evaluation of corn inbreds and advanced breeding lines for resistance to aflatoxin contamination in developing corn kernels, *Plant Dis.*, 86(3), 232–234, 2002.

13. Widstrom, N.W., McMillian, W.W., Beaver, R.W., and Wilson, D.M., Weather-associated changes in aflatoxin contamination of preharvest maize, *J. Prod. Agric.*, 3(2), 196–199, 1990.

14. Lillehoj, E.B., Kwolek, W.F., Zuber, M.S., Bockholt, A.J., Calvert, O.H., Findley, W.R., Guthrie, W.D., Horner, E.S., Josephson, L.M., King, S., Manwiller, A., Sauer, D.B., Thompson, D., Turner, M., and Widstrom, N.W., Aflatoxin in corn before harvest: interaction of hybrids and locations, *Crop Sci.*, 20(6), 731–734, 1980.

15. Lillehoj, E.B., Kwolek, W.F.., Horner, E.S., Widstrom, N.W., Josephson, L.M., Franz, A.O., and Castalano, E.A., Aflatoxin contamination of preharvest corn: role of *Aspergillus flavus* inoculum and insect damage, *Cereal Chem.*, 57(4), 255–257, 1980.

16. Barry, D., Widstrom, N.W., Darrah, L.L., McMillian, W.W., Riley, T.J., Scott, G.E., and Lillehoj, E.B., Maize ear damage by insects in relation to genotype and aflatoxin contamination of maize grain, *J. Econ. Entomol.*, 85(6), 2492–2495, 1992.

17. Windham, G.L., Williams, W.P., and Davis, F.M., Effects of southwestern corn borer on *Aspergillus flavus* kernel infection and aflatoxin accumulation in maize hybrids, *Plant Dis.*, 83(6), 535–540, 1999.

18. King, S.B. and Scott, G.E., Field inoculation techniques to evaluate maize hybrids for reaction to kernel infection by *Aspergillus flavus*, *Phytopathology*, 72(7), 782–785, 1982.

19. Tucker, D.H., Trevathan, L.E., King, S.B., and Scott, G.E., Effect of four inoculation techniques on infection and aflatoxin concentration of resistant and susceptible corn hybrids inoculated with *Aspergillus flavus*, *Phytopathology*, 76(3), 290–293, 1986.

20. Zummo, N. and Scott, G.E., Evaluation of field inoculation techniques for screening maize genotypes against kernel infection by *Aspergillus flavus* in Mississippi, *Plant Dis.*, 73(4), 313–316, 1989.

21. Scott, G.E. and Zummo, N., Preharvest kernel infection by *Aspergillus flavus* for resistant and susceptible maize hybrids, *Crop Sci.*, 30(2), 381–383, 1990.

22. Scott, G.E., Zummo, N., Lillehoj, E.B., Widstrom, N.W., Kang, M.S., West, D.R., Payne, G.A., Cleveland, T.E., Calvert, O.H., and Fortnum, B.A., Aflatoxin in corn hybrids field inoculated with *Aspergillus flavus*, *Agron. J.*, 83(3), 595–598, 1991.

23. Scott, G.E. and Zummo, N., Registration of Mp313E parental line of maize, *Crop Sci.*, 30(6), 1378, 1990.

24. Scott, G. E. and Zummo, N., Registration of Mp420 germplasm line of maize, *Crop Sci.*, 32(5), 1296, 1992.

25. Windham, G.L. and Williams, W.P., *Aspergillus flavus* infection and aflatoxin accumulation in resistant and susceptible maize hybrids, *Plant Dis.*, 82(3), 281–284, 1998.

26. Scott, G.E. and Zummo, N., Sources of resistance in maize to kernel infection by *Aspergillus flavus* in the field, *Crop Sci.*, 28(3), 504–507, 1988.

27. Williams, W.P. and Windham, G.L., Registration of maize germplasm line Mp715, *Crop Sci.*, 4(4), 1374–1375, 2001.

28. Williams, W.P. and Davis, F.M., Registration of maize germplasm line Mp716, *Crop Sci.*, 42(2), 671–672, 2002.

29. Williams, W.P. and Davis, F.M., Registration of maize germplasms Mp713 and Mp714, *Crop Sci.*, 40(2), 584, 2000.

30. McMillian, W.W., Widstrom, N.W., and Wilson, D.M., Registration of GT-MAS:gk maize germplasm, *Crop Sci.*, 33(4), 882, 1993.

31. Griffing, B., Concept of general and specific combining ability in relation to diallel systems, *Aust. J. Biol. Sci.*, 9, 463–493, 1956.

19 Identifying Sources of Resistance to Aflatoxin and Fumonisin Contamination in Corn Grain: History and Progress from the University of Illinois

Michael J. Clements and Donald G. White

CONTENTS

19.1 INTRODUCTION

Aspergillus flavus Link:Fr, *Fusarium verticillioides* (Sacc.) Nirenb. (Syn = *F. moniliforme* J. Sheld.), and *F. proliferatum* (Matsushima) Nirenb. are economically important pathogens to U.S. corn (*Zea mays* L.) producers. *Aspergillus flavus* is associated with *Aspergillus* ear rot of corn and the synthesis of aflatoxin in grain, while *F. verticillioides* and *F. proliferatum* are associated with *Fusarium* ear and kernel rot of corn and the synthesis of fumonisin in grain. Studies have linked consumption of corn grain contaminated with either aflatoxin or fumonisin to a number of detrimental health effects in animals and humans.[1-3] Interstate commerce of aflatoxin-contaminated corn grain is restricted by the U.S. Food and Drug Administration (FDA) at an action level of 20 ng/g,[4] and FDA guidance levels for fumonisin have been suggested at 2 to 4 µg/g for various cleaned and dry milled corn products.[3]

Fumonisin or aflatoxin accumulation in preharvest grain is most prevalent when plants are predisposed to disease development by heat, drought, damage from insects, and other stresses.[5–8] Proactive breeding programs aimed at improving commercial germplasm with genetic resistance to disease and insects as well as genetic tolerance to environmental stress are generally considered to be the most effective means of minimizing aflatoxin and fumonisin contamination in grain prior to harvest.

This chapter reviews over a decade of research from the University of Illinois on resistance to mycotoxin accumulation in corn grain. Researchers at the University of Illinois seek to identify sources of resistance that contribute alleles for low mycotoxin accumulation in grain and low ear rot severity to commercial inbreds. Successes in the program have been due, in part, to adherence to four basic guidelines. First, one of the greatest barriers to breeding for resistance is the significant variation in ear rot severity and mycotoxin accumulation in grain brought about by the environment;[9] genotypes should be evaluated in multiple years and locations, and, where possible, plants should be inoculated to minimize variation encountered in studies that rely on natural infection. Second, the severity of ear rot and the mycotoxin concentration in grain are not well correlated;[10–17] inferences about mycotoxin concentration in grain based solely on ear rot severity should be made with caution or avoided, and selection for resistance to mycotoxin accumulation in grain should be made directly. Third, the majority of inbred seed parents developed for commercial hybrid production in the United States share common ancestry in the forms of Reid Yellow Dent (including Stiff Stalk Synthetic), the inbred B73, or other related B73-type lines;[18–21] genotypes that contribute alleles for resistance to hybrids developed with B73-type lines should improve the resistance of a large number of seed parents used to produce commercial hybrids in the United States. Fourth, high levels of resistance may be developed by pyramiding alleles for resistance from multiple loci and diverse sources into commercially used inbreds; numerous genotypes must be evaluated to identify novel genes that improve the resistance of commercial inbred lines.

19.2 SOURCES OF RESISTANCE TO AFLATOXIN CONTAMINATION IN CORN GRAIN

In the summer of 1988, drought and above-average temperatures contributed to severe *Aspergillus* ear rot and aflatoxin contamination of corn grain produced throughout much of the midwestern United States. Interest in mycotoxins in food and feed intensified, and then Illinois Representative Dick Durbin sponsored a "special grant" for research aimed at minimizing aflatoxin contamination in grain. Adequate funding provided researchers at the University of Illinois the opportunity to initiate what has become a pragmatic breeding program for resistance.

Work during the first 3 years of the program focused on developing hybrid crosses for a preliminary evaluation of resistance, collecting isolates of *Aspergillus flavus* that are suitable for evaluating corn genotypes in inoculated trials in the Midwest, and identifying an inoculation technique that efficiently differentiates resistant and susceptible corn inbreds and hybrids in the Midwest. By 1990, over 2100 F_1 hybrids had been developed with a large, genetically diverse collection of inbred lines and the historically important inbreds Mo17 and B73.[11] Also, four isolates of *A. flavus* had been identified that synthesize aflatoxin in grain and induce severe ear rot on susceptible genotypes in Illinois (D. White, original study unpublished). By 1991, F_2 and backcross-to-the-susceptible-parent (BC_1) generations were developed from F_1 hybrids produced in 1990, the optimal timing of inoculation in Illinois was determined,[10] and a pinboard inoculation device was developed that efficiently differentiates resistant and susceptible corn genotypes in Illinois.[10] Also in 1991, F_1 crosses of 1189 inbreds with Mo17 and 978 inbreds with B73 were pinboard inoculated and evaluated for resistance to *Aspergillus* ear rot in two replicates in central Illinois.[11,22] From this preliminary work, 31 genotypes (inbreds 33-16, 75-RO12, B9, B37Ht2, B40, CH66-17, CI2, CO158, F486, FR809, H103, KYS, KY-58, LB31, L317, MI82, MS214, N6, N8, NC232, ND363, OH513, OH516, SD18, SDP031, SDP262, SP292, T115, Tex6, TR213, and Y7) were selected for further study.[11]

From 1992 to 1993, the focus of the program shifted from preliminary work to studies of the inheritance of resistance. During this time, a serological procedure was developed that rapidly and inexpensively quantifies aflatoxin concentration in grain.[11] Genotypes selected in 1991 were evaluated for ear rot severity, incidence of kernels infected with *Aspergillus flavus*, and aflatoxin concentration in grain in multiple environments and experiments that included parental lines, F_1, F_2, F_3, and backcross generations.[11,12] Genotypes not associated with adequate levels of resistance across populations and environments were dropped from the program. Heritability, a measure of the efficiency with which parental performance is transferred to offspring, for resistance to *Aspergillus* ear rot ranged from 12 to 68% among several of the remaining genotypes. Also among the remaining genotypes, up to eight effective factors, here defined as genes or tightly linked polygenes associated with a trait, were estimated to be involved in resistance.[12] Over 90% of ears from F_2 plants developed with the inbreds Tex6 and Mo17 had aflatoxin concentration in grain at or below 20 ng/g. Over 55% of ears from F_2 plants developed with inbreds CI2, Oh513, 75-R001, and N6 and the inbreds B73 or Mo17 had aflatoxin concentration in grain at or below 20 ng/g. Frequency distributions for aflatoxin concentration in grain from F_2 plants and from F_3 families developed with several of the resistant genotypes were skewed toward the resistant parents.[12] The sum total cumulative influence of alleles from multiple loci (additive genetic effects) and the influence of allelic interactions at individual loci (dominance genetic effects) on the severity of *Aspergillus* ear rot were determined for the resistant genotypes. Magnitudes of additive and dominance genetic effects associated with *Aspergillus* ear rot were dependent on the cross studied.[12] Based on this information, researchers concluded that selection for low aflatoxin accumulation in grain among families in segregating populations should be an effective means of developing resistant inbred lines.[12]

In 1993, inbred LB31 was chosen as the first of several candidates for studies of the types and magnitudes of gene action associated with resistance to ear rot severity and aflatoxin accumulation in grain.[23] Inbred LB31 (PI561695) was developed by M.E. Smith and V.E. Gracen from the International Synthetic population at Pennsylvania State University.[24] Resistance from LB31 to aflatoxin accumulation in grain was associated with additive and dominant genetic effects in crosses with B73.[23] Treatment means of aflatoxin concentration in grain from inbred LB31 were 98 and 40 ng/g in inoculated experiments done in central Illinois in 1993 and 1994, respectively.[23] Treatment means of aflatoxin concentration in grain from inbred B73 were 367 and 133 ng/g, respectively, during the same experiments in 1993 and 1994. Aflatoxin concentration in grain from F_3 families developed with LB31 and B73 ranged from less than 20 to greater than 400 ng/g.[23] Heritability for resistance to aflatoxin accumulation in grain from LB31 was 66% among F_3 families developed with B73. Soon to follow the study of LB31 were evaluations of inbreds Tex6,[13] CI2,[14] MI82,[15] and Oh516.[25] All of these inbreds were selected based on low aflatoxin concentration in grain and low ear rot severity when evaluated in inoculated trials as inbreds per se or in hybrid combination with B73 or Mo17.[11,12,26]

Inbred Tex6 is an unreleased line developed by D.G. White from "Whitemaster Hybrid" (PI401763), a southern corn variety from Texas.[11,27] Resistance to aflatoxin accumulation in grain from Tex6 was primarily associated with additive genetic effects in crosses with B73 or Mo17, although some dominant effects were apparent.[13] Treatment means of aflatoxin concentration in grain from Tex6 ranged from 2 to 39 ng/g in inoculated experiments done in central Illinois from 1994 to 1996.[13] Treatment means of aflatoxin concentration in grain from inbreds B73 and Mo17 ranged from 70 to 271 ng/g during the same experiments. Researchers determined that one cycle of selection for resistance to aflatoxin accumulation in grain among F_3 families developed with Tex6 and B73 would reduce aflatoxin concentration in grain by 19 ng/g.[13] Heritability for resistance to aflatoxin accumulation in grain from Tex6 ranged from 63 to 65% in crosses developed with Mo17 or B73, respectively. Kernels from Tex6 contain proteins that inhibit aflatoxin accumulation in grain and the growth of *Aspergillus flavus* in culture.[28] Kernels from Tex6 also exhibit activity of β-1,3-glucanase[29] and chitinase,[30] two enzymes that degrade fungal cell walls and possibly minimize kernel infection by *A. flavus*. Kernels from Tex6 support minimal fungal growth and low aflatoxin accumulation when endosperms are or are not wounded prior to inoculation.[31]

Inbred CI2 was developed by the U.S. Department of Agriculture (USDA) in Missouri from the backcross [(CI23 × CI4-8) × CI23].[18,27] CI23 is a self from the open-pollinated variety "U.S. Selection 119" with origins in "Boone County White."[18] CI4-8 is a selection from "Lancaster Surecrop."[18] Agronomic performance and aflatoxin accumulation in grain were confounded within environments during a study of generations developed with CI2 and B73 in central Illinois.[14] In that study, seed set on inbred CI2 was poor, and differences in aflatoxin accumulation between resistant (CI2) and susceptible (B73) inbred lines were not apparent in one of two environments. Adequate estimates of genetic effects associated with resistance to aflatoxin accumulation in grain from CI2 were available only from one environment in which mean separation between resistant and susceptible inbred lines was apparent. In an inoculated experiment in 1999, treatment means of aflatoxin concentration in grain were 39 ng/g for inbred CI2 and 285 ng/g for inbred B73.[14] Like Tex6, resistance to aflatoxin accumulation in grain from CI2 is primarily associated with additive genetic effects.[14] Broad-sense heritability for resistance from CI2 to aflatoxin accumulation in grain ranged from 32% for F_3 families to 26% for backcross-to-the-susceptible-parent-selfed (BC_1S_1) families developed with B73.[14] In a laboratory study, growth of *Aspergillus flavus* and aflatoxin accumulation in grain from CI2 were low when kernels were not wounded prior to inoculation.[31] In the same study, however, growth of *A. flavus* and aflatoxin accumulation were great in wounded kernels from CI2.[31] Researchers have hypothesized that intact pericarp, aleurone layer, or other kernel structures may function as important components of resistance from CI2.[14,31]

Inbred MI82 is an unreleased line developed by D.G. White from a hybrid commercially used in India.[15] Resistance to aflatoxin accumulation in grain from MI82 was primarily associated with dominant genetic effects in crosses with B73, although some additive effects were apparent.[15] Differences in aflatoxin concentration in grain between resistant (MI82) and susceptible (B73) parents were not significant in inoculated experiments in 2000 and 2001, but differences among BC_1S_1 families developed with MI82 and B73 were apparent.[15] Aflatoxin concentration in grain ranged from less than 10 to greater than 200 ng/g, and from less than 200 to greater than 2000 ng/g among BC_1S_1 families in 2000 and 2001, respectively. In 2001, generation means for aflatoxin concentration in grain were the highest values recorded since research on aflatoxin resistance began at the University of Illinois. Heritability for resistance to aflatoxin accumulation in grain from MI82 was 74% in crosses developed with B73. Kernels from MI82 support minimal fungal growth and moderate to low aflatoxin accumulation when endosperms are or are not wounded prior to inoculation.[31,32] Kernels from MI82 support acute fungal growth and high aflatoxin concentration when embryos are wounded prior to inoculation.[32] A 14-kDa protein quantified in kernels of MI82[33] may limit the growth of *Aspergillus flavus* by inhibiting α-amylase production in the kernel endosperm,[34,35] and may aid in minimizing concentration of aflatoxin in kernels with an intact embryo.

Inbred Oh516 was developed by Bill Findley at The Ohio State University from the backcross [(B14 × L97) × B14]. B14 is a selection out of Iowa Stiff Stalk Synthetic, and L97 is a selection out of Tuxpan, an open-pollinated variety from the southwestern United States.[18] Resistance to aflatoxin accumulation in grain from Oh516 was primarily associated with dominant genetic effects in crosses with B73, although additive effects were apparent.[25] Treatment means of aflatoxin concentration in grain from inbred Oh516 were 193 and 274 ng/g in inoculated experiments done in central Illinois in 2001 and 2002, respectively.[25] Treatment means of aflatoxin concentration in grain from inbred B73 were 541 and 477 ng/g in the same experiments in 2001 and 2002, respectively. Heritability for resistance to aflatoxin accumulation in grain was between 1 and 29% from test crosses developed with inbred LH185 (Holden's Foundation Seeds, Inc.; Williamsburg, IA) and 217 BC_1S_1 families derived from the cross of Oh516 and B73.[25] Aflatoxin concentration in grain of the 217 test crosses ranged from 100 to 6400 ng/g across inoculated experiments at Urbana, IL, Ganado, TX, and Batesville, TX, and averaged 162, 525, and 2469 ng/g at the three locations, respectively.

The current focus of the aflatoxin resistance program is on identification of QTL associated with resistance to aflatoxin accumulation in grain and on incorporation of alleles for resistance into a commercial inbred line. Genetic mapping of BC_1S_1 families developed with inbreds Oh516 and B73 is underway as a collaborative project with Monsanto. Genetic mapping populations comprised of $F_{2:3}$ or BC_1S_1 families developed with inbreds Tex6 and B73 were inoculated and evaluated in 1996 and 1997 in central Illinois.[36] Aflatoxin concentration in grain averaged 48 and 329 ng/g across $F_{2:3}$ families in 1996 and 1997, respectively. Aflatoxin concentration in grain averaged 50 and 208 ng/g across BC_1S_1 families in 1996 and 1997, respectively. Low aflatoxin accumulation in grain was associated with alleles from Tex6 and B73. Regions within chromosomes bin 3.05–06, 4.07–08, 5.01–02, 5.04–05, and 10.05–07 explained 13, 7, 16, 18, and 15% of the variation in aflatoxin concentration in grain among $F_{2:3}$ and BC_1S_1 families in 1997. Narrow-sense heritability for resistance to aflatoxin accumulation in grain was 29% among $F_{2:3}$ families and 19% among BC_1S_1 families. Multiple quantitative trait loci (QTL) with small effects on resistance were detected; however, very few molecular markers were associated with QTL for resistance to aflatoxin accumulation in grain across populations and environments. Researchers concluded that aflatoxin accumulation in grain is likely affected by multiple gene/environment associations and that alleles from multiple sources of resistance should be incorporated into elite lines.

Resistance to aflatoxin accumulation in grain from inbred Tex6 and inbred Mp313E (PI539859), a line released by the USDA-ARS and Mississippi State University,[37] is currently being incorporated into the commercial inbred FR1064, a widely-used, B73-type line sold by Illinois Foundation Seeds, Inc. (Champaign, IL).[18] Mp313E was developed by Gene Scott and Natale Zummo from Tuxpan and was selected primarily for resistance to kernel infection by *Aspergillus flavus*.[37] Genetic mapping of an $F_{2:3}$ population developed from the cross of Mp313E and B73 has been completed by the USDA-ARS at Mississippi State, MS.[38] Aflatoxin concentrations in grain ranged from less than 20 to 16,400 ng/g across $F_{2:3}$ families at Mississippi State and Stoneville, MS, from 2000 to 2002. QTL on chromosomes 2 (bin 2.05) and 4 (bin 4.06) were associated with resistance to aflatoxin accumulation in grain from Mp313E in 3 of 4 and 4 of 4 environments, respectively. Additional QTL for resistance from Mp313E were identified on chromosomes 3, 5, and 6, but effects from these regions were not consistent across environments. The QTL for resistance from Mp313E on chromosome 2 is different from QTL identified in a study of resistance from Tex6;[36] therefore, pyramiding resistance from Tex6 and Mp313E into a B73-type commercial background should be beneficial.

19.3 SOURCES OF RESISTANCE TO FUMONISIN ACCUMULATION IN CORN GRAIN

Fusarium ear and kernel rot of corn has only recently become a significant concern of corn producing and processing industries in the United States.[3,39,40] Few sources of resistance to fumonisin accumulation in corn grain have been identified, largely because the public is generally unaware of fumonisin and federal guidelines do not yet regulate its presence in food or feed. To address concerns of industry, researchers at the University of Illinois initiated a program to identify sources of resistance to *Fusarium* ear rot and fumonisin accumulation in grain in 1999. Progress in the program has been rapid, due principally to the application of experience gained through the study of resistance to aflatoxin in grain and financial support provided by the National Research Institute.

In 1999, we developed over 1500 F_1 hybrids with a large, genetically diverse collection of inbred lines and the inbred FR1064. In 2000, we proactively developed F_2 and BC_1 generations from all of the F_1 hybrids,[41] with hopes that several genotypes might be useful in studies of inheritance of resistance and the identification of molecular markers associated with resistance. Also by 2000, we had identified six isolates of *Fusarium verticillioides* and *F. proliferatum* that produce severe *Fusarium* ear rot and high fumonisin concentration in grain of susceptible genotypes in the Midwest;[41] adapted an enzyme-linked immunosorbent assay to rapidly and inexpensively quantify concentration of fumonisins B_1, B_2, and B_3 in grain;[17] identified an inoculation technique for *Fusarium* ear rot that differentiates resistant or susceptible corn inbreds and hybrids in the Midwest;[17] and evaluated F_1 hybrids developed in 1999 for resistance to *Fusarium* ear rot and fumonisin accumulation in grain in inoculated trials in Central Illinois and naturally infected trials provided by Syngenta Seeds, Inc., in Eastern North Carolina.[42] From this research, 35 genotypes (inbreds A131, A635Rpld, B8, B66, BC555, CM5, CQ201, FR36, FR2114, GE440, H117, J2705TV, L289, M14, M162W, MI925, ND302, RN28Htrhm, SDp2A, SP228, SQ18, SU80-1, TBA76125, TIE84, TrTrf, Va46, W438, W627C, Y5, A188, CG1, CK31, NY302, T236, Va24) were selected for further study. Grain from F_1 hybrids developed with the 35 genotypes and FR1064 had 5 μg fumonisin per gram in two trials or 4 μg fumonisin per gram when data from only one trial were available.[42]

In 2001, F_3 and BC_1S_1 generations were developed with the 35 genotypes selected in 2000. Genotypes selected in 2000 were inoculated and evaluated for resistance to ear rot and fumonisin concentration in grain in experiments that included parental lines, F_1, F_2, and backcross generations.[42] Thirty-five of the genotypes were evaluated at Urbana, IL, and 29 of the genotypes were evaluated at Haubstadt, IN, in plots provided by Monsanto. In general, alleles for resistance from these genotypes were dominant in crosses with FR1064. Fumonisin concentration in grain from the F_2 and BC_1 generations developed with many of the genotypes was low.[42] Alleles associated with fumonisin accumulation in grain within these generations should segregate among plants; therefore, if a small number of alleles was associated with fumonisin accumulation in grain, then plants within these generations would segregate for resistance and susceptibility, and many plants would be susceptible to fumonisin accumulation in grain. In this case, mean fumonisin concentration in grain of these generations would be moderate. Because the mean fumonisin concentration in grain of these generations was low, the majority of plants within these generations were resistant. Multiple alleles associated with low fumonisin accumulation in grain are likely segregating among plants, and multiple loci are likely associated with resistance.

From 2002 to the present, focus of the program has been on studies of types and magnitudes of gene action associated with resistance and on identification of QTL associated with resistance. Studies of inheritance of resistance from genotypes CG1, CQ201, GE440, and TBA76125 are in progress, and genetic mapping populations based on crosses of GE440 or TBA76125 and FR1064 are currently being evaluated.

Inbred CG1 was developed at the University of Guelph, Ontario, Canada, from "Funk's G10."[18] Inbred CQ201 was selfed from the backcross [(Minnesota No.13 × Wf9) × Wf9] at Macdonald College, Quebec, Canada.[18] Minnesota No. 13 was selected by W. Hays out of the open-pollinated variety "Pride of the North,"[18,20] and Wf9 is a selection out of an Indiana strain of Reid Yellow Dent.[18] Inbred GE440 is a line of unknown lineage possibly developed in the southeastern United States, and inbred TBA76125 was developed by Limagrain (BP1-63 720 Chappes, France) from a synthetic population of "flint-type" lines in the Danube river area of Western Europe.

A mapping population comprised of 215 BC_1S_1 families produced with FR1064 and one of the most promising genotypes, GE440, was inoculated and evaluated in replicated trials at Mt. Olive, NC, and Haubstadt, IN, in 2002. Plots in North Carolina were provided by North Carolina State University, and the plots in Indiana were provided by Monsanto. Families and parental lines were genotyped with SSR markers by L. Robertson, J. Holland, and G. Payne at North Carolina State University. Heritability for resistance from GE440 to fumonisin accumulation in grain was estimated to be 34% among BC_1S_1 families.[43] Two QTL located on chromosome 5 were associated with resistance to fumonisin accumulation in grain and resistance to *Fusarium* ear rot.[43] Additional QTL associated with resistance to *Fusarium* ear rot were identified on chromosomes 1, 3, 6, and 10. In 2003, researchers from North Carolina State University reevaluated the mapping population at Clayton, NC, and Plymouth, NC. Data from these experiments are forthcoming.

19.4 CURRENT DIRECTION

Although sources of resistance to *Aspergillus* and *Fusarium* ear rots and aflatoxin and fumonisin accumulation in corn grain have been identified, resistance has not been successfully incorporated into commercial hybrids. This is largely because of difficulties encountered in identifying resistance that is stable in multiple environments and in maintaining high yield and favorable agronomics while integrating resistance into elite lines. Researchers in Illinois have identified several sources of resistance and are now identifying and incorporating chromosome regions associated with resistance into commercial inbred lines via marker-assisted selection (MAS).

Molecular marker technology has vastly improved since the advent of isozymic analyses and restriction fragment length polymorphisms (RFLP) in the early 1980s. Refinement of the DNA polymerase chain reaction (PCR) and simple sequence repeats (SSR) from the late 1980s to the present has led to rapid, safe, and simple varietal profiling and has made genetic mapping accessible and practical for plant breeders worldwide. At the University of Illinois, traditional breeding for resistance to aflatoxin and fumonisin accumulation in grain by backcrossing has required many cycles of selection and has resulted in the development of inbreds that impart superior resistance and poor yield to hybrid performance. Molecular markers are necessary to transfer alleles for resistance from multiple loci and multiple, nonadapted sources into elite commercial inbreds that impart high yield to hybrid performance.

Marker-assisted selection in the backcross breeding program has eliminated the need to evaluate genotypes for mycotoxin accumulation in grain during every cycle of selection and facilitated selection of resistant genotypes from winter or summer nurseries from which phenotypic data are not available. MAS has expedited transfer of alleles for resistance into agronomically favorable genetic backgrounds by hastening recovery of commercial phenotypes and has aided in pyramiding alleles from multiple sources of resistance into a commercial inbred. MAS also has minimized the number of genotypes that must be evaluated with determinative tests for mycotoxins in grain and has vastly improved efficiency of the breeding program in Illinois.

Many commercial seed companies and public institutions have in-house or collaborative access to technology necessary for MAS. With continued funding, agronomically favorable sources of resistance along with information on molecular markers associated with QTL for resistance soon may be released. Also with continued funding, isolines of resistant inbreds will be developed with MAS to study effects of specific chromosome regions on mechanisms of resistance.

ACKNOWLEDGMENTS

The authors thank J. Dudley, University of Illinois, and R. Brown, USDA–ARS, for critical review of this chapter. The authors also thank T. Brooks, USDA–ARS; K. Busboom and K. Kleinschmidt, University of Illinois; and L. Robertson, J. Holland, and G. Payne, North Carolina State University. This chapter is a joint contribution of the USDA–ARS and the University of Illinois.

REFERENCES

1. Moreno, O.J. and Kang, M.S., Aflatoxins in maize: the problem and genetic solutions, *Plant Breeding*, 118, 1–16, 1999.
2. Castegnaro, M. and McGregor, D., Carcinogenic risk assessment of mycotoxins, *Rev. Med. Vet.*, 149(6), 671–678, 1998.
3. CFSAN, *Background Paper in Support of Fumonisin Levels in Corn and Corn Products Intended for Human Consumption*, Docket Number 00D-1277, Center for Food Safety and Applied Nutrition, U.S. Food and Drug Administration, Rockville, MD, 2001 (http://www.cfsan.fda.gov/~dms/fumonbg3.html).
4. ORA Division of Compliance Policy, Section 555.400, Foods: Adulteration with Aflatoxin (CPG 7120.26), in *FDA/ORA Compliance Policy Guides Manual*, Office of Regulatory Affairs, U.S. Food and Drug Administration, Rockville, MD, 2000, p. 268.
5. Jones, R.K., Duncan, H.E., and Hamilton, P.B., Planting date, harvest date and irrigation effects on infection and aflatoxin production by *Aspergillus flavus* in field corn, *Phytopathology*, 71(8), 810–816, 1981.
6. Lillehoj, E.B., Fennell, D.I., Kwolek, W.F., Adams, G.L., Zuber, M.S., Horner, E.S., Widstrom, N.W., Warren, H., Guthrie, W.D., Sauer, D.B., Findley, W.R., Manwiller, A., Josephson, L.M., and Bockholt, A.J., Aflatoxin contamination of corn before harvest: *Aspergillus flavus* association with insects collected from developing ears, *Crop Sci.*, 18, 921–924, 1978.
7. Payne, G.A., Aflatoxin in maize, *CRC Crit. Rev. Plant Sci.*, 10(5), 423–440, 1992.
8. Widstrom, N.W., McMillian, W.W., Beaver, R.W., and Wilson, D.M., Weather-associated changes in aflatoxin contamination of preharvest maize, *J. Prod. Agric.*, 3(2), 196–199, 1990.

9. Zuber, M.S., Darrah, L.L., Lillehoj, E.B., Josephson, L.M., Manwiller, A., Scott, G.E., Gudauskas, R.T., Horner, E.S., Widstrom, N.W., Thompson, D.L., Bockholt, A.J., and Brewbaker, J.L., Comparison of open-pollinated maize varieties and hybrids for preharvest aflatoxin contamination in the southern United States, *Plant Dis.*, 67, 185–187, 1983.

10. Campbell, K.W. and White, D.G., An inoculation device to evaluate maize for resistance to ear rot and aflatoxin production by *Aspergillus flavus*, *Plant Dis.*, 78(8), 778–781, 1994.

11. Campbell, K.W. and White, D.G., Evaluation of corn genotypes for resistance to *Aspergillus* ear rot, kernel infection, and aflatoxin production, *Plant Dis.*, 79, 1039–1045, 1995.

12. Campbell, K.W. and White, D.G., Inheritance of resistance to *Aspergillus* ear rot and aflatoxin in corn genotypes, *Phytopathology*, 85, 886–896, 1995.

13. Hamblin, A.M. and White, D.G., Inheritance of resistance to *Aspergillus* ear rot and aflatoxin production of corn from Tex6, *Phytopathology*, 90(3), 292–296, 2000.

14. Walker, R.D. and White, D.G., Inheritance of resistance to *Aspergillus* ear rot and aflatoxin production of corn from CI2, *Plant Dis.*, 85(3), 322–327, 2001.

15. Maupin, L.M., Clements, M.J., and White, D.G., Evaluation of the MI82 corn line as a source of resistance to aflatoxin in grain and use of BGYF as a selection tool, *Plant Dis.*, 87(9), 1059–1066, 2003.

16. Clements, M.J., Campbell, K.W., Maragos, C.M., Pilcher, C., Pataky, J.K., and White, D.G., Influence of Cry1Ab protein and hybrid genotype on fumonisin contamination and *Fusarium* ear rot of corn, *Crop Sci.*, 43, 1283–1293, 2003.

17. Clements, M.J., Maragos, C.M., Kleinschmidt, C.E., Pataky, J.K., and White, D.G., Evaluation of inoculation techniques for *Fusarium* ear rot and fumonisin contamination of corn, *Plant Dis.*, 87, 147–153, 2002.

18. Gerdes, J.T., Behr, C.F., Coors, J.G., and Tracy, W.F., *Compilation of North American Maize Breeding Germplasm*, Tracy, W.F., Coors, J.G., and Geadelmann, J.L., Eds., Crop Science Society of America, Madison, WI, 1993, 202 pp.

19. Troyer, A.F., Background of U.S. hybrid corn, *Crop Sci.*, 39, 601–626, 1999.

20. Troyer, A.F., Origins of modern corn hybrids, in *Proc. 55th Annual Corn and Sorghum Research Conference*, Chicago, IL, December, 2000, pp. 27–42.

21. Troyer, A.F. and Rocheford, T.R., Germplasm ownership: related corn inbreds, *Crop Sci.*, 42, 3–11, 2002.

22. Campbell, K.W., White, D.G., Toman, J., and Rocheford, T., Sources of resistance in F_1 corn hybrids to ear rot caused by *Aspergillus flavus*, *Plant Dis.*, 77, 1169, 1993.

23. Campbell, K.W., Hamblin, A.M., and White, D.G., Inheritance of resistance to aflatoxin production in the cross between corn inbreds B73 and LB31, *Phytopathology*, 87(11), 1144–1147, 1997.

24. Smith, M.E. and Gracen, V.E., Registration of LYLB31 and NYRD4058 parental lines of maize, *Crop Sci.*, 33, 361, 1993.

25. Busboom, K.N. and White, D.G., Oh516 as a source of resistance to *Aspergillus* ear rot and aflatoxin production, in *Proc. Aflatoxin/ Fumonisin Elimination and Fungal Genomics Workshop*, Savannah, GA, October 13–15, 2003.

26. Naidoo, G., Forbes, A.M., Paul, C., White, D.G., and Rocheford, T.R., Resistance to *Aspergillus* ear rot and aflatoxin accumulation in maize F_1 hybrids, *Crop Sci.*, 42, 360–364, 2002.

27. GRIN, *USDA-ARS National Genetic Resources Program: Germplasm Resources Information Network*, National Germplasm Resources Laboratory, Beltsville, MD, 2001 (http://www.ars-grin.gov).

28. Huang, Z., White, D.G., and Payne, G.A., Corn seed proteins inhibitory to *Aspergillus flavus* and aflatoxin biosynthesis, *Phytopathology*, 87, 622–627, 1997.
29. Lozovaya, V.V., Waranyuwat, A., and Widholm, J.M., β-1,3-glucanase and resistance to *Aspergillus flavus* infection in maize, *Crop Sci.*, 38(5), 1255–1260, 1998.
30. Moore, K.G., Boston, R.S., Price, M.S., Weissinger, A.K., and Payne, G.A., A chitinase from Tex6 maize kernels inhibits growth of *Aspergillus flavus*, *Phytopathology*, 94(1), 82–87, 2004.
31. Brown, R.L., Cleveland, T.E., Payne, G.A., Woloshuk, C.P., Campbell, K.W., and White, D.G., Determination of resistance to aflatoxin production in maize kernels and detection of fungal colonization using an *Aspergillus flavus* transformant expressing *Escherichia coli* β-glucuronidase, *Phytopathology*, 85, 983–989, 1995.
32. Brown, R.L., Cleveland, T.E., Payne, G.A., Woloshuk, C.P., and White, D.G., Growth of an *Aspergillus flavus* transformant expressing *Escherichia coli* beta-glucuronidase in maize kernels resistant to aflatoxin production, *J. Food Protect.*, 60(1), 84–87, 1997.
33. Chen, Z.Y., Brown, R.L., Lax, A.R., Guo, B.Z., Cleveland, T.E., and Russin, J.S., Resistance to *Aspergillus flavus* in corn kernels is associated with a 14-kDa protein, *Phytopathology*, 88(4), 276–281, 1998.
34. Chen, Z.Y., Brown, R.L., Russin, J.S., Lax, A.R., and Cleveland, T.E., A corn trypsin inhibitor with antifungal activity inhibits *Aspergillus flavus* alpha-amylase, *Phytopathology*, 89(10), 902–907, 1999.
35. Fakhoury, A.M. and Woloshuk, C.P., *Amy*1, the α-amylase gene of *Aspergillus flavus*: involvement in aflatoxin biosynthesis in maize kernels, *Phytopathology*, 89, 908–914, 1999.
36. Paul, C., Naidoo, G., Forbes, A., Mikkilineni, V., White, D., and Rocheford, T., Quantitative trait loci for low aflatoxin production in two related maize populations, *Theor. Appl. Genet.*, 107(2), 263–270, 2003.
37. Scott, G.E. and Zummo, N., Registration of Mp313E parental line of maize, *Crop Sci.*, 30, 1378, 1990.
38. Brooks, T.D., Williams, W.P., Windham, G.L., and Abbas, H.K., Molecular characterization of resistance to aflatoxin accumulation in Mp313E, in *Proc. Aflatoxin/Fumonisin Elimination and Fungal Genomics Workshop*, Savannah, GA, October 13–15, 2003.
39. Gelderblom, W.C.A., Jaskiewicz, K., Marasas, W.F.O., Thiel, P.G., Horak, R.M., Vleggaar, R., and Kriek, N.P.J., Fumonisins: novel mycotoxins with cancer-promoting activity produced by *Fusarium moniliforme*, *Appl. Environ. Microbiol.*, 54, 1806–1811, 1988.
40. Marasas, W.F.O., Kellerman, T.S., Gelderblom, W.C.A., Coetzer, J.A.W., and Thiel, P.G., Leukoencephalomalacia in a horse induced by fumonisin B$_1$ isolated from *Fusarium moniliforme*, *Onderstepoort J. Vet. Res.*, 55, 197–203, 1988.
41. Clements, M.J., Resistance to Fumonisins and *Fusarium* Ear Rot of Corn, Ph.D. thesis, UMI No. 3070279, University of Illinois, Urbana, 2002, 144 pp.
42. Clements, M.J., Maragos, C.M., Pataky, J.K., and White, D.G., Sources of resistance to fumonisin accumulation in grain and *Fusarium* ear rot of corn, *Phytopathology*, 94, 251–260, 2003.
43. Robertson, L.A., Payne, G.A., White, D.G., and Holland, J.B., Identifying QTLs for fumonisin accumulation and ear rot resistance in maize, in *Proc. Aflatoxin/Fumonisin Elimination and Fungal Genomics Workshop*, Savannah, GA, October 13–15, 2003.

20 Techniques Used to Identify Aflatoxin-Resistant Corn*

*Gary L. Windham, W. Paul Williams,
Paul M. Buckley, Hamed K. Abbas,
and Leigh K. Hawkins*

CONTENTS

20.1 INTRODUCTION

Field studies in 1971 and 1972 first established aflatoxin contamination as a preharvest problem in corn.[1] Results of these studies initiated the evaluation of corn genotypes for sources of resistance to *Aspergillus flavus* kernel infection and aflatoxin contamination.[2,3] Because aflatoxin contamination is sporadic from growing season to growing season, inoculation techniques were developed to uniformly infect corn ears with *A. flavus*.[4,5] The development of effective inoculation techniques is

---

* Mention of trade names or commercial products in this chapter is solely for the purpose of providing specific information and does not imply recommendation or endorsement by the U.S. Department of Agriculture.

difficult because *A. flavus* is a weak pathogen. Also, environmental conditions have a significant impact on kernel infection and aflatoxin accumulation.[6] The inoculation techniques first developed could not identify corn genotypes that were resistant to *A. flavus* with any consistency. Thus, progress in developing resistant germplasm was slowed. Significant progress has been made in the last 15 years in developing inoculation techniques that can be used in the field or laboratory to identify corn genotypes with resistance to *A. flavus* and aflatoxin contamination. Several reports are available on a myriad of techniques used to artificially inoculate corn ears with *A. flavus*.[1–11] This chapter discusses inoculation techniques that are currently being used to evaluate corn genotypes for resistance to *A. flavus* and aflatoxin in corn in the southern and midwestern United States. Inoculum production and factors that have an impact on field evaluations are also discussed.

20.2 EVALUATION OF AFLATOXIN RESISTANCE IN THE FIELD

Inoculation techniques used in field evaluations can be classified as wounding or nonwounding types. Nonwounding techniques mimic natural infection and allow the identification of corn germplasm that may have resistance mechanisms found on kernel surfaces such as waxes or thickened pericarps. Wounding techniques are generally more consistent in producing kernel infection and subsequent aflatoxin production; however, because kernels are damaged during inoculations, only genotypes with internal (physiological) mechanisms of resistance can be identified.

20.2.1 NONWOUNDING INOCULATION TECHNIQUES

One of the more commonly used nonwounding inoculation techniques in field studies involves spraying or atomizing small volumes of *Aspergillus flavus* conidial suspensions on silks exposed from the husks of ears.[12,13] In a North Carolina study, silks were spray inoculated when they had turned yellow-brown in an effort to monitor aflatoxin contamination during ear development.[13] After inoculation, ears were covered with a plastic bag for 3 days. Spray inoculations have been successfully used in studies in West Africa to identify aflatoxin-resistant genotypes.[14] Progeny of cycles of selection of four maize genotypes were inoculated by atomizing conidia on to the silks and covering the ears with pollination bags. A spray technique has also been developed that can be used to inoculate large field tests.[15] Hybrids were evaluated for resistance to aflatoxin accumulation using a Solo® backpack sprayer (Solo; Newport News, VA). A conidial suspension containing 9×10^7 conidia/mL was sprayed on silks and husks when silks began emerging, and spray treatments continued weekly for 5 weeks. The mean level of aflatoxin contamination for 45 commercial hybrids inoculated with this method was 2208 ppb. Hybrids inoculated with the backpack sprayer had aflatoxin contamination at levels similar to hybrids inoculated with a wounding inoculation technique. Spray inoculation techniques have also been used to study the interactions of southwestern corn borer (*Diatraea grandiosella* Dyar) and *A. flavus*.[16] Conidia were sprayed on silks using an Idico®

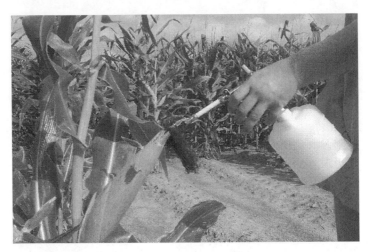

FIGURE 20.1 Spraying *Aspergillus flavus* conidia onto silks of a developing ear using a tree marking gun.

tree-marking gun (Idico Products; New York, NY) fitted with a spray nozzle (Figure 20.1). High levels of aflatoxin were found in ears inoculated with *A. flavus* and infested with southwestern corn borer.

Another nonwounding inoculation technique is the silk channel technique.[17] An Idico® tree-marking gun fitted with a 14-gauge needle was used to inject *Aspergillus flavus* conidia into the silk channel 6 days after midsilk (50% of the plants in a plot had silks emerged). Kernel infection of inbreds inoculated with the silk channel technique was similar in inbreds inoculated using wounding inoculation techniques. The silk channel technique is an excellent inoculation method to use in field studies on evaluating corn genotypes for aflatoxin resistance when no kernel damage is desired.[18]

Applications of granular material infected with *Aspergillus flavus* has been used to inoculate corn ears in field studies.[19] Corn seed infected with *A. flavus* and spread within plots to inoculate developing ears has been used successfully in field evaluations in the Coastal Bend of Texas (G. Odvody, pers. comm.). Various formulations of alginate pellets containing *A. flavus* mycelia were evaluated for seeding agricultural fields.[20] Atoxigenic isolates of *A. flavus* cultured on long-grain rice were applied to fields to control aflatoxin in corn and peanut.[21,22] Wheat seed infected with an atoxigenic isolate of *A. flavus* has been successfully used to control aflatoxin contamination in cottonseed in the southwestern United States.[23,24] Preliminary studies are being conducted by the authors to adapt this technology to inoculate corn in field studies with toxigenic strains of *A. flavus*.[25] Applications of wheat infected with toxigenic isolates of *A. flavus* have been as effective as spray techniques in producing high levels of aflatoxin contamination. Applications of *A. flavus*-infected granular material are less labor intensive than other inoculation techniques and provide a more natural method of infection of the developing corn ears.

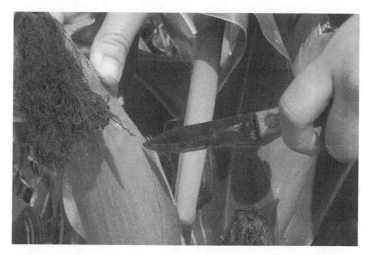

FIGURE 20.2 Inoculating a corn ear using the knife inoculation technique. A grafting or paring knife dipped into suspensions of *Aspergillus flavus* conidia is inserted through the husk and into the midsection of a corn ear.

20.2.2 WOUNDING INOCULATION TECHNIQUES

Wounding inoculation techniques commonly used to evaluate corn genotypes include the knife, pinbar, modified pinbar, pinboard, side-needle, toothpick, and punch drill/pipe cleaner techniques. The knife technique (Figure 20.2) has been the inoculation method of choice for evaluating corn genotypes for resistance in south Georgia.[3,6,26–28] This involves dipping the tip of a grafting or paring knife into a conidial suspension and inserting the blade through the husk and into the mid-section of an ear approximately 20 days after silking.[3,6] In one study, ears inoculated with the knife technique had higher levels of aflatoxin contamination than ears inoculated with a needle or a multiple puncture technique.[6] Tropical hybrids inoculated with the knife technique had lower levels of aflatoxin contamination than adapted hybrids in field evaluations.[28] In North Carolina, ears of a commercial hybrid inoculated with the knife technique had aflatoxin levels during ear development comparable to ears that were inoculated by spraying spores on silks.[13]

The pinbar technique (Figure 20.3) utilizes a single 100-mm-long row of 35 to 36 sewing needles mounted in wood or a plastic bar with approximately 6 mm of the points exposed.[4] The needles are dipped in an *Aspergillus flavus* conidial suspension (2×10^7 conidia/mL), aligned parallel with the ear axis, and pressed through the husk and into the kernels. Resistance to *A. flavus* can be quantified by determining kernel infection of kernels in rows adjacent to the wounded kernels[4,5] or by bulking wounded kernels with nonwounded kernels for aflatoxin analyses.[29,30] This technique is used by researchers at Louisiana State University for field evaluations. Environmental conditions favorable to disease development may result in extremely high aflatoxin contamination levels that limit the ability to separate resistant from susceptible genotypes. A modified pinbar (Figure 20.4), consisting of four needles

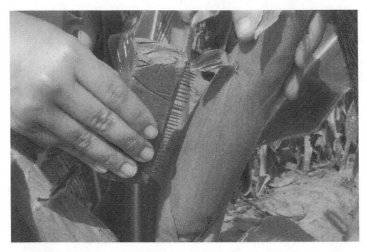

FIGURE 20.3 The pinbar technique is effective in producing high levels of aflatoxin contamination. Pins are dipped into suspensions of *Aspergillus flavus* conidia and inserted through the husk into the kernels.

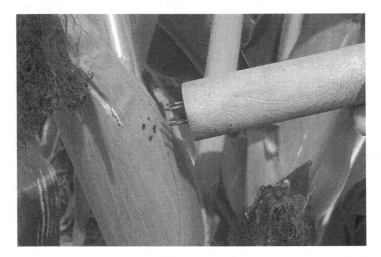

FIGURE 20.4 Inoculation with the modified pinbar provides a point source for *Aspergillus flavus* inoculum dispersal and allows the movement of the fungus in the ear to be monitored.

mounted in a large dowel, has been used by the authors to study movement of *Aspergillus* spp. in developing ears of corn. Inoculation with the modified pinbar provides a point source for inoculum dispersal and allows the movement of *Aspergillus* spp. in the ear to be monitored.[31]

The pinboard technique was developed to evaluate corn genotypes for resistance in the midwestern United States,[32] where the environment is often not conducive to *Aspergillus flavus* development and subsequent aflatoxin contamination. The pinboard inoculator was developed at the University of Illinois and consists of a

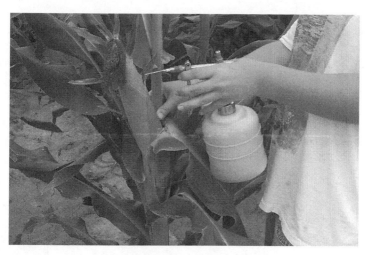

FIGURE 20.5 The side-needle technique is a reliable method for inoculating ears with *Aspergillus flavus*. This technique utilizes a tree-marking gun fitted with a 14-gauge needle.

pinboard of 7 rows of 23 steel pins. The pinboard is attached to a spray gun, which is connected to a Solo® backpack sprayer. To inoculate a developing corn ear, the pinboard is aligned with the ear axis, the pins are pushed through the husk into the kernels, and 5 mL of *A. flavus* inoculum (2×10^5 conidia/mL) are injected under the husk. A large number of kernels are damaged using this technique. Ear rot ratings of ears inoculated with the pinboard are highest when ears are inoculated 14 to 23 days after midsilk.[32] The pinboard inoculator was used to evaluate corn inbreds in Illinois and Mississippi.[33] The mean levels of aflatoxin contamination in Illinois and Mississippi were 363 and 2844 ppb, respectively. The pinboard inoculator severely wounds ears and may be impractical for use in the hot, humid South; however, it does provide a reliable method to evaluate corn genotypes in the temperate conditions of the Midwest.[33–36]

The side-needle technique (Figure 20.5) has been used for 16 years in Mississippi to evaluate corn germplasm for resistance to *A. flavus*.[17] This technique is a reliable method for inoculating corn ears in the field with minimal damage to developing kernels.[37] The side-needle technique utilizes an Idico® tree-marking gun fitted with a 14-gauge needle. Inoculations made with the side-needle technique are most effective 6 days after midsilk as opposed to 12 or 18 days.[38] Multiple inoculations do not increase the amount of kernel infection or aflatoxin contamination.[38] To inoculate ears using this technique, the needle is inserted under the husks on the upper third of the ear, and 3.4 mL of an *A. flavus* conidial suspension (9×10^7 conidia/mL) is injected over the kernels. When compared with ears inoculated with the pinbar and silk channel techniques, ears inoculated with the side-needle technique had similar levels of *A. flavus* kernel infection.[17] An advantage of the side-needle technique over the pinbar and silk channel techniques is the speed and ease of making the inoculations. The side-needle technique has recently been used in Mississippi to identify corn inbreds and advanced breeding lines with resistance to aflatoxin contamination.[39,40] Although labor intensive, this technique has proven superior to other wounding and nonwounding inoculation techniques in field evaluations.[17,25]

The toothpick-under-husk (TUH) and punch drill/pipe cleaner (PDPC) techniques have also been used to evaluate the resistance of corn genotypes.[41,42] Inoculum for the TUH technique is increased on toothpicks placed on a growth medium and then inoculated with *Aspergillus flavus*. Developing ears are inoculated by making an incision in the husks in the middle of the ear and inserting a toothpick. In field studies in Louisiana, the TUH technique produced higher levels of aflatoxin contamination with less variability than three nonwounding inoculation techniques;[42] however, in a Mississippi study, ears inoculated with *A. flavus* using the TUH technique had lower levels of kernel infection than ears inoculated with the pinbar or side-needle technique.[17] The PDPC technique has been used in hybrid evaluations at Weslaco, TX.[41] Pipe cleaners inoculated with *A. flavus* were placed in holes drilled into the cob of developing ears. At harvest, nonwounded kernels were harvested from around the drilled holes and evaluated for aflatoxin contamination to determine resistance of Corn Belt hybrids.

Insect vectors have also been used to inoculate developing ears with *Aspergillus flavus*.[16,43] In a study in Mississippi, a hand-operated dispenser previously developed to infest plants with lepidopterans was used to apply corn cob grits containing *A. flavus* conidia onto corn silks inside a shoot bag.[16] This application was followed 24 hours later by an application of southwestern corn borer neonate larvae. Inoculating the fungus and infesting silks with the insect dispenser worked well in producing high levels of aflatoxin contamination. This inoculation technique may also be useful in studying *A. flavus* interactions with other ear-feeding insects.

20.2.3 INOCULUM

The *Aspergillus flavus* isolate and the conidial concentration of inoculum are both critical in providing adequate kernel infection in field evaluations. *A. flavus* isolates vary in their ability to infect corn kernels on developing ears in the field.[44] The NRRL 3357 isolate of *A. flavus* infected a higher percentage of kernels than an *A. parasiticus* isolate and other *A. flavus* isolates.[44] This isolate is a reliable producer of aflatoxin under field conditions and has been used in field studies for over 25 years at different locations.[4,17,18,26,38,40,45] New NRRL 3357 cultures should be started every year prior to the growing season from freeze-dried mycelial plugs that can be obtained from the USDA Agricultural Research Service, Northern Regional Research Laboratory, Peoria, IL. To ensure adequate infection of corn genotypes in the Midwest, mixtures of toxigenic isolates of *A. flavus* have been used in field evaluations.[33,34] The amount of kernel infection of corn genotypes in field evaluations is dependent on the conidial concentrations of the inoculum. Ears inoculated with wounding and nonwounding techniques had the highest levels of kernel infection when a conidial concentration of 10^6/mL was used compared to concentrations of 10^4/mL and 10^5/mL.[17] *A. flavus* inoculum can be increased on a V8 Vegetable Juice® medium or on Czapek solution agar amended with NaCl.[23,24] Toxigenic isolates of *A. flavus* should not be repeatedly transferred in culture in the laboratory. Serial transfers often result in the degeneration of cultures and the loss of aflatoxin production.[46] Large amounts of *A. flavus* inoculum can be produced on sterilized wheat or on sterilized corn cob grits (Grit-O-Cobs®, Maumee, OH).[17,23] Conidia in liquid suspensions can be quantified using a turbidity meter or a hemacytometer. Tween® 20 or a spreader sticker (Hi-Yield Chemical Co., Bonham, TX) should be added to conidial suspensions to reduce surface tension and disperse the conidia.

Color mutants of *Aspergillus flavus* (white, tan) and *A. parasiticus* (reddish-brown) have been used in field studies to evaluate corn for aflatoxin resistance.[45,47] These isolates are easily recognizable from wild-type isolates, which are predominantly yellow-green or olive-green. *Aspergillus* species have been identified that produce norsolorinic acid (NOR) which is a visible orange intermediate of aflatoxin.[48] An *A. parasiticus* isolate that produces NOR has been used in field evaluations to identify resistant corn genotypes (D.M. Wilson, pers. comm.). Ears inoculated with this NOR mutant were visually screened for fungal infection by counting kernels that had a reddening of the aleurone layer. The NOR mutant was used to identify highly susceptible genotypes in the initial stages of mass screenings in an effort to reduce aflatoxin analyses and expenses. Transformants of *A. flavus* containing the green fluorescent protein (GFP) gene from the jellyfish *Aequorea victoria* have been developed and may be useful for identifying resistant corn genotypes in future studies.[49]

20.2.4 HARVEST, SAMPLE PREPARATION, TOXIN ANALYSES, AND FUNGAL INFECTION

After inoculations have been completed in the field, steps must be taken to obtain samples that accurately and precisely measure aflatoxin contamination in experimental plots. Developing ears of corn are typically inoculated with *Aspergillus flavus* 7 to 20 days after midsilk.[6,17,29,40] Aflatoxin levels reach relatively high levels by 35 days after midsilk and increase until harvest (Figure 20.6). Ears from plots are hand harvested 63 days after midsilk, dried at 38°C for 7 days, and then either hand or machine shelled. Grain samples should then be cleaned with a forced air cleaner, poured into a sample splitter twice to thoroughly mix the grain, and ground in a Romer Series II Mill (Union, MO) or equivalent. The Romer Series II Mill will simultaneously grind and split the grain sample. Proper grinding and mixing increases the chances of detecting aflatoxin especially in samples with low levels of contamination.

Aflatoxin contamination can be determined using a variety of methods. The Vicam AflaTest® (Watertown, MA) has been used to quantify aflatoxin in 50-g subsamples from plots. The AflaTest® P column has been certified by the Association of Analytical Communities (AOAC International) for aflatoxin determination.[50] This procedure can detect aflatoxins (B_1, B_2, G_1, G_2) at concentrations as low as 1 ppb. Enzyme-linked immunosorbent assay (ELISA) kits (Neogen, Inc.; Lansing, MI) have also been used by researchers to quantify aflatoxin contamination in field plots.[51,52] Because of the large variability associated with the quantification of aflatoxin in grain samples, aflatoxin data should be transformed to equalize variances prior to data analysis.

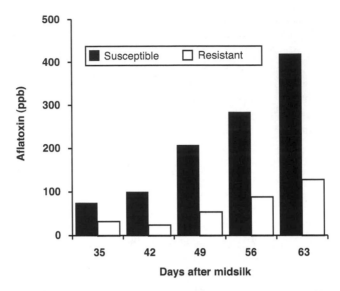

FIGURE 20.6 Aflatoxin accumulation in resistant and susceptible corn hybrids at five harvest dates. Ears were inoculated with *Aspergillus flavus* using the side-needle technique.

The amount of *Aspergillus flavus* infection in corn ears can be determined by plating surface-sterilized kernels on agar plates. An effective method of surface sterilization involves dipping kernels momentarily (5 seconds) in 70% ethanol, soaking for 3 minutes in 1.5% NaOCl, and rinsing in sterile distilled water.[17] Surface-sterilized kernels should then be placed in 100-mm Petri dishes (13 kernels per dish) containing Czapek solution agar amended with 7.5% NaCl. The salt amendment restricts the growth of bacteria and other fungi. After 7 days at 28°C, kernels can be examined for *A. flavus* growth. A sample size of 200 to 390 kernels per plot has been determined to be adequate to detect *A. flavus* infection.[53]

20.2.5 ENVIRONMENTAL EFFECTS

Three major factors are associated with preharvest contamination of corn by aflatoxin: environment, insect damage, and hybrid susceptibility.[54] Several studies illustrate the great influence of variations in weather-related factors in screening for aflatoxin response from year to year and among locations.[55–57] Environmental factors that favor the production of aflatoxin in preharvest corn include high temperatures, low humidity, drought stress, and net evaporation rates.[3,56,58] Higher than normal ambient temperatures and drought conditions have shown the most consistent association with high levels of aflatoxin contamination.[57] Hybrids can be exposed to an increased risk of aflatoxin contamination when environmental stress occurs during the flowering and grain filling periods.[18,57,58,59] Aflatoxin production in ears artificially inoculated with *Aspergillus flavus* can also be influenced by environmental conditions, and huge fluctuations of aflatoxin contamination from year to year may result.[16,40] It is imperative to choose an inoculation technique that will allow researchers to distinguish between resistant and susceptible genotypes consistently from year to year regardless of the environmental conditions. Wounding inoculation techniques are generally less susceptible to environmental influences than nonwounding techniques. Ears inoculated by spraying conidia on silks may have low levels of *A. flavus* infection and little aflatoxin contamination when growing conditions do not favor fungal development. Also, inoculum deposited on the exterior surface of the ear may be exposed to unfavorable conditions such as high temperatures during mid-day. Spray inoculations made in late afternoon have been successful in establishing the fungus in developing kernels.[14]

20.3 EVALUATION OF AFLATOXIN RESISTANCE IN THE LABORATORY

Laboratory evaluations for detecting aflatoxin resistance in corn genotypes have been developed.[60–63] The advantages of using laboratory evaluations include: (1) they can be used to screen material year-round, (2) they are less expensive compared to field evaluations, and (3) fewer kernels are required for evaluations. A kernel-screening assay (KSA) has been used to quantify aflatoxin contamination and fungal growth in mature kernels.[61,62] Kernels evaluated in KSA are surfaced sterilized, dipped into an *Aspergillus flavus* conidial suspension, and incubated in 100% relative humidity at 31°C for 7 days. Aflatoxin contamination and fungal infection of kernels can then be quantified. An *A. flavus* β-glucuronidase (GUS) transformant was used in KSA studies to evaluate corn inbreds for resistance to fungal infection.[62] The kernel-screening assay has also been used to confirm resistance identified in field studies and to identify potential new sources of resistance.[61,62] This technique has also been used with wounding and nonwounding inoculation techniques to study resistance mechanisms.[64,65]

20.4 SAFETY PRECAUTIONS

Aspergillus flavus isolate NRRL 3357 is classified as a "Biosafety Level 1" agent by the American Type Culture Collection (www.atcc.org). Level 1 agents are microorganisms not known to consistently cause diseases in healthy adult humans;[66] however, these organisms may cause infections in the young, the aged, and immunodeficient or immunosuppressed individuals. When working with level 1 agents, a basic level of containment that relies on standard microbiological practices with no special primary or secondary barriers is recommended, other than a sink for handwashing. It is recommended that laboratory personnel wear a long-sleeved laboratory coat and gloves. A number of field inoculation techniques involve the use of sharp pins, needles, or knifes. Personnel inoculating ears with *Aspergillus flavus* in the field should wear a long-sleeved shirt, long pants, a hat, and gloves. It is recommended that personnel wear a dust mask or respirator when harvesting *A. flavus*-inoculated corn ears and when removing harvested ears from driers. Shelling, cleaning, mixing, and grinding operations should be carried out in a well-ventilated room, and workers should wear dust masks or respirators.

20.5 SUMMARY

Although tremendous progress has been made in developing inoculation techniques that can be used to identify aflatoxin resistant corn genotypes, an inoculation technique that could be used at multiple locations regardless of the environmental conditions is still needed. Inoculation techniques that require minimal labor and produce uniform levels of infection would be useful to private and public scientists in the development of resistant hybrids. Research on factors that affect *Aspergillus flavus* infection and aflatoxin contamination in the field must continue in order to develop efficient evaluation procedures. Continued improvement of laboratory techniques for evaluating corn genotypes is also necessary. The use of *A. flavus* transformants containing GUS and GFP reporter genes may lead to improved inoculation and evaluation techniques.

ACKNOWLEDGMENTS

This manuscript is a joint contribution of USDA–ARS and the Mississippi Agricultural and Forestry Experiment Station, Mississippi State, MS.

REFERENCES

1. Anderson, H.W., Nehring, E.W., and Wichser, W.R., Aflatoxin contamination of corn in the field, *Agric. Food Chem.*, 23(4), 775–782,1975.
2. Lillehoj, E.B., Kwolek, W.F., Manwiller, A., Durant, J.A., LaPrade, J.C., Horner, E.S., Reid, J., and Zuber, M.S., Aflatoxin production in several corn hybrids grown in South Carolina and Florida, *Crop Sci.*, 16(4), 483–485, 1976.
3. Widstrom, N.W., Wilson, D.M., and McMillian, W.W., Aflatoxin contamination of preharvest corn as influenced by timing and method of inoculation, *Appl. Environ. Microbiol.*, 42(2), 249–251, 1981.
4. King, S.B. and Scott, G.E., Field inoculation techniques to evaluate maize for reaction to kernel infection by *Aspergillus flavus*, *Phytopathology*, 72(7), 782–785, 1982.
5. Tucker, D.H., Tevathan, L.E., King, S.B., and Scott, G.E., Effect of four inoculation techniques on infection and aflatoxin concentration of resistant and susceptible corn hybrids inoculated with *Aspergillus flavus*, *Phytopathology*, 76(3), 290–293, 1986.
6. Widstrom, N.W., McMillian, W.W., Beaver, R.W., and Wilson, D.M., Weather-associated changes in aflatoxin contamination of preharvest maize, *J. Product. Agric.*, 3(2), 196–199, 1990.
7. Kang, M.S. and Moreno, O.J., Maize improvement for resistance to aflatoxins: progress and challenges, in *Crop Improvement: Challenges in the Twenty-First Century*, Kang, M.S., Ed., Food Products Press, New York, 2002, pp. 75–108.
8. King, S.B. and Wallin, J.R., Methods for screening corn for resistance to kernel infection and aflatoxin production by *Aspergillus flavus*, in *Aflatoxin and Aspergillus flavus in Corn*, Diener, U.L., Asquith, R.L., and Dickens, J.W., Eds., Southern Cooperative Series Bulletin No. 279, Southern Association of Agricultural Experiment Station Directors, Raleigh, NC, 1983, pp. 77–80.

9. Scott, G.E. and Zummo, N., Host-plant resistance: screening techniques, in *Aflatoxin in Maize*, Zuber, M.S., Lillehoj, E.B., and Renfro, B.L., Eds., CIMMYT, Mexico City, 1987, pp. 221–233.

10. Wilson, D.M., Widstrom, N.W., McMillian, W.W., and Beaver, R.W., Aflatoxins in corn, in *Proc. 44th Annual Corn and Sorghum Research Conference*, Chicago, IL, 1989, pp. 1–26.

11. Moreno, O.J. and Kang, M.S., Aflatoxin in maize: the problem and genetic solutions, *Plant Breed.*, 118(1), 1–16, 1999.

12. Jones, R.K., Duncan, H.E., Payne, G.A., and Leonard, K.J., Factors influencing infection by *Aspergillus flavus* in silk-inoculated corn, *Plant Dis.*, 64(9), 859–863, 1980.

13. Payne, G.A., Hagler, W.M., and Adkins, C.R., Aflatoxin accumulation in inoculated ears of field-grown maize, *Plant Dis.*, 72(5), 422–424, 1988.

14. Cardwell, K.F., Kling, J.G., Maziya-Dixon, B., and Bosque-Perez, N.A., Interaction between *Fusarium verticilliodes*, *Aspergillus flavus*, and insect infestation in four maize genotypes in lowland Africa, *Phytopathology*, 90(3), 276–284, 2000.

15. Windham, G.L. and Williams, W.P., *Aflatoxin Accumulation in Commercial Corn Hybrids in 1998*, Research Report 22(8), Mississippi Agricultural and Forestry Experimental Station, Mississippi State University, Mississippi State, MS, 1999, pp. 1–4.

16. Windham, G.L., Williams, W.P., and Davis, F.M., Effects of the southwestern corn borer on *Aspergillus flavus* kernel infection and aflatoxin accumulation in maize hybrids, *Plant Dis.*, 83(6), 535–540, 1999.

17. Zummo, N. and Scott, G.E., Evaluation of field inoculation techniques for screening maize genotypes against kernel infection by *Aspergillus flavus* in Mississippi, *Plant Dis.*, 73(4), 313–316, 1989.

18. Betran, F.J. and Isakeit, T., Aflatoxin accumulation in maize hybrids of different maturities, *Agron. J.*, 96(2), 565–570, 2004.

19. Olanya, O.M., Hoyos, G.M., Tiffany, L.H., and McGee, D.C., Waste corn as a point source of inoculum for *Aspergillus flavus* in the corn agroecosystem, *Plant Dis.*, 81(6), 576–581, 1997.

20. Daigle, D.J. and Cotty, P.J., Formulating atoxigenic *Aspergillus flavus* for field release, *Biocontrol Sci. Technol.*, 5, 175–184, 1995.

21. Dorner, J.W., Cole, R.J., and Blankenship, P.D., Effect of inoculum rate of biological control agents on preharvest aflatoxin contamination of peanuts, *Biol. Control*, 12(3), 171–176, 1998.

22. Dorner, J.W., Cole, R.J., and Wicklow, D.T., Aflatoxin reduction in corn through field application of competitive fungi, *J. Food Protect.*, 62(6), 650–656, 1999.

23. Bock, C.H. and Cotty, P.J., Wheat seed colonized with atoxigenic *Aspergillus flavus*: characterization and production of a biopesticide for aflatoxin control, *Biocontrol Sci. Technol.*, 9, 529–543, 1999.

24. Cotty, P.J., Influence of field application of an atoxigenic strain of *Aspergillus flavus* on the populations of *A. flavus* infecting cotton bolls and on the aflatoxin content of cottonseed, *Phytopathology*, 84(11), 1270–1277, 1994.

25. Windham, G.L., Williams, W.P., Buckley, P.M., Abbas, H.K., and Hawkins, L.K., A comparison of inoculation techniques for *Aspergillus flavus* on corn, in *Proc. Aflatoxin Elimination Workshop*, San Antonio. TX, 2002, p. 139.

26. Widstrom, N.W., Wilson, D.M., and McMillian, W.W., Evaluation of sampling methods for detecting aflatoxin contamination in small test plots of maize inoculated with *Aspergillus flavus*, *J. Environ. Qual.*, 11(4), 655–657, 1982.

27. Widstrom, N.W., Wilson, D.M., and McMillian, W.W., Differentiation of maize genotypes for aflatoxin concentration in developing kernels, *Crop Sci.*, 26(5), 935–937, 1986.

28. Widstrom, N.W., Forster, M.J., Martin, W.K., and Wilson, D.M., Agronomic performance in the southeastern United States of maize hybrids containing tropical germplasm, *Maydica*, 41, 59–63, 1996.

29. Tubajika, K.M. and Damann, K.E., Sources of resistance to aflatoxin production in maize, *J. Agric. Food Chem.*, 49(5), 2652–2656, 2001.

30. Tubajika, K.M., Mascagni, Jr., H.J., Damann, K.E., and Russin, J.S., Susceptibility of commercial corn hybrids to aflatoxin contamination in Louisiana, *Cereal Res. Comm.*, 28(4), 463–467, 2000.

31. Windham, G.L., Williams, W.P., Brown, R.L., Cleveland, T.E., and Payne, G.A., Spread of genetically altered *Aspergillus* species in resistant and susceptible corn kernels, in *Proc. Aflatoxin Elimination Workshop*, St. Louis, MO, 1998, p. 83.

32. Campbell, K.W. and White, D.G., An inoculation device to evaluate maize for resistance to ear rot and aflatoxin production by *Aspergillus flavus*, *Plant Dis.*, 78(8), 778–781, 1994.

33. Campbell, K.W. and White, D.G., Evaluation of corn genotypes for resistance to *Aspergillus* ear rot, kernel infection, and aflatoxin production, *Plant Dis.*, 79(10), 1039–1045, 1995.

34. Campbell, K.W. and White, D.G., Inheritance of resistance to *Aspergillus* ear rot and aflatoxin in corn genotypes, Phytopathology, 85(8), 886–896, 1995,

35. Naidoo, G., Forbes, A.M., Paul, C., White, D.G., and Rocheford, T.R., Resistance to *Aspergillus* ear rot and aflatoxin accumulation in maize F_1 hybrids, *Crop Sci.*, 42(2), 360–364, 2002.

36. Walker, R.D. and White, D.G., Inheritance of resistance to *Aspergillus* ear rot and aflatoxin production of corn from C12, *Plant Dis.*, 85(3), 322–327, 2001.

37. Windham, G.L. and Williams, W.P., *Aspergillus flavus* infection and aflatoxin accumulation in resistant and susceptible maize hybrids, *Plant Dis.*, 82(3), 281–284, 1998.

38. Scott, G.E. and Zummo, N., Kernel infection and aflatoxin production in maize by *Aspergillus flavus* relative to inoculation and harvest dates, *Plant Dis.*, 78(2), 123–125, 1994,

39. Williams, W.P. and Windham, G.L., Registration of maize germplasm line Mp715, *Crop Sci.*, 41(4), 1374–1375, 2001.

40. Windham, G.L. and Williams, W.P., Evaluation of corn inbreds and advanced breeding lines for resistance to aflatoxin contamination in the field, *Plant Dis.*, 86(3), 232–234, 2002.

41. Wicklow, D.T., Miles, M., and Dunlap, J., Aflatoxin contamination of resistant and susceptible corn belt hybrids grown at Weslaco, Texas, 1993, in *Proc. Aflatoxin Elimination Workshop*, St. Louis, MO, 1994, p. 3.

42. Zhang, Y., Simonson, J.G., Wang, G., Kang, M.S., and Morris, H.F., A reliable field-inoculation method for identifying aflatoxin-resistant maize, *Cereal Res. Comm.*, 26(3), 45–251, 1998.

43. Barry, D., Zuber, M.S., Lillehoj, E.B., McMillian, W.W., Adams, N.J., Kwolek, W.F., and Widstrom, N.W., Evaluation of two arthropod vectors as inoculators of developing maize ears with *Aspergillus flavus*, *Environ. Entomol.*, 14(5), 634–636, 1985.

44. Zummo, N. and Scott, G.E., Pathogenicity of *Aspergillus flavus* group isolates in inoculated maize ears in Mississippi, *Biodeterioration Res.*, 4, 217–224, 1994.

45. Zummo, N., Concurrent infection of individual corn kernels with white and green isolates of *Aspergillus flavus*, *Plant Dis.*, 75(9), 910–913, 1991.

46. Horn, B.W. and Dorner, J.W., Effect of competition and adverse culture conditions on aflatoxin production by *Aspergillus flavus* through successive generations, *Mycologia*, 94(5), 741–751, 2001.

47. Wilson, D.M., McMillian, W.W., and Widstrom, N., Use of *Aspergillus flavus* and *A. parasiticus* color mutants to study aflatoxin contamination of corn, in *Biodeterioration VI: The 6th International Biodeterioration Symposium*, Washington, D.C., August, 1984, Barry, S., Houghton, D. R., Eds., CAB International, London, 1986, pp. 284–288.

48. Keller, N.P., Butchko, R.A.E., Sarr, B., and Phillips, T.D., A visual pattern of mycotoxin production in maize kernels by *Aspergillus* spp., *Phytopathology*, 84(5), 483–488, 1994.

49. Du, W., Huang, Z., Flaherty, J.E., Wells, K., and Payne, G.A., Green fluorescent protein as a reporter to monitor gene expression and food colonization by *Aspergillus flavus*, *Appl. Environ. Microbiol.*, 65(2), 834–836, 1999.

50. Trucksess, M.W., Committee on natural toxins: mycotoxins, *J. AOAC*, 79(1), 200–205, 1996.

51. Abbas, H.K., Williams, W.P., Windham, G.L., Pringle, III, H.C., Xie, W., and Shier, W.T., Aflatoxin and fumonisin contamination of commercial corn (*Zea mays*) hybrids in Mississippi, *J. Agric. Food Chem.*, 50(18), 5246–5254, 2002.

52. Abbas, H.K., Zablotowicz, R.M., Weaver, M.A., Horn, B.W., Xie, W., and Shier, W.T., Comparison of cultural and analytical methods for determination of aflatoxin production by Mississippi delta *Aspergillus* isolates, *Can. J. Microbiol.*, 50(3), 193–199, 2004.

53. Scott, G.E. and Zummo, N., Size of maize sample needed to determine percent kernel infection by *Aspergillus flavus*, *Plant Dis.*, 79(8), 861–864, 1995.

54. Lillehoj, E.B., Kwolek, W.F., Zuber, M.S., Bockholt, A.J., Calvert, O.H., Findley, W.R., Guthrie, W.D., Horner, E.S., Josephson, L.M., and King, S.B., Aflatoxin in corn before harvest: interaction of hybrids and locations, *Aspergillus flavus*, mycotoxin, corn insects, *Crop Sci.*, 20(6), 731–734, 1980,

55. Betran, F.J., Isakeit, T., and Odvody, G., Aflatoxin accumulation of white and yellow maize inbreds in diallel crosses, *Crop Sci.*, 42(6), 1894–1901, 2002.

56. Payne, G.A., Aflatoxin in maize, *CRC Crit. Rev. Plant Sci.*, 10, 423–440, 1992.

57. Widstrom, N.W., The aflatoxin problem with corn grain, *Adv. Agron.*, 56, 219–280, 1996.

58. Widstrom, N.W., Aflatoxin in developing maize: interactions among involved biota and pertinent econiche factors, in *Handbook of Applied Mycology*, Vol. 5, Bhatnagar, D., Lillehoj, E.B., and Arora, D.K., Eds., Marcel Dekker, New York, 1992, pp. 23–58.

59. Smith, M.S. and Riley, T.J., Direct and interactive effects of planting date, irrigation, and corn earworm (Lepidoptera: Noctuidae) damage on aflatoxin production in preharvest field corn, *J. Econ. Entomol.*, 85(3), 998–1106, 1992.

60. Adams, N.J., Scott, G.E., and King, S.B., Quantification of *Aspergillus flavus* growth on inoculated excised kernels of corn genotypes, *Agron. J.*, 76(1), 98–102, 1984.

61. Brown, R.L., Cleveland, T.E., Payne, G.A., Woloshuk, C.P., Campbell, K.W., and White, D.G., Determination of resistance to aflatoxin production in maize kernels and detection of fungal colonization using an *Aspergillus flavus* transformant expressing *Escherichia coli* β-glucuronidase, *Phytopathology*, 85(9), 983–989, 1995.

62. Brown, R.L., Chen, Z.-Y., Menkir, A., Cleveland, T.E., Cardwell, K., Kling, J., and White, D.G., Resistance to aflatoxin accumulation in kernels of maize inbreds selected for ear rot resistance in West and Central Africa, *J. Food Protect.*, 64(3), 396–400, 2001.

63. Wallin, J.R., Production of aflatoxin in wounded and whole maize kernels by *Aspergillus flavus*, *Plant Dis.*, 70(5), 429–430, 1986.

64. Brown, R.L., Cleveland, T.E., Payne, G.A., Woloshuk, C.P., and White, D.G., Growth of an *Aspergillus flavus* transformant expressing *Escherichia coli* β-glucuronidase in maize kernels resistant to aflatoxin production, *J. Food Protect.*, 60(1), 84–87, 1997.

65. Brown, R.L., Chen, Z.-Y., Cleveland, T.E., and Russin, J.S., Advances in the development of host resistance in corn to aflatoxin contamination by *Aspergillus flavus*, *Phytopathology*, 89(2), 113–117, 1999.

66. Richmond, J.Y. and McKinney, R.W., Eds., *Biosafety in Microbiological and Biomedical Laboratories*, HHS Publication No. (CDC) 93-8395, Centers for Disease Control and Prevention, National Institutes of Health, U.S. Department of Health and Human Services, U.S. Government Printing Office, Washington, D.C., 1999.

21 Marker-Assisted Breeding for Host Resistance to Mycotoxin Contamination

Leilani A. Robertson, Gary A. Payne, and James B. Holland

CONTENTS

21.1 INTRODUCTION

Naturally occurring fungal toxins, such as aflatoxin, produced by *Aspergillus flavus*, and fumonisin, produced by *Fusarium verticillioides*, are chronic contaminants of maize grain in the United States. Similarly, barley grain is often contaminated with deoxynivalenol (DON), produced by *Fusarium graminearum*.[1] Cultural practices such as early harvest, planting adapted cultivars, managing nutrient inputs, and optimizing planting dates may help reduce the level of aflatoxin and fumonisin contamination of maize grain in most growing seasons;[2–5] however, when environmental conditions are conducive for the production of these mycotoxins, cultural practices alone are not sufficient to prevent mycotoxin contamination that exceeds the standards established by the United States and its foreign trading partners.[5–7]

Even though genetic resistance to plant diseases has been proven to be one of the most effective disease control strategies, especially for grain crops that require minimum production inputs, at present, for example, no commercial maize hybrids are completely resistant to mycotoxin contamination; however, maize genotypes differ in resistance to mycotoxin contamination,[8] indicating the existence of genetic components of resistance that can be selected for. Also, resistance to mycotoxin contamination and visible disease symptoms, such as resistance to fumonsin contamination and ear and kernel rot, have the potential for being distinct phenotypes.[5] The ultimate breeding goal is to develop cultivars that are resistant to mycotoxin contamination as well as visible disease symptoms while having commercially valuable agronomic characteristics.

The first challenge to implementing marker-assisted breeding (MAB) for reduced mycotoxin contamination is to find sources of resistance and to accurately identify the genome regions containing resistance loci. Because resistance to mycotoxin accumulation varies quantitatively among genotypes, we expect that resistance is controlled by multiple quantitative trait loci (QTL). Identifying DNA markers linked to resistance QTL will allow breeders to track the inheritance of resistance QTL throughout each generation of a breeding program. Using this MAB approach, resistance QTL can be introduced and fixed in the genetic background of an agronomically elite cultivar, providing growers with a commercially competitive product.

Marker-assisted breeding has proven in some cases to be a strategy for breeding resistant cultivars more quickly and more efficiently, and it should be an effective strategy for breeding for resistance to mycotoxin contamination for four main reasons. First, when markers linked to resistance genes have been identified, the need for performing inoculations, which are time consuming, labor intensive, and expensive, can be greatly reduced. Second, screening plants with markers associated with known resistance genes is more cost efficient than phenotypically evaluating mycotoxin levels each season throughout a breeding program, because phenotypic evaluations require costly lab techniques such as high-performance liquid chromatography (HPLC) or enzyme-linked immunosorbent assay (ELISA) to quantify toxin levels. Third, selection for marker alleles linked to resistance genes can be performed on individual plants, unlike mycotoxin assays, which usually require multiple plants and multiple replications to obtain accurate data. Finally, MAB can be performed in environments that are not conducive to disease; thus, MAB can be implemented in greenhouses or in off-season nurseries, permitting multiple generations of selection each year and speeding up the development of a resistant cultivar.

Because using MAB as a tool for breeding for reduced mycotoxin contamination is in its preliminary stages, for the purposes of this paper we have examined the uses of MAB for the selection of other traits, and we have identified the benefits and challenges associated with using MAB. We also discuss some preliminary studies of breeding for resistance to mycotoxin accumulation. By also examining the use of MAB for traits other than resistance to mycotoxin contamination, we can better understand the conditions under which MAB is likely to be more efficient than traditional breeding.

21.2 STRATEGY FOR MARKER-ASSISTED BREEDING

The first step in breeding for resistance to mycotoxin contamination, either through conventional selection or marker-assisted breeding techniques, is to identify sources of resistance. When dealing with the fungi that produce mycotoxins, inoculation procedures that will provide equal coverage of all experimental units are crucial so no plants escape contact with the pathogen. Even if the pathogen is present in sufficient populations to produce disease naturally, artificial inoculation will provide a more uniform coverage of fungal spores, minimizing the nongenetic differences among plots. Application of inoculum is also important to induce a greater amount of disease and mycotoxin contamination than might occur naturally. Several experiments have been performed to identify the inoculation techniques that yield the best results.[9-11]

Inoculation of maize with mycotoxin-producing fungi has been shown to reduce the error variance associated with mycotoxin level estimates and to lead to better separation between resistant and susceptible genotypes. Low levels of within-line variation combined with high levels of between-line variation results in more accurate and precise phenotyping of resistant and susceptible genotypes within a segregating population. This facilitates correct identification of resistant sources. Proper inoculation techniques will promote accurate phenotyping in segregating mapping populations, which will allow QTL to be identified more easily.

Whereas many disease resistances can be identified on juvenile plants, mycotoxin accumulation resistance can only be evaluated on grain produced by mature plants. Similarly, whereas many other disease resistances can be scored by simple visual inspections of plants, evaluation of mycotoxin accumulation resistance requires time-consuming and expensive toxin assays. Despite these difficulties, maize genotypes that can serve as sources of resistance to aflatoxin accumulation[12,13] and to fumonisin accumulation[14] have been identified through careful and extensive evaluation. Once resistance sources have been identified, they must be tested in multiple environments to ensure they confer resistance even in environments that are most conducive to disease and toxin development. After this is accomplished, the actual breeding program can begin.

Understanding the genetic basis of toxin accumulation resistance will help to effectively plan a marker-assisted breeding program. Levels of resistance to mycotoxin contamination display continuous variation among different genotypes, suggesting that they are due to the joint effects of multiple genes. This quantitative form of resistance is distinct from gene-for-gene types of disease resistance, which often are mediated by hypersensitive responses, segregate as discrete phenotypes controlled by single-gene differences, and can confer complete resistance to a disease.[15] In contrast, quantitative resistance is conferred by multiple genes, or quantitative trait loci. QTL involved in quantitative resistance may be comprised of many loci, each with small effects, or a few major-effect loci along with many smaller effect loci. In typical mapping studies, estimates of QTL positions are not sufficiently precise to determine whether an identified QTL region consists of one gene or a cluster of genes.[16]

In order to identify QTL associated with a reduction in mycotoxins, a mapping population needs to be developed that is segregating for resistance QTL. This is often achieved by crossing a resistant parent line to a susceptible parent line and developing a population of progeny lines that can be replicated through self-fertilization. At harvest, each line or family within the segregating population is evaluated to determine the concentration of the mycotoxin. Genotypic variability for resistance must be sufficient to permit the accurate identification of QTL.

DNA markers that are polymorphic between the two parents must be chosen. Markers should be evenly distributed throughout the genome in order to ensure accurate coverage. Many options are available when choosing the type of marker, and each marker type has different advantages and disadvantages such as the amount of polymorphism, ease of use, cost, labor, and time.[17,18] DNA markers are then used to genotype each family or line within the mapping population. To test if a QTL is linked to a marker locus, the population is classified into two groups. One group consists of progeny lines that have the same genotype as the first parent at the locus being tested. The other group consists of progeny lines that have the same genotype as the second parent at that locus. If no significant difference between the mean phenotypic values of the two classes is observed, then we accept the null hypothesis that the marker is not associated with a QTL. If, however, the means of the families of one genotypic class have a significantly lower toxin level than the means of the families with the other genotypic class, then we conclude that a QTL is genetically linked to the marker locus. This type of test can be repeated for each marker locus that has been scored in the population, leading to identification of regions of the genome that contain resistance QTL. Statistical advances in QTL mapping techniques have refined this method to identify the most likely position of QTL in intervals between markers, to estimate QTL effects while simultaneously controlling for segregation of QTL at other chromosomal regions, and to account for epistatic interactions among QTL.[16,19,20] Even with the best available statistical procedures, however, identifying QTL is time consuming and expensive. In addition, false-positive and false-negative errors can occur, and these can only be minimized by carefully controlling experimental conditions and using large mapping population sizes.[16]

21.3 CHALLENGES IN QTL IDENTIFICATION

Many challenges, when not overcome, can hinder the identification of QTL for toxin-accumulation resistance, such as genotype by environment interaction, low heritabilities, low power of QTL detection, and low correlation between disease symptoms and toxin concentration. If markers that are consistently associated with resistance QTL could be identified, however, they could be used in future generations of selection to more easily select resistant lines, thus avoiding the difficulties of accurately measuring resistance phenotypes. For the markers to be useful, such associations must be made, requiring highly accurate phenotypic evaluations at least for the identification of the QTL.

Quantitatively inherited traits tend to be highly influenced by the environment, and mycotoxin contamination resistance seems to be particularly sensitive to environmental conditions. For example, hot and dry conditions contribute to high levels of both aflatoxin and fumonisin production, with heat stress alone being able to significantly influence the production of high concentrations of mycotoxins.[2,21]

Because mycotoxin contamination is highly influenced by the environment, the environment must be considered when designing experiments in order to accurately and efficiently identify QTL. Such experiments should be performed in a sample of environments that are representative of those where the resulting cultivars are eventually to be grown. This is important, because QTL alleles that are beneficial in one location may have no effect or even be unfavorable in another location with different environmental conditions. Also, if the environment is not conducive to disease and mycotoxin production every season, more seasons of phenotyping may need to be performed to ensure that the data sufficiently support the accurate identification of QTL. Paul et al.[22] conducted experiments to identify loci associated with reduced aflatoxin production in maize in $F_{2:3}$ and BC_1S_1 generations of the cross between a more resistant parent line, Tex6, and a more susceptible parent line, B73. They found that the large genotype by environment interaction observed for aflatoxin content hindered the accurate characterization of QTL positions and effects. They were not able to identify any QTL regions consistently associated with mycotoxin levels across years within either generation, nor were QTL regions consistent across populations in the first year of the study. In the second year, though, one marker on chromosome 10 was found to be significant across both populations. This marker locus, BMC1185 (more commonly named BNLG1185), was associated with about 14% of the phenotypic variation for aflatoxin content in the $F_{2:3}$ population and with about 5% of the variation in the BC_1S_1 population.

Another example of genotype by environment interaction for mycotoxin accumulation was observed by Zhu et al.,[1] who identified QTL associated with so-called type III resistance (i.e., degradation of the mycotoxin DON) in a barley mapping population. They identified potential QTL for type III resistance in two of four environments. Of these two environments, two QTL were identified in a low-disease environment, and four QTL were identified in a high-disease environment. Only one of these QTL was consistent across environments, and the consistent QTL was associated with between 7 and 13% of the variation in the population.

Heritability (the proportion of observed phenotypic variation that is due to genetic, rather than environmental, effects) is another key determinant of the probability of successful QTL identification. Detecting QTL and accurately estimating their effects is more difficult for traits of low heritability.[23] For example, blackmold resistance QTL were mapped in an interspecific cross between a wild species of tomato, *Lycopersicon cheesmanii*, and cultivated tomato, *Lycopersicon esculentum*.[24] The heritability of blackmold resistance in this mapping population was estimated to be only 16%. Robert et al.[24] reported that with such a low heritability, QTL could not be mapped accurately, and that two of the five resistance QTL identified, when introgressed into the cultivated tomato line using MAB, did not confer resistance. These results illustrate how a low heritability can result in errors in the detection of QTL which can reduce the effectiveness of MAB; however, the loss of wild-species QTL effects following their introgression into cultivated tomato could also have been due to their dependence on their original genetic background (i.e., epistasis).[24]

Heritability of resistance to aflatoxin accumulation has been estimated in numerous maize populations. Campbell et al.[25] estimated heritability of aflatoxin production on a progeny mean basis in F_3 families to be 66%. Hamblin and White[26] estimated aflatoxin production heritability on a progeny mean basis for a Mo17 × Tex6 population as 63% and for a B73 × Tex6 population as 65%. Walker and White[27] estimated aflatoxin production heritabilities in the broad sense (i.e., including dominance effects in the estimated genetic variance) of a B73 × CI2 population to be 32 and 26% for F_3 and BC_1S_1 families, respectively, and heritability in the narrow sense (i.e., including only heritable additive effects in the genetic variance estimate) to be 25 and 17% for F_3 and BC_1S_1 families, respectively. Paul et al.[22] found that, in their experimental populations, heritability for aflatoxin content was low (ranging from 19 to 29%), indicating that much of the phenotypic variation observed was due to environmental or genotype-by-environment interaction effects, rather than direct genetic effects. In addition to the studies in maize, Urrea et al.[28] estimated the heritability of the accumulation of deoxynivalenol to be 46% and *Fusarium* head blight resistance to be 65% in barley. Heritabilities represent the upper limit on the amount of phenotypic variation due to genetics (the joint effects of QTL).

The variation in heritability among these experiments may be due in part to different levels of segregation of resistance QTL, leading to different amounts of additive genetic variance among populations. Probably more important is the fact that heritability of line means is a function of the experimental design, with heritability of family means increasing with increasing numbers of replications and environments in which data are collected.[29] Thus, one can increase the line mean heritability of a trait by phenotyping the population in more environments, and this will lead to greater power to detect QTL for the trait.

To illustrate how heritabilities can affect the identification of QTL, simulation studies indicate that if ten loci affect a trait with 30% heritability, mapping in a population of 100 F_2 progeny will result in detection of a true quantitative trait locus with only 9% probability, and the variance explained by each true quantitative trait locus will be overestimated 5.6 times.[23] Increasing the number of progenies tested will improve the power of QTL detection for any level of heritability. Increasing the number of replications and the number of testing environments in the mapping stage will increase the family mean heritability for any sample size. Thus, mapping population sample sizes and the extent of replication within and across environments must be sufficient to permit accurate identification of QTL positions and effects, which will lead to effective MAB. Simulation studies suggest that population sample sizes should be substantially greater than 100 and line mean heritabilities greater than 30% to achieve reasonable power and accuracy in QTL detection studies.[23]

van Berloo and Stam[30] compared MAB and conventional selection in breeding for the extreme phenotypes of early and late flowering time in *Arabidopsis thaliana*. They found that, with a highly heritable trait such as flowering time, both methods were equally successful. The high heritability of the trait allowed them to accurately identify QTL. Flowering time is very easy to phenotype accurately, and with its high heritability it is not necessary to use MAB; however, for resistance to mycotoxin accumulation, if QTL could be identified accurately, MAB might be more economically efficient than phenotypic selection if the cost of DNA marker assays is less than the cost of biochemical assays required to inoculate and assay toxin concentrations, or if MAB could be implemented in additional generations grown in greenhouses or winter nurseries, where phenotypic selection is inaccurate. Thus, if resources are available to conduct extensive and accurate phenotypic evaluations of mycotoxin accumulation for the initial QTL identification experiment, the heritability of resistance can be made to be high enough to permit accurate QTL identification, at which point MAB could be used instead of the more costly phenotypic selection.

The number of loci conditioning a trait also influences the potential efficiency of MAB. Bernardo[31] used computer simulation to determine the usefulness of marker-assisted selections assuming that all of the QTL positions affecting yield were known. He found that it is more advantageous to make selections on the basis of known QTL if only a few loci controlled the trait (e.g., 10 loci). With many loci controlling the trait (e.g., 50 loci), estimates of QTL effects become imprecise, and selections based on gene information can become less and less useful and may even become detrimental as more and more QTL are discovered. This result implies that QTL mapping studies for mycotoxin accumulation resistance should be focused on accurately identifying the most important 10 or fewer QTL for resistance, rather than trying to detect all possible QTL that might have only small effects on resistance.

Many plant pathologists and plant breeders have argued that if disease symptoms, such as ear rot on maize, can be eliminated, then mycotoxin contamination will also be eliminated, assuming that no disease implies the absence of the fungus, which means that no mycotoxin can be produced. An example of this would be breeding for resistance to aflatoxin contamination by breeding for resistance to *Aspergillus* ear and kernel rot; however, the assumption that reducing ear rot will also reduce mycotoxin contamination is not necessarily correct. This assumption can be tested by estimating correlations between disease symptom levels and mycotoxin levels, or more precisely by testing if QTL map positions for both disease and mycotoxin levels are congruent.

Campbell et al.[32] found only a limited correlation ($r = 0.49$) between aflatoxin contamination and ear rot in progeny of a B73 × LB31 cross. Using the same mapping population, Kaufman et al.[33] identified three QTL regions significantly associated with ear rot resistance and four QTL regions significantly associated with resistance to aflatoxin production, with only one QTL region significantly associated with resistance to both ear rot and aflatoxin production. Walker and White[27] found that, in the progeny of a B73 × CI2 cross, no significant relationship existed between *Aspergillus* ear rot and aflatoxin production in the 1998 growing season, and only a slight but statistically significant relationship in the 1999 growing season was observed, indicating that the relationship between ear rot and aflatoxin contamination is inconsistent across environments. Clements et al.[14] found moderately high correlations between ear rot and fumonisin concentration in two environments ($r = 0.54$ and $r = 0.60$). In barley, Zhu et al.[1] found that levels of *Fusarium graminearum* penetration and mycotoxin (DON) concentrations measured in the same environment were correlated ($r = 0.40$ to 0.67); however, they found few coincident QTL for these two traits that would explain these correlations. As more QTL studies are performed, we will be able to further elucidate the relationship between visual fungal symptoms and mycotoxin contamination by gaining more knowledge about the consistency of QTL associated with one or both of these traits. Until we understand more of the genetics of resistance, we must assume, based on the data from studies such as these, that breeding strictly for ear rot or other symptoms of infection will not necessarily result in improved resistance to mycotoxin contamination.

21.4 APPLICATIONS OF
MARKER-ASSISTED BREEDING

Resistance alleles are often found in lines and plant introductions that are not commercially desirable. MAB can be used to select for rare progeny in which recombination events near the target gene have produced chromosomes that contain the target allele and as little possible surrounding DNA from the donor parent. Young and Tanksley[34] demonstrated that large amounts of donor parent chromosomal material may remain around a target gene even after many generations of conventional backcrossing. Because this surrounding material may contribute to linkage drag, especially if the donor parent is a wild relative or exotic germplasm source, minimizing the size of the introgressed segment from the donor parent is often critical to the successful backcross breeding of a new cultivar.

An experiment with wheat demonstrated that, if MAB is used in the first backcross generation, plants containing the gene of interest from the donor parent and 50% or less of the donor parent's chromosome on which that gene resides could be selected.[35] In contrast, if traditional selection methods were used, the length of the donor segment could be up to 94% of the chromosome containing the donor gene. In general, selection for parental alleles at markers unlinked to the target gene being introgressed can reduce the number of generations of backcrossing required to obtain progeny that are very similar (say 98% or more identical) to the recurrent parent,[36] thus recovering the genes that confer the favorable parent phenotype. Therefore, using DNA markers can increase the speed of backcrossing programs, even when the target alleles from the donor parent can be easily selected.

Marker-assisted breeding is not only useful in backcrossing breeding programs but can also be implemented in forward-crossing programs (i.e., breeding programs using mainly crosses between already elite germplasm). The examples where MAB has been, or is expected to soon be, an important part of mainstream forward-crossing breeding programs have two important factors in common. First, the markers are associated with a small number of genes with relatively large effects on traits that are difficult or costly to accurately phenotype. Second, specific marker alleles are associated with desired alleles at target genes consistently across multiple breeding populations.[37] This second point is key as it eliminates the need to establish the linkage phase between the marker and the target alleles in every population. If this were not the case, then MAB could not be easily implemented in forward-crossing programs where many crosses are made annually between constantly changing sets of breeding parents. It is important to note that these two situations are not expected to be generally applicable for most traits and most populations.[38] Wheat *Fusarium* head blight (FHB) resistance illustrates this principle. The most important source of FHB resistance currently being used by North American wheat breeders is a Chinese cultivar, Sumai3. Various resistant lines are being used in different breeding programs, but most trace their resistance back to Sumai3;[39] therefore, markers developed for resistance derived from Sumai3 tend to be consistent across all populations that use a derivative of Sumai3 as the resistant parent.[40]

21.5   CONVENTIONAL BREEDING
VS. MARKER-ASSISTED BREEDING

Several studies have compared conventional breeding with MAB. Willcox et al.[41] transferred regions associated with resistance to first-generation southwestern maize borer into an elite line using backcrossing. Their objective was to compare marker-assisted backcrossing with conventional backcrossing. When the results of the three trials were combined, they found no significant differences between the two selection methods, and both methods produced lines that were significantly improved over the original lines. Ultimately, MAB resulted in 8% more fixed recurrent parent background after several rounds of selection. The researchers estimated that their MAB program would cost three times as much as a conventional breeding program, with their phenotyping expenses being limited to the cost of rating leaf damage and weighing larva. Inferring this result to breeding for reduced mycotoxin contamination, a critical issue is how much more time and money would be required for a conventional breeding program if inoculations had to be performed and their phenotyping had consisted of running HPLC or ELISA on each experimental line, relative to genotyping costs?

Another study comparing the cost of marker-assisted backcrossing with conventional backcrossing was conducted by Morris et al.[42] They compared costs of marker-assisted and traditional backcrossing of a single major gene into an elite line, and found that marker-assisted backcrossing was faster but cost more than traditional selection. They concluded that deciding whether or not to use MAB depends on the difference in cost between phenotypic and genotypic screening, the amount of time saved, the distribution of benefits associated with accelerated release of improved lines, and the availability of a large enough budget to handle a MAB program. This result supports the use of MAB for developing cultivars resistant to mycotoxin contamination, because phenotypic screening for mycotoxins is very expensive. Also, if the environment does not consistently favor disease development or if a breeder wishes to utilize a winter nursery, MAB could reduce the number of growing seasons needed to release a resistant cultivar.

21.6   ARGUMENT FOR MARKER-ASSISTED BREEDING

In a MAB program, QTL conferring resistance to mycotoxin contamination must first be successfully identified. Once the positions of the QTL are known, MAB can provide an easier and more reliable method to breed for resistance. MAB works by successfully identifying a marker closely linked to a locus associated with resistance. The inheritance of the identified marker can then be followed throughout the breeding program, with only plants containing the marker and, therefore, with a high probability the resistance locus, being used to create the next generation. Presumably, multiple QTL for reduced mycotoxin contamination can be identified, and the inheritance of each quantitative trait locus would then be tracked based on its associated marker genes.

Because no inoculation step is required and because environment is not important for tracking the presence of resistance QTL, MAB can be conducted in any environment, including winter nurseries and greenhouses, and at any stage in the development of a plant. Furthermore, marker-based selection can be applied to individual plants, whereas accurate phenotypic selection would require evaluation of a family or line containing multiple progeny that can be replicated within and across environments. These two factors would reduce the number of generations required to breed resistant lines with MAB compared to conventional breeding methods.

In order for MAB to move from the academic exercise of identifying QTL to becoming a truly useful tool for breeding for mycotoxin resistance, several factors must come together. QTL identified for mycotoxin accumulation resistance must remain functional resistance alleles when transferred from their donor parent into an elite breeding line, whether through a backcrossing or a forward-crossing breeding program. If reduced effectiveness of a gene in a different genetic background occurs, then the QTL will have limited utility. Identification of QTL whose functions are conserved in many different backgrounds will greatly increase their use in multiple breeding crosses.

When we have an estimate of the heritability and number of QTL involved in mycotoxin accumulation resistance, the relative effect of each quantitative trait locus, and the relative costs of phenotypic and genotypic analyses, we can decide if applying the MAB approach is worth the cost. If many genes confer resistance, each with a small effect, it could be very difficult to transfer resistance alleles at each of those genes into the same elite line, as seems to be the case for *Fusarium* ear rot resistance in tropical maize.[43] MAB will, however, markedly improve the likelihood of identifying a line with many of the resistance QTL; furthermore, it may permit the pyramiding of resistance QTL from multiple sources.

If many QTL control resistance, it will be difficult to select progeny with all of the resistance QTL without also selecting a larger than desired proportion of the donor genome linked to these loci. If the resistance source is exotic or otherwise unadapted, then the linkage drag — often yield reduction or a loss of other quality traits — that accompanies this introgression can counteract much of the value gained from the addition of the resistance gene. Thus, although MAB provides the opportunity to introgress QTL while selecting for plants with minimal linkage drag, this becomes increasingly difficult as selection is applied to more QTL.

Marker-assisted breeding is a tool that when used correctly will allow plant breeders to move resistance QTL into useful breeding material more quickly and more efficiently. It will allow growers to obtain high-quality resistant seed more quickly than with conventional selection methods. With genotyping supplies and equipment becoming less expensive as the technology continues to develop, more public plant breeders and pathologists will be able to take part in the identification of resistance QTL along with the movement of these loci into breeding lines, which can then either be used by the public breeders themselves or passed on to private companies, for the development of resistant cultivars.

REFERENCES

1. Zhu, H., Gilchrist, L., Hayes, P., Kleinhofs, A., Kudrna, D., Liu, Z., Prom, L., Steffenson, B., Toojinda, T., and Vivar, H., Does function follow form? Principal QTLs for *Fusarium* head blight (FHB) resistance are coincident with QTLs for influorescence traits and plant height in a doubled haploid population of barley, *Theor. Appl. Genet.*, 99, 1221–1232, 1999.
2. Payne, G.A., Aflatoxins in maize, *CRC Crit. Rev. Plant Sci.*, 10, 423–440, 1992.
3. Widstrom, N.W., The aflatoxin problem with corn grain. In *Advances in Agronomy*, Vol. 56, Academic Press, San Diego, CA, 1996, pp. 220–280.
4. Munkvold, G.P., Cultural and genetic approaches to managing mycotoxins in maize, *Annu. Rev. Phytopathol.*, 41, 99–116, 2003.
5. Bush, B.J., Carson, M.L., Cubeta, M.A., Hagler, W.M., and Payne, G.A., Infection and fumonisin production by *Fusarium verticillioides* in developing maize kernels, *Phytopathology*, 94, 88–93, 2004.
6. FDA, *Guidance for Industry: Fumonisin Levels in Human Foods and Animal Feeds*, U.S. Food and Drug Administration, Washington, D.C., 2001 (http://www.cfsan.fda.gov/~dms/fumongu2.html).
7. CAST, *Mycotoxins: Risks in Plant, Animal, and Human Systems*, Report No. 139, Council for Agricultural Science and Technology, Ames, IA, 2003.
8. Shelby, R.A., White, D.G., and Bauske, E.M., Differential fumonisin production in maize hybrids, *Plant Dis.*, 75, 582–584, 1994.
9. Zummo, N. and Scott, G.E., Evaluation of field inoculation techniques for screening maize genotypes against kernel infection by *Aspergillus flavus* in Mississippi, *Plant Dis.*, 73, 313–316, 1989.
10. Scott, G.E., Zummo, N., Lillehoj, E.B., Widstrom, N.W., Kang, M.S., West, D.R., Payne, G.A., Cleveland, T.E., Calvert, O.H., and Fortnum, B.A., Aflatoxin in corn hybrids field inoculated with *Aspergillus flavus*, *Agron. J.*, 83, 595–598, 1991.
11. Clements, M.J., Kleinschmidt, C.E., Maragos, C.M., Pataky, J.K., and White, D.G., Evaluation of inoculation techniques for *Fusarium* ear rot and fumonisin contamination of corn, *Plant Dis.*, 87, 147–153, 2003.
12. Windham, G.L. and Williams, W.P., Evaluation of corn inbreds and advanced breeding lines for resistance to aflatoxin contamination in the field, *Plant Dis.*, 86, 232–234, 2002.
13. Williams, W.P., Windham, G.L., and Buckley, P.M., Enhancing maize germplasm with resistance to aflatoxin contamination, *J. Toxicol. Toxin Rev.*, 22, 175–193, 2003.
14. Clements, M.J., Maragos, C.M., Pataky, J.K., and White, D.G., Sources of resistance to fumonisin accumulation in grain and *Fusarium* ear and kernel rot of corn, *Phytopathology*, 94, 251–260, 2004.
15. Holland, J.B., Enhancing disease resistance of crops through breeding and genetics, in *Dealing with Genetically Modified Crops*, Wilson, R.F., Hou, C.T., and Hildebrand, D.F., Eds., AOCS Press, Champaign, IL, 2001, pp. 60–83.
16. Asíns, M.J., Present and future of quantitative trait locus analysis in plant breeding, *Plant Breeding*, 121, 281–291, 2002.
17. Gupta, P.K., Varshney, R.K., Sharma, P.C., and Ramesh, B., Molecular markers and their applications in wheat breeding, *Plant Breeding*, 118, 369–390, 1999.

18. Smith, J.S.C., Chin, E.C.L., Shu, H., Smith, O.S., Wall, S.J., Senior, M.L., Mitchell, S.E., Kresovich, S., and Ziegle, J., An evaluation of the utility of SSR loci as molecular markers in maize (*Zea mays L.*): comparisons with data from RFLPs and pedigree, *Theor. Appl. Genet.*, 95, 163–173, 1997.

19. Kao, C., Zeng, Z., and Teasdale, R.D., Multiple interval mapping for quantitative trait loci, *Genetics*, 152, 1203–1216, 1999.

20. Doerge, R.W., Mapping and analysis of quantitative trait loci in experimental populations, *Nat. Rev. Genet.*, 3, 43–52, 2002.

21. Abbas, H.K., Williams, W.P., Windham, G.L. et al., Aflatoxin and fumonisin contamination of commercial corn (*Zea mays*) hybrids in Mississippi, *J. Agric. Food Chem.*, 50, 5246–5254, 2002.

22. Paul, C., Naidoo, G., Forbes, A., Mikkilineni, V., White, D., and Rocheford, T., Quantitative trait loci for low aflatoxin production in two related maize populations, *Theor. Appl. Genet.*, 107, 263–270, 2003.

23. Beavis W.D., QTL analyses: power, precision, and accuracy, in *Molecular Dissection of Complex Traits*, Paterson, A.H., Ed., CRC Press, Boca Raton, FL, 1998, pp. 145–162.

24. Robert, V.J.M., West, M.A.L., Inai, S., Caines, A., Arntzen, L., Smith, J.K., and St.Clair, D.A., Marker-assisted introgression of blackmold resistance QTL alleles from wild *Lycopersicon cheesmanii* to cultivated tomato (*L. esculentum*) and evaluation of QTL phenotypic effects, *Mol. Breeding*, 8, 217–233, 2001.

25. Campbell, K.W., Hamblin, A.M., and White, D.G., Inheritance of resistance to aflatoxin production in the cross between corn inbreds B73 and LB31, *Phytopathology*, 87, 1144–1147, 1997.

26. Hamblin, A.M. and White, D.G., Inheritance of resistance to *Aspergillus* ear rot and aflatoxin production of corn from Tex6, *Phytopathology*, 90, 292–296, 2000.

27. Walker, R.D. and White, D.G., Inheritance of resistance to *Aspergillus* ear rot and aflatoxin production of corn from CI2, *Plant Dis.*, 85, 322–327, 2001.

28. Urrea, C.A., Horsely, R.D., Steffenson, B.J., and Schwarz, P.B., Heritability of *Fusarium* head blight resistance and deoxynivalenol accumulation from barley accession CIho 4196, *Crop Sci.*, 42, 1404–1408, 2002.

29. Holland, J.B., Nyquist, W.E., and Cervantes-Martinez, C.T., Estimating and interpreting heritability for plant breeding: and update, *Plant Breeding Rev.*, 22, 9–112, 2003.

30. van Berloo, R. and Stam, P., Comparison between marker-assisted selection and phenotypical selection in a set of *Arabidopsis thaliana* recombinant inbred lines, *Theor. Appl. Genet.*, 98, 113–118, 1999.

31. Bernardo, R., What if we knew all the genes for a quantitative trait in hybrid crops?, *Crop Sci.*, 41, 1–4, 2001.

32. Campbell, K.W. and White, D.G., Inheritance of resistance to *Aspergillus* ear rot and aflatoxin in corn genotypes, *Phytopathology*, 85, 886–896, 1995.

33. Kaufman, B., Campbell, K.W., White, D.G., and Rocheford, T.R., Maize RFLPs associated with resistance to fungal growth and aflatoxin production, in *Abstracts of the Annual Meeting of the American Society of Agronomy*, American Society of Agronomy, Madison, WI, 1995, pp. 174–175.

34. Young, N.D. and Tanksley, S.D., RFLP analysis of the size of chromosomal segments retained around the Tm-2 locus of tomato during backcross breeding, *Theor. Appl. Genet.*, 77, 353–359, 1989.

35. Salina, E., Dobrovolskaya, O., Efremova, T., Leonova, I., and Roder, M.S., Microsatellite monitoring of recombination around theVrn-B1 locus of wheat during early backcross breeding, *Plant Breeding*, 122, 116–119, 2003.

36. Frisch, M., Bohn, M., and Melchinger, A.E., Comparison of selection strategies for marker-assisted backcrossing of a gene, *Crop Sci.*, 39, 1295–1301, 1999.
37. Holland, J.B., Implementation of molecular markers for quantitative traits in breeding programs: challenges and opportunities, in *Proc. 4th International Crop Science Congress*, Brisbane, Australia, 2004 (www.cropscience.org/av/icsc2004/).
38. Luby, J.J. and Shaw, D.V., Does marker-assisted selection make dollars and sense in a fruit breeding program?, *HortScience*, 36, 872–879, 2001.
39. Kolb, F.L., Bai, G.H., Muehlbauer, G..J., Anderson, J.A., Smith, K.P., and Fedak, G., Host plant resistance genes for *Fusarium* head blight: mapping and manipulation with molecular markers, *Crop Sci.*, 41, 611–619, 2001.
40. Zhou, W.C., Kolb, F.L., Bai, G.H., Domier, L.L., Boze, L.K., and Smith, N.J., Validation of a major QTL for scab resistance with SSR markers and use of marker-assisted selection in wheat, *Plant Breeding*, 122, 40–46, 2003.
41. Willcox, M.C., Khairallah, M.M., Bergvinson, D., Crossa, J., Deutsch, J.A., Edmeades, G.O., Gonzalez-de-Leon, D., Jiang, C., Jewell, D.C., Mihm, J.A., Williams, W.P., and Hoisington, D., Selection for resistance to southwestern corn borer using marker-assisted and conventional backcrossing, *Crop Sci.*, 42, 1516–1528, 2002.
42. Morris, M., Dreher, K. Ribaut, J.M., and Khairallah, M., Money matters. II. Costs of maize inbred line conversion schemes at CIMMYT using conventional and marker-assisted selection, *Mol. Breeding*, 11, 235–247, 2003.
43. Pérez-Brito, D., Jeffers, D., González-de-León, D., Khairallah, M., Cortés-Cruz, M., Velázquez-Cardelas, G., Azpíroz-Rivero, S., and Srinivasan, G., QTL mapping of *Fusarium moniliforme* ear rot resistance in highland maize, Mexico, *Agrociencia*, 35, 181–196, 2001.

22 Prevention of Preharvest Aflatoxin Contamination: Integration of Crop Management and Genetics in Corn

Baozhu Z. Guo, Neil W. Widstrom, Dewey R. Lee, David M. Wilson, and Anton E. Coy

CONTENTS

22.1 INTRODUCTION

The fungal metabolites called aflatoxins are among the most potent naturally occurring carcinogens and are produced primarily by *Aspergillus* spp. fungi.[1] Its production in corn (*Zea mays* L.) can be dramatically influenced by several environmental factors,[2] some of which are beyond the control of producers: rainfall, ambient temperatures, humidity, and soil type.[2] Although considered uncontrollable, even these factors may be modified by appropriate management practices, such as irrigation, site selection, and crop rotation.[3] The importance of crop management to reduce contamination by aflatoxin became apparent when research revealed that most of the components that influence *Aspergillus* spp. infection and aflatoxin contamination are those that can be controlled by the producer.[2] A listing of these components would include planting date selection,[3] fertilization,[4] tillage,[5] irrigation,[6,7] choice of an appropriate hybrid,[8–10] and control of insects,[11–14] diseases,[15,16] and weeds.[17] Each factor mentioned above, whether controlled or not, is inextricably related to plant stress in some manner. In general, a healthy, nonstressed plant will be less likely to have high levels of infection or contamination than one subjected to stress; however, when conditions are favorable for aflatoxin contamination, no plant has been found to be immune.

Host plant resistance to biological and environmental factors has been the subject of much research. Such factors as insects, diseases, weeds, and drought cause plant stress and sometimes contribute directly to the infection process. The early studies on host plant resistance were conducted prior to 1980,[8,18,19] but others have followed since then.[20–22] These studies have clearly demonstrated that resistance in hybrids does in a real sense provide a protective barrier against the development of stress in the plant. That resistance is influenced by environmental and biological factors that can contribute to ear infection and aflatoxin contamination.[2,23,24] Host plant resistance is the most effective, efficient, and dependable tool for protecting corn from the preharvest infection and aflatoxin contamination processes.[10,12,25] Our efforts are focused on identification of the most important and effective environmental factors and development through genetic improvement of chemical and physical traits in hybrids that reduce plant stress and contribute to host plant resistance. Our goal is to combine the major genetic traits using marker-assisted selection (MAS) and to incorporate them into a management system that includes manipulation of critical environmental factors to minimize the risk of preharvest contamination by aflatoxin.[26] This chapter outlines progress made to date, describes a plan for continued research, and projects expected outcomes.

22.2 ENVIRONMENTAL FACTORS

Numerous environmental components were mentioned in the previous section. In addition to their identification, each of the environmental and nongenetic components must be critically assessed to determine which are the most important in their influence on aflatoxin contamination. The field environment is a logical place to search for clues that will assist in the identification of causes for poor plant health, reduced vigor, and other symptoms of abnormal development expressed by the growing plant. Identification of specific individual causes is often achieved with great difficulty due to the myriad of interactions that occur among the factors imposing effects on plant environment. The major environmental influences are discussed here individually with the intent of assessing the relative importance of each, fully realizing that all are intricately interrelated in the imposition of stress on the plant and in the development of aflatoxin contamination of the corn crop.

22.2.1 TEMPERATURE

Drought is defined in terms of dry conditions that induce plant stress and is usually associated with higher than normal temperatures. Such weather is usually accompanied by insect injury and fungus infection of the corn ear.[27] *Aspergillus flavus* is uniquely thermo-tolerant and fits ideally into the environmental niche that produces drought and heat stress in the corn field. The optimal temperature for production of aflatoxin is approximately 30°C,[28,29] while that for the growth of corn is about 27°C,[30,31] although it is lower still when the plant is subjected to drought conditions.[32] Average daily temperatures during grain fill reach or exceed this value in several southern states;[32] therefore, during years with even short periods of temperatures above 27°C, the fungus will increase its aflatoxin production activity while the plant reduces its capacity for growth and grain filling and thus is less able to defend against fungal infection.

The establishment of temperature as an important component of infection by *Aspergillus flavus* and subsequent aflatoxin contamination has been clearly demonstrated under controlled greenhouse conditions.[33,34] The concept was corroborated by several field studies in which temperatures were monitored.[35,36] Some efforts to illustrate a relationship between temperature and aflatoxin contamination were unsuccessful.[37] The reason for this phenomenon can be traced to a detectable relationship that exists only during years when aflatoxin contamination is high. McMillian et al.[38] conducted a 6-year study in which the 3 years with the highest contamination also had the highest average daily temperatures during the growing season. Similarly, in a 5-year study, a significant positive correlation between aflatoxin contamination and temperature was obtained only during the 2 years with exceptionally high concentrations of aflatoxin.[39] We conclude, therefore, that high temperatures do significantly contribute to the fungal infection process and the ultimate amount of aflatoxin produced.

22.2.2 RAINFALL

The interrelationship of climatic factors such as temperature and precipitation cannot be ignored, but each has its own unique contribution to the aflatoxin contamination problem. It has been suggested that differences in precipitation amounts from region to region contribute to contamination.[40] If so, this has especially important implications for the producer who grows dryland corn, while the effect can, to a large extent, be ignored if irrigation is available. Seasons with very low rainfall produce stress conditions for dryland corn and the high temperatures that usually accompany low rainfall are related to the severity of aflatoxin contamination. When late-season rainfall prevents timely harvest of the corn crop, the grain obtained from the delayed harvest can be expected to have increased aflatoxin.[41]

22.2.3 RELATIVE HUMIDITY AND NET EVAPORATION

Relative humidity and net evaporation are intricately interrelated, as these two traits themselves are a result of the interaction between water and temperature. Lillehoj[2] discussed these interrelationships in terms of water activity and pointed out that water activity of 0.9 and above is ideal for *Aspergillus flavus* growth and aflatoxin synthesis while water activity less than 0.85 severely reduces aflatoxin production. Significant amounts of aflatoxin are not generated in inoculated samples of corn when incubated for 7 days at relative humidities less than 91%.[42] The determination and application of environmental limits for fungus growth and elaboration of aflatoxin in laboratory studies can be misleading if the information is extrapolated directly for use in to field but is vital to initiating experiments to study those factors under highly variable field conditions.[2] Sisson[43] monitored field conditions in several corn-growing states, and determined that high humidity and high temperatures are both conducive to high concentrations of aflatoxin contamination. The common occurrence of heavy dews in the southern United States, simulated by ear wetting at least three times each week during grain fill, can also significantly increase aflatoxin concentrations in mature ears.[44] Field measurements of mean temperature and net evaporation are significantly correlated with aflatoxin concentrations of grain samples taken at harvest. These measurements are both judged to be more important than relative humidity or total precipitation in determining contamination.[38]

22.2.4 SOIL TYPE

Crop history affecting the amount and kinds of plant refuse in the soil profile and on the soil surface does influence the mycobiota available and the microenvironment for fungal development.[45] Soil types can also exert great influence on aflatoxin contamination of crops grown on them. Preharvest samples obtained from corn grown on sandy Coastal Plain soils had higher aflatoxin contamination than those sampled from the crop grown on heavier clay soils.[46] The difference was attributed to additional plant stresses incurred from reduced water availability from the lighter soils. It has been demonstrated that both soil type and cultivation practices influence spore load and crop contamination by aflatoxin.[47] The sandy soils of the southeastern United States have less than one half the water-holding capacity of most soils in the corn belt, thus increasing the probability of drought stress during the growing season.[25] Though conservation tillage reduces the loss of water from soils, conventional wisdom suggests that such practices increase the *Aspergillus flavus* spore load available for infection of the crop following the rotation.[47]

22.3 CROP MANAGEMENT FACTORS

Crop management has not been considered to be an efficient approach to control preharvest aflatoxin contamination, although the influence of crop environment has been known since aflatoxin was first recognized as a preharvest problem.[48] Crop management practices can alter the environmental effects and their influence on preharvest aflatoxin contamination.[2,5,23] The use of these practices to modify or manipulate toxin formation, however, has not been the primary consideration for control of preharvest aflatoxin contamination. More recently, the use of crop management to prevent or limit aflatoxin contamination of the preharvest crop has been recommended.[4,49] The relative impact on aflatoxin contamination and ease of manipulation of each management component require additional assessment before an effective plan for control can be initiated. Additionally, the economics of the application of control measures will greatly influence their integration into an overall management system.[50]

22.3.1 PLANTING DATE

Choosing a planting date to avoid plant stress during the critical grain-fill period was first suggested by Zuber and Lillehoj.[24] Studies that supported this concept were reported shortly thereafter.[41,46,51] The data were conflicting, however, in that Lillehoj et al.[51] reported that an early planting had the highest amount of aflatoxin while Jones et al.[46] suggested that early plantings had reduced amounts of aflatoxin in North Carolina. The most comprehensive study was conducted on planting dates with data accumulated over a 5-year period.[39] A study demonstrated a reduction in aflatoxin contamination for plantings as late as June or July on the coastal plain soils at Tifton, GA. Normal planting months are March and April. Unfortunately, late plantings are also associated with increasing reductions in yield. The study did confirm the importance of temperature and net evaporation during the critical grain-fill period.[38] Significant correlations between aflatoxin contamination and both temperature and net evaporation[39] were quite similar to those reported earlier[38] and discussed in the previous section on environmental factors. In most years, corn planted in early April in North Carolina was less drought stressed, and as planting dates were delayed past middle of April yield reductions were observed. Late planting shifted the ear-development phase, which was accompanied by increased temperatures during ear development.[41,46]

22.3.2 IRRIGATION

Many environmental components are responsible for imposing stress on the corn plant during development and maturation. The most common, and possibly the most significant of these, is drought.[24] The obvious remedy is irrigation, especially in areas where rainfall is limited or soils are sandy, providing little water-holding capacity,[2] although irrigation does not always prevent aflatoxin contamination of the corn crop.[52] The amount of contamination is normally reduced to some extent when irrigation is applied to alleviate drought conditions,[46] and irrigation effects have been described as being similar to adequate rainfall in reducing the incidence and amount of aflatoxin in the grain.[5] Irrigation not only alleviates the moisture stress in the plant but also changes the overall environment in the field, creating cooler temperatures in the plant canopy. The influence of irrigation in modifying temperature, a factor considered by many to be the most important factor in reducing preharvest aflatoxin contamination,[23] cannot be ignored. Finally, a net beneficial effect of irrigation has been demonstrated by most research on the subject, as indicated in several published research reports.[6,7,53] A major concern in many areas where corn is grown and aflatoxin is a problem is that irrigation is not available. More than one half of the corn acreage in the southeastern United States is corn grown under dryland conditions.[53]

22.3.3 TILLAGE

The recent trends toward conservation tillage and organically grown crops may have some impact on the risk for aflatoxin contamination of corn. Deep tillage or subsoiling is regularly practiced on sandy soils of the Coastal Plain in the southeastern United States as a means of breaking up the subsurface hardpan layers that develop.[54] This practice probably has its greatest effect in reducing drought stress by promoting good root development and penetration.[5] Burying crop residue has obvious advantages such as covering inoculum sources for disease in high-risk, monoculture rotations.[55] Individual tillage effects on aflatoxin contamination of the crop have not been verifiable, possibly because of interaction with other more significant factors, such as moisture availability.

22.3.4 FERTILIZATION

The first definitive research reporting preharvest aflatoxin contamination of corn also reported that stressed growing conditions, such as low nitrogen level, appeared to increase the incidence of aflatoxin contamination.[48] Conflicting results were reported for 1976 and 1977 when interpreting the influence of nitrogen fertilization on the amount of field contamination.[5,24] Adequate fertilization has been suggested as a cultural practice that will alleviate plant nutrient stress and reduce aflatoxin contamination.[24,49] Similar recommendations advocating sufficient nitrogen fertilization to minimize aflatoxin contamination have been proposed by several other researchers.[2,5,17,49,53] Research specifically addressing the effects of nitrogen has been the basis for most of these recommendations;[4,41,57] however, a recent study in Mexico failed to show any effect on aflatoxin contamination due to fertilization.[58] A word of caution was given by Wilson et al.,[4] who warned against applying excess nitrogen, which can increase plant stress and aflatoxin concentration. This precaution probably only applies to those attempting to maximize rather than optimize their yields.

22.3.5 WEED CONTROL

Weed infestation of corn fields was a predisposing factor studied by Anderson et al.[48] in terms of the way weed populations contribute to plant stress. The suggested consideration of weeds as potential contributors to field contamination[5] is obvious because their control often requires additional tillage practices and always involves a crop management decision that will alleviate plant stress through a reduction in competition for water and nutrients.[24] These competition effects have been directly linked to amounts of aflatoxin found in kernels.[59] The influence of herbicides on aflatoxin contamination and the interaction of weed populations have not been investigated extensively.[2] Research to measure aflatoxin concentration in corn grown under three cultivation rates for weed control was inconclusive.[60] Because most producers practice effective weed control by chemical or other means, it has not been demonstrated to be a critical consideration in an aflatoxin management program.[3]

22.3.6 FUNGAL COMPETITION

The concept of introducing fungal competitors into the field has been considered because studies have demonstrated a reduction in aflatoxin produced by *Aspergillus* spp. when other fungi are present.[61] Calvert et al.[62] reported this phenomenon using mixed inocula of *A. flavus* and *A. parasiticus*. Similar results were obtained when *A. niger* was used as a competitive species.[63] *Fusarium moniliforme* was also identified as a fungus that could effectively suppress aflatoxin synthesis by *A. flavus*.[64] The development of hybrids with the ability to support nontoxin-producing microbes that could effectively compete with toxin-producing *Aspergilli* was suggested by Lillehoj.[65] *A. flavus* has been shown to be better adapted to infection of the corn ear than *A. parasiticus*.[66] It was discovered that *A. flavus* and *F. moniliforme* invade different parts of the ear but that infection by one fungus does influence colonization of the ear by the other fungus.[67] The production of aflatoxin by *A. flavus* in the field was reduced when placed in competition with *F. moniliforme* in a subsequent study.[68] Similar results were obtained by Widstrom et al.[69] when *A. flavus* was observed to be a competitor with *F. moniliforme* and by Choudhary[70] for *A. flavus* against other toxigenic molds. The effective use of other toxigenic fungi to suppress aflatoxin production by *A. flavus*[71] or even the use of nontoxigenic strains of the same fungus, as suggested by Brown et al.,[72] still represents a potentially serious ear rot problem. Most, if not all, of the fungi that effectively reduce aflatoxin production by *A. flavus* are ear-rotting organisms that reduce the quality and yield of the grain crop.

22.4 GENETIC CONTROL STRATEGIES

22.4.1 CONVENTIONAL

The establishment of the aflatoxin contamination problem in preharvest corn alerted plant breeders to the need for germplasm development with genetically controlled resistance.[48] A series of review papers on genetic control of field contamination suggests various approaches for development of hybrids with (1) resistance to insects, (2) resistance to plant stress (adapted hybrids), and (3) resistance based on a relationship to other plant traits.[24,32,49,73,74] Even before these reports appeared in print, breeders were busy screening germplasm in a search for resistance among commercial hybrids,[19,74,75] experimental hybrids,[8,19,77,78] and varieties.[79,80] Results from early screening were inconclusive in that significant differences were not always found among germplasm entries. Zuber[10] had proposed a genetic solution to the aflatoxin problem, and this led to the establishment of procedures for identification of resistant types. While initial screening was being conducted, several other studies were initiated to determine the best methods for field inoculation and evaluation.[77,81–84] The ensuing genetic experiments provided convincing evidence of the potential for genetic control of resistance to aflatoxin contamination and a genetic solution to the contamination problem;[21,36,85–89] consequently, several sources of resistance were identified and released for use by public and private breeders.[90–93]

22.4.2 RELATED PLANT RESISTANCE FACTORS

22.4.2.1 Insects

Ear-feeding insects have been implicated as a contributing factor in aflatoxin contamination from the first substantiated instance of preharvest contamination of corn.[48] Fennell et al.[94–96] reported an association between insect damage and aflatoxin contamination in stored samples, and these investigations were followed by the confirmation of aflatoxin contamination as a preharvest problem associated with insect feeding damage.[13,75,97,98] McMillian et al.[38] demonstrated a consistent association between insect damage and field aflatoxin contamination. Several insects have been found to be associated with contamination of corn kernels. Among these are the corn earworm (*Helicoverpa zea*),[97,99] the maize weevil (*Sitophilus zeamais*),[11,100] and the European corn borer (*Ostrinia nubilalis*).[101,102] The European corn borer is not yet a serious problem in the southeastern United States, where aflatoxin contamination is chronic. The other two insects will be discussed in conjunction with husk coverage.

22.4.2.2 Silk Maysin

The report of a "lethal silk" factor in corn by Walter[103] and subsequent studies to investigate these claims[104–106] led to the isolation and identification of maysin, a flavone glycoside in corn silks[107] that has biological activity against the corn earworm.[108] Snook et al.[109] found numerous germplasm sources for this compound, some which have been selected for extremely high maysin concentrations and have been publicly released.[110,111] The inheritance of silk-maysin concentration is known, so its transfer to commercial germplasm will not be difficult.[112,113] Molecular studies have located numerous quantitative trait loci (QTL) that influence maysin concentration in corn silks,[114–116] several of which are associated with loci found by conventional methods.[117] Butron et al.[118] outlined a program of marker-assisted selection to improve resistance to the corn earworm, but it must be remembered that insect resistance is only one necessary link in solving the problem of aflatoxin contamination in corn.

22.4.2.3 Husk Coverage

Both the length and tightness of husk coverage around the ear appear to be important in aflatoxin contamination. Research supports the concept that complete and tight husk coverage helps protect the ear against invasion by ear-feeding insects and against *Aspergillus flavus* infection with or without the presence of insect damage.[98] The importance of husk traits to prevent ear damage by insects has been emphasized in the literature,[119,120] and when it was discovered that insecticide treatments reduced but did not eliminate aflatoxin contamination, it was concluded that differences in husk protection also reduced contamination. Wiseman et al.[121] determined that husk coverage beyond the ear tip was not sufficient to provide resistance, but that husk tightness was a necessary condition to prevent ear damage by corn earworm. Similarly, husk coverage and tightness are necessary to protect the ear from invasion and damage by the maize weevil.[11,100,122] Two loose-husked hybrids were contaminated with more than twice as much aflatoxin as two tight-husked hybrids in an inoculation study.[81] Five hybrids, each with a different level of husk tightness, had significantly reduced aflatoxin contamination concentrations as husk tightness increased.[122] Widstrom et al.[123,124] concluded that many corn hybrids depend heavily on husk protection for their resistance against aflatoxin contamination, although none gives complete or consistent protection. Finally, high silk-maysin concentrations will not protect the ear against corn earworm unless husk coverage is sufficient to force the insect to feed on silks when entering the ear.[125,126]

22.4.3 PLANT RESISTANCE TO AFLATOXIN FORMATION

22.4.3.1 Plant Stress

Plant stress was recognized as a factor that enhances aflatoxin contamination in the field even prior to the firm establishment of hybrid differences as being important.[24] Stress is most often associated with periods of extreme drought which, in turn, have been associated with aflatoxin contamination.[2] Several of the factors already discussed are responsible for imposing stress on the plant,[73] complicating the interpretation of research data.[49,74] Plant stress is sometimes equated with adaptation, thus the recommendation for planting adapted hybrids with the ability to buffer against local stresses.[32] Efforts are now being made to identify drought-stress-resistant germplasm and incorporate that trait into other germplasms in addition to resistance to insect and aflatoxin contamination.[127]

22.4.3.2 Kernel Resistance

The search for resistance to contamination began shortly after it was defined as a preharvest problem.[48] Differences among germplasm sources were often inconsistent,[10,49] causing some to be skeptical as to whether genetic differences existed for aflatoxin accumulation.[128] In 1980, two types of kernels, distinctly different in appearance, were selected from the same open-pollinated ear on a hybrid plant and used to generate two different breeding populations.[87] These populations were tested extensively in the field and laboratory and found to be distinctly different in their resistance to aflatoxin production and their phenotypic appearance. The differences persisted when tested in experimental crosses to several southern inbred lines.[53] The resistant population, called GT-MAS:gk, was released in 1992 and registered as a germplasm source of resistance in 1993.[92] Four years of experimentation on kernels of commercial hybrids and varied endosperm types indicated that sweet or sugary endosperm types supported greater colonization by *Aspergillus flavus* and higher aflatoxin production than starchy endosperm types.[129] Inconsistent results had been obtained in previous testing of endosperm types; however, sugary endosperm types were not included in those tests.[130,131]

Brown et al.[132] attributed differences between wounded and unwounded kernels of certain resistant genotypes to the presence of something in the maize living embryo. Some of the resistance in the same genotypes was attributed to the wax and cutin layers on the kernel pericarp,[133] a finding that was confirmed by Russin et al.[134] Guo et al.[42] concluded that an aflatoxin inhibitor was induced during germination of the seed and later determined that a zeamatin-like kernel protein and at least one ribosome-inactivating protein (RIP), present in the kernel, were capable of inhibiting growth of *Aspergillus flavus*.[135] Studies of the protein profiles of kernels revealed that several proteins were found in resistant types in greater concentrations than in susceptible types, and others were present only in susceptible types.[136] Additional research determined that RIP is primarily in the aleurone layer of the endosperm, and zeamatin occurs mainly in the embryo.[137] Both proteins uniquely protect kernels from pathogens and may provide important aspects of resistance to *A. flavus* and aflatoxin contamination in corn.

22.4.3.3   Genetic Studies and Selection

Genetic experiments were conducted before adequate screening techniques for resistance to aflatoxin were developed and available.[78] The first genetic parameter estimates were made among single crosses, among which some inbreds gave large estimates of general combining ability (GCA), and the crosses provided evidence for resistance being recessively inherited.[24] Some of the earliest screening was conducted among adapted southern open-pollinated varieties that were grown widely prior to the transition to hybrid corn production.[36] The test failed to reveal exceptional resistance in any of the open-pollinated varieties when compared to popular hybrids being grown in the 1980s. General combining ability effects were determined to be responsible for primary control of aflatoxin contamination among southern dent and sweet corn inbreds when tested as single crosses.[86] Controlled environment experiments by Thompson et al.[85] revealed the importance of replication in detecting differences among genotypes. Gardner et al.,[138] using the same germplasm tested by Zuber et al.,[78] concluded that experiments with eight replications provided a good compromise between controlling the variance estimates in an experiment and the cost for aflatoxin analyses. The germplasm evaluated by Zuber et al.[78] and Gardner et al.[138] was again evaluated in a five-state experiment.[20] The tests effectively accentuated the difficulties in repeating results in different environments and under varied inoculation techniques. Evaluations among genetically diverse varieties also illustrated difficulties in identifying germplasm with the most resistance in any given test.[139]

The most efficient time to sample from field tests was determined to be at physiological maturity, as susceptible genotypes tend to accumulate aflatoxin at a higher rate than resistant genotypes.[82] Widstrom et al.[87] also demonstrated that two separate populations, generated from kernels collected off the same open-pollinated ear, were different in their ability to inhibit elaboration of aflatoxin by *A. flavus*. Kernel infection percentages have been used to identify resistant germplasm.[88,140] When kernel infection percentages are compared to identifications made by other traits, such as total aflatoxin concentrations, the same germplasm sources are usually identified as resistant,[22] regardless of the inoculation technique. The same problems of interaction with environments and large sampling variances, however, continue to plague all genetic experiments and germplasm evaluation procedures.

Some of the most recent genetic research efforts on *Aspergillus flavus* infection and aflatoxin contamination have been focused on ear rot symptoms and aflatoxin production.[21,141,142] In general, these studies have produced conflicting results in that resistance is sometimes attributed to additive effects, sometimes to dominance, and sometimes to both. An encouraging common thread through all of these studies seems to be that the same hybrids and inbreds always fall into resistant and susceptible categories. Recurrent selection studies have been in progress for two breeding populations during the last 10 to 15 years.[143] One breeding population was generated by random mating of plants in a cross made between two released resistance sources, GT-MAS:gk and Mp313E. Two cycles of selection based on S_1 progeny performance have now been completed in this population. Replicated experiments for evaluation of selection progress reveal an aflatoxin contamination of 175 ng/g for the original population compared with only 67 ng/g for the C2 population. A slight reduction in husk tightness occurred in the C2, causing a large standard error for aflatoxin and preventing the decrease in contamination from being statistically significant. A second breeding population was generated by random mating of multiple crossings among eight dent single crosses and seven commercial hybrids, all of which had demonstrated some resistance to aflatoxin contamination. Four cycles of selection based on S_1 progeny performance have now been completed in that population, and a replicated experiment to evaluate progress indicated that contamination of the original population has been decreased an average of 30 ng/g per cycle, as determined by the regression of cycle means on selection cycles. The original population had an average aflatoxin concentration of more than 220 ng/g, and the fourth selection cycle (C4) population was contaminated with 114 ng/g aflatoxin. Plant and ear height were reduced as a result of the selection, and the C4 population also matured 4 days later than the original breeding population.

22.4.3.4 Molecular Breeding

Conventional breeding has been proposed as a genetic solution to preharvest aflatoxin contamination.[21,87,89,144] Recombination was unclear to breeders who must make selections based on phenotypic variation. Breeders increase genetic variation by crossing complementary lines with different desirable traits and attempting to detect individuals with the desirable traits as identified by phenotype. Because of recombination events that occur, progenies are carrying chromosomal segments from both parents. The method of using genetic markers to tag useful traits or characters could provide tremendous potential when used in marker-assisted selection (MAS) and overcome many difficulties of conventional breeding.[145,146] Because of the complexity of the interactions between *Aspergillus* and corn and the factors affecting aflatoxin formation, molecular breeding and MAS methods should enhance or improve general genetic resistance to fungal aflatoxin formation, ear-feeding insects, and drought stress. Molecular procedures have been proposed to develop southern-adapted corn hybrids that control or prevent preharvest aflatoxin contamination in corn.[144,147] Markers based on DNA restriction fragment length polymorphism (RFLP) are being used extensively to build detailed genetic maps for a wide variety of crop species. RFLP has been proposed as a powerful analytical tool that has many practical applications in plant breeding.[148] A sufficient number of difficult quantitative traits have been mapped to suggest that RFLP technology will have substantial utility in this area.[146,149–151]

Mapping studies to reveal the complexity of QTL have been used frequently to identify important chromosomal regions linked to agronomical important traits.[152] Molecular marker profiles should help improve the heritability or power of selection and may also help to more efficiently and effectively organize, combine, and select new genotypic combinations.[153,154] Butrón et al.[155] conducted genetic mapping of the loci associated with reduced aflatoxin contamination from an F_2 population derived from GT-A1 × GT119. A major QTL for maysin was identified on chromosome 1S[151], and QTL for husk tightness were located on chromosomes 4L and 7S. The recombination of progenies with chromosome region 1S from GT-A1 and 2L from GT119 gave the lowest aflatoxin concentrations. A two-loci model accounted for 24.7% of the phenotypic variance for aflatoxin concentrations. Further fine-mapping will be necessary in conducting marker-assisted selection in a corn population with the purpose of pyramiding the resistance to *Aspergillus* spp. infection and ear-feeding insects in an elite inbred source.

22.5　CONCLUSIONS

Aflatoxin contamination in corn is chronic problem in the southern United States but sporadic in the corn belt. Aflatoxin contamination of corn in the field is influenced by numerous factors, abiotic or biotic. We have sufficient knowledge of the contamination process to establish guidelines and management practices that will minimize the probability of contamination under certain environment conditions, but long-term solutions are needed if the problem is to be adequately controlled or resolved. The genetic strategies, conventional or molecular, are vital in the long-term effort to develop hybrids resistant to infection by *Aspergillus flavus* and subsequent aflatoxin contamination. In the southern or southeastern United States, the condition of high temperature coupled with drought is favorable to *A. flavus* infection and aflatoxin production. Loose-husked hybrids used in the south are open invitations to ear-feeding insects and fungal spores. When grown in the south, these corn-belt type hybrids with loose or open husks accentuate insect damage and aflatoxin contamination. The development and breeding of southern-type hybrids with good husk coverage and flint-hard kernel character are important factors for the control of preharvest aflatoxin contamination. In fact, several research programs in the southern states are conducting genetic manipulation of southern-type corn and introducing tropic and subtropic corn genetics with hard-type kernels and drought tolerance into U.S. germplasm to develop southern-type hybrids in order to constrain the problem of aflatoxin contamination.[156]

REFERENCES

1. Squire, R.A., Ranking animal carcinogens: a proposed regulatory approach, *Science*, 214, 877, 1981.
2. Lillehoj, E.B., Effect of environmental and cultural factors on aflatoxin contamination of developing corn kernels, in *Aflatoxin and* Aspergillus flavus *in Corn*, Diener, U.L., Asquith, R.L., and Dickens, J.W., Eds., Southern Coop Series Bull. No. 279, Alabama Agricultural Experiment Station, Auburn AL, 1983, pp. 27–34.
3. Widstrom, N.W., The aflatoxin problem with corn grain, in *Advances in Agronomy*, Sparks, D.L., Ed., Academic Press, New York, 1996, pp. 219–280.
4. Wilson, D.M., Widstrom, N.W., McMillian, W.W., and Beaver, R.W., Aflatoxins in corn, in *Proc. 44th Annual Corn and Sorghum Research Conference*, Chicago, IL, December 1989, pp. 1–26.
5. Jones, R.K., The influence of cultural practices on minimizing the development of aflatoxin in field maize, in *Aflatoxin in Maize*, Zuber, M.S., Lillehoj, E.B., and Renfro, B.L., Eds., CIMMYT, Mexico, 1987, pp. 136–144.
6. Payne, G.A., Cassel, D.K., and Adkins, C.R., Reduction of aflatoxin contamination in corn by irrigation and tillage, *Phytopathology*, 76, 679–684, 1986.
7. Smith, M.S. and Riley, T.J., Direct and interactive effects of planting date, irrigation, and corn earworm (Lepidoptera: Noctuidae) damage on aflatoxin production in preharvest field corn, *J. Econ. Entomol.*, 85, 998–1006, 1992.
8. LaPrade, J.C. and Manwiller, A., Aflatoxin production and fungal growth on single cross corn hybrids inoculated with *Aspergillus flavus*, *Phytopathology*, 66, 675–677, 1976.
9. Lillehoj, E.B., Manwiller, A, Whitaker, T.B., and Zuber, M.S., South Carolina corn yield trial samples as probes for the natural occurrence of aflatoxin in preharvest kernels, *Cereal Chem.*, 59, 136–138, 1982.
10. Zuber, M.S., Influence of plant genetics on toxin production in corn, in *Mycotoxins in Human and Animal Health*, Rodericks, J.V., Hesseltine, C.W., and Mehlman, M.A., Eds., Pathotox Publishers, Park Forest South, IL, 1977, pp. 173–179.
11. McMillian, W.W., Widstrom, N.W., Wilson, D.M., and Hill, R.A., Transmission by maize weevils of *Aspergillus flavus* and its survival on selected corn hybrids, *J. Econ. Entomol.*, 73, 793–794, 1980.
12. Lillehoj, E.B., Kwolek, W.F., Horner, E.S., Widstrom, N.W., Josephson, L.M., Franz, A.O., and Catalano, E.A., Aflatoxin contamination of preharvest corn: role of *Aspergillus flavus* inoculum and insect damage, *Cereal Chem.*, 57, 255–257, 1980.
13. Widstrom, N.W., Sparks, A.N., Lillehoj, E.B., and Kwolek, W.F., Aflatoxin and Lepidopteran insect injury on corn in georgia, *J. Econ. Entomol.*, 68, 855–866, 1975.
14. Wilson, D.M., Widstrom, N., W., Marti, L.R., and Evans, B.D., *Aspergillus flavus* group, aflatoxin, and bright greenish yellow fluorescence in insect-damaged corn in georgia, *Cereal Chem.*, 58, 40–42, 1981.
15. Campbell, K.W., White, D.G., and Toman, J., Sources of resistance in F_1 corn hybrids to ear rot caused by *Aspergillus flavus*, *Plant Dis.*, 77, 778–781, 1993.
16. Doupnik, B., Maize predisposed to fungal invasion and aflatoxin contamination by *Helminthsporium maydis* ear rot, *Phytopathology*, 62, 1367–1368, 1972.
17. Glover, J.W. and Krenzer, Jr., E., *Practices to Minimize Aflatoxin in Corn*, AG-234, North Carolina Cooperative Extension Service, Raleigh, NC, 1980, 2 pp.
18. Lillehoj, E.B., Kwolek, W.F., Manwiller, A., DuRant, J.A., LaPrade, J.C., Horner, E.S., Reid, J., and Zuber. M.S., Aflatoxin production in several corn hybrids grown in South Carolina and Florida, *Crop Sci.*, 16, 483–485, 1976.

19. Widstrom, N.W., Wiseman, B.R., McMillian, W.W., Kwolek, W.F., Lillehoj, E.B., Jellum, M.D., and Massey, J.H., Evaluation of commercial and experimental three-way corn hybrids for aflatoxin B₁ production potential, *Agron, J.*, 70, 9886–988, 1978.

20. Darrah, L.L., Inheritance of aflatoxin B₁ levels in maize kernels under modified natural inoculation with *Aspergillus flavus*, *Crop Sci.*, 27, 869–872, 1987.

21. Naidoo, G., Forbes, A.M., Paul, C., White, D.G., and Rocheford, T.R., Resistance to *Aspergillus* ear rot and aflatoxin accumulation in maize F₁ hybrids, *Crop Sci.*, 42, 360–364, 2002.

22. Scott, G.E., Zummo, N., Lillehoj, E.B., Widstrom, N.W., Kang, M.S., West, D.R., Payne, G.A., Cleveland, T.E., Calvert, O.H., and Fortnum, B.A., Aflatoxin in corn hybrids field inoculated with *Aspergillus flavus*, *Agron. J.*, 83, 595–598, 1991.

23. Fortnum, B.A., Effect of environment on aflatoxin development in preharvest maize, in *Aflatoxin in Maize*, Zuber, M.S., Lillehoj, E.B., and Renfro, B.L., Eds., CIMMYT, Mexico, 1987, pp. 145–151.

24. Zuber, M.S. and Lillehoj, E.B., Status of the aflatoxin problem in corn, *J. Environ. Qual.*, 8, 1–5, 1979.

25. Widstrom, N.W., Aflatoxin in developing maize: interactions among involved biota and pertinent econiche factors, in *Handbook of Applied Mycology: Mycotoxins in Ecological Systems*, Vol. 5, Bhatnager, D., Lillehoj, E.B., and Arora, D.K., Eds., Marcel Dekker, New York, 1992, pp. 23–58.

26. Widstrom, N., Butron, A., Guo, B., Wilson, D., Snook, M., Cleveland, T., and Lynch, R., Control of preharvest aflatoxin contamination in maize through pyramiding resistance genes to ear-feeding insects and invasion by *Aspergillus* spp., in *Proc. 3rd International Crop Science Congress: Book of Abstracts*, Hamburg, Germany, August 17–22, 2000, Christen, O. and Ordon, F., Eds., European Society of Agronomy, Hamburg, 2000, p. 89.

27. Taubenhaus, J.J., *A Study of the Black and Yellow Molds of Ear Corn*, Bull. No. 270, Texas Agriculture Experiment Station, 1920, 38 pp.

28. Boller, R.A. and Schroeder, H.W., Influence of temperature on production of aflatoxin in rice by *Aspergillus parasiticus*, *Phytopathology*, 64, 283, 1974.

29. Sorenson, W.G., Hesseltine, C.W., and Shotwell, O.L., Effect of temperature on production of aflatoxin on rice by *Aspergillus flavus*, *Mycopathol. Mycol. Appl.*, 33, 49, 1967.

30. Aldrich, S.R., Scott, W.O., and Leng, E.R., *Modern Corn Production*, A & L Publications, Champaign, IL, 1975.

31. Shaw, R.H., Climatic requirement, in *Corn and Corn Improvement*, Sprague, G.F.. Ed., American Society of Agronomy, Madison, WI, 1977, p. 591.

32. Zuber, M.S. and Lillehoj, E.B., Aflatoxin contamination in maize and its biocontrol, in *Biocontrol of Plant Diseases*, Vol. 2, Murkerji, K.G. and Garg, K.L., Eds., CRC Press, Boca Raton, FL, 1987, pp. 85–102.

33. Payne, G.A., Thompson, D.L., Lillehoj, E.B., Zuber, M.S., and Adkins, C.R., Effect of temperature on the preharvest infection of maize kernels by *Aspergillus flavus*, *Phytopathology*, 78, 1376–1380, 1988.

34. Thompson, D.L., Lillehoj, E.B., Leonard, K.J., Kwolek, W.F., and Zuber, M.S., Aflatoxin concentration in corn as influenced by kernel development stage and post-inoculation temperature in controlled environments, *Crop Sci.*, 20, 609–612, 1980.

35. Jones, R.K., Duncan, H.E., Payne, G.A., and Leonard, K.G., Factors influencing infection by *Aspergillus flavus* in silk-inoculated corn, *Plant Dis.*, 64, 859–863, 1980.

36. Zuber, M.S., Darrah, L.L., Lillehoj, E.B., Josephson, L.M., Manwiller, A., Scott, G.E., Gudauskas, R.T., Horner, E.S., Widstrom, N.W.,Thompson, D.L., Bockholt, A.J., and Brewbaker, J.L., Comparison of open-pollinated maize varieties and hybrids for preharvest aflatoxin contamination in the southern United States, *Plant Dis.*, 67, 185–187, 1983.

37. Stoloff, L. and Lillehoj, E.B., Effect of genotype (open pollinated vs. hybrid) and environment on preharvest aflatoxin contamination of maize grown in southeastern United States, *J. AOCS*, 58, 976A–980A, 1981.

38. McMillian, W.W., Wilson, D.M., and Widstrom, N.W., Aflatoxin contamination of preharvest corn in Georgia: a six-year study of insect damage and visible *Aspergillus flavus*, *J. Environ. Qual.*, 14, 200–202, 1985.

39. Widstrom, N.W., McMillian, W.W., Beaver, R.W., and Wilson, D.M., Weather-associated changes in aflatoxin contamination of preharvest maize, *J. Prod. Agric.*, 3, 196–199, 1990.

40. Lillehoj, E.B., Kwolek, W.F., Zuber, M.S., Calvert, O.H., Horner, E.S., Widstrom, N.W., Guthrie. W.D., Scott, G.E., Thompson, D.L., Findley, W.R., and Bockholt, A.J., Aflatoxin contamination of field corn: evaluation of regional test plots for early detection, *Cereal Chem.*, 55, 1007–1013, 1978.

41. Jones, R.K. and Duncan, H.E., Effect of nitrogen fertilizer, planting date, and harvest date on aflatoxin production in corn inoculated with *Aspergillus flavus*, *Plant Dis.*, 65, 741–744, 1981.

42. Guo, B.Z., Russin, J.S., Brown, R.L., Cleveland, T.E., and Widstrom, N.W., Resistance to aflatoxin contamination in corn as influenced by relative humidity and kernel germination, *J. Food. Prot.*, 59, 276–281, 1996.

43. Sisson, P.F., The effect of climatic conditions on the incidence and severity of aflatoxin in the USA, in *Aflatoxin in Maize*, Zuber, M.S., Lillehoj, E.B., and Renfro, B.L., Eds., CIMMYT, Mexico, 1987, pp. 172–177.

44. McMillian, W.W., Widstrom, N.W., and Wilson, D.M., Insect damage and aflatoxin contamination in preharvest corn: influence of genotype and ear wetting, *J. Entomol. Sci.*, 20, 66–68, 1985.

45. Martyniuk, S. and Wagner, G.H., Quantitative and qualitative examination of soil microflora associated with different management systems, *Soil Sci.*, 125, 343–350, 1978.

46. Jones, R.K., Duncan, H.E., and Hamilton, P.B., Planting date, harvest date, and irrigation effects on infection and aflatoxin production by *Aspergillus flavus* in field corn, *Phytopathology*, 71, 810–816, 1981.

47. Angle, J.S., aflatoxin and aflatoxin-producing fungi in soil, in *Aflatoxin in Maize*, Zuber, M.S., Lillehoj, E.B., and Renfro, B.L., Eds., CIMMYT, Mexico, 1987, pp. 152–163.

48. Anderson, H.W., Nehring, E.W., and Wichser, W.R., Aflatoxin contamination of corn in the field, *Agric. Food Chem.*, 23, 775–782, 1975.

49. Widstrom, N.W., McMillian, W.W., and Wilson, D.M., Contamination of preharvest corn by aflatoxin, in *Proc. 39th Annual Corn and Sorghum Research Conference*, Chicago, IL, 1984, pp. 68–83.

50. Widstrom, N.W., Lamb, M.C., and Williams, R.G., Economic input for an "expert management system" to minimize risk of aflatoxin contamination of maize, in *Proc. Aflatoxin/Fumonisin Workshop 2000*, Robens, J., Cary, J.W., and Campbell, B.C., Eds., Yosemite, CA, October 25–27, 2000, p. 64.

51. Lillehoj, E.B., Kwolek, W.F., Zuber, M.S., Bockholt, A.J., Calvert, O.H., Findley, W.R., Guthrie. W.D., Horner, E.S., Josephson, L.M., King, S., Manwiller, A., Sauer, D.B., Thompson, D.L., Turner, M., and Widstrom, N.W., Aflatoxin in corn before harvest: interaction of hybrids and locations, *Crop Sci.*, 20, 731–734, 1980.

52. Fortnum. B.A. and Manwiller, A., Effects of irrigation and kernel injury on aflatoxin B_1 production in selected maize hybrids, *Plant Dis.*, 69, 262–265, 1985.

53. McMillian, W.W., Widstrom, N.W., Beaver, R.W., and Wilson, D.M., Aflatoxin in Georgia: factors associated with its formation in corn, in *Iowa Agric. Home Econ. Exp. Stn. Res. Bull.*, 599, 329–334, 1991.

54. Griffin, G.J., Garren, K.H., and Taylor, J.D., Influence of crop rotation and minimum tillage on the population of *Aspergillus flavus* group in peanut field soil, *Plant Dis.*, 65, 898–900, 1981.

55. Cole, R.J., Hill, R.A., Blankenship, P.D., Sanders T.H., and Gurren, J.H., Influence of irrigation and drought stress on invasion of *Aspergillus flavus* of corn kernels and peanut pods, *Dev. Industr. Microbiol.*, 23, 229–236, 1982.

56. Wilson, D.M., McMillian, W.W., and Widstrom, N.W., Field aflatoxin contamination of corn in South Georgia, *J. AOCS*, 56, 798–799, 1979.

57. Payne, G.A., Kamprath, E.J., and Adkins, C.R., Increased aflatoxin contamination in nitrogen-stressed corn, *Plant Dis.*, 73, 556–559, 1989.

58. Bucio-Villalobos, C.M., Guzman-de-Pena, D., and Pena-Cabriales, J.J., Aflatoxin synthesis in corn fields in Guanajuato, *Mexico. Rev. Iberoam Micol.*, 18, 83–87, 2001.

59. Cobb, W.Y., Aflatoxin in the southeastern United States: was 1977 exceptional?, *Q. Bull. Assoc. Food Drug Off.*, 43, 99–107, 1979.

60. Bilgrami, K.S., Ranjan, K.S., and Masood, A., Influence of cropping pattern on aflatoxin contamination in preharvest Khrif (Monsoon) maize crop (*Zea mays*), *J. Sci, Food Agric.*, 58, 101–106, 1992.

61. Ehrlich, K., Ciegler, A., Klich, M., and Lee, L., Fungal competition and mycotoxin production in corn, *Experientia*, 41, 691–693, 1985.

62. Calvert, O.H., Lillehoj. E.B., Kwolek, W.F., and Zuber, M.S., Aflatoxin B_1 and G_1 production in developing *Zea mays* kernels from mixed inocula of *Aspergillus flavus* and A. *parasiticus*, *Phytopathology*, 68, 501–506, 1978.

63. Horn, B.W. and Wicklow, D.T., Factors influencing the inhibition of aflatoxin production in corn by *Aspergillus niger*, *Can, J. Microbiol.*, 29, 1087–1091, 1983.

64. Wicklow, D.T., Horn, B.W., Shotwell, O.L., Hesseltine, C.W, and Caldwell, R.W., Fungal interference with *Aspergillus flavus* infection and aflatoxin contamination of maize grown in a controlled environment, *Phytopathology*, 78, 68–74, 1988.

65. Lillehoj, E.B., The aflatoxin-in-maize problem: the historical perspective, in *Aflatoxin in Maize*, Zuber, M.S., Lillehoj, E.B., and Renfro, B.L., Eds., CIMMYT, Mexico, 1987, pp. 152–163.

66. Zummo, N. and Scott, G.E., Relative aggressiveness of *Aspergillus flavus* and A. *parasiticus* on maize in Mississippi, *Plant Dis.*, 74, 978–981, 1990.

67. Zummo, N. and Scott, G.E., Cob and kernel infection by *Aspergillus flavus* and *Fusarium moniliforme* in inoculated, field-grown maize ears, *Plant Dis.*, 74, 627–631, 1990.

68. Zummo, N. and Scott, G.E., Interaction of *Fusarium moniliforme* and *Aspergillus flavus* on kernel infection and aflatoxin contamination in maize ears, *Plant Dis.*, 76, 771–773, 1992.

69. Widstrom, N.W., McMillian, W.W., Wilson, D.M., Richard, J.L., Zummo, N., and Beaver, R.W., Preharvest aflatoxin contamination of maize inoculated with *Aspergillus flavus* and *Fusarium moniliforme*, *Mycopathologia*, 14, 119–123, 1994.

70. Choudhary, A.K., Influence of microbial co-habitants on aflatoxin synthesis of *Aspergillus flavus* on maize kernels, *Lett. Appl. Microbiol.*, 14, 143–147, 1992.

71. Dorner, J.W., Cole, R.J., and Wicklow, D.T., Aflatoxin reduction in corn through field application of competitive fungi, *J. Food. Prot.*, 62, 650–656, 1999.

72. Brown, R.L., Cotty, P.J., and Cleveland, T.E., Reduction in aflatoxin content of maize by atoxigenic strains of *Aspergillus flavus*, *J. Food Prot.*, 54, 623–626, 1991.

73. Widstrom, N.W. and Zuber, M.S., Prevention and control of aflatoxin in corn: sources and mechanisms of genetic control in the plant, in *Aflatoxin and* Aspergillus flavus *in Corn*, Diener, U.L., Asquith, R.L., and Dickens, J.W., Eds., Southern Coop Series Bull. No. 279, Alabama Agricultural Experiment Station, Auburn AL, 1983, pp. 72–76.

74. Widstrom, N.W., Breeding strategies to control aflatoxin contamination of maize through host plant resistance, in *Aflatoxin in Maize*, Zuber, M.S., Lillehoj, E.B., and Renfro, B.L., Eds., CIMMYT, Mexico, 1987, pp. 212–220

75. LaPrade, J.C. and Manwiller, A., Relation of insect damage, vector, and hybrid reaction to aflatoxin B$_1$ recovery from field corn, *Phytopathology*, 67, 544–547, 1977.

76. Manwiller, A. and Fortnum, B.A., *A Comparison of Aflatoxin Levels in Preharvest Corn from the South Carolina Coastal Plain for 1977–78*, Agronomy and Soils Research Series No. 101, South Carolina Agricultural Experiment Station, Clemson, SC, 1979.

77. King, S.B. and Scott, G.E., Field inoculation techniques to evaluate maize for reaction to kernel infection by *Aspergillus flavus*, *Phytopathology*, 72, 782–785, 1982.

78. Zuber, M.S., Calvert, O.H., Kwolek, W.F., Lillehoj, E.B., and Kang, M.S., Aflatoxin B$_1$ production in an eight-line diallel of *Zea mays* infected with *Aspergillus flavus*, *Phytopathology*, 68, 1346–1349, 1978.

79. Priyadarshini, E. and Tulpule, P.G., Relationship between fungal growth and aflatoxin production in varieties of maize and groundnut, *J. Agric Food Chem.*, 26, 249–252, 1978.

80. Tulpule, P.G., Bhat, R.V., Nagarajan, V., and Priyadarshini, E., Variations in aflatoxin production due to fungal isolates and crop genotypes and their scope in prevention of aflatoxin production, *Arch. Instit. Pasteur Tunis.*, 54, 187–193, 1977.

81. Widstrom, N.W., Wilson, D.M., and McMillian, W.W., Aflatoxin contamination of preharvest corn as influenced by timing and method of inoculation, *Appl. Environ. Microbiol.*, 42, 249–251, 1981.

82. Widstrom, N.W., Wilson, D.M., and McMillian, W.W., Differentiation of maize genotypes for aflatoxin concentration in developing ears, *Crop Sci.*, 26, 935–937, 1986.

83. Tucker, D.H., Trevathan, L.E., King, S.B., and Scott, G.E., Effect of four inoculation techniques on infection and aflatoxin concentration of resistant and susceptible corn hybrids inoculated with *Aspergillus flavus*, *Phytopathology*, 76, 290–293, 1986.

84. Campbell, K.W. and White, D.G., An inoculation device to evaluate maize for resistance to ear rot and aflatoxin production by *Aspergillus flavus*, *Plant Dis.*, 78, 778–781, 1994.

85. Thompson, D.L., Rawlings, J.O., Zuber, M.S., Payne, G.A., and Lillehoj, E.B., Aflatoxin accumulation in developing kernels of eight maize single crosses after inoculation with *Aspergillus flavus*, *Plant Dis.*, 68, 465–467, 1984.

86. Widstrom, N.W., Wilson, D.M., and McMillian, W.W., Ear resistance of maize inbreds to field aflatoxin contamination, *Crop Sci.*, 24, 1155–1157, 1984.

87. Widstrom, N.W., McMillian, W.W., and Wilson, D.M., Segregation for resistance to aflatoxin contamination among seeds on an ear of hybrid maize, *Crop Sci.*, 27, 961–963, 1987.

88. Scott, G.E. and Zummo, N., Sources of resistance in maize to kernel infection by *Aspergillus flavus* in the field, *Crop Sci.*, 28, 504–507, 1988.

89. Gorman, D.P., Kang, M.S., Cleveland, T.E., and Hutchinson, R.I., Combining ability for resistance to field aflatoxin accumulation in maize grain, *Plant Breed.*, 109, 296–303, 1992.

90. Scott, G.E. and Zummo, N., Registration of Mp313E parental line of maize, *Crop Sci.*, 30, 1378, 1990.

91. Scott, G.E. and Zummo, N., Registration of Mp420 germplasm line of maize, *Crop Sci.*, 32, 1296, 1992.

92. McMillian, W.W., Widstrom, N.W., and Wilson, D.M., Registration of GT-MAS:gk maize germplasm, *Crop Sci.*, 33, 882, 1993.

93. William, W.P. and Windham, G.L., Registration of maize germplasm line Mp715, *Crop Sci.*, 41, 1374–1375, 2001.

94. Fennell, D.I., Lillehoj, E.B., and Kwolek, W.F., *Aspergillus flavus* and other fungi associated with insect-damaged field corn, *Cereal Chem.*, 52, 314–321, 1975.

95. Fennell, D.I., Kwolek, W.F., Lillehoj, E.B., Adams, G.A., Bothast, R.J., Zuber, M.S., Calvert, O.H., Guthrie, W.D., Bockholt, A.J., Manwiller, A., and Jellum, M.D., *Aspergillus flavus* presence in silks and insects from developing and mature corn ears, *Cereal Chem.*, 54, 770–778, 1977.

96. Fennell, D.I., Lillehoj, E.B., Kwolek, W.F., Guthrie, W.D., Sheeley, R., Sparks, A.N., Widstrom, N.W., and Adams, G.L., Insect larval activity on developing corn ears and subsequent aflatoxin contamination of seed, *J. Econ. Entomol.*, 71, 624–628, 1978.

97. McMillian, W.W., Wilson, D.M., and Widstrom. N.W., Insect damage, *Aspergillus flavus* ear mold, and aflatoxin contamination in South Georgia corn fields in 1977, *J. Environ. Qual.*, 7, 564–566, 1978.

98. Lillehoj, E.B., Fennell, D.I., Kwolek, W.F., Adams, G.L., Zuber, M.S., Horner, E.S., Widstrom, N.W., Warren, H., Guthrie, W.D., Sauer, D.B., Findley, W.R., Manwiller, A., Josephson, L.M., and Bockholt, A.J., Aflatoxin contamination of corn before harvest: *Aspergillus flavus* association with insects collected from developing ears, *Crop Sci.*, 18, 921–924, 1978.

99. McMillian, W.W., Widstrom, N.W., Wilson, D.M., and Evans, B.D., Annual contamination of *Heliothis zea* (Lepidoptera: Noctuidae) moths with *Aspergillus flavus* and incidence of aflatoxin contamination in preharvest corn in the Georgia Coastal Plain, *J. Entomol. Sci.*, 25, 123–124, 1990.

100. Barry, D., Zuber, M.S., Lillehoj, E.B., McMillian, W.W., Adams, N.J., Kwolek, W.F., and Widstrom, N.W., Evaluation of two Arthropod vectors as inoculators of developing maize ears with *Aspergillus flavus*, *Environ. Entomol.*, 14, 634–636, 1985.

101. Guthrie, W.D., Lillehoj, E.B., McMillian, W.W., Barry, D., Kwolek, W.F., Franz, A.O., Catalano, E.A., Russell, W.A., and Widstrom, N.W., Effect of hybrids with different levels of susceptibility to second-generation European corn borers on aflatoxin contamination in corn, *J. Agric. Food Chem.*, 29, 1170–1172, 1981.

102. McMillian, W.W., Widstrom, N.W., Barry, D., and Lillehoj, E.B., Aflatoxin contamination in selected corn germplasm classified for resistance to European corn borer (Lepidoptera: Noctuidae), *J. Entomol. Sci.*, 23, 240–244, 1988.

103. Walter, E.V., Corn earworm lethal factor in silks of sweet corn, *J. Econ. Entomol.*, 50, 105–106, 1957.

104. Wann, E.V. and Hills, W.A., Earworm resistance in sweet corn at two stages of development, *Proc. Am. Soc. Hort. Sci.*, 89, 491–486, 1966.

105. Chambliss, O.L. and Wann, E.V., Antibiosis in earworm resistant sweet corn, *J. Am. Soc. Hort. Sci.*, 96, 273–277, 1971.

106. Widstrom, N.W., Wiseman, B.R., and McMillian, W.W., Responses of corn earworm larvae to maize silks, *Agron, J.*, 69, 815–817, 1977.

107. Waiss, Jr., A.C., Chan, B.G., Elliger, C.A., Wiseman, B.R., McMillian, W.W., Widstrom, N.W., Zuber, M.S., and Keaster, A.J., Maysin, a flavone glycoside from corn silks with antibiotic activity toward corn earworm, *J. Econ. Entomol.*, 72, 256–258, 1979.

108. Elliger, C.A., Chan, B.G., Waiss, Jr., A.C., Lundin, R.E., and Haddon, W.F., C-Glyco-sylflavones from *Zea mays* that inhibit insect development, *Phytochemistry*, 19, 293–297, 1980.

109. Snook, M.E., Gueldner, R.C., Widstrom, N.W., Wiseman, B.R., Himmelsbach, D.S., Harwood, J.S., and Costello, C.E., Levels of maysin and maysin analogues in silks of maize germplasm, *J. Agric. Food Chem.*, 41, 1481–1485, 1993.

110. Widstrom, N.W. and Snook, M.E., Registration of EPM6 and SIM6 maize germplasm, high silk-maysin sources of resistance to corn earworm, *Crop Sci.*, 41, 2009–2010, 2001.

111. Widstrom, N.W., Wiseman, B.R., Snook, M.E., Nuessly, G.S., and Scully, B.T., Regis-tration of the maize population Zapalote Chico 2451F, *Crop Sci.*, 42, 444–445, 2003.

112. Widstrom, N.W. and Snook, M.E., Inheritance of maysin content in silks of maize inbreds resistant to the corn earworm, *Plant Breed.*, 112, 120–126, 1994.

113. Widstrom, N.W. and Snook, M.E., Genetic variation for maysin and its analogues in crosses among corn inbreds, *Crop Sci.*, 38, 372–375, 1998.

114. Byrne, P.F., McMullen, M.D., Snook, M.E., Musket, T.A., Theuri, J.M., Widstrom, N.W., Wiseman, B.R., and Coe, E.H., Quantitative trait loci and metabolic pathways: genetic control of the concentration of maysin, a corn earworm resistance factor, in maize silks, *Proc. Natl. Acad. Sci. USA*, 93, 8820–8825, 1996.

115. Byrne, P.F., McMullen, M.D., Wiseman, B.R., Snook, M.E., Musket, T.A., Theuri, J.M., Widstrom, N.W., and Coe, E.H., Identification of maize chromosome regions associated with antibiosis to corn earworm (Lepidoptera: Noctuidae) larvae, *J. Econ. Entomol.*, 90, 1039–1045, 1997.

116. Byrne, P.F., McMullen, M.D., Wiseman, B.R., Snook, M.E., Musket, T.A., Theuri, J.M., Widstrom, N.W., and Coe, E.H., Maize silk maysin concentration and corn earworm antibiosis QTLs and genetic mechanisms, *Crop Sci.*, 38, 461–471, 1998.

117. Widstrom, N.W. and Snook, M.E., Congruence of conventional and molecular studies to locate genes that control flavone synthesis in maize silks, *Plant Breed.*, 120, 143–147, 2001.

118. Butron, A., Guo, B.Z., Widstrom, N.W., Snook, M.E., and Lynch, R.E., Use of markers for maize silk antibiotic polyphenol compounds to improve resistance to corn earworm, *Rec. Res. Devel. Agric. Food Chem.*, 4, 193–201, 2000.

119. Lillehoj, E.B. and Zuber, M.S., Aflatoxin problem in corn and possible solutions, in *Proc. 30th Annual Corn and Sorghum Research Conference*, Chicago, IL, December 1975, pp. 230–250.

120. Widstrom, N.W., Lillehoj. E.B., Sparks, A.N., and Kwolek, W.F., Corn earworm damage and aflatoxin B_1 on corn ears protected with insecticide, *J. Econ. Entomol.*, 69, 677–679, 1976.

121. Wiseman, B.R., Widstrom, N.W., and McMillian, W.W., Ear characteristics and mecha-nisms of resistance among selected corns to corn earworm, *Fla. Entomol.*, 60, 97–103, 1977.

122. Barry, D., Lillehoj, E.B., Widstrom, N.W., McMillian, W.W., Zuber, M.S., Kwolek, W.F., and Guthrie, W.D., Effect of husk tightness and insect (Lepidoptera) infestation on aflatoxin contamination of preharvest maize, *Environ. Entomol.*, 15, 1116–1118, 1986.

123. Widstrom, N.W., Zummo, N., Richard, J.L., and Wilson, D.M., *Fungal Competition, Plant Injury and Husk Effects on Preharvest Contamination of Corn Grain*, Agronomy Abstracts, Madison, WI, 1993, p. 105.

124. Widstrom, N.W., Wilson, D.M., Richard, J.L., and McMillian, W.W., Resistance in maize to preharvest contamination by aflatoxin, *Plant Pathol. Trends Agric. Sci.*, 1, 49–54, 1993.

125. Widstrom, N.W. and Snook, M.E., Recurrent selection for maysin, a compound in maize silks, antibiotic to earworm, *Plant Breed.*, 120, 357–359, 2001.

126. Rector, B.G., Snook, M.E., and Widstrom, N.W., Effect of husk characters on resistance to corn earworm (Lepidoptera: Noctuidae) in high-maysin maize populations, *J. Econ. Entomol.*, 95, 1303–1307, 2002.

127. Li, H., Butron, A., Jiang, T., Guo, B.Z., Coy. A.E., Lee, R.D., Widstrom, N.W., and Lynch, R.E., Evaluation of corn germplasm tolerance to drought stress and effects on aflatoxin production, in *Proc. Aflatoxin/Fumonisin Workshop 2000*, Robens, J., Cary, J.W., and Campbell, B.C., Eds., Yosemite, CA, October 25–27, 2000, p. 161.

128. Davis, N.D., Currier, C.G., and Diener, U.L., *Response of Corn Hybrids to Aflatoxin Formation by Aspergillus flavus*, Bull. No. 575, Alabama Agricultural Experiment Station, Auburn, AL, 1985.

129. Widstrom, N.W., McMillian, W.W., Wilson, D.M., Garwood, D.L., and Glover, D.V., Growth characteristics of *Aspergillus flavus* on agar infused with maize kernel homogenates and aflatoxin contamination of whole kernel samples, *Phytopathology*, 74, 887–890, 1984.

130. Lillehoj, E.B., Kwolek, W.F., Vandegraft, E.E., Zuber, M.S., Calvert, O.H., Widstrom, N.W., Futrell, M.C., and Bockholt, A.J., Aflatoxin production in *Aspergillus flavus* inoculated ears of corn grown at diverse locations, *Crop Sci.*, 15, 267–270, 1975.

131. Lillehoj, E.B., Zuber, M.S., Darrah, L.L., Kwolek, W.F., Findley, W.R., Horner, E.S., Scott, G.E., Manwiller, A., Sauer, D.B., Thompson, D.L., Warren, H., West, D.R., and Widstrom, N.W., Aflatoxin occurrence and levels in preharvest corn kernels with varied endosperm characteristics grown at diverse locations, *Crop Sci.*, 23, 1181–1184, 1983.

132. Brown, R.L., Cotty, P.J., Cleveland, T.E., and Widstrom, N.W., Living maize embryo influences accumulation of aflatoxin in maize kernels, *J. Food Prot.*, 56, 967–971, 1993.

133. Guo, B.Z., Russin, J.S., Cleveland, T.E., Brown, R.L., and Widstrom, N.W., Wax and cutin layers in maize kernels associated with resistance to aflatoxin production by *Aspergillus flavus*, *J. Food Prot.*, 58, 296–300, 1995.

134. Russin, J.S., Guo, B.Z., Tubajika, K.M., Brown, R.L., Cleveland, T.E., and Widstrom, N.W., Comparison of kernel wax from corn genotypes resistant or susceptible to *Aspergillus flavus*, *Phytopathology*, 87, 529–533, 1997.

135. Guo, B.Z., Chen, Z.Y., Brown, R.L., Lax, A.R, Cleveland, T.E., Russin, J.S., Mehta, A.D., Selitrennikoff, C.P., and Widstrom, N.W., Germination induces accumulation of specific proteins and antifungal activities in corn kernels, *Phytopathology*, 87, 1174–1178, 1997.

136. Guo, B.Z., Brown, R.L., Lax, A.R., Cleveland, T.E., Russin, J.S., and Widstrom, N.W., Protein profiles and antifungal activities of kernel extracts from corn genotypes resistant and susceptible to *Aspergillus flavus*, *J. Food Prot.*, 61, 98–102, 1998.

137. Guo, B.Z., Cleveland, T.E., Brown, R.L., Widstrom, N.W., Lynch, R.E., and Russin, J.S., Distribution of antifungal proteins in maize kernel tissues using immunochemistry, *J. Food Prot.*, 62, 295–299, 1999.

138. Gardner, C.A.C., Darrah, L.L., Zuber, M.S., and Wallin, J.R., Genetic control of aflatoxin production in maize, *Plant Dis.*, 71, 426–429, 1987.

139. Kang, M.S., Lillehoj, E.B., and Widstrom, N.W., Field aflatoxin contamination of maize genotypes of broad genetic base, *Euphytica*, 51, 19–23, 1990.

140. Scott, G.E. and Zummo, N., Preharvest kernel infection by *Aspergillus flavus* for resistant and susceptible maize hybrids, *Crop Sci.*, 30, 381–383, 1990.

141. Campbell, K.W. and White, D.G., Inheritance of resistance to *Aspergillus* ear rot and aflatoxin in corn genotypes, *Phytopathology*, 85, 886–896, 1995.

142. Hamblin, A.M. and White, D.G., Inheritance of resistance to *Aspergillus* ear rot and aflatoxin production of corn from Tex6, *Phytopathology*, 90, 292–296, 2000.

143. Widstrom, N.W. and Snook, M.E., Recurrent selection for maysin, a compound in maize silk, antibiotic to corn earworm, *Crop Sci.*, 120, 357–359, 2001.

144. Widstrom, N.W., Butrón, A., Guo, B.Z., Wilson, D.M., Snook, M.E., Cleveland, T.E., and Lynch, R.E., Control of preharvest aflatoxin contamination in maize through pyramiding QTL involved in resistance to ear-feeding insects and invasion by *Aspergillus* spp., *Eur. J. Agron.*, 19, 563–572, 2003.

145. Dudley, J.W., Molecular markers in plant improvement: manipulation of genes affecting quantitative traits, *Crop Sci.*, 33, 660–668, 1993.

146. Ribaut, J.M. and Hoisington, D., Marker-assisted selection: new tools and strategies, *Trends Plant Sci.*, 3, 236–239, 1998.

147. Guo, B.Z., Widstrom, N.W., Cleveland, T.E., and Lynch, R.E., Control of preharvest aflatoxin contamination in corn: fungus-plant-insect interactions and control strategies, *Rec. Res. Devel. Agric. Food Chem.*, 4, 165–176, 2000.

148. Tanksley, S.D., Young, N.D., Paterson, A.H., and Bonierbale, M.W., RFLP mapping in plant breeding: new tools for an old science, *Bio/Technology*, 7, 257–264, 1989.

149. Guo, B.Z., Butron, A., Li, H., Widstrom, N.W., and Lynch, R.E., Restriction fragment length polymorphism assessment of the heterogeneous nature of maize population GT-MAS:gk and field evaluation of resistance to aflatoxin production by *Aspergillus flavus*, *J. Food Product.*, 65, 167–171, 2002.

150. Guo, B.Z., Zhang, Z.J., Li, R.G., Widstrom, N.W., Snook, M.E., Lynch, R.E., and Plaisted, D., Restriction fragment length polymorphism markers associated with silk maysin, antibiosis to corn earworm larvae (Lepidoptera: Noctuidae), in a dent and sweet corn cross, *J. Econ. Entomol.*, 94, 564–571, 2001.

151. Butrón, A., Li, R.G., Guo, B.Z., Widstrom, N.W., Snook, M.E., Cleveland, T.E., and Lynch, R.E., Molecular markers to increase corn earworm resistance in a maize population, *Maydica*, 46, 117–124, 2001.

152. Agrama, H.A.S. and Moussa, M.E., Mapping QTLs in breeding for drought tolerance in maize (*Zea mays* L.), *Euphytica*, 91, 89–97, 1996.

153. Inukai, T., Zeigler, R.S., Sarkarung, S., Bronson, M., Dung, L.V., Kinoshita, T., and Nelson, R.J., Development of pre-isogenic lines for rice blast-resistance by marker-aided selection from a recombinant inbred population, *Theor. Appl. Genet.*, 93, 560–567, 1996.

154. Visscher, P.M., Haley, C.S., and Thompson, R., Marker-assisted introgression in backcross breeding programs, *Genetics*, 144, 1923–1932, 1996.

155. Butrón, B., Guo, B.Z., Widstrom, N.W., Snook, M.E., Wilson, D.M., and Lynch, R.E., Markers associated with silk antibiotic compounds, husk coverage, and aflatoxin concentrations in two maize mapping populations, in *Proc. Aflatoxin/Fumonisin Workshop 2000*, Robens, J., Cary, J.W., and Campbell, B.C., Eds., Yosemite, CA, October 25–27, 2000, p. 160.

156. Guo, B.Z., Yu, J., Lee, R.D., Holbrook, C.C., and Lynch, R.E., Application of differential display RT-PCR and EST/microarray technologies to the analysis of gene expression in response to drought stress and elimination of aflatoxin contamination in corn and peanut, *J. Toxicol. Toxin Rev.*, 22, 291–316, 2003.

23 Bt Corn and Mycotoxin Reduction: An Economic Perspective

Felicia Wu, J. David Miller,
and Elizabeth A. Casman

CONTENTS

23.1 INTRODUCTION

The 2003 Council for Agricultural Science and Technology (CAST) Mycotoxin Report identifies the "economics of mycotoxin contamination" as one of seven major research and policy needs in this century. *Bacillus thuringiensis* (Bt) corn is genetically modified to produce a delta-endotoxin that is insecticidal to several lepidopteran pests. Corn infested with these insects often has increased levels of various mycotoxins, particularly deoxynivalenol (DON) and fumonisin.[1] Aflatoxin is another mycotoxin that contaminates corn, but correlation with insect damage is weaker, so claims cannot be made for reduction of aflatoxins in Bt corn varieties at this time. The economic consequence of mycotoxin reduction in Bt corn is the subject of this chapter.

Mycotoxins that accumulate in corn — particularly fumonisin, aflatoxin, and deoxynivalenol — can cause damage in the hundreds of million dollars annually in the United States alone.[2] These costs result primarily from market losses through rejection of contaminated grain and toxicity to livestock. In developing nations, such losses are even more severe and include human health problems, particularly in those parts of the world where corn is a staple in the diet. Export losses in the developing world are also expected to be severe due to increasingly stringent mycotoxin standards in Europe.[3]

Several factors predispose mycotoxin accumulation in corn. Preharvest and postharvest conditions are both important. In preharvest corn, high temperatures, drought stress, and unsuitability of the corn hybrid for the region in which it is planted, insect damage, and other fungal diseases increase mycotoxin levels.[4,5] High temperature may be the most important weather factor in determining formation and accumulation of fumonisins. Drought stress increases insect herbivory on corn, so it is not really possible to separate these two factors.[1] In any case, insect damage is well recognized as a collateral factor in fumonisin development. Insects also play a role, both by creating wounds on the corn kernels (leaf feeding may not be important for increasing mycotoxin contamination) and by acting as vectors for certain types of fungal spores.[5–8] In postharvest corn, storage conditions such as high humidity, preharvest presence of mycotoxin-producing fungi, and the presence of stored grain insects contribute to further fungal development and accumulation of mycotoxins in corn.[6,9]

Hybrid Bt corn and other genetically modified crops are undergoing intense scientific and political scrutiny. Though numerous potential benefits and risks have been discussed, one impact that has been virtually ignored in genetically modified organism (GMO) policy debates is mycotoxin reduction, an effect that could improve human and animal health and potentially relieve some food market asymmetries. This study evaluates the losses caused by three mycotoxins that develop commonly in corn (fumonisins, aflatoxins, and deoxynivalenol) and the potential impact Bt corn may have on reducing these losses. Estimates are made of the monetary benefits of the role of Bt corn in reducing fumonisin and deoxynivalenol.

23.2 MYCOTOXINS IN CORN

23.2.1 AFLATOXINS

Aflatoxins, perhaps the most well-known class of mycotoxins, are mainly produced by the fungus *Aspergillus flavus*. Aflatoxins are the most potent chemical liver carcinogens known. Moreover, the combination of aflatoxin with hepatitis B and C, which is prevalent in Asia and sub-Saharan Africa, is synergistic, raising more than tenfold the risk of liver cancer compared with either exposure.[10] Aflatoxins are also associated with stunting in children[11] and possibly immune system disorders.[12]

TABLE 23.1
FDA Action Levels for Aflatoxins in Human and Animal Foods

Product or Animal	Total Aflatoxin Action Level (ppb)
Human food	20
Milk	0.5
Beef cattle	300
Swine over 100 lb	200
Breeding beef cattle, swine, or mature poultry	100
Immature animals	20
Dairy animals	20

Source: FDA, *Section 683.100: Action Levels for Aflatoxins in Animal Feeds*, CPG 7126.33, U.S. Food and Drug Administration, Rockville, MD, 1994 (www.fda/gov/ora/compliance_ref/cpg/cpgvet/cpg683-100.html).

Aflatoxin B_1, the most toxic of the aflatoxins, causes a variety of adverse effects in different animal species, especially chickens. In poultry, these include liver damage, impaired productivity and reproductive efficiency, decreased egg production in hens, inferior eggshell quality, inferior carcass quality, and increased susceptibility to disease.[13] Swine are somewhat less sensitive than poultry species. Aflatoxin is hepatotoxic, and its acute and chronic effects in swine are largely attributable to liver damage.[14] In cattle, the primary symptom is reduced weight gain as well as liver and kidney damage. Milk production is reduced,[15] and aflatoxin M_1 is excreted in the milk.

Because moldy grain often cannot be sold, some farmers feed it to their livestock. Aflatoxin in poor-quality grain reduces animal productivity and decreases the food supply in developing nations. The loss of income from lower animal production leads to greater poverty, thus reinforcing the conditions conducive to poor human health.[16,17]

Although almost all aflatoxin-related costs in the United States are associated with market losses, the aflatoxin-related costs in many parts of the developing world are associated with losses to human and animal health. In a comprehensive economic assessment, Lubulwa and Davis[18] found that the annual social costs of aflatoxin in Indonesia, Thailand, and the Philippines, including losses to human and animal health and market impacts, totaled almost 1 billion in 2003 U.S. dollars. In sub-Saharan Africa, where aflatoxin levels are roughly comparable to or worse than those in these three Asian nations, health losses are likely to be more severe because corn is a staple in people's diets.

The presence of aflatoxins in foods is restricted in the United States to the minimum levels practically attainable by modern processing techniques. Aflatoxins are regulated by the U.S. Food and Drug Administration (FDA) at the action level, meaning that the food processing industry is held liable if its food products are found to contain aflatoxins above the FDA tolerances shown in Table 23.1. Many other

TABLE 23.2
National Maximum Tolerated Levels
for Aflatoxins in Human Food

Nation	Total Aflatoxin Standard in Human Food (ppb)
Argentina	20
Australia	5
Canada	15
China	20
Denmark	4
Germany	4
Guatemala	20
India	30
Ireland	30
Kenya	20
Malaysia	35
Taiwan	50

Note: A more complete list can be found in CAST.[20]

nations have established maximum tolerated levels of aflatoxin in food and feed. A sampling of worldwide regulations for aflatoxins in human food is provided in Table 23.2.

23.2.2 FUMONISINS

Fumonisins are a recently discovered class of mycotoxins produced by the fungi *Fusarium verticillioides* (formerly *F. moniliforme*), *Fusarium proliferatum*, and some related species.[21] The disease in corn caused by these fungi is called *Fusarium* kernel rot. The first report implicating fumonisins in human disease was in connection with high human esophageal cancer rates in Transkei, South Africa, in 1988. The following year, interest in these mycotoxins increased dramatically after unusually high horse and swine death rates in the United States were linked to contaminated feed.[22] Since then, more than ten types of fumonisins have been isolated and characterized. Of these, fumonisin B_1 (FB_1) is the most common in corn worldwide.[21]

While there have been no confirmed cases of acute fumonisin toxicity or carcinogenicity in humans, epidemiological studies have associated the consumption of fumonisin-contaminated grain with elevated human esophageal cancer incidence in various parts of Africa, Central America, and Asia[22] and among the African American population in Charleston, South Carolina.[23] Fumonisin is listed as an International Agency for Research on Cancer (IARC) *possible* human carcinogen,* and the Joint

---

* This category is lower than "known" or "probable" carcinogen categories and means there is currently limited evidence of carcinogenicity in animals and an absence of conclusive human data.

TABLE 23.3
FDA Guidelines for Fumonisin Concentrations in Food and Feed

Product	Recommended Total Fumonisin Maximum Level (mg/kg)
Human food products	
Degermed dry-milled corn products	2
Whole or partially degermed dry-milled corn products	4
Dry-milled corn bran	4
Cleaned corn intended for *masa*	3
Cleaned corn intended for popcorn	3
Animal feeds[a]	
Equids (horses) and rabbits	5
Catfish, swine	20
Ruminants	60
Poultry	100
Ruminant, mink, and poultry breeding stock	30
All other livestock species and pets	10

[a] It was assumed, when developing these guidelines, that corn made up no more than 20% of horse and rabbit feed and no more than 50% of other animals' feed.

Source: Data from the U.S. Food and Drug Administration.[30,31]

FAO/WHO Expert Committee on Food Additives set a provisional tolerable daily intake for fumonisin in 2000.[21,24] Because FB_1 reduces the uptake of folate in different cell lines, fumonisin consumption has been implicated in connection with neural tube defects in human infants.[25,26] Increased rates of neural tube birth defects in Cameron County in Texas were associated with high but undocumented corn consumption after a year of high fumonisin in the crop.[27]

Elevated levels of fumonisins in animal feed cause diseases such as equine leukoencephalomalacia (ELEM) in horses and porcine pulmonary edema (PPE) and liver damage in swine.[28–30] Horses have been shown to exhibit symptoms of ELEM after feeding on grain containing 10.56 mg/kg total fumonisins for 92 to 122 days, and swine have exhibited liver injury at 23 mg/kg total fumonisins for 14 days.[30] Fumonisins have been shown to cause liver and kidney cancer in rats.[21] Because of these potential impacts on animal and human health, the FDA has set guidelines to industry for levels of fumonisin acceptable in human food and animal feed (Table 23.3). At the moment, very few regulations exist in other nations regarding acceptable fumonisin levels. The 1999 Joint FAO/WHO Expert Committee on Food Additives (JECFA) has, however, recommended a provisional maximum tolerable daily intake (PMTDI) of 2 µg/kg body weight per day. In some parts of the world, such as Latin America and sub-Saharan Africa, corn is a staple in the human diet; thus, meeting the PMTDI for fumonisin would be considerably more difficult in these regions than in the United States or Europe, where corn consumption is much lower.

TABLE 23.4

FDA Guidelines to Industry for Deoxynivalenol Concentrations in Food and Feed

Product	Recommended Deoxynivalenol Maximum Level (mg/kg)
Human food products	1
Animal feeds:[a]	
Swine	5
Ruminants	10
Poultry	10
All other livestock species and pets	5

[a] It was assumed, when developing these guidelines, that grains vulnerable to deoxynivalenol contamination made up no more than 20% of swine feed, no more than 50% of ruminant and poultry feed, and no more than 40% of other animals' feed.

Source: Data from FDA.[35]

23.2.3 DEOXYNIVALENOL

Deoxynivalenol (DON, or vomitoxin), the most common mycotoxin in cereals, is produced by the fungus *Fusarium graminearum* and the related species *Fusarium culmorum* in cooler climates. It is a significant contaminant of corn, wheat, and barley in generally more temperate regions of the world, such as the United States, Canada, and Europe.[32] It causes *Fusarium* head blight in wheat, and *Gibberella* or pink ear rot in corn.[8] Epidemics of *F. graminearum* infection in crops can occur worldwide when relatively warm temperatures and rain coincide with corn silk emergence.[20] In the 1990s, DON was a major problem in the northern United States (primarily in wheat). Because of a near-zero tolerance policy for DON, grain buyers and food processors refuse to purchase crops from highly contaminated regions. As a result, crop market losses around the Great Lakes due to DON contamination were significant.[33] DON is an inhibitor of protein biosynthesis and causes human and animal effects ranging from feed refusal, vomiting, and nausea to immunosuppression and loss of productivity.[34] Table 23.4 lists the FDA's guidelines for DON content in human food and in feed. Aside from the United States, only three nations have established DON standards in food. These standards are outlined in Table 23.5.

23.3 BT CORN

Hybrid Bt corn is one of the most commonly grown genetically modified crops in the world today. Genetically modified (GM), or *transgenic*, crops contain genes from unrelated organisms that are introduced into the plant genome through a variety of

**TABLE 23.5
National Maximum Tolerated
Levels for Deoxynivalenol in
Human Food**

Nation	Total DON Standard in Food (mg/kg)
Austria	0.5
Brazil	0.2
Canada	2
France	2
Russia	1
Uruguay	0.5

Source: Data from CAST,[20] FAO,[37] and Rosner and Egmond.[37]

nonsexual methods. Bt corn contains a gene from the soil bacterium *Bacillus thuringiensis*. A common Bt gene in Bt corn is for a delta-endotoxin (crystal or Cry protein) Cry1Ab. This protein is toxic to certain members of the order Lepidoptera, including the common corn pests European corn borer *Ostrinia nubilalis* (ECB), southwestern corn borer *Diatraea grandiosella* (SWCB), and corn earworm *Helicoverpa zea* (CEW),* but is harmless to vertebrates and non-lepidopteran insects. Over 100 types of Bt toxins exist, but only a few have been used in Bt corn. Other Bt toxins are effective against insects in the orders Diptera (mosquitoes) and Coleoptera (beetles). The alkaline environment of the insect gut solubilizes the Cry protoxin, which is activated by proteolytic cleavage into the active core toxin. The active toxin binds to high-affinity receptors found only on the midgut epithelial cell membranes of susceptible insects. The activated Cry protein inserts into the midgut epithelial cell membrane causing lysis of the cells. The insect stops eating and eventually dies within a few days.[38,39]

Non-genetically modified microbial Bt pest control agents containing Bt Cry proteins, living spores, and formulating agents were first registered for pesticidal use in the United States in 1961.[38] Commercial liquid and dust "natural" insecticides all contain Bt[40] and are often referred to as *microbial Bt sprays*. Microbial Bt sprays are highly regarded by organic farmers and other growers, as they are safe to mammals and birds and safer to nontarget insects than conventional insecticides. These microbial Bt sprays remain in use to control various pest populations in agriculture and forestry; however, they have limited residual action following foliar spraying due to their rapid inactivation by sunlight and removal from leaf surfaces by rain and wind, so spraying may have to be repeated. Also, Bt spray and other

---

* A new variety of Bt corn has recently been registered with the EPA (February 2003) that protects against the corn rootworm. This type of Bt corn is not included in this study.

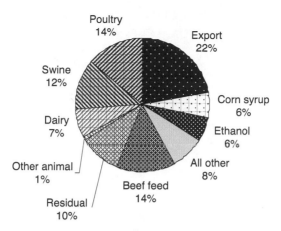

FIGURE 23.1 Uses of field corn in the United States. (From Munkvold, G.P., in *Mycotoxins: The Cost of Achieving Food Security and Food Quality*, APSnet Feature Story, American Phytopathological Society, St. Paul, MN, 2001 [www.apsnet.org/online/feature/mycotoxin/top.html]. With permission.)

sprayed insecticides do not reach some of the most pest-susceptible interior parts of the corn plant. Varieties of Bt corn, on the other hand, can produce the Cry insect control protein constitutively throughout the plant throughout the growing season, including tissues that are difficult to protect with surface-applied insecticides.

Although the technology of Bt corn was first envisioned in the 1980s, the seed was not commercially available until 1996. The toxins in currently registered Bt corn events are nearly 100% effective against the European corn borer and southwestern corn borer and to a more limited extent also control corn earworm. (*Event* is trade jargon for a transgenic variety.) This is a marked improvement over previous pest management strategies such as conventional insecticide sprays, which provide at best 40 to 80% protection against ECB. Although ECB can cause $1 to 2 billion annual damage in the United States,[41,42] the majority of field corn growers do not use any pest management strategy at all because of low infestation levels, the cost of conventional pesticides, or their mediocre performance against ECB. Food-grade corn, however, may be treated with insecticides as needed.

In 2003, Bt corn was grown on about 25% of U.S. field corn acres.[43] Currently, as U.S. regulations do not require segregation of genetically modified grains, Bt corn and traditional grain corn are treated as identical for almost all commercial uses in the United States, with the exception of a small number of food companies that will not use genetically modified food (such as Gerber in its baby food; D. Kendra, pers. comm.). The majority of harvested Bt corn is used as animal feed. A small percentage and specific varieties of corn are designated "food grade" for human consumption. In most cases, however, corn intended for both food and feed are treated equally from the planting stage through to the grain elevator (D. Kendra, pers. comm.). Other uses include nonfood items such as paper, adhesives, and pharmaceuticals (Figure 23.1).

23.4 EVIDENCE THAT BT CORN REDUCES MYCOTOXIN LEVELS

The corn pests European corn borer, southwestern corn borer, and corn earworm all have been shown to contribute to the occurrence of mycotoxins in corn.[45] Even when the larvae do not directly carry the fungi to the corn wounds, spores falling later on the wounded tissue are more likely to infect the plant.[7] Insect-damaged corn is also prone to aflatoxin accumulation in storage.[6] Stored grain insects are the problem in this case, creating grain wounds and spreading fungal spores to cause further post-harvest accumulation of mycotoxins.

23.4.1 AFLATOXIN

Insect damage is not well correlated with aflatoxin concentrations, as multiple factors predispose corn to accumulation of this mycotoxin. The lepidopteran insects that are controlled by the Cry1Ab protein in existing Bt hybrids are not as important in predisposing plants to infection by *Aspergillus flavus* as they are for *Fusarium verticillioides* and *F. graminearum*;[8] *A. flavus* can infect corn not just through kernel wounds caused by insects but also through the silks. This may explain why the effect of Bt corn (which reduces insect damage) on aflatoxin concentration is inconsistent.

Indeed, the experimental record is mixed. Depending on the predominant insect pests in different regions of the United States, Bt corn may or may not have lower levels of aflatoxin than its non-Bt isogenic counterparts. A few success stories have been reported. Benedict et al.[46] found that in two locations in Texas, under conditions of both artificial and natural infection with *A. flavus*, the events of Bt corn still registered today consistently had between 2.5 and 53% lower levels of aflatoxin than the non-Bt isolines. In all cases, however, aflatoxin levels were above the 20 ppb action level for aflatoxin in food. Windham et al.[47] examined the relationship between insect damage and aflatoxin concentration in different corn hybrids, including a Bt11 hybrid. When corn was manually infested with southwestern corn borer, which is well controlled by Bt corn, aflatoxin concentration was significantly lower in Bt11 than in conventional corn. In one field test, the concentration of aflatoxin in conventional corn averaged 41 ppb compared with 5 ppb in Bt11, and in another test that ratio was 19 ppb to 4 ppb; however, in the controls (natural insect infestation), both Bt corn and conventional corn had aflatoxin concentrations below the FDA action level. In a follow-on study, Williams et al.[48] found that the relationship between Bt corn and aflatoxin reduction depends on the *A. flavus* inoculation technique. The nonwounding technique (spraying *A. flavus* inoculum on young ears) and control case resulted in significantly lower aflatoxin levels in Bt corn, while the wounding technique (damaging the kernels) resulted in no difference in aflatoxin levels between Bt and non-Bt corn.

Other studies show either no significant effect of Bt corn or mixed results. Buntin et al.[49] observed that, while Bt11 and MON810 had significantly lower pest damage than non-Bt corn, no significant difference in aflatoxin levels between the two groups was observed. Their study also confirmed that *Aspergillus* ear rot and aflatoxin contamination can be less dependent than *Fusarium* species on insect damage.

TABLE 23.6

Link Between Bt Corn and Aflatoxin Reduction in Various Field Studies

Study	Significant Aflatoxin Reduction?	Details
Benedict et al.[46]	Yes	Texas — Of the Bt corn events still registered today, all exhibited lower aflatoxin levels than their non-Bt isolines under natural and artificial infection of *Aspergillus flavus*.
Windham et al.[47]	Yes	Mississippi — When infested with Southwestern corn borer *Diatraea grandiosella* (SWCB), Bt corn had significantly lower aflatoxin levels.
Williams et al.[48]	Yes/No	Mississippi — Depends on *A. flavus* inoculation technique; nonwounding technique and control result in significantly lower aflatoxin levels in Bt corn.
Buntin et al.[49]	No	Georgia
Odvody et al.[50]	Yes/No	Texas — At some sites in some years, Bt corn had significantly lower *or* higher levels of aflatoxin than non-Bt isolines; in others, no significant difference was observed.
Dowd[52] [a]	No	Illinois
Masoero et al.[53] [a]	No	Italy
Maupin et al.[54] [a]	No	Illinois
Munkvold et al.[55] [a]	No	Iowa
Pietri, and Piva[56] [a]	No	Italy

[a] See Munkvold.[51]

Odvody et al.[50] found significantly lower levels of insect damage in Bt corn in regions of Texas but inconsistent comparative results on aflatoxin levels in Bt and non-Bt corn. In one field test, MON810 actually exhibited higher levels of aflatoxin than non-Bt corn, which the authors attributed to poor adaptability of the MON810 hybrid used in the experiment. In another field test, the situation was reversed, and MON810 had significantly lower aflatoxin levels than non-Bt isolines. The authors concluded that other factors, such as drought stress and individual hybrid vulnerability, are more important in determining aflatoxin contamination levels than insect damage. Munkvold[51] compiled a summary of studies linking Bt hybrids and mycotoxin reduction and found that in six studies, with the exception of Odvody et al.,[50] no significant aflatoxin reduction was achieved in Bt hybrids. Table 23.6 summarizes the literature examining the link between Bt corn and aflatoxin concentrations.

23.4.2. FUMONISINS

Field studies indicate that when insect damage from European corn borer (ECB) or southwestern corn borer is high, fumonisins are substantially lower in Bt corn

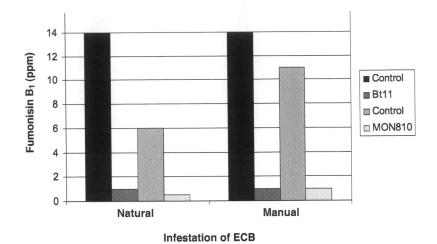

FIGURE 23.2 Differences in fumonisin concentration in Bt and non-Bt corn pairs. (From Munkvold, G.P. and Hellmich, R.L., *Plant Dis.*, 83(2), 130–138, 1999. With permission.)

compared with conventional corn. Munkvold and Hellmich[7] found that in cases of both a natural ECB infestation and a manual ECB infestation, the amount of *Fusarium* kernel rot and concentration of fumonisin B_1 were significantly lower in Bt corn events Bt11 and MON810 than in their near-isogenic, nontransgenic counterparts (Figure 23.2). Of the Bt events tested, only these two are still planted today. Perhaps more importantly, in this study, fumonisins in these two events were reduced to safe levels for human consumption. As can be seen in Figure 23.2, the reductions afforded by Bt11 and MON810 brought FB_1 levels well below 2 mg/kg in these tests, which indicates that total fumonisins in Bt corn would be lower than the FDA's lowest total fumonisin guideline (see Table 23.1). It has been pointed out that a single year's results should not be generalized, as years vary in their corn borer and other insect pressure, which has a major influence on Bt performance trials. Even though these results represent a best-case year, such years are still relevant.

Dowd[57] also showed a 1.8- to 15-fold reduction of fumonisins in Bt corn over conventional corn, depending on the control level of pest damage. He noted, however, that the greatest reductions in fumonisins in Bt corn occur where European corn borer is the predominant insect pest. Where corn earworm, fall armyworm, western bean cutworm, or other pests are predominant, there is greater skepticism about fumonisin reductions in Bt corn, which does not achieve complete control of these pests. Thus, in regions such as the southeastern United States or Texas where very high fumonisin levels occur, fumonisin may not be controlled by Bt corn because of damage by Bt-resistant caterpillars. No studies have been published comparing Bt with non-Bt isolines in these regions.

Hammond et al.[58] found consistently lower levels of fumonisin in Bt hybrids when compared to controls in 288 separate test sites in Argentina, France, Italy, Turkey, and the United States. Fumonisin concentrations in Bt grain were often lower than 4 mg/kg, with a significant proportion of these below 2 mg/kg. Likewise,

Bakan et al.[59] found lower levels of fumonisin B_1 contamination in Bt corn than in non-Bt isolines grown in France and Spain.

Alternative methods for preventing fumonisin accumulation in corn are few. Some currently available corn hybrids are less susceptible to *Fusarium* kernel rot, probably due to better adaptation, insect resistance, or other factors.[1] This tolerance is not sufficient to consistently prevent fumonisin contamination. At the moment, Bt corn is considered to be more effective in reducing fumonisins in preharvest corn.[60]

23.4.3 DEOXYNIVALENOL

Although *Fusarium graminearum* is similar to *Aspergillus flavus* in that it can infect corm without insect damage, the evidence for lower levels of deoxynivalenol in Bt corn is more solid. Schaafsma et al.[61] found that where European corn borer pressure was high, the use of Bt hybrids reduced the level of DON by 88% compared with non-Bt isolines. In these cases, Bt corn consistently had levels of DON that were acceptable by FDA standards (i.e., below 1 mg/kg). Where ECB pressure was low, however, no significant difference was found between DON levels in Bt vs. non-Bt hybrids (which were below 1 mg/kg in either case). Aulrich et al.[62] found that, in animal feed, the only nutritional difference between Bt and non-Bt corn feeds was that Bt corn had lower levels of DON and another mycotoxin, zearalenone; however, in a central European field study, the association between European corn borer damage and DON concentrations was not consistent across years.[63]

23.5 ECONOMIC ANALYSIS OF THE IMPACT OF BT CORN ON MYCOTOXIN REDUCTION

To date, few analyses of the costs mycotoxins pose to society have been performed. Lubulwa and Davis[18] calculated the total social costs of aflatoxin in three developing Asian nations, the Philippines, Thailand, and Indonesia, to be on the order of nearly US$1 billion (1994). These costs included losses in market return and from compromised animal and human health. A recent World Bank study[3] found that compliance with an aflatoxin standard of 2 ppb could cost African nations $720 million through lost exports alone. Within the United States, Vardon et al.[2] estimated the costs of three mycotoxins in various crops and found that total annual costs within the United States were close to $1 billion. Annual losses through aflatoxin contamination were estimated to be close to $300 million of this total cost. In addition, Robens and Cardwell[64] estimated that the costs to manage mycotoxins in the United States, including research and testing, are in the tens of millions of dollars.

In this study, we characterize the economic losses associated with the major fumonisins and DON in field corn in the United States. We also estimate the value the benefits that Bt corn provides through reduced mycotoxins. Conceptually, we identify three classes of impact: market, animal health, and human health:

$$\text{Mycotoxin losses} = Loss_{Market} + Loss_{Animal} + Loss_{Human\ Health} \qquad (23.1)$$

High-quality corn can be sold as human-food-grade corn at the highest market price. Corn contaminated with levels of mycotoxins between the highest permitted levels of food and feed can be sold for animal feed at a lower price, and corn with high levels of mycotoxins is either sold for non-food and non-feed uses at an even lower price or rejected outright. This framework is similar to the approach adopted by Vardon et al.[2] but makes the distinction that feed for horses must meet a stricter standard than feed for other animals. The proportions of the total crop that are rejected at each of these levels depend on the national or international standards for mycotoxins in food and feed; thus,

$$Loss_{Market} = M_{crop} * [dP_{food}Q_{food}R_{food} + dP_{feed}Q_{equine}R_{equine} + dP_{feed}Q_{other}R_{other}] \quad (23.2)$$

where M_{crop} is the proportion of total corn harvest sold; dP_{food} is the price difference between food-grade and feed-grade corn; dP_{feed} is the price difference between feed-grade and lowest grade corn; Q_{food}, Q_{equine}, Q_{other} are the quantities intended for food, equine feed, and other feed grade corn, respectively; and R_{food}, R_{equine}, R_{other} are the proportions of corn found to be above mycotoxin guidelines.

Animal health as a function of mycotoxin contamination is dependent on three factors: the number of animals experiencing mortality or morbidity as a result of mycotoxin ingestion, the cost of treatment for sick animals, and the market value of each animal:

$$Loss_{Animal} = \sum_{a} \left[\left(A_{mort(a)} * \left[V_{animal(a)} + Treat_a \right] + A_{morb(a)} * Treat_a \right) \right] \quad (23.3)$$

where A_{mort} and A_{morb} are the number of animals experiencing mortality or morbidity, respectively; V_{animal} is the market value per animal; $Treat_a$ is the medical treatment cost per animal; and the subscript a indicates the affected species of animals, where $a = \{cattle, horses, swine, poultry\}$.

Finally, human health impacts are calculated in a manner similar to the animal health impact calculations. In addition, a value of pain and suffering is included in the human calculation but not in the animal calculation:

$$Loss_{Human} = H_{mort} * [V_{human} + P_{mort} + T_{mort}] + H_{morb} * [P_{morb} + T_{morb}] \quad (23.4)$$

where H_{mort} and H_{morb} are the number of humans experiencing mortality or morbidity, respectively, from mycotoxins in corn; V_{human} is the statistical value of a human life; P_{mort} and P_{morb} are the value of pain and suffering per human death or illness; T_{mort} and T_{morb} are the medical treatment costs per human death or illness. We make several important assumptions:

- The calculations here are made for Bt field corn, not for Bt sweet corn.
- We assume that in the best case, in Texas and southeastern states aflatoxin in Bt corn will be reduced to FDA-safe levels for human consumption

50% of the time, when aflatoxin concentrations would otherwise be too high to be sold for food.*

- We assume that Bt corn only has this level of effect on aflatoxin in Texas and the southeastern states (not corn belt states) and that 80% of the aflatoxin problems that lead to food and feed rejection occur in these states.
- We assume that fumonisins in Bt corn will be reduced to FDA-safe levels for human consumption 80 to 95% of the time, when fumonisin concentrations would otherwise be too high to be sold for food. This is based on the greater than 99% control of ECB that Bt corn provides.[40] We assume this is also true of SWCB, but not of corn earworm or fall armyworm, which are more important pests in Texas and Southeastern states (see footnote).
- We assume that DON in Bt corn will be reduced to FDA-safe levels for human consumption 50 to 75% of the time, when DON concentrations would otherwise be too high to be sold for food.
- We assume that food and feed purchased in the market have safe mycotoxin levels in the United States.
- We assume that corn rejected for food is used for feed and that corn rejected for horse feed can still be used in the feed of other animals.
- Because mycotoxin testing and management will take place in the United States regardless of whether Bt corn is planted, we assume that testing and management costs will be same even if Bt corn is introduced. (In practice, these costs may vary year to year and are partly dependent on whether buyers receive information about favorable conditions for a good clean crop as opposed to a contaminated one.)
- Because the human health loss in the United States is presumed to be negligible, it is omitted from our calculation.

Key parameters, descriptions, and references relevant to fumonisins are summarized in Table 23.7. Uncertainties are estimated from the literature. Many inputs to this calculation are uncertain, in the sense that they are not known with precision. Also, many natural sources of uncertainty and variability exist for the case of Bt corn, such as weather conditions that would lead to changes in pest infestation. Economic uncertainties include the price of corn in a given year or the acceptability of genetically modified corn in various parts of the world. Quality of data is yet another source of uncertainty and variability.

In this study, uncertainties are estimated by reviewing the literature available on the particular benefit or risk parameter, giving weight to the quality of the work, and fitting a distribution to the available data based on its quality and measurements of uncertainty. The model was run in Monte Carlo mode with 1000 iterations, using Analytica® software (http://www.lumina.com).

---

* The total corn planting in Texas, Alabama, Florida, Georgia, Louisiana, and Mississippi makes up about 5% of total U.S. corn planting.[43] Most of the significant aflatoxin contamination takes place in these states.

TABLE 23.7
Key Parameters, Descriptions, Values, and References for Empirical Model of Bt Corn and Mycotoxin Reduction

Parameter	Description	Value[a]	Refs.
dP_{food}	Cost to grower (dollars per bushel) of reduced value of food corn with high mycotoxin contamination	Uniform [0.82, 1]	2
dP_{feed}	Cost to grower (dollars per bushel) of reduced value of feed corn with high mycotoxin contamination	Lognormal [1.50, 1.4]	2, D. Wittenauer (pers. comm.)
Q_{food}	Quantity of corn intended for food (million bushels)	Uniform [900, 1000]	66
Q_{equine}	Quantity of corn intended for equine feed (million bushels)[b]	Uniform [43, 86]	67, R. Wright (pers. comm.)
Q_{other}	Quantity of corn intended for other animal feed (million bushels)	Uniform [4000, 5000]	66
$R_{food(a)}$	Proportion of corn with aflatoxins >20 ppb	Uniform [0.01, 0.066]	2, 68, 69
$R_{feed(a)}$	Proportion of corn with aflatoxins >300 ppb	Uniform [0, 0.036]	2, 68, 69
$R_{food(f)}$	Proportion of corn with fumonisins >2 mg/kg[c]	Lognormal [0.05, 2]	45, 68, 69, 70
$R_{equine(f)}$	Proportion of corn with fumonisins >5 mg/kg	Lognormal [0.01, 2]	45, 68, 69, 70
$R_{other(f)}$	Proportion of corn with fumonisins >10 mg/kg	Assumed to be negligible in the United States due to generally high-quality corn and blending practices	—
A_{mort} (for horses)	Estimated number of horse mortalities in United States due to fumonisins in corn feed	Uniform [4,100]	28, 29, P. Constable (pers. comm.), J. Robens (pers. comm.)
V_{animal} (for horses)	Value per horse in the United States	Lognormal [3600, 2]	67

[a] The parameters in the uniform distributions represent upper and lower bounds on the value. The parameters in the lognormal distributions represent, respectively, the mean and the geometric standard deviation.

[b] This value was derived by multiplying the total number of horses in the United States by the number of pounds corn consumed daily per horse, then dividing by the pound-to-bushel ratio (56 lb shelled corn per bushel).

[c] This value and the value for proportion of corn with fumonisins >5 mg/kg are based on fumonisin levels in corn from 1990 to 2000.

23.6 RESULTS

23.6.1 AFLATOXINS

We estimate that in the United States, the total annual loss due to aflatoxins in corn is about $163 million ($73M to $332M; here and following, the values in parentheses represent the 95% confidence levels).* The annual market loss through corn rejected for food is about $31 million ($10M to $54M), while the loss through corn rejected for feed and through livestock losses is estimated at $132 million ($14M to $298M). While these estimated losses fall within the range of the estimates by Vardon et al.,[2] ours are slightly lower, particularly for feed losses, because we assume that contaminated corn may in some cases be blended with clean corn to achieve an overall safe level for animals. (Blending is not useful, however, in regions and in years in which aflatoxin concentrations are so high that insufficient clean corn is available to blend to achieve a safe level.)

Bt corn would reduce aflatoxin in cases where insect damage from Bt-sensitive insects was the main determinant of aflatoxin development. This is difficult to estimate, so we offer instead an approximate upper bound on this benefit. This means we think the benefits would not exceed this number and could be considerably less. Given the current level of Bt corn planting in this region at about 17%[43] and our assumptions that Bt corn is partly effective in reducing aflatoxin only in Texas and the southeastern United States, where 80% of the aflatoxin contamination problems occur, the upper bound of the current benefit is about $11 million ($5.0M to $22M): at best, a 7% (3 to 14%) reduction in total annual costs due to aflatoxin in field corn. As the mixed results of previous field studies have shown, it must be emphasized that aflatoxin reductions in Bt corn are not by any account guaranteed, and the effective reduction may be zero. The actual benefit depends on many things that are not well delineated, so we use this calculation guardedly to indicate the order of magnitude of the benefit, not the actual amount.

23.6.2 FUMONISINS

We estimate that, in the United States, the *average* total annual loss due to fumonisins in corn is about $40 million ($14M to $88M). The annual market loss in the United States from corn rejected either for food or for feed makes up most of this loss: roughly $39 million ($14M to $86M). Of this amount, about $38 million of the estimated losses is due to corn being rejected for food, and slightly less than $1 million of the losses is due to corn being rejected for feed. The expected loss from corn rejected for feed is relatively low, because the proportion of corn consumed by horses (the animal group most sensitive to fumonisin) is small because United States corn is generally of high enough quality to meet standards for other feed and because contaminated corn may be blended with clean corn to achieve a safe level for feed. Assuming that Bt corn contains fumonisins at or below the FDA standard for human

---

* The values of the 2.5th and 97.5th percentile of the 1000 iterations approximate the 95% confidence interval.

consumption 80 to 95% of the time,* the savings to U.S. farmers from increased market acceptance is estimated at $8.8 million annually ($2.3M to $31M).

The total value of animal mortality from fumonisin consumption is relatively small in the United States. This is because in most years, fumonisin levels are sufficiently low that few, if any, animals are affected in most regions of the United States. We estimate that the annual loss from fatal fumonisin-induced ELEM in horses is $270,000 ($51,000 to $2 million). In swine, the annual expected losses from fumonisin-induced PPE are on the order of several tens of thousands of U.S. dollars. These deaths occur on farms that grow their own corn rather than buying commercial feed, which presumably has safe fumonisin levels. The benefit of planting Bt corn to prevent swine and horse mortality is estimated to be $67,000 annually ($13,000 to $500,000).

Human health benefits from reducing fumonisin in food through Bt corn in the United States are currently impossible to calculate meaningfully, because of weaknesses of the epidemiological literature and the lack of a reliable biomarker for fumonisin exposure. More research in these areas is necessary to clear the uncertainties in human health impacts. In any case, it is expected that, in the United States, human health losses due to fumonisin consumption are negligible due to the diligence of the food production industry and adherence to the FDA guidelines.

23.6.3 DEOXYNIVALENOL

We estimate that the total annual loss in the United States due to deoxynivalenol in corn is $52 million ($17M to $120M), all from market losses due to corn being rejected for food and used instead for feed, as DON levels in U.S. corn are rarely so high that any of it is rejected for animal feed.[2] With current levels of Bt corn planting, assuming that DON in Bt corn will be reduced to FDA-safe levels for human consumption 50 to 75% of the time, the benefit that Bt corn provides through DON reduction is estimated at $8.1 million ($2.6M to $16M). We assume that no substantial animal health loss is associated with DON in corn, that 6.9% of corn intended for food has DON levels exceeding 1 mg/kg[2], and that DON concentrations in Bt corn are consistently safe for human consumption. Table 23.8 summarizes our estimates for economic losses due to fumonisin and DON in corn in the United States and benefits that Bt corn currently provides in terms of reducing mycotoxin contamination.

23.7 DISCUSSION

23.7.1 THE UNITED STATES

Where Bt corn is planted, depending on the severity of other impacts such as weather conditions, it may significantly reduce fumonisin and DON when pest infestation would otherwise cause high levels of these mycotoxins. In the United States, where

---

* Based on corn fumonisin concentrations in the United States from 1990 to 2000.

TABLE 23.8
Estimated Losses Due to Mycotoxins in U.S. Corn and the Benefit from Use of Bt Corn

	Fumonisin ($US million)		Deoxynivalenol ($US million)		Aflatoxin ($US million)	
	Average	Range	Average	Range	Average	Range
Market loss	39	14 to 86	52	17 to 120	163	73 to 332
Animal health loss	0.27	0.051 to 2	0	—	N/A	N/A
Total U.S. loss	40	14 to 88	52	17 to 120	163	73 to 332
Benefit from planting Bt corn	8.8	2.3 to 31	8.1	2.6 to 16	14	6.2 to 28

Note: 95% confidence intervals.

roughly a quarter of total field corn acreage is planted with Bt corn, the annual benefits that Bt corn provides in terms of lower fumonisin and DON contamination are estimated at about $17 million. This calculation does not include other benefits of Bt corn, such as improved yield and reduced pesticide use, nor losses, such as the technology fee (seed premium cost to Bt corn growers) or market rejection of transgenic crops. Though in the United States the fumonisin and DON problems are usually not large enough to affect price, this may change as demand for high-quality corn increases in the United States. Bt corn, by its effect on fumonisin and DON, may be a useful tool enabling farmers and food producers to meet the increasing demand for high-quality corn.

It appears that Bt corn influences aflatoxin contamination only under certain conditions, when aflatoxin risk factors other than insect damage from European corn borer and southwestern corn borer are absent. Damage from insects controlled by Bt typically is not the most important predisposing factor in aflatoxin development. A generous estimate of the amount of aflatoxin contamination related to these conditions produces a high estimate of the savings that Bt corn could provide through reduced market losses due to aflatoxin — about $11 million annually. The uncertainty around this number means that the maximum benefit could be as low as $5 million or as high as $22 million. Because the preponderance of studies found no reduction in aflatoxins, the actual benefit may be zero dollars in terms of mycotoxin-related reduced market rejection. Importantly, though Bt corn may not always exhibit aflatoxin levels below the FDA food and feed standards in the regions with high aflatoxin contamination, the level of reduction it may afford could be helpful if additional control or decontamination methods are available. Moreover, Bt corn may encourage farmers to produce corn in areas where production would otherwise have been discouraged because of high aflatoxin levels.

23.7.2 THE DEVELOPING WORLD

It is likely that the animal and human health benefits of Bt corn would be more prominent than market gains in areas such as Latin America and sub-Saharan Africa, where corn is a staple in animal and human diets and mostly exchanged locally. In developing nations, many individuals are not only malnourished but also chronically exposed to high levels of mycotoxins in their diet.[70] Aflatoxin consumption, particularly in sub-Saharan Africa, has been associated with liver cancer, immune suppression, vitamin A malnutrition, and stunted growth in humans. Moreover, aflatoxin consumption among livestock reduces animal productivity and decreases the food supply in developing nations, reinforcing the conditions conducive to poor human health.[17] The impacts of Bt corn on reducing aflatoxin contamination in developing nations have not yet been explored.

Fumonisins are a serious problem in corn grown in Africa and Asia, and options for control have thus far been few in those nations. Where Bt corn has been tested in various regions of the world compared with their non-Bt isolines, fumonisins have decreased,[58,59] suggesting that the effectiveness of Bt corn at controlling fumonisin extends beyond the United States to possibly benefit regions with high fumonisin contamination. DON seems to be less of a problem than fumonisins in corn from Africa, Latin America, and Asia.[24] In developing nations as a whole, evidence does not suggest that DON contamination of corn is a significant problem; however, it does occur where corn is grown in temperate areas of Africa, Asia, and South America.[71-73] While Bt corn tested against non-Bt isolines has shown lower DON concentrations in North America, it has not yet been tested on these other continents.

It is premature to recommend Bt corn for the developing world as a solution to mycotoxin problems. Bt corn only controls a few insect pests, and insect damage is not the only and perhaps not the most important factor in mycotoxin accumulation in corn. Field tests would be required to settle this issue, but, because of fears that genetically modified crops are not safe to humans or the environment or that they may face export barriers, some developing nations have rejected Bt corn and other genetically modified crops.[74,75] Thus, some countries with the greatest potential benefit of mycotoxin reduction through genetically modified corn are least interested in it.

ACKNOWLEDGMENTS

Drs. Scott Farrow, Granger Morgan, Benoit Morel, and Christopher Wozniak provided much helpful advice in the early stages of this paper. Support for this work was provided by RAND, an EPA STAR Fellowship, and the Center for Study and Improvement of Regulation, Carnegie Mellon University. We thank Drs. Hamed Abbas, Bruce Hammond, David Kendra, Gary Munkvold, Jane Robens, Arthur Schaafsma, and W. Paul Williams and our anonymous reviewers for their substantive, helpful comments. The opinions expressed here are those of the authors only.

REFERENCES

1. Miller, J.D., Factors that affect the occurrence of fumonisins, *Environ. Health Perspect.*, 109(Suppl. 2), 321–324, 2001.
2. Vardon, P., McLaughlin, C., and Nardinelli, C., Potential economic costs of mycotoxins in the United States, in *Mycotoxins: Risks in Plant, Animal, and Human Systems*, Task Force Report No. 139, Council for Agricultural Science and Technology, Ames, IA, 2003.
3. Otsuki, T., Wilson, J.S., and Sewadeh, M., What price precaution? European harmonization of aflatoxin regulations and African groundnut exports, *Eur. Rev. Agric. Econ.*, 28(2), 263–283, 2001.
4. Shelby, R.A., White, O.G., and Burke, E.M., Differential fumonisins production in maize hybrids, *Plant Dis.*, 78(6), 582–584, 1994.
5. Wicklow, D.T., Preharvest origins of toxigenic fungi in stored grain, in *Stored Product Protection: Proc. 6th International Working Conference on Stored-Product Protection*, Highley, E., Wright, E.J., Banks, H.J., and Champ, B.R., Eds., CAB International, Wallingford, 1994, pp. 1075–1081.
6. Sinha, A.K., The impact of insect pests on aflatoxin contamination of stored wheat and maize, in *Stored Product Protection: Proc. 6th International Working Conference on Stored-Product Protection*, Highley, E., Wright, E.J., Banks, H.J., and Champ, B.R., Eds., CAB International, Wallingford, 1994, pp. 1059–1063.
7. Munkvold, G.P. and Hellmich, R.L., Comparison of fumonisin concentrations in kernels of transgenic Bt maize hybrids and nontransgenic hybrids, *Plant Dis.*, 83(2), 130–138, 1999.
8. Miller, J.D., Fungi and mycotoxins in grain: implications for stored product research, *J. Stored Prod. Res.*, 31, 1–6, 1995.
9. Wilson, D.M. and Abramson, D., Mycotoxins, in *Storage of Cereal Grains and Their Products*, Sauer, D.B., Ed., American Association of Cereal Chemists, St. Paul, MN, 1992.
10. Turner, P.C., Sylla, A., Diallo, M.S., Castegnaro, J.J., Hall, A.J., and Wild, C.P., The role of aflatoxins and hepatitis viruses in the etiopathogenesis of hepatocellular carcinoma: a basis for primary prevention in Guinea-Conakry, West Africa, *J. Gastroenterol. Hepatol.*, 17(Suppl.), S441–S448, 2002.
11. Gong, Y.Y., Cardwell, K., Hounsa, A., Egal, S., Turner, P.C., Hall, A.J., and Wild, C.P., Dietary aflatoxin exposure and impaired growth in young children from Benin and Togo: cross-sectional study, *Br. Med. J.*, 325, 20–21, 2000.
12. Turner, P.C., Moore, S.E., Hall, A.J., Prentice, A.M., and Wild, C.P., Modification of immune function through exposure to dietary aflatoxin in Gambian children, *Environ. Health Perspect.*, 111(2):217–20, 2003.
13. Wyatt, R.D., Poultry, in *Mycotoxins and Animal Foods*, Smith, J.E. and Henderson, R.S., Eds., CRC Press, Boca Raton, FL, 1991, pp. 553–606.
14. Armbrecht, B.H., Aflatoxicosis in swine, in *Mycotoxic Fungi, Mycotoxins, Mycotoxicoses*, Vol. 2, Wyllie, T.D. and Morehouse, L.G., Eds., Marcel Dekker, New York, 1978, pp. 227–235.
15. Keyl, A.C., Aflatoxicosis in cattle, in *Mycotoxic Fungi, Mycotoxins, Mycotoxicoses*, Vol. 2, Wyllie, T.D. and Morehouse, L.G., Eds., Marcel Dekker, New York, 1978, pp. 9–27.
16. Bhat, R.V. and Miller, J.D., Mycotoxins and the food supply, *Food Nutr. Agric.*, 1, 27–31, 1991.
17. Miller, J.D. and Marasas, W.F.O., Ecology of mycotoxins in maize and groundnuts, *LEISA Mag.*, (Suppl.), 23–24, 2002.

18. Lubulwa, A.S.G. and Davis, J.S., Estimating the social costs of the impacts of fungi and aflatoxins in maize and peanuts, in *Stored Product Protection: Proc. 6th International Working Conference on Stored-Product Protection*, Highley, E., Wright, E.J., Banks, H.J., and Champ, B.R., Eds., CAB International, Wallingford, 1994, pp. 1017–1042.

19. FDA, Section 683.100: Action Levels for Aflatoxins in Animal Feeds, CPG 7126.33, U.S. Food and Drug Administration, Rockville, MD, 1994 (www.fda.gov/ora/compliance_ref/cpg/cpgvet/cpg683-100.html.)

20. CAST, *Mycotoxins: Risks in Plant, Animal, and Human Systems*, Task Force Report No. 139, Council for Agricultural Science and Technology, Ames, IA, 2003.

21. IARC, *Some Traditional Herbal Medicines: Some Mycotoxins, Naphthalene and Styrene*, IARC Monographs No. 82, International Agency for Research on Cancer, Lyon, 2002 (http://monographs.iarc.fr/htdocs/indexes/vol82index.html).

22. Marasas, W.F.O., Fumonisins: history, world-wide occurrence and impact, in *Fumonisins in Food*, Jackson, L., Ed., Plenum Press, New York, 1996.

23. Sydenham, E.W., Shephard, G.S., Thiel, P.G., Marasas, W.F.O., and Stockenstrom, S., Fumonisin contamination of commercial corn-based human foodstuffs, *J. Agric. Food Chem.*, 39, 2014–2018, 1991.

24. JECFA, *Safety Evaluation of Certain Mycotoxins in Food*, WHO Food Additives Series 47, FAO Food and Nutrition Paper 74, Joint FAO/WHO Expert Committee on Food Additives, Geneva, 2001.

25. Carratù, M.R., Cassano, T., Coluccia, A. et al., Antinutritional effects of fumonisin B_1 and pathophysiological consequences, *Toxicol. Lett.*, 140–141, 459–463, 2003.

26. Marasas, W.F.O., Riley, R.L., Hendricks, K.A., Stevens, V.L., Sadler, T.W., Gelineau-van Waes, J., Missmer, S.A., Cabrera, J., Torres, O., Gelderblom, W.C.A., Allegood, J., Martinez, C., Maddox, J., Miller, J.D., Starr, L., Sullards, M.C., Roman, A.V., Voss, K.A., Wang, E., and Merrill, Jr., A.H., Fumonisins disrupt sphingolipid metabolism, folate transport, and neural tube development in embryo culture and *in vivo*: a potential risk factor for human neural tube defects among populations consuming fumonisin-contaminated maize, *J. Nutrition*, 134, 711–716, 2004.

27. Hendricks, K., Fumonisins and neural tube defects in south Texas, *Epidemiology*, 10, 198–200, 1999.

28. Ross, P.F., Rice, L.G., Osweiler, G.D., Nelson, P.E., Richard, J.L., and Wilson, T.M., A review and update of animal toxicoses associated with fumonisin-contaminated feeds and production of fumonisins by Fusarium isolates, *Mycopathologia*, 117, 109–114, 1992.

29. Kellerman, T.S., Marasas, W.F., Thiel, P.G., Gelderblom, W.C., Cawood, M., and Coetzer, J.A., Leukoencephalomalacia in two horses induced by oral dosing of fumonisin B_1, *Onderstepoort J. Vet. Res.*, 57(4): 269–275, 1990.

30. FDA, *Background Paper in Support of Fumonisin Levels in Animal Feed*, U.S. Food and Drug Administration, Rockville, MD, 2000 (http://vm.cfsan.fda.gov/~dms/ fumonbg2.html).

31. FDA, *Background Paper in Support of Fumonisin Levels in Corn and Corn Products Intended for Human Consumption*, U.S. Food and Drug Administration, Rockville, MD, 2000 (http://www.cfsan.fda.gov/~dms/fumonbg3.html).

32. IARC, *Some Naturally Occurring Substances: Food Items and Constituents, Heterocyclic Aromatic Amines and Mycotoxins*, IARC Monographs No. 56, International Agency for Research on Cancer, Lyon, 1993 (http://monographs.iarc.fr/htdocs/indexes/vol56index.html).

33. Schaafsma, A.W., Economic changes imposed by mycotoxins in food grains: case study of deoxynivalenol in winter wheat, *Adv. Exp. Med. Biol.*, 504, 271–276, 2002.

34. Miller, J.D., ApSimon, J.W., Blackwell, B.A., Greenhalgh, R., and Taylor, A., Deoxynivalenol: a 25-year perspective on a trichothecene of agricultural importance, in *Fusarium*, Summerell, B.A., Leslie, J.F., Backhouse, D., Bryden, W.L., and Burgess, L.W., Eds., APS Press, St. Paul, MN, 2001, pp. 310–320.

35. FDA, *Mycotoxins in Domestic Foods. Food and Cosmetic Compliance Programs*, U.S. Food and Drug Administration, Rockville, MD, 2003 (http://www.cfsan.fda.gov/~comm/cp07001.html).

37. FAO, *Worldwide Regulations for Mycotoxins*, Food and Nutrition Paper 64, Food and Agricultural Organization, Rome, 1995.

38. Rosner, J. and van Egmond, H.P., Mykotoxin-Hoechstmengen in Lebensmitteln, *Bundesgesundheitsblatt*, 12, 467–473, 1995.

39. IPCS, *Microbial Pest Control Agent* Bacillus thuringiensis, Environmental Health Criteria 217, International Programme on Chemical Safety, World Health Organization, Geneva, 1999.

40. Federici, B.A., Case study: Bt crops — a novel mode of insect control, in *Genetically Modified Crops: Assessing Safety*, Vol. 22, Atherton, K.T., Ed., Taylor & Francis, New York, 2002, 164–200.

41. Ostlie, K., Hutchison, W., and Hellmich, R., *Bt Corn and European Corn Borer*, NCR Publ. No. 602, University of Minnesota, St. Paul, 1997.

42. Hyde, J., Martin, M.A., Preckel, P.V., and Edwards, C.R., The economics of Bt corn: valuing protection from the European corn borer, *Rev. Agric. Econ.*, 21, 442–454, 1999.

43. Levidow, L., Regulating Bt maize in the United States and Europe: a scientific-cultural comparison, *Environment*, 41(10), 10–22, 1999.

44. USDA, *Acreage*, National Agricultural Statistics Service, Agricultural Statistics Board, U.S. Department of Agriculture, Washington, D.C., 2003.

45. Munkvold, G.P., Potential impact of FDA guidelines for fumonisins in foods and feeds, in *Mycotoxins: The Cost of Achieving Food Security and Food Quality*, APSnet Feature Story, American Phytopathological Society, St. Paul, MN, 2001 (www.apsnet.org/online/feature/mycotoxin/top.html).

46. Dowd, P.F. The involvement of arthropods in the establishment of mycotoxigenic fungi under field conditions, in *Mycotoxins in Agriculture and Food Safety*, Sinha, K.K. and Bhatnagar, D., Eds., Marcel Dekker, New York, 1998.

47. Benedict, J., Fromme, D., Cosper, J., Correa, C., Odvody, G., and Parker, R., *Efficacy of Bt Corn Events MON810, Bt11, and E176 in Controlling Corn Earworm, Fall Armyworm, Sugarcane Borer and Aflatoxin*, Texas A&M University System, College Station, TX, 1998 (http://lubbock.tamu.edu/ipm/AgWeb/r_and_d/1998/Roy%20Parker/Bt%20Corn/BtCorn.html).

48. Windham, G.L., Williams, W.P., and Davis, F.M., Effects of the southwestern corn borer on *Aspergillus flavus* kernel infection and aflatoxin accumulation in maize hybrids, *Plant Dis.*, 83(6), 535–540, 1999.

49. Williams, W.P., Windham, G.L., Buckley, P.M., and Daves, C.A., Aflatoxin accumulation in conventional and transgenic corn hybrids infested with southwestern corn borer (Lepidoptera: Crambidae), *J. Agric. Urban Entomol.*, 19(4), 227–236, 2002.

50. Buntin, G.D., Lee, R.D., Wilson, D.M., and McPherson, R.M., Evaluation of YieldGard transgenic resistance for control of fall armyworm and corn earworm (Lepidoptera: Noctuidae) on corn, *Fla. Entomol.*, 84(1), 37–42, 2001.

51. Odvody, G.N., Chilcutt, C.F., Parker, R.D., and Benedict, J.H., Aflatoxin and insect response of near-isogenic Bt and non-Bt commercial corn hybrids in south Texas, in *Proc. 2000 Aflatoxin/Fumonisin Workshop*, J.F. Robens, Ed., U.S. Department of Agriculture, Agricultural Research Service, Beltsville, MD, 2000.

52. Munkvold, G.P., Cultural and genetic approaches to managing mycotoxins in maize, *Annu. Rev. Phytopathol.*, 41, 99–116, 2003.
53. Dowd, P.F., Indirect reduction of ear molds and associated mycotoxins in *Bacillus thuringiensis* corn under controlled and open field conditions: utility and limitations, *J. Econ. Entomol.*, 93, 1669–1679, 2000.
54. Masoero, F., Moschini, M., Rossi, F., Prandini, A., and Pietri, A., Nutritive value, mycotoxin contamination and *in vitro* rumen fermentation of normal and genetically modified corn (Cry1Ab) grown in northern Italy, *Maydica*, 44, 205–209, 1999.
55. Maupin, L.M., Clements, M.J., Walker, S.L., and White, D.G., Effects of Cry1Ab on *Aspergillus* ear rot in commercial corn hybrids, *Phytopathology*, 91, S59, 2001.
56. Munkvold, G.P., Hellmich, R.L., and Biggerstaff, C.M., Interactions among *Fusarium verticillioides*, insect pests, *Aspergillus flavus* in transgenic and conventional maize hybrids, in *Proc. 2000 Aflatoxin/Fumonisin Workshop*, J.F. Robens, Ed., U.S. Department of Agriculture, Agricultural Research Service, Beltsville, MD, 2000.
57. Pietri, A. and Piva, G., Occurrence and control of mycotoxins in maize grown in Italy, *Proc. 6th International Feed Products Conference*, Piacenza, Italy, 2000, pp. 226–236.
58. Dowd, P.F., Biotic and abiotic factors limiting efficacy of Bt corn in indirectly reducing mycotoxin levels in commercial fields, *J. Econ. Entomol.*, 94(5), 1067–1074, 2001.
59. Hammond, B., Campbell, K., Pilcher, C., Robinson, A., Melcion, D., Cahagnier, B., Richard, J., Sequeira, J., Cea, J., Tatli, F., Grogna, R., Pietri, A., Piva, G., and Rice, L., Reduction of fumonisin mycotoxins in Bt corn, *Toxicologist*, 72(S-1), abstract 1217, 2003.
60. Bakan, B., Melcion, D., Richard-Molard, D., and Cahagnier, B., Fungal growth and *Fusarium* mycotoxin content in isogenic traditional maize and genetically modified maize grown in France and Spain, *J. Agric. Food Chem.*, 50(4), 728–731, 2002.
61. Munkvold, G.P., Statement to U.S. Environmental Protection Agency FQPA Scientific Advisory Panel: Public Meeting on Bt Plant Insecticides Risk and Benefit Assessments, Docket #OPP-00678, Arlington, VA, 2000.
62. Schaafsma, A.W., Hooker, D.C., Baute, T.S., and Illincic-Tamburic, L., Effect of Bt-corn hybrids on deoxynivalenol content in grain at harvest, *Plant Dis.*, 86(10), 1123–1126, 2002.
63. Aulrich, K., Bohme, H., Daenicke, R., Halle, I., and Flachowsky, G., Genetically modified feeds (GMOs) in animal nutrition: *Bacillus thuringiensis* (Bt) corn in poultry, pig and ruminant nutrition, *Arch. Animal Nutr.*, 54, 183–195, 2001.
64. Magg, T., Melchinger, A.E., Klein, D., and Bohn, M., Relationship between European corn borer resistance and concentration of mycotoxins produced by *Fusarium* spp. in grains of transgenic Bt maize hybrids, their isogenic counterparts, and commercial varieties, *Plant Breeding: Zeitschrift für Pflanzenzuchtung*, 121(2), 146–154, 2002.
65. Robens, J. and Cardwell, K., The costs of mycotoxin management to the USA: management of aflatoxins in the United States, *J. Toxicol. Toxin Rev.*, 22(2–3), 143–156, 2003.
66. USDA, *Crop Values: 2002 Summary*, PR 2(03), National Agricultural Statistics Service, U.S. Department of Agriculture, Washington, D.C., 2003.
67. USDA, *Equine*, Agricultural Statistics Board, National Agricultural Statistics Service, U.S. Department of Agriculture, Washington, D.C., 1999.
68. USDA, *Mycotoxin Levels in the 1995 Midwest Preharvest Corn Crop*, Animal and Plant Health Inspection Service, U.S. Department of Agriculture, Washington, D.C., 1996 (www.aphis.usda.gov/vs/ceah/cahm/mycotxt.htm).
69. USDA, *Mycotoxin Levels in the 1996 Midwest Preharvest Corn Crop*, Animal and Plant Health Inspection Service, U.S. Department of Agriculture, Washington, D.C., 1997 (www.aphis.usda.gov/vs/ceah/cahm/mycotx96.htm).

70. USDA, *Fumonisin B₁ Mycotoxin in Horse Grain/Concentrate on U.S. Horse Operations*, Veterinary Services Info Sheet, Animal and Plant Health Inspection Service, U.S. Department of Agriculture, Washington, D.C., 2000 (www.aphis.usda/gov/vs/ceah/cahm/Equine/eq98fumonisin.htm).

71. Cardwell, K.F., Desjardins, A., Henry, S.H., Munkvold, G., and Robens, J., *Mycotoxins: The Cost of Achieving Food Security and Food Quality*, APSnet Feature Story, American Phytopathological Society, St. Paul, MN, 2001 (www.apsnet.org/online/feature/mycotoxin/top.html).

72. Beardall, J. and Miller, J.D., Natural occurrence of mycotoxins other than aflatoxin in Africa, Asia and South America, *Mycotoxin Res.*, 10, 21–24, 1994.

73. Ngoko, Z., Marasas, W.F.O., Rheeder, J.P., Shephard, G.S., Wingfield, M.J., and Cardwell, K.F., Fungal infection and mycotoxin contamination of maize in the humid forest and the western highlands of Cameroon, *Phytoparasitica*, 29(4), 352–360. 2001.

74. Placinta, C.M., D'Mello, J.P.F., and Macdonald, A.M.C., Review of worldwide contamination of cereal grains and animal feed with *Fusarium* mycotoxins, *Animal Feed Sci. Technol.*, 78(1–2), 21–37, 1999.

75. Paarlberg, R., African famine, made in Europe [editorial], *Wall Street J.*, 240(39), August 23, 2002.

76. Wu, F., Explaining consumer resistance to genetically modified corn: an analysis of the distribution of benefits and risks, *Risk Anal.*, Best Paper Issue, 24(3), 717–728, 2004.

24 Advances in Reducing Aflatoxin Contamination of U.S. Tree Nuts

Bruce C. Campbell, Russell J. Molyneux, and Thomas F. Schatzki

CONTENTS

24.1 INTRODUCTION

Aflatoxins are secondary metabolites produced by various species of *Aspergillus*. *Aspergillus flavus* Link and *A. parasiticus* Speare are the most significant species from an agronomic and food safety perspective.[1–3] Aflatoxin B_1 (AFB_1) and related difuranocoumarins are a concern to public health as potential carcinogens to humans and their proven toxicity to animals.[4-6] AFB_1 is generally considered to be hepato- toxic and a potent human liver carcinogen. Its mechanism of genotoxicity results from liver cytochrome P-450 epoxidation of AFB_1 to AFB_1 *exo*-8,9-epoxide (AFBO). This epoxide reacts with DNA at the guanyl N^7 atom after intercalation, forming a genotoxic DNA adduct.[7-9] Consumption of agricultural products contaminated with aflatoxins could result in acute hepatotoxicity and theoretically lead to chronic hepatocellular carcinoma (HCC) and mutagenesis in humans; however, Stoloff[10] questions the hepatocellular pathology caused by exposure to aflatoxin. Additionally, aflatoxin M_1 (AFM_1), a metabolite of AFB_1 found in milk of dairy cattle or lactating mothers exposed to aflatoxin, is of concern because of potential hepatotoxic and immunotoxic effects in infants and children. The likelihood of hepatotoxicity and hepatocarcinogenicity is greatly increased in developing countries where hepatitis B and C viruses (HBV and HCV) are endemic.[11-13] The incidence of HBV and HCV has been increasing in the United States which has added to concerns about aflatoxins in the domestic food supply. In 1994, the U.S. Food and Drug Administration (FDA) set guideline threshold levels for total aflatoxins in foods for domestic consumption at 20 ng/g (ppb);[14] however, the European Union (EU) and Japan are also quite concerned over the issue of aflatoxin contamination. These countries have set their threshold levels for imported commodities at least five times lower than the United States, at 4 ppb and below.

24.1.1 THE TREE NUT INDUSTRY

A number of agricultural commodities are affected by contamination with aflatox- ins.[15] The principal U.S. crops of concern include corn, peanuts, cottonseed, and, relevant to this chapter, tree nuts. The primary commercial tree nut crops affected by the threat of aflatoxin contamination are almonds, *Prunus dulcis* (Mill.) D.A. Webb; walnuts, *Juglans regia* L.; and pistachios, *Pistacia vera* L. Essentially, the entire commercial U.S. almond, pistachio, and walnut crops are produced in Cal- ifornia. Of this domestically produced crop, approximately 60% are exported to other nations. The total U.S. commercial value of the three tree nut crops has steadily increased over the last 2 decades and currently stands at an annual value of about $2 billion (harvested crop). California produces 75% of the world's almonds. Almost 400,000 metric tons were harvested in 2001, a value of close to $1 billion. Almonds, the number one horticultural export from the United States, approached $700 million in value in 2000, followed by wine. Spain is the world's second largest producer of almonds, with a harvest about five times less than California. The chief importers of U.S. almonds are countries of the EU, India, and Japan. Domestic walnut production is also overwhelmingly performed in California. The annual harvested value of walnuts has steadily increased over the past decade and fluctuates around $300 million per year. The U.S. produces over 30% of the world's walnuts. China is actually the top producer, but the United States is the top exporter of walnuts, exporting close to 60% of its domestic production. Again, countries of the EU and Japan are the main importers of U.S. walnuts, followed by Canada. Iran is the world's largest producer and exporter of pistachios. The value of the U.S. pistachio crop, almost entirely from California, is around $250 million per year, with about 50% of the harvest exported overseas. The main importers of U.S. pistachios are Hong Kong, countries of the EU, and Canada.[16] In addition to the actual value of harvested and processed-shelled nuts, tree nuts have a substantial added value as components of a variety of edible consumer products. In fact, almost 40% of tree nuts consumed domestically are from breakfast cereals. Other types of value-added products include marzipan and other types of nut pastes, ice creams, candies, and bakery products.[16]

24.1.2 TRADE AND FOOD SAFETY ISSUES

Aflatoxin contamination of tree nuts has become a growing international food safety concern for over a two-decade period.[17-22] A repercussion of this increasing concern has become the arguably very low threshold levels required to comply with Codex Alimentarius standards on imported tree nuts. The low thresholds for aflatoxin contamination have significantly increased the probability for rejection of tree nut shipments by the major importing nations of the EU and Japan. The EU initially rejected shipments of Iranian pistachios in 1998 and almonds from the United States in 1999. Because of current heightened concerns in the EU about aflatoxin, a continuing embargo has been placed on the importation of pistachios from Iran. The embargo, while leading to more pistachio exports from the United States, has increased awareness of potential for contamination of other tree nuts. In 1999, almost 70 tons of U.S. almonds were rejected by the EU. These rejections have increased pressure to ensure that U.S. shipments of tree nuts are below mandated contamination action-levels for aflatoxin. The total loss of tree nut sales from aflatoxin contamination averages around $50 million/year but can be much higher in years of greater insect damage.[23] The impact of the potential for aflatoxin contamination in almonds, pistachios, and walnuts, as food safety and international trade issues, has created a heightened desire to develop methods and strategies for reducing aflatoxins in pre- and post-harvest tree nut products.

Aflatoxin could possibly be used for agroterrorism. Following the Persian Gulf War, the United Nations Special Commission discovered a number of Iraqi missiles with payloads of aflatoxin. In view of the nonacute toxicity of aflatoxin to humans, it is difficult to surmise what tactical military advantage aflatoxin-bombardment of opposing forces might confer to a military campaign. Exposure to aflatoxin might increase the incidence of human liver cancer, but years after exposure.[24] Alternative targets of these weapons may have been agricultural commodities, such as the pistachio industry of Iran, where contamination would render them unexportable.

24.1.3 MECHANISMS FOR AFLATOXIN CONTAMINATION OF TREE NUTS

Insect-feeding damage is a principal factor leading to preharvest fungal infection of nut kernels of almonds, pistachios, and walnuts which may lead to subsequent aflatoxin contamination. Wounds to the protective layers surrounding nut kernels (hull, shell, and seedcoat) provide avenues for infection by windborne spores of aflatoxigenic aspergilli.[25-29] The principal insect pests of tree nuts are larvae of the navel orangeworm (NOW), *Amyelois transitella* Walker (Lepidoptera: Pyralidae), which infests kernels of almonds, walnuts, and pistachios; the peach twig borer (PTB), *Anarsia lineatella* Zell. (Lepidoptera: Gelechiidae), which infests meristem leaf shoots, husks, and kernels of almonds; and the codling moth (CM), *Cydia pomonella* (L.) (Lepidoptera: Tortricidae), which infests the husks and kernels of walnuts. Infestation of tree nuts by these insects entails a sequence of insect behaviors.[30,31] NOW females lay eggs on "mummy" nuts (stick-tight nuts from the previous season) in the fall through early summer.[32] NOW females do not normally lay eggs on immature nuts of the current season crop until those nuts mature at hull-split in August through early October;[33] however, NOW females will lay eggs on a current season crop before hull-split if nuts are already damaged by feeding of other insects (e.g., CM in walnuts and PTB in almonds)[34-36] or in pistachios if nuts have prematurely split open (so-called early splits [ESs]). Aflatoxin contamination of split-hull pistachios, without evidence of insect presence, has been reported, however.[34]

Alternate routes for fungal infection may occur during development of the nut kernel or through natural breaks in the protective layers during kernel maturation; for example, the stem end of the developing pistachio fruit hardens at a later point in development than the remaining tissues.[37] While surrounding tissues are still soft, the pistachio kernel is vulnerable to being pierced by sucking-insects possessing stylet-like mouthparts. These insects are mainly various heteropterans such as leaf-footed and stink bugs, common to pistachio and almond orchards.[37,38] In addition to proteolytic and hydrolyzing enzymes in their saliva, the stylets of such insects can also harbor a variety of microorganisms, including fungal spores, that can be coinjected into plant tissues along with the saliva.[39] Fungal infection by this type of injection presents a problem because no telltale signs of damage to the nut are apparent externally. Without such telltale indicators it is difficult to detect and remove such nuts from the processing stream. Pistachio nuts damaged externally by NOW or other chewing insects and later infected by fungi generally show some form of discoloration around the suture of the split hull. In pistachios, discoloration of the suture may occur without insect damage. This type of discoloration is readily detectable, and such nuts can be removed from the processing stream;[40] however, spores of a number of species of *Aspergillus*, including *A. flavus*, can be detected in the internal tissues of pistachios, almonds, and walnuts that exhibit no exterior damage.[41] Although such nuts may not be contaminated with aflatoxin, proper postharvest handling and storage of such tree nuts is required to prevent further colonization of internal tissues.

A major reservoir of *Aspergillus* spores in tree nut orchards can occur in the leaf, hull, and unharvested litter surrounding the trees. This type of litter presents a special problem to pistachios where *Aspergillus* frequently infects and sporulates on fallen fruit and male flowers. Aflatoxin-producing strains of *A. flavus* and *A. parasiticus* can be found in such litter. While it is not known whether direct infection of arboreal fruits occurs, litter infected with these fungi contributes to increased probability of wounded nuts becoming infected by wind-blown fungal spores.[42]

24.2 RESEARCH EFFORTS

The economic return to tree nut producers and processors is directly related to the quality of their product. Contamination by aflatoxins disrupts efficient marketing of tree nuts and results in extra costs passed to the consumer. In some instances, after costs of harvesting, processing, and shipping have been incurred, the product may be rejected from domestic or foreign markets. Currently available methods of removing aflatoxins from tree nuts after contamination are impractical and expensive.[43] Moreover, use of fungicides to control aflatoxigenic aspergilli can have an opposite effect in that sublethal doses may actually induce aflatoxin production.[44] There is a need to design new and environmentally safe methods of reducing infection of tree nuts by aflatoxigenic aspergilli and to inhibit aflatoxin biosynthesis. The main thrust of research to reduce aflatoxin contamination of tree nuts is being performed by two groups of collaborating scientists in California whose research is funded by the U.S. Department of Agriculture (USDA) Agricultural Research Service (ARS). One group includes a team of scientists in the Plant Mycotoxin Research Unit, Western Regional Research Center, USDA, ARS, Albany, CA. The other group includes scientists at the University of California, Davis (UCD), in the Department of Pomology and at the Kearney Agriculture Center. Efforts by these scientists focus on insect control, fungal control, orchard management, and postharvest sampling, detection, and removal of contaminated nuts. These teams of scientists include individuals with expertise in insect biology, ecology, microbiology, molecular biology, plant pathology, natural product chemistry, plant breeding, risk assessment analysis, and agricultural engineering.

24.2.1 REDUCING PREHARVEST CONTAMINATION

24.2.1.1 Insect Control

Developing new methods of insect control in tree nut orchards is gaining more attention as a result of increased insect resistance to currently available pesticides.[45–48] Moreover, recent regulations by the Environmental Protection Agency (EPA) require phasing out the use of specific organophosphorous pesticides. This EPA regulation is in response to the Food Quality Protection Act, which mandates strict reductions in pesticide use. This act also mandates the eventual ban of some pesticides used for the control of tree nut pests in the Central Valley of California. In spite of insecticide usage, harvested nuts have an annual rejection rate of 4 to 12% due to insect and associated mold damage.[49] Research and development of new methods to curtail insect-feeding damage to tree nuts have involved a variety of approaches. Semiochemicals, chemical cues insects use for communication and discerning their environment, are being exploited to disrupt insect migratory, reproductive, and host-finding behaviors. Plant breeding is developing almonds with better shell integrity and an improved suture seal that prevent infestation of the nut kernel by insects. Genetic engineering has developed transgenic walnuts that manufacture the insect-specific CRYL1A(c) endotoxin of *Bacillus thuringiensis*.[50,51] Improved methods for orchard management have been developed to remove mummies, unharvested nuts that remain on trees that act as overwintering reservoirs for insects, and to reduce early-split in pistachios that frequently become infested by NOW.[52]

24.2.1.1.1 Semiochemical-Based Insect Control

Many insect behaviors, including feeding, mating, egg-laying, and dispersal, are mediated by semiochemicals.[53] The dependency of insects on semiochemicals provides a unique means of control through monitoring pest populations and disrupting normal behavior. Implementing the use of semiochemicals is increasingly relevant in view of the tree nut industry's environmental and food safety concerns over restrictions in use of pesticides. One category of semiochemicals includes sex pheromones. While multicomponent sex pheromones for PTB[54] and CM[55] have been identified, the identification of components of the pheromone of NOW are incomplete. Synthetic reproductions of these pheromones have been effective on a commercial level for monitoring populations, but their use as mating disruptants has been unreliable. The potential exists to attain requisite effectiveness of mating disruption by combining host plant volatiles (HPVs) with pheromones.[56] PTB and CM vastly prefer fruit hosts to nuts. Some success has been achieved at exploiting pome fruit and stone fruit HPVs in tree nuts. Commercial mating disruption systems for both species have had limited success and must be augmented with insecticide sprays.[57]

The main constituent of the sex pheromone of PTB was identified as Z-5-decen-1-yl acetate;[58] however, using this compound for mating disruption met with little success.[57] It was later determined that PTB sex pheromone contains the Z-5-decen-1-yl acetate and a Z-5-decen-1-ol, where the acetate was represented by >80% relative to the alcohol.[54] After some initial indications of success, this formulation did not function fully as a mating disruptant.[59] Examination of the pheromone of both a wild strain and a laboratory strain of PTB revealed two main components, (E)-5-decenyl acetate and (E)-5-decen-1-ol; however, the ratios of these components varied between the two strains, with the major component being the alcohol at 98% in the wild strain and 89% in the lab strain.[60] The much greater presence of the alcohol component is opposite to that reported previously[54] and may explain the failure of the currently used formulation.

Chemical cues governing insect host-finding and ovipositioning in differing tree nut conditions are largely unknown. A number of volatiles from almond[61–63] and walnut[64–70] have been identified in past reports, but none of these reports examined all tree nut tissues. A single preliminary analysis of volatile constituents of larval frass of NOW has been published.[71] Also, many of the pest insects of tree nuts have other host plants (e.g., CM on pome fruits) whose volatiles might be effective in a tree nut orchard. CM is attracted to the odor of apples.[72,73] One apple volatile, (E,E)-α-farnesene, was found to be an attractant to CM based exclusively on laboratory bioassays[74] and also to CM larvae.[75] The instability and rapid chemical breakdown of (E,E)-α-farnesene limits its use for controlling CM.[76] Gas chromatographic/mass spectrometric (GC-MS) analyses of HPVs of walnut leaves,[67,77] pear leaves,[78,79] apples,[80] walnut husks,[81] and unripe apple or pear fruits[82] showed a preponderance of mono-, sesqui-, and oxygenated-terpenoids. By contrast, HPVs of ripe fruits of apple and pear are predominantly aliphatic esters, a few short chain-length aliphatic alcohols, and several sesquiterpenes.[82–84] CM prefer pome fruits over walnuts.[85] In view of this preference for pome fruits, an array of volatile blends and individual HPVs of pome fruits were tested for attractancy to CM in a walnut orchard environment.[86] A pear-derived volatile, ethyl (2E,4Z)-2,4-decadienoate, was discovered that is CM specific and stable and attracts male CM at an equivalent level of activity as commercial female pheromone; however, the CM pheromone is of limited utility in that it only attracts male moths. In contrast, the newly discovered kairomone attracts female CM, both virgin and mated. Such a lure that can attract female moths is of particular value in that it can be exploited to control the egg-laying life stage of the pest insect.

The discovery of a potent kairomone for female moths is rare. Male lures are generally common and usually based on sex pheromones. The pear-based attractant to CM provides a biorational alternative to conventional insecticide applications while simultaneously ensuring food safety and reducing negative impact to the environment. Potential novel uses of this CM attractant in integrated pest management (IPM) include: (1) monitoring female flight patterns for prudential scheduling of insecticide applications; (2) monitoring pest emergence in orchards undergoing sex pheromone-based mating disruption, where accurate monitoring of the moth population with pheromone traps is not feasible; (3) assessing whether female moths have mated; and (4) direct control of CM by mass trapping, disrupting CM mating and ovipositional behaviors, or killing CM by using the lure as an attracticide, where the lure is combined with a pesticide. Another attracticide-like approach currently being tested is the use of trap trees, where adults are attracted to baited walnut trees genetically transformed with Bt toxin.[50,87] In view of its unique properties to control one of the major agricultural pests in the United States, the pear-based kairomone has received a patent.[88]

Dispensing egg traps in tree nut orchards is the most commonly used method of monitoring NOW populations. Such monitoring is needed for timing application of insecticides.[89] The bait in NOW egg traps is a crude almond press cake impregnated with almond oil.[90] Effectiveness of these traps is variable because of the crude, unrefined nature of the bait.[91] Evidence suggests that the attractiveness of the bait involves long-chain fatty acids, especially oleic and linoleic acids;[63] however, more precise analysis of chemical composition is necessary to improve the bait as a monitoring lure, attracticide, or ovipositional disruptant. A single-component sex pheromone of NOW has been identified but is not effective as a mating disruptant. Additional minor components of the female pheromonal emission of NOW have been identified; however, a new two-component blend has had mixed results in mating disruption trials.[92,93]

24.2.1.1.2 Other Strategies for Insect Control

Additional nonpesticidal approaches to controlling insect pests of tree nuts include one that entails the discovery of and augmenting the constitutive natural products of tree nuts that deter insect feeding. For example, almonds possess low levels of cyanogenic compounds that could deter feeding by NOW.[94] One such cyanogenic compound, amygdalin, can produce small amounts of hydrogen cyanide upon hydrolysis. Many lepidopterous insects, such as NOW, possess gut β-glucosidases that can perform this hydrolysis.[95] One approach now being undertaken is augmenting amygdalin levels in certain almond tissues.[96] Another strategy to reduce insect damage to tree nut kernels has involved a breeding program to improve the integrity of the endocarp (shell) surrounding the nut kernel. California almonds typically possess a more papery shell as compared to the relatively more peach-pit type of shell inherent to Asian and European varieties. The thinner shells of California varieties increase the probability of becoming damaged during mechanical harvesting or of penetration by chewing or sucking insects, especially along the suture seal. Such damage can lead to fungal infection of the kernel. The weakened suture area was found to be associated with the developing funiculus. This discovery now allows trait selection for breeding almonds that will be more resistant to shell split.[38]

24.2.1.1.3   Insect Pests and Aflatoxin Interactions

The role of insects in facilitating the infection of tree nuts by aflatoxigenic *Aspergillus* is well documented for pistachios and almonds. An interesting observation, however, is that many tree nut pests feed and develop normally on tree nuts that are heavily infected with fungi. Because these insects thrive in a highly fungal- and mycotoxin-contaminated environment, understanding the mechanisms for their survival might provide either biological or metabolic clues to detoxification or avoiding toxicosis by mycotoxins. Efforts have been made in the past to identify microbial agents or products that degrade or inhibit synthesis of AFB_1;[97–99] however, degradation products or products within the aflatoxin biosynthetic pathway that might accumulate in lieu of the final aflatoxin product are frequently overlooked. Some degradative or preaflatoxin products, such as sterigmatocystin, can also be cytotoxic or carcinogenic.[100–102]

Metabolism of aflatoxins is intimately linked with toxic and carcinogenic effects. Accordingly, interspecies variations in AFB_1-induced carcinogenesis or mutagenesis appear to be reflected in differences in metabolism, particularly in terms of cytochrome P-450 (Cyt P-450) and glutathione *S*-transferase (GST) activities. Cyt P-450 monooxygenases are microsomal, membrane-bound enzymes located in the endoplasmic reticulum of eucaryotic cells; for example, in humans, the family of CYP3 cytochromes P-450 catalyzes epoxidation reactions of the terminal furan ring of AFB_1 to AFBO. AFBO is a highly reactive epoxide and is responsible for nucleic acid alkylation.[7,103] GST, on the other hand, efficiently conjugates tripeptide glutathione (GSH) with the lipophilic electrophile, AFBO.[104] This conjugation reaction is believed to be the primary detoxification pathway of AFBO. The significance of the interplay of enzymatic activities and respective biotransformation products is demonstrated in mice. Mice are much less likely to develop hepatocarcinoma than rats when exposed to AFB_1 because of higher rates of GST activity and conjugation of AFBO with GSH in mice than in rats.[105]

Though the chronic and acute lethal and mutagenic effects of AFB_1 are reported, little is known about the actual metabolism of aflatoxin by insects and respective biotransformation products. Aflatoxins have insecticidal, larvicidal, chemosterilizing, and genotoxic properties against many insect species.[106–110] AFL was the major *in vitro* metabolite identified in 12 genetically distinct strains of *Drosophila melanogaster* Meigen.[111] In this *Drosophila* study, the Hikone-R strain, a strain selected for insecticidal resistance, produced mostly aflatoxicol (AFL) and small amounts of

AFM_1 and aflatoxin B_{2a} (AFB_{2a}). The relative amounts of these metabolites varied significantly among the strains of *D. melanogaster* examined. AFB_1 can induce recessive lethal mutations in *D. melanogaster*.[112] This insect possesses a Cyt P-450 (CYP6a2) homologous to human CYP3a.[113] AFM_1 was found to be a DNA-damaging agent in certain flies, but with an activity approximately threefold lower than AFB_1.[110] Several species of cockroaches are less sensitive to aflatoxins than other insects.[114,115] Because cockroaches have varied diets, it is possible that they evolved mechanisms of resistance toward naturally occurring aflatoxins routinely present in decaying matter or developed as a means of excreting or sequestering the toxin in an inactive form. Infection of the sugarcane mealybug, *Saccharicoccus sacchari*, by either *Aspergillus parasiticus* or *A. flavus* has demonstrated no entomopathogenic effects from aflatoxins.[116]

With regard to insects infesting tree nuts, larvae of NOW are often in a microenvironment that includes mycelia, hyphae, and spores of aflatoxigenic fungi.[28,42,117] Despite contact with these fungal tissues, this insect pest continues to develop and complete its life cycle. Larvae of CM, however, while frequently inhabiting walnut kernels that are highly infected with various fungi, have a lower potential for exposure to aflatoxin because walnut kernels are relatively antiaflatoxigenic compared with other tree nuts.[118] The aflatoxin biotransformation products produced by these two insects were examined and compared to those produced by mouse and chicken.[119] A field strain of NOW produced three main AFB_1 biotransformation products, chiefly AFL and minor amounts of AFB_{2a} and AFM_1. With AFL as a substrate, NOW larvae produced AFB_1 and aflatoxicol M_1 ($AFLM_1$). A laboratory strain of CM larvae exposed to AFB_1 showed no detectable levels of any AFB_1 biotransformation products in comparison to a field strain that produced trace amounts of only AFL. Neither NOW nor CM produced AFBO, the principal carcinogenic metabolite of AFB_1. In comparison, metabolism of AFB_1 by chicken liver yielded mainly AFL, whereas mouse liver produced mostly AFM_1 at a rate eightfold greater than AFL. Mouse liver also produced AFBO.

The relatively high production of AFL by NOW compared to CM may reflect an adaptation to detoxify AFB_1. NOW larvae frequently inhabit environments highly contaminated with fungi and, hence, aflatoxin. Only low amounts, if any, of this mycotoxin occur in the chief CM hosts, walnuts and pome fruits. Lee and Campbell[119] concluded that NOW larvae do not possess particular cytochromes P-450 for epoxidation of AFB_1; however, biotransformation of AFB_1 to AFL by NOW is generated by a cytosolic NADPH-dependent reductase. This study also suggested AFB_1 reductase activity found in NOW larvae may result from a novel enzyme in view of involvement of GSH as an electron donor for AFL formation. The absence of the mutagenic biotransformation product of AFB_1 in these insects, as compared to its production in mammals and birds,[120,121] may have some eco-evolutionary basis. Both CM and NOW are major pests of tree nuts. The kernels of these nuts, if damaged, are prone to infection by fungi; thus, these insects have consistently evolved in an environment of intimate contact with fungi, with the potential exposure to mycotoxins during larval development being quite high. This interaction between nut-kernel-inhabiting insects and fungi may have existed for tens if not hundreds of millions of years as opposed to more recent interactions between mammals and aflatoxins.

24.2.1.2 Fungal Control

24.2.1.2.1 Fungal Associations with Tree Nuts

The association of infection by the fungus *Aspergillus flavus* with contamination of tree nuts by aflatoxin has been reported on numerous occasions beginning in the 1970s.[19,25,122–125] Surveys to further understand microbial ecology with regard to fungal communities inhabiting tree nut orchards have also been undertaken for pistachios in Turkey[126,127] and California[42,117] and almonds in California.[128,129] A comprehensive survey of the fungal flora found in California almonds, pistachios, walnuts, and figs, collected from orchards and purchased from supermarkets, was also performed.[41,130] These studies found that different tree nuts maintained a different set of fungal species as microflora, both on the surface and in internal tissues. Spores of *A. flavus* were found on internal tissues of some tree nuts that had no visible cracks in hull or shell. The fact that spores of *A. flavus* were found in internal tissues, kernels in some cases, reinforces the need for proper postharvest handling of tree nuts. Such spores could serve as an inoculum should a favorable postharvest environment for germination arise. A further implication from this study may provide some knowledge with regard to the biological control of *A. flavus* or aflatoxigenesis. These studies also identified another toxin-producing fungus, *A. alliaceus*, on tree nuts. This fungus is the chief species responsible for ochratoxin contamination of figs[130] and had been previously identified on tree nuts.[117] Moreover, two other aspergilli reported to produce ochratoxin, *A. ochraceus* and *A. melleus*, were also identified on some tree nuts, but none of the strains identified produced ochratoxin.

Current effective efforts at the biological control of *Aspergillus flavus* involve the use of atoxigenic strains as biocompetitors of toxigenic strains in cotton fields.[131] Bayman et al.[41] were able to identify a number of fungal associations native to tree nut orchards where populations of *A. flavus* were reduced. The strategy of using microorganisms native to tree nut orchards as biological control agents has also resulted in identification of a number of saprophytic yeasts.[132] These yeasts do not have a pathology associated with humans. One of the yeast isolates reduced aflatoxin production 100-fold relative to controls in *in vitro* studies.

24.2.1.2.2 Constitutive Natural Products

Current approaches to applying fungicides for preventing growth of microorganisms or chemical treatments to destroy aflatoxins are not feasible for ensuring that shipments of tree nuts are within tolerance levels. A more fruitful strategy, therefore, may be to find natural products within the crop that confer resistance to colonization by *Aspergillus* or prevent aflatoxin biosynthesis. These two classes of protective natural factors exist in nature. One includes phytoalexins that are inducible metabolites, formed after invasion *de novo* (e.g., by activation of latent enzyme systems). The other is phytoanticipins, which are constitutive metabolites present *in situ*, either in the active form or easily generated from a precursor. Because phytoalexins are produced only in response to fungal attack, their presence would lag behind the infection, and levels capable of suppressing aflatoxin contamination might be difficult to regulate. In contrast, phytoanticipins are always present and such factors offer the potential for enhancement through breeding and selection of more resistant cultivars, or even genetic manipulation to introduce or enhance their levels. When such compounds have been identified, it is only necessary to ensure that they are present in large enough quantities and in tissues from which fungal growth and aflatoxin deposition must be excluded. It would also have to be determined that such compounds do not affect taste or other qualities of the product and that they are not harmful to consumers.

As mentioned above, tree nuts appear to be shielded against infection by a series of protective layers that provide chemical or physical barriers to microorganisms. Despite these barriers, tree nuts may nevertheless become contaminated with aflatoxins. These barriers include the husk or hull, consisting of the outer (epicarp) and inner (mesocarp) layers; the shell (endocarp); and the pellicle, which is a thin, paper-like tissue (seed coat) surrounding the kernel. While the shell provides a physical barrier, it is not entirely impervious to penetration by insects that may introduce fungal spores through the shell suture or the stem end, where the shell is less dense. Protection from infection in the softer tissues such as the husk, pellicle, and possibly the kernel itself are more likely to be dependent upon the presence of natural constituents.

The triterpenoids betulinic acid, oleanolic acid, and ursolic acid have been shown to occur in high concentrations in almond hulls,[133] but preliminary tests failed to show any significant antiaflatoxigenic activity. In addition, 3-prenyl-4-*O*-*b*-D-glu-copyranosyloxy-4-hydroxybenzoic acid, together with the ubiquitous phytochemicals, catechin and protocatechuic acid, have been isolated,[134] but these compounds have not been tested. Anacardic acids, natural constituents of the hulls of pistachios, have been shown to be capable to some extent of suppressing the biosynthesis of aflatoxins by *Aspergillus flavus* under laboratory conditions;[135] however, hulls of walnuts are most highly resistant to *A. flavus* growth in comparison with other tree nuts, such as pistachios and almonds.

A series of naphthoquinones in walnuts have also been shown to be potent inhibitors of aflatoxin biosynthesis. It is well established that *Juglans* species contain a series of structurally related naphthoquinones and that these compounds occur in particularly high concentrations in the fleshy husk surrounding the nut.[68] Moreover, leaves of the pecan *Carya illinoensis* (Wangenh) K. Koch, another member of the Juglandaceae but in a different subfamily from *Juglans*, contain the naphthoquinone juglone, which inhibits mycelial growth of *Cladosporium caryigenum* (Ellis & Langl.) Gottwald (= *Fusicladium effusum* G. Winter), the causative agent of pecan scab.[136] Pure juglone and a crude extract from green walnut hulls have been tested for their activity against a wide range of microorganisms, including a variety of bacteria, filamentous bacteria, algae, and dermatophytes.[137] Although juglone has been evaluated against a number of plant pathogens[138] and juglone and plumbagin have been shown to be fungitoxic at high concentrations to 24 different fungi, including *A. flavus*,[139] the effect of juglone and related naphthoquinones on aflatoxigenesis has not been investigated. We have therefore studied the activity of a series of these compounds in order to establish whether or not they are factors in the resistance of walnuts to contamination by aflatoxins and, if so, the structural features contributing to such activity.

Fungal viability and aflatoxigenesis as affected by the four major naphthoquinones present in walnut husks — 1,4-naphthoquinone, juglone (5-hydroxy-1,4-naphthoquinone), 2-methyl-1,4-naphthoquinone, and, plumbagin (5-hydroxy-2-methyl-1,4-naphthoquinone) — were studied *in vitro*. The quinones delayed germination of the fungus and were capable of completely inhibiting growth at higher concentrations. 2-Methyl-1,4-naphthoquinone and plumbagin had similar activity and were much more effective than the other two quinones, with germination delayed to 40 hours at 20 ppm and no growth at 50 ppm, whereas a control sample with no quinones present germinated in 16 hours. The effect on aflatoxin levels was highly dependent on the concentration of individual naphthoquinones in the media. At higher concentrations, aflatoxin production was decreased or completely inhibited, but at lower concentrations a stimulatory effect on aflatoxin biosynthesis was observed, with a greater than threefold increase at 20 ppm of 2-methyl-1,4-naphthoquinone. Structural features associated with decreased fungal viability and greatest effect on aflatoxigenesis were the presence of a 5-hydroxyl or 2-methyl substituent, but no significant additive effect was observed when both of these substituents were present.[118] Of particular interest is the influence of these compounds in enhancing aflatoxin production at lower concentrations while reducing it at higher concentrations. It can be hypothesized that the naphthoquinones have a regulatory effect on certain genes in the gene cluster responsible for aflatoxin biosynthesis. The molecular biology of aflatoxin biosynthesis has been investigated in detail, and the genes controlling specific steps of the pathway have been identified.[3,140] It may be significant that the early stages of aflatoxin biosynthesis, proceeding from norsolorinic acid to versicolorin A, involve hydroxylated anthraquinones that have structural moieties common also to juglone and plumbagin. Because of this structural similarity, naphthoquinones and the anthraquinone precursors may similarly affect domains of regulatory receptors which can upregulate or downregulate aflatoxin biosynthesis. Alternatively, *aflR* encodes for a zinc-containing, DNA-binding protein, and it is possible that the naphthoquinones act as chelators of this metal ion through sequestration by the 5-hydroxyl group adjacent to the quinonoid keto group. In any event, the effect of juglone and other walnut naphthoquinones on specific genes involved in aflatoxin biosynthesis warrants further investigation.

In vitro laboratory experiments using 5% ground kernels in agar have shown a significant difference in the capacity to which almonds and walnuts support aflatoxin production, with walnuts being much less susceptible to contamination. Only one variety of pistachio, "Kerman," is in commercial production, and it fell between walnuts and almonds in the capacity to support aflatoxin production. On average, using a specific bioassay regimen, *Aspergillus flavus* spores inoculated onto various walnut varieties produced 0 to 28 mg/plate, the pistachio produced 40 mg/plate, and various almond varieties produced 20 to 192 mg/plate. Moreover, the varietal differences within the 34 varieties and breeding lines of almonds showed a 10-fold range in aflatoxin levels while 26 walnut cultivars exhibited a 1400-fold range.[141] The "Tulare" variety of walnut completely suppressed aflatoxin production. This is the first example of any known crop plant affected by issues of aflatoxin contamination that possesses complete inhibition of aflatoxin biosynthesis. Several other commercial walnut varieties, including "Vina," "Howard," "Eureka," and "Payn," all produced <5mg/plate aflatoxin, whereas "Chico" produced 27 mg/plate. Black walnut (*Juglans nigra*) was the least inhibitory, with an aflatoxin output of 44 mg/plate. These results indicate a heritable natural resistance to aflatoxigenesis in walnuts and possibly to a lesser extent in almonds. These findings further suggest that selections of breeding lines for this characteristic can be made.

The particularly potent inhibition of aflatoxin biogenesis by the "Tulare" walnut indicated that attention should be focused on this variety when attempting to elucidate the nature of the resistance factor. Sampling of the kernels over their period of development from June to September established that they had little resistance when first formed, with aflatoxin at 94% of control in June, but this level declined rapidly to 13% in July and was only 0.6% at maturity in September. Additional studies showed that the kernel resistance was not affected by rootstock or growing location and was therefore a trait of the "Tulare" cultivar. In order to determine whether the resistance factor was localized in the seed coat or in the kernel without seed coat, these were physically separated and all of the activity was found to reside in the seed coat. At a level of 0.5% seed coat in agar, the aflatoxin produced amounted to only 2% of control, whereas the kernels without seed coat produced no inhibition; at levels above 1% incorporation in agar, the aflatoxin levels rapidly increased, attaining 410% of control at 4% incorporation. This is probably a consequence of an increased supply of lipid and carbohydrate nutrients to the fungus.

Based on these observations, it appeared that the resistance factors are entirely located in the seed coat.[141] Extraction of seed coat material with a series of solvents of increasing polarity and incorporation of the residual tissue after extraction into agar showed that nonpolar solvents removed very little of the antiaflatoxigenic activity, but substantial amounts were extracted by polar solvents such as methanol and water; however, some activity remained unextractable, suggesting bioactivity resided in a complex of hydrolyzable tannins.[142] Such tannins can be hydrolyzed by a tannase present in *Aspergillus flavus*,[143] yielding gallic acid and ellagic acid. Testing showed that only gallic acid had potent inhibitory activity towards aflatoxin biosynthesis.[142] Comparison of gallic and ellagic acid contents between "Tulare" and "Chico" cultivars, over two growing seasons, showed gallic acid content increased rapidly during nut maturation. Moreover, the gallic acid content in "Tulare" was 1.5 to 2 times higher than in "Chico." Levels of gallic acid in pellicles of a number of commercial English walnuts and two species of black walnut (*J. nigra* and *J. hindsii*) correlated with their potential for inhibition of aflatoxigenesis. By using deletion mutants of *Saccharomyces cerevisiae* as a model system, the antiaflatoxigenic mode of action of gallic acid appears to be the result of amelioration of oxidative stress in the fungus.[144] For example, the negative effects on yeasts lacking the antioxidative stress gene *cta1* exposed to hydrogen peroxide were reversed when these mutants were treated with gallic acid. Another deletion mutant lacking the signal transduction gene *yap1*, which induces downstream expression of at least four antioxidative stress genes, showed results similar to those of the *cta1* deletion mutant. Gallic acid also appears to affect the mitogen-activated protein (MAP) kinase signaling pathway of the fungus, as well.[144] Regulation of gallic acid levels in hydrolyzable tannins of walnuts through conventional breeding or some other form of genetic manipulation could potentially provide new cultivars highly inhibitory to aflatoxigenesis.

A number of compounds have been identified in almond kernels, primarily as a consequence of a search for healthful food constituents. These include a sphingolipid, sterols (β-sitosterol and daucosterol), and nucleosides (uridine and adenosine).[145] It is doubtful whether any of these compounds would have activity against aflatoxin biosynthesis, and a strategy is now underway to search for antiaflatoxigenic constituents patterned on the successful approach used with walnuts. Different varieties of almond kernels bred for different oleic and linoleic acid balance showed varying degrees of supporting aflatoxigensis when inoculated with a toxigenic strain of *A. flavus*; however, the level of aflatoxin production could not be correlated with oil content.[146]

24.2.1.3   Cultural Practices

Irrigation practices can also have a profound effect on risks associated with aflatoxin contamination of pistachios. Deficit irrigation of pistachio trees early in the growing season can lead to a phenomenon known as "early-split nuts."[52] In such cases, the shell and hull split open prior to harvest. Such splitting exposes the pistachio kernel to infestation by insects, especially NOW, and infection by aflatoxigenic aspergilli. Typically, the rate of early splitting in commercial pistachio orchards in California averages around 2 to 3% in a growing season. Experimental procedures using differently sized microsprinklers determined that the level of deficit irrigation in April or May, a period contemporaneous with shell growth, influences the incidence of early splits. Deficit irrigation at later stages during nut development does not appear to affect incidence of early splits; hence, growers need to be aware of providing sufficient irrigation to pistachio orchards in early spring.[52]

24.2.2   Reducing Postharvest Contamination

24.2.2.1   Rehydration

Practices involved in the production and processing of tree nuts can have profound effects on levels of aflatoxin in the finished product. Natural dehiscence (shell splitting) is a desirable feature of pistachios because most of the crop is marketed in-shell and the separation enables the shell to be easily removed by the consumer. If they are to be marketed, the undehisced portion of the crop must be sorted out and the shells removed before marketing as kernels.[147] Closed-shell pistachios are generally reprocessed overseas by water-soaking and artificial opening using low-cost labor.[148] The potential therefore exists for any nuts sequestering aflatoxigenic *Aspergillus* spores or aflatoxins to contaminate the batch during the rehydration process. In order to investigate the conditions under which such contamination could occur, a study was undertaken to assess the extent of fungal propagation during reprocessing and to attempt to define the point of entry of *A. flavus* giving rise to aflatoxins in closed-shell pistachios.

Inoculation of fresh, or dried and rehydrated, closed-shell pistachios at the stem end of the shell with spores of *Aspergillus flavus* resulted in aflatoxin contamination of the kernel after incubation. The proportion of contaminated nuts was 48% for the fresh pistachios and 35% for the dried pistachios, with 18 and 4%, respectively, having kernels containing aflatoxin levels in excess of 90 µg/kernel, sufficient to contaminate a 10-lb test lot at the 20-ppb guidance level. Closed-shell pistachios batch-rehydrated for 3 hours in a bath inoculated with *A. flavus* spores showed aflatoxin levels in the kernels of 170 ppb after 2 days of incubation and the extraordinarily high level of 87,500 ppb after 6 days.[149] This demonstrates that the kernels of closed-shell pistachios can become highly contaminated with aflatoxin, even though the shell would appear to provide a physical barrier to the fungus. It has been shown that the stem end of the fruit remains relatively soft later in the season compared to the rest of the shell. This area is vulnerable to being pierced by the stylet-like mouthparts of heteropteran insects, which feed preferentially at this site.[37] It therefore seems probable that any fungal attack by aflatoxigenic *Aspergillus* species would also be most likely to occur through penetration of the stem end of the shell. These results strongly indicate that the practice of rehydration prior to mechanical splitting should be avoided.

24.2.2.2 Sampling Theory

When nuts, or other granular materials, are sampled for contaminants or other chemical inclusions, samples of a preselected number of nuts are withdrawn. These samples are then homogenized in some way and the contaminant concentration (c) is established by chemical or physical analysis. If this experiment is repeated a number of times, using the same sample size (N nuts) each time, the results will not be identical in general but will form a *sample distribution*: $P(N,C)$. P will depend strongly on N, particularly in its breadth (standard deviation, s). For most nut products and practical sample sizes, s is often quite large, as large or larger then the mean m of all the samples. Because we commonly want the mean of the lot from which the samples are chosen and which is represented by the sample mean m, such large standard deviations pose a serious problem in testing.

In addition to the sample distribution is a more fundamental one, the *lot distribution* (p), which describes the probability that a single nut or granule, chosen from the lot at random, contains a concentration (c) of contaminant. This probability will generally depend on c; that is, there may be more nuts at one concentration than another. We write p as $p(c)$. The lot distribution $p(c)$ is, of course, simply the sample distribution $P(1, C)$ when the sample size is 1; however, sample sizes of 1 are not practical. In typical nut lots, the chance of any single nut being contaminated is exceedingly small (on the order of 1 in 10,000 to 100,000 nuts), thus it would take an extraordinary number of samples and analyses to obtain any positive results. What is needed is to relate sample distributions and lot distributions directly, so one can be derived from the other. In what follows, we shall use capital letters when referring to sample values (which will depend on N) and lower case when referring to lot values.

To understand the relation between $p(c)$ and $P(N, C)$ the following analogy might be helpful. Imagine a barrel of black beans among which are a small number of beans of differing colors, say white, red, blue, etc. The colors will be indexed by a subscript, i. These colored beans are assumed to be well mixed in but to be present in differing amounts (p_i), where p_i is the fraction of all beans of color i. Each colored bean is associated with a value, depending on its color: nothing for black ones but with widely different amounts for the colored ones — say, \$1 for white ones and \$1,000,000 for the most expensive color. We are, however, totally color blind; all the beans look exactly the same to us. When we remove a sample of a fixed size N from the barrel, we can measure the total value (c) of the sample, but we cannot establish how many beans are colored or of which color they are. What we can do, however, is calculate the *probability* that the sample we have chosen will have the value C, as long as we know the p_i for each color. This is so because each color will form its own sample probability distribution, independently of the other colors. This distribution is the Poisson distribution, which depends solely on Np_i. It tells us the chance that a sample of size N will contain exactly none, or one, or two, etc. beans of color i. (To be precise, the probability of drawing a sample of k beans of color i is given by $P_k = \exp(-Np_i)(Np_i)^k/k!$.) If $Np_i \ll 1$, this probability drops off rapidly with k, so the probability of having no contaminated beans in the sample is approximately unity, of having a single bean by Np_i, while the chance of finding more than one may be ignored. This situation remains if we have beans of many colors but of varying concentrations, given by p_j, p_n, etc. Each forms its own Poisson, and the probability of having several beans of different colors present is simply the product of the appropriate terms in the Poissons. As before, if $Np_i \ll 1$ for all i, only combinations containing a single colored bean of whatever color must be considered. To apply the situation to tree nuts, we replace the beans with nut kernels, the colors with concentrations.

To estimate a sample distribution from a lot distribution, we choose N and pick at random an N-size collection of kernels of all contamination levels (including uncontaminated ones), each according to its own probability $p(c_i) = p_i$. For this, we calculate the concentration of the sample C by summing over all the kernels. We then repeat this process a large number of times to obtain an estimate of the frequency for which the random N sample falls into a set of limited ranges of C, which we designate C_i. This frequency is precisely the sample distribution $P(N,C_i)$. This method is called the Monte Carlo method and is commonly carried out by computer. The restriction $Np_i \ll 1$ for all i is not required here, but it does speed up the calculation.

To do the reverse, to estimate the lot distribution from the sample distribution, is, in general, much more difficult. One approach has been taken by Whitaker and coworkers.[150–152] They assume a parametric form for the lot distribution and use it to compute sample distributions in the manner discussed above. The calculated distributions depend on the parameters, of course. They then measure sample distributions by measuring many samples of the same size and, using standard statistical methods, compare these with their calculated ones. From "best fit" they obtain an estimate of the best parameters and thus the best lot distribution. This approach has a couple of disadvantages. First, the tests are rather insensitive to the parameters, so we obtain rather poor estimates. Along with this comes the fact that certain resulting values, in particular the estimated mean concentration m, is particularly sensitive to the actual lot distribution, especially at high concentration. Again, such values are estimated poorly by these methods. Second, local manifestations of the lot distribution (location of maxima and minima, limits in the concentration, and the like) can be very revealing of the processes causing the contamination in the first place. Such aspects are generally not part of any functional form of a previously studied distribution and are missed entirely if we use a standard parametric form. For these reasons, it is much preferable to use a method that is totally empirical and can adapt to any shape of lot distribution.

On the other hand, if the restriction $Np_i \ll 1$ for all i is maintained, this approach allows the evaluation of the lot distribution from the sample distribution in straightforward manner.[153] To do so, we estimate the sample distribution for an appropriate N by making several hundred sample measurements. (The value of N is chosen so $Np(c_i) < 0.1$ but not much less. This ensures that the probability of obtaining a sample with two contaminated nuts is less than 5% of that of a single nut, but the chance of getting at least some contamination in the range of C of interest is not much less than 10%. The appropriate value of N is chosen on the basis of a few trial experiments.) Because we now have at most a single significantly contaminated nut per sample at concentration c_i, we know that the frequency of contaminated samples at concentration C_i is given by $P(N,C_i) = Np_i$, on the basis of the Poisson distribution, while the sample concentration C_i is given by $C_i = c_i/N$, by dilution. Thus, p_i and c_i, which constitute the distribution of aflatoxin among single nuts in the lot, can be computed from the sample distribution and N. Interestingly enough, $P(N,C_i)$ on a log P vs. log C plot is just the lot distribution $p(c_i)$, shifted by log N in both axes. (The index i indicates binning in the log C axis, typically of half-decade width.) Any lot distribution, regardless of functional form or parameters, may be estimated. To cover the usual range of interest, say 10^2 to 10^6 ng/g, a few hundred measurements will suffice, rather than the several hundred thousand that would have been needed had we measured $P(1,C_i)$ instead.

24.2.2.3 Sampling Applications, Results, and Use

The above methods have been applied to lots of various types of nuts susceptible to aflatoxin contamination. Among U.S.-grown nuts are mainly pistachios and almonds and occasionally walnuts and peanuts. The most common foreign grown nuts include Brazil nuts. Lot distributions have been calculated from sample distributions reported by others which the number of samples and the sample size N and were adequate to allow reliable estimates of the sample probabilities $P(N,C_i)$ and conversion to lot distributions ($P(N,C_i) < 0.1$). In all cases, $P(N,C_i)$ is expressed as the probability of a sample falling into a log C interval one half decade in size. Additional results were measured in our laboratory for other lots of interest. Typical results are shown in Figure 24.1,[154–156] Figure 24.2,[29,157] and Figure 24.3.[158] Each curve represents 200 to 400 samples in our work, up to 700 samples in work of others.

The figures in most cases show lot distributions for lots expected to have high aflatoxin contamination and are not representative of high-quality product in commerce. The latter might show levels 10 times or more lower. Distributions will differ, depending on production and processing history and, of course, commodity. By and large, the distributions have been found to be rather flat from around 1000 ng/g to an upper limit, around 10^5 to 10^6 ng/g. At this point they suddenly seem to fall to zero (no samples occur above the limit, suggesting that there is a limit to the nutrient

500 Aflatoxin and Food Safety

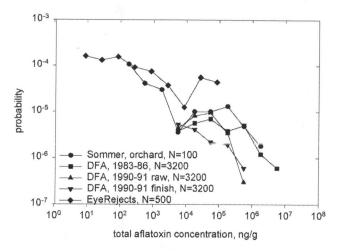

FIGURE 24.1 Total aflatoxin lot distributions computed from assorted pistachio sample distributions.[156] Aflatoxin lot distribution is the probability of a single kernel in a lot having aflatoxin content in a 3.16-fold range of aflatoxin concentration. Sample distribution is the probability of a sample from a group of samples of fixed size falling in such a range. Sample distribution will depend on sample size.

supply for the fungus). Note that this uniform limit applies only to lot distributions, for sample distributions the limit appears at 10^5 to $10^6/N$ ng/g, as each positive sample contains but one "hot" nut. For $c < 1000$ ng/g, the distribution rises rapidly. The distributions cannot be tracked beyond $P(N,C_i) = 0.1$ without a change of N. We have generally not done so, as it increases the work substantially. There is little

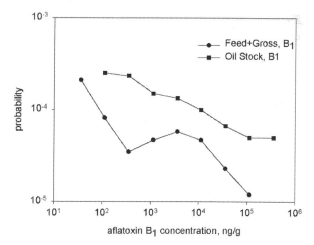

FIGURE 24.2 B_1 Aflatoxin lot distributions of insect damaged almonds.[29] Feed = insect damage is indicated as feeding damage (removed kernel meat, not tunnels). Gross = insect damage is indicated by the presence of insect fragments or other filth. Oil stock = severely damaged almonds, based largely on insect damage.

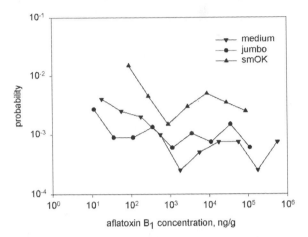

FIGURE 24.3 B_1 Aflatoxin lot distributions for lots of dry-farmed Florunner peanuts of various nut sizes.[158] Jumbo and medium: Peanut sizes are large enough to be acceptable for human consumption (>0.95 cm). SmOK: Peanuts fall through a 0.56-cm screen.

interest in that part of the distribution function because the lot mean m is given by $\%_i p(c_i) c_i$ and thus is dominated by the high end of the distribution. (Conversely, a much larger N might elucidate data above 10^5 to 10^6 ng/g.)

When lots of similar provenance, but differing processing severity or production constraints are compared we find that the lot distributions differ in height but have a similar shape. An example is seen in Figure 24.3 for three peanut sublots of the same dry-farmed Florunner peanut lot.[157] The original lot was sorted for peanut size and those of the smallest size (smOK) show a lot distribution significantly higher but of similar shape than the sublots consisting of larger nuts. The medium size distribution lies slightly higher than that of the larger jumbos but extends to higher concentration, which accounts in this case for its higher aflatoxin level. In peanuts it is well known that the smaller the nuts the higher the aflatoxin level tends to be. The smaller size sublots (such as smOK) are restricted from sale for human consumption, so in this case size sorting serves as aflatoxin sorting as well.

When the lot distribution is known, the sample distribution may be computed for any sample size N. This may be exploited when the sampling distribution is desired for a lot of very small p_i, when a large N is required. Such large N would require laborious and expensive sample measurements to construct a sample distribution directly. The difficulty can be avoided by obtaining the lot distribution, deriving the sampling distributions by random sampling by computer. The situation may be illustrated by an actual problem arising in connection with the testing protocol established by the EU for acceptance of pistachios.[159] This protocol (the details of which will be avoided here for brevity) involves samples of 10 kg ($N = \sim 9000$), which must not exceed 2 ng/g of aflatoxin B_1 (4 ng/g total). Even such large samples are not adequate to represent a lot, and the sampling distribution shows extensive variance. As a result, it is entirely possible that a sample drawn from a lot having a mean m well below 2 ng/g will still fail the acceptance test, resulting in great cost to the shipper (costs exceeding $100,000/shipped lot). The shipper asks: "What are the chances a lot for which I know the mean will be rejected?" or, better yet, "How clean does my lot have to be so I can expect a 95% acceptance rate?" Similarly, the buyer demands: "Given that a lot passes acceptance, is there at least a 95% probability that such a lot will pass possible subsequent tests, such as occur when a consumer group pulls retail samples?" Such questions can be answered, using the calculations given here.

We proceed as follows. We measure the sample distribution of a lot of reasonably high contamination with aflatoxin but otherwise similar to the lot to be sold. This might be accomplished by a sample size of $N = 200$ (adequate for $200p_i < 0.1$) and perhaps 400 samples. From the resulting set of $p(c_i)$, we derive first the sample average concentration m as $\%_i p(c_i)c_i$. We next establish the sample distribution $P(9000,C_i)$ by Monte Carlo. We then compute the probability of acceptance from the integral:

$$\int_0^{2ng/g} P(9000, C_i)dC_i$$

by simply establishing what fraction of the sample distribution fell below 2 ng/g. We will express that as $P(10 \text{ kg} < 2 \text{ ng/g}|m)$, given m. We now multiply all the p_i by an arbitrary factor λ (which represents the lot distribution at a different level of contamination) and repeat the entire process, obtaining $P(10 \text{ kg} < 2 \text{ ng/g}|m)$, the probability of acceptance at this new contamination level. We keep changing λ, and so map out the probability of acceptance at all values of contamination of interest as a function of λm, as we have done for the decreasing curve in Figure 24.4. (More

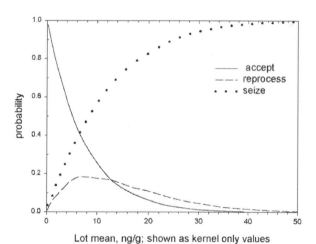

Lot mean, ng/g; shown as kernel only values

FIGURE 24.4 Probability of acceptance, required reprocessing, and seizure for unshelled pistachios as a function of the lot mean aflatoxin concentration, using the EU acceptance levels.[159] "Accept" = acceptance of lot as is; each of three 10-kg samples tests as <2 ng/g total aflatoxin. "Reprocess" = a resorting of the lot is allowed; a 30-kg sample tests as <5 ng/g total aflatoxin. "Seize" = lot is confiscated; aflatoxin levels other than above.

precisely, we map out $(P[10 \text{ kg} < 2 \text{ ng/g}|\lambda m])^3$, because of details of the protocol.) As expected, the probability of acceptance drops as the lot average increases, reaching about 50% at $m = 2$. Surprisingly, a lot must have an average aflatoxin level as low as 0.12 ng/g to be acceptable 95% of the time. American producers now produce a product at such levels for the European trade.

Lot distributions can also be made use of in designing sorting equipment. Because the lot mean m is dominated by the $p(c_i)$ at high levels of c, knowledge of $p(c_i)$ in that region determines how much product needs to be discarded to reduce by a preset number. This is discussed in detail below.

Finally, the lot distribution curves can be used to directly guide cultural practices. Inspection of Figure 24.1 shows that the aflatoxin contamination is not entirely independent of concentration for $c > 10^3$ ng/g but shows a slight intermediate minimum, with a similar shape for all curves. This shape may be directly associated with the onset of *Aspergillus flavus* contamination. It is only necessary to realize that production of aflatoxin occurs at an exponential rate as the mold grows and that henceforth the log C axis should be colinear with time since fungal attack. Furthermore, aflatoxin is only observed in pistachios for which the hull splits prior to harvest (which may vary from 1% to 8–10%, depending on the orchard) with additional contribution due to insect injury. Because early hull splitting commences about 6 weeks prior to harvest, peaks about 2 weeks later, and ceases about 2 weeks prior to harvest, the lot distribution curve reflects this splitting, with the minimum corresponding to 6 weeks, the final drop-off to 2 weeks prior to harvest. The nuts splitting at the earliest time generate the most aflatoxin, and good cultural practices suggest that insecticides should be applied at that time. The time constants derived from Figure 24.1 may be directly applied to Figure 24.2, where a similar shaped curve is observed in insect damaged almonds. The derived times, here 4 weeks and immediately prior to harvest, match the observed hull splitting in that commodity.

24.2.2.4 Sorting

Although aflatoxin content is of major concern in tree nuts, particularly in pistachios and almonds, little sorting to reduce this toxin occurs commercially. The reason is that extensive sorting already occurs for quality, resulting in a number of process streams, and it is found that aflatoxin is associated only with a few low-volume process streams. Removal of the pertinent streams, plus hand sorting in certain cases, can result in low aflatoxin counts. In pistachios, major sorting steps are, in order, trash removal, water flotation to segregate empty-shell and immature nuts, hull removal, drying to 5 to 6% water content, sorting to remove closed-shell (again somewhat immature) nuts, electronic color sorting to segregate and remove stained shell nuts, and, if required, hand sorting to complete the electronic process and also remove nuts with visible insect damage. Finally, nuts are size sorted. In addition, closed-shell nuts are sent overseas for rehydration and manual cracking; however, this process is becoming outdated for U.S. sales. Tests have shown[148] that high aflatoxin is found primarily in: (1) nut meats that have fallen freely from the shell, (2) very small nuts (>40 nuts/oz.), (3) nuts showing insect damage or severe staining, (4) large "floaters," and (5) rehydrated nuts (presumably postharvest, due to insufficient drying after cracking). Streams 1 to 4 are generally due to preharvest effects. Most of these substreams are of small enough volume that such nuts can be removed from commerce, either optionally or through marketing orders.

In the 1970s, it was believed that the well-known bright greenish-yellow (BGY) fluorescence seen in aflatoxin-contaminated corn could be used to detect aflatoxin in pistachios.[160] On this basis, Farsaie and McClure[161] developed a prototype sorter that performed well in removing such nuts; however, it was later realized that the BGY fluorescence indicated kojic acid, a cometabolite of aflatoxin, and that aflatoxin itself in tree nuts was of too low a concentration to allow the use of BGY for the selection of aflatoxin-contaminated nuts. A second approach to removing such nuts from process streams was based on the realization that toxin contamination was commonly higher in insect-damaged nuts. Accordingly, considerable effort went into x-ray imaging of pistachios[162,163] followed by the development of algorithms[164,165] that could discern the presence of insect-caused holes in the image. The difficulty of obtaining x-ray images at a fast enough rate (single-channel sorting rates of 40 nuts/second were required to match other commercial sorting equipment) and the emergence of better methods to detect nuts containing aflatoxin caused abandonment of this approach. The most successful method was based on the work of Sommer,[34] which indicated that only nuts in which the hull and shell split prior to harvest (ES, about 2% of the total) showed aflatoxin. This level would increase if insect damage occurred as well.[34,117] Such splitting would allow access to the kernel and thus infection by *Aspergillus flavus*, required for aflatoxin to appear. This hull splitting resulted in a recognizable tannin stain of the shell that remained after process hulling and drying.[166] This stain pattern was utilized by Pearson,[40,167] who developed an image-based sorter that could remove all aflatoxin-contaminated nuts (up to 2% of total) at commercial rates and with acceptable false-positive rejection. The sorter failed to perform satisfactorily during the occasional year when insect damage was so high that 2% removal was inadequate. So far, this sorter has not yet found wide commercial acceptance.

In the case of almonds, commercial sorting for quality results in rejects and a number of process streams of differing value. The higher value product consists of natural almonds — that is, almonds still in the brown skin of the kernel (in-shell almonds have little market). Blanching results in lower value of manufacturing stock. Within each class, increasing damage or cutting or grinding reduces value. Ostensibly, all nuts showing insect (or bird or rodent) damage are rejected. A survey was carried out of results on all 1993 California crop material for which results and grade were recorded.[168] It was found that aflatoxin was found essentially only on chopped or ground manufacturing stock, with concentrations increasing as the chop or grind became finer. This suggested that at least some lots with insect or similar damage (holes or broken surfaces) had been commutated to hide such damage and that aflatoxin occurred only following insect damage. Subsequent work on hand picking out insect-damaged nuts indicated that only a certain type of insect damage (gross and feeding) was associated with aflatoxin.[29] Such damage is easily detected in natural almonds by color sorters; thus, removal of this single stream should eliminate aflatoxin contamination in almonds. A method of detecting pinholes in almonds from x-ray imaging, similar to the work in pistachios discussed above, was carried out as well,[169] but in light of the pinhole results discussed earlier further research was abandoned. For walnuts, the main commercial sorting is carried out to separate the light-colored (high-value) shells from the darker shells that develop during late harvest. The dark shells contain shriveled or darkened kernels. Work is currently in progress to relate such dark skin kernels to aflatoxin content.

24.3 SUMMARY AND CONCLUSIONS

The research efforts outlined above indicate the steady progress in producing tangible strategies and products for reducing aflatoxin contamination of tree nuts. New approaches to control insect pests of tree nuts are under development and some have already achieved success under field conditions. Additionally, a group of natural products associated with hydrolysable tannins has been identified from walnut that could render aflatoxin-producing aspergilli as virtually atoxigenic. Moreover, the discovery of these compounds, the availability of an expressed sequence tag (EST) library for *Aspergillus flavus* from scientists at the USDA's Southern Regional Research Center, and high throughput methods of functional genomics being development by scientists in the Plant Mycotoxin Research Unit at WRRC will allow the discovery of genes to be targeted for preventing mycotoxin biosynthesis or fungal development. Mathematical models have been developed that assess ways to balance the rigors required to detect aflatoxin contamination in tree nut samples juxtaposed against the amount of shipped nuts that must be sacrificed as a result of reliable sampling. Finally, commercially viable sorters have been or are under development that will improve removal of contaminated products from the processing stream.

In conclusion, because one of the fundamental factors promoting preharvest contamination of tree nuts by aflatoxins is insect-feeding damage, identification of natural compounds present in tree nuts that deter insect feeding would be of additional value to the research efforts outlined above. Some volatile compounds affecting insect behavior may also have antifungal activity toward *Aspergillus* or be antiaflatoxigenic. Third, because aflatoxin genotoxicity results from its enzymatic transformation, mainly by a certain family of cytochrome P-450, antioxidants may inhibit this process. Anti-insect, antifungal, antiaflatoxigenic, and antioxidant properties would directly lower contamination levels of aflatoxins in tree nut commodities, reduce risk to human consumers, and lower the chances of exported shipments being rejected. All of these properties exist in tree nut natural products. Identifying these natural products (e.g., gallic acid as the "Tulare" walnut factor) could be followed by augmenting their amounts and optimizing respective bioactivities through modification of chemical structures. These procedures could be achieved using either conventional tree nut-breeding techniques or possibly through direct genetic engineering.[50,87,170–173] As outlined above, constitutive natural products can directly nullify aflatoxin biosynthesis, and the use of microbial-based antifungal natural products, such as iturins, is also promising.[174] Finally, as we gain more knowledge about the molecular biology of aflatoxin biosynthesis, interrupting the pathway, either genetically or with endogenous natural products, will become ever more achievable.[175,176]

ACKNOWLEDGMENTS

We thank PMR scientists J. Baker, P. Bayman, R. Buttery, K. Chan, S. Hua, J.H. Kim, S.-E. Lee, D. Light, N. Mahoney, G. Merrill, and J. Roitman and University of California, Davis, scientists A. Dandekar, M. Doster, T. Gradziel, C. Leslie, G. Mcgranahan, and T. Michailides for their contributions to this chapter. We also thank M. Hurley, Dried Fruit Association of California; M. Jacobs, Almond Board of California; R. Klein, California Pistachio Commission; G. Gray, Blue Diamond; D. Ramos, Walnut Board of California; and J. Robens, National Program Leader, ARS, for their continued interest in this research effort.

REFERENCES

1. Diener, U.L., Cole, R.J., Sanders, T.H., Payak, G.A., Lee, L.S., and Klich, M.A., Epidemiology of aflatoxin formation by *Aspergillus flavus*, *Ann. Rev. Phytopathol.*, 25, 249–270, 1987.

2. Lewis, C.W., Anderson, J.G., and Smith, J.E., Health related aspects of the genus *Aspergillus*, in *Aspergillus*, Smith, J.E., Ed., Plenum Press, New York, 1994, pp. 219–261.

3. Payne, G.A. and Brown, M.P., Genetics and physiology of aflatoxin biosynthesis, *Ann. Rev. Phytopathol.*, 36, 329–362, 1998.

4. Fujimoto, Y., Hampton, L.L., Wirth, P.J., Wang, N.J., Xie, J.P., and Thorgeirsson, S.S., Alternations of tumor suppressor genes and allelic losses in human hepatocellular carcinomas in China, *Cancer Res.*, 54, 281–285, 1994.

5. Hosono, S., Chou, M.J., Lee, C.S., and Shih, C., Infrequent mutation of $p53$ gene in hepatitis B virus positive primary hepatocellular carcinomas, *Oncogene*, 8, 491–496, 1993.

6. Aguilar, F., Hussain, S.P., and Cerutti, P., Aflatoxin B_1 induces the transversion of G→T in codon 249 of the $p53$ tumor suppressor gene in human hepatocytes, *Proc. Nat. Acad. Sci. USA*, 90, 8586–8590, 1993.

7. Essigmann, J.M., Croy, R.G., Nadzan, Jr., A.M., Reinhold, V.N., Buchi, G., and Wogan, G.N., Structural identification of the major DNA adduct formed by aflatoxin B_1 *in vitro*, *Proc. Natl. Acad. Sci. USA*, 74, 1870–1874, 1977.

8. Lin, J.K., Miller, J.A., and Miller, E.C., 2,3-dihydro-2-(guan-7-yl)-3-hydroxy-aflatoxin B_1, a major acid hydrolysis product of aflatoxin B_1-DNA or -ribosomal RNA adducts formed in hepatic microsome-mediated reactions and in rat liver *in vivo*, *Cancer Res.*, 37, 4430–4438, 1977.

9. Johnson, W.W. and Guengerich, F.P., Reaction of aflatoxin B_1 *exo*-8,9-epoxide with DNA: kinetic analysis of covalent biding and DNA-induced hydrolysis, *Proc. Natl. Acad. Sci. USA*, 94, 6121–6125, 1997.

10. Stoloff, L., Aflatoxin is not a probable carcinogen: the published evidence is sufficient, *Regulat. Toxicol. Pharmacol.*, 10, 272–283, 1989.

11. Barraud, L., Guerret, S., Chevailler, M.B.C., Jamard, C., Trepo, C., Wild, C.P., and Cova, L., Enhanced duck hepatitis B virus gene expression following aflatoxin B_1 exposure, *Hepatology*, 29, 1317–1323, 1999.

12. Stuver, S.O., Towards global control of liver cancer?, *Semin. Cancer Biol.*, 8, 299–306, 1998.

13. Henry, S.H., Bosch, X.F., Troxell, T.C., and Bolger, P.M., Reducing liver cancer: global control of aflatoxin, *Science*, 286, 2453–2454, 1999.

14. FDA, *Compliance Program Guidance 683: Action Levels for Aflatoxins in Animal Feeds*, CPG 7126.33, Office of Regulatory Affairs, U.S. Food and Drug Administration, Washington, D.C., 1994.
15. Robens, J.F. and Richard, J.L., Aflatoxins in animal and human health, *Rev. Environ. Contamin. Toxicol.*, 127, 69–93, 1992.
16. NAS, *Noncitrus Fruits and Nuts: 2001 Preliminary Summary*, National Agricultural Statistics Service, U.S. Department of Agriculture, Washington, D.C., 2002.
17. CAST, *Aflatoxin and Other Mycotoxins: An Agricultural Perspective*, Council for Agricultural Science and Technology, Ames, IA, 1979, pp. 1–56.
18. ABC, *Twenty Years of Discovery: A Review of Almond Board of California Production Research 1972–1992*, The Almond Board of California, Sacramento, 1993.
19. Fuller, G., Spooncer, W.W., King, A.D.J., Schade, J., and Mackey, B., Survey of aflatoxin in California tree nuts, *J. AOCS*, 54, 231A–234A, 1977.
20. Phillips, D.J., Purcell, S.L., and Stanley, G.I., *Aflatoxins in Almonds*, Agricultural Reviews and Manuals ARM-W-20, U.S. Department of Agriculture, Washington, D.C., 1980.
21. Buchanan, J.R., Sommer, N.F., and Fortlage, R.J., *Aspergillus flavus* infection and aflatoxin production in fig fruits, *Appl. Microbiol.*, 30, 238–241, 1975.
22. Morton, S.G., Eadie, T., and Llewellyn, G.C., Aflatoxigenic potential of dried figs, apricots, pineapples and raisins, *J. AOAC*, 62, 958–962, 1979.
23. Cardwell, K.F., Desjardins, A., Henry, S.H., Munkvold, G., and Robens, J.M., The cost of achieving food security and food quality, APSnet Feature Story, American Phytopathological Society, St. Paul, MN, 2001, pp. 1–27.
24. Zilinskas, R.A., Iraq's biological weapons: the past as future?, *J. Am. Med. Assoc.*, 278, 418–424, 1997.
25. Phillips, D.J., Uota, M., Monticelli, D., and Curtis, C., Colonization of almond by *Aspergillus flavus*, *J. Am. Soc. Hort. Sci.*, 101, 19–23, 1976.
26. Klonsky, K., Zalom, F.A., and Barnett, W., California's almond IPM program, *Calif. Agric.*, 44, 21–24, 1990.
27. Doster, M.A. and Michailides, T.J., The relationship between date of hull splitting and decay of pistachio nuts by *Aspergillus* species, *Plant Dis.*, 79, 766–769, 1995.
28. Doster, M.A. and Michailides, T.J., Relationship between shell discoloration of pistachio nuts and incidence of fungal decay and insect infestation, *Plant Dis.*, 83, 259–264, 1999.
29. Schatzki, T.F. and Ong, M.S., Dependence of aflatoxin in almonds on the type and amount of insect damage, *J. Agric. Food Chem.*, 49, 4513–4519, 2001.
30. Curtis, C.E. and Barnes, M.M., Oviposition and development of the navel orangeworm in relation to almond maturation, *J. Econ. Entomol.*, 70, 395–398, 1977.
31. Kuenen, L.P.S. and Barnes, M.M., Spatial and temporal development of maturation of nonpareil almonds and infestation by the navel orangeworm, *Amyelois transitella* (Walker), *Environ. Entomol.*, 10, 673–675, 1981.
32. Sibbett, G.S. and Van Steenwyk, R.A., Shedding "mummy" walnuts is key to destroying navel orangeworm in winter, *Calif. Agric.*, 47, 26–28, 1993.
33. Barnes, M.M., Oviposition and development of the navel orangeworm in relation to almond maturation, *J. Econ. Entomol.*, 70, 395–398, 1977.
34. Sommer, N.F., Buchanan, J.R., and Fortlage, R.J., Relation of early splitting and tattering of pistachio nuts to aflatoxin in the orchard, *Phytopathology*, 76, 692–694, 1986.
35. Connell, J.H., Labavitch, J.M., Sibbett, G.S., Reil, W.O., Barnett, W.H., and Heintz, C., Early harvest of almonds to circumvent late infestation by navel orangeworm, *J. Am. Soc. Hort. Sci.*, 114, 595–599, 1989.
36. Andrews, K.L. and Barnes, M.M., Differential attractiveness of infested and uninfested mummy almonds to navel orangeworm moths, *Environ. Entomol.*, 11, 280–282, 1982.

37. Michailides, T.J., The "Achilles Heel" of pistachio fruit, *Calif. Agric.*, 43, 10–11, 1989.
38. Gradziel, T.M. and Dandekar, A.M., Field performance of seed and endocarp based resistance to preharvest aflatoxin contamination in almond, in *Proc. 14th Aflatoxin Elimination Workshop*, Tucson, AZ, 2001, 125 pp.
39. Campbell, B.C.and Nes, W.D., A reappraisal of sterol biosynthesis and metabolism in aphids, *J. Insect Physiol.*, 29, 149–156, 1983.
40. Pearson, T.C., Machine vision system for automated detection of stained pistachio nuts, *Lebensmittel-Wissensch, U. Techn.*, 29, 203–209, 1996.
41. Bayman, P.B., Baker, J.L., and Mahoney, N.E., *Aspergillus* on tree nuts: incidence and associations, *Mycopathologia*, 155(3), 161–169, 2002.
42. Doster, M.A. and Michailides, T.J., Development of *Aspergillus* molds in litter from pistachio trees, *Plant Dis.*, 78, 393–397, 1994.
43. Scott, P.M., Industrial and farm detoxification processes for mycotoxins, *Rev. Med. Vet.*, 149, 543–548, 1998.
44. D'Mello, J.P.F., Macdonald, A.M.C., Postel, D., Dijksma, W.T.P., Dujardin, A., and Placinta, C.M., Pesticide use and mycotoxin production in *Fusarium* and *Aspergillus* phytopathogens, *Eur. J. Plant Pathol.*, 104, 741–751, 1998.
45. Varela, L.G., Welter, S.C., Jones, V.P., Brunner, J.F., and Riedl, H., Monitoring and characterization of insecticide resistance in codling moth (Lepidoptera: Tortricidae) in four western states, *J. Econ. Entomol.*, 86, 1–10, 1993.
46. Blomefield, T., Codling moth resistance: is it here, and how do we manage it?, *Deciduous Fruit Grower*, 44, 130–132, 1994.
47. Knight, A.L., Brunner, J.F., and Alston, D., Survey of azinphosmethyl resistance in codling moth (Lepidoptera: Tortricidae) in Washington and Utah, *J. Econ. Entomol.*, 87, 285–292, 1994.
48. Sauphanor, B. and Bouvier, J.C., Cross-resistance between benzoylureas and benzoyl-hydrazines in the codling moth, *Cydia pomonella* L., *Pest. Sci.*, 45, 369–375, 1995.
49. Bentley, W., A look at a decade of almond rejects in Kern county, in *Kern Nut Crops*, University of California, Berkeley, 1993, pp. 6–7.
50. Dandekar, A.M., McGranahan, G.H., Vail, P.V., Uratsu, S.L., Leslie, C.A., and Tebbets, J.S., High levels of expression of full-length *cryIA(c)* gene from *Bacillus thuringiensis* in transgenic somatic walnut embryos, *Plant Sci.*, 13, 181–193, 1998.
51. Leslie, C.A., McGranahan, G.H., Dandekar, A.M., Uratsu, S.L., Vail, P.V., and Tebbets, J.S., Development and field-testing of walnuts expressing the *CRYIA(c)* gene for lepidopteran insect resistance, *Acta Hort.*, 544, 195–199, 2001.
52. Doster, M.A., Michailides, T.J., Goldhamer, D.A., and Morgan, D.P., Insufficient spring irrigation increases abnormal splitting of pistachio nuts, *Calif. Agric.*, 55, 28–31, 2001.
53. Bell, W.J. and Cardé, R.T., *Chemical Ecology of Insects*, Sinauer, Sunderland, MA, 1984, 524 pp.
54. Millar, J.G. and Rice, R.E., Reexamination of the sex pheromone of the peach twig borer: field screening of minor constituents of pheromone gland extracts and of pheromone analogs, *J. Econ. Entomol.*, 85, 1709–1716, 1992.
55. McDonough, L.M., Davis, H.G., Chapman, P.S., and Smithhisler, C.L., Codling moth, *Cydia pomonella*, (Lepidoptera: Tortricidae): is its sex pheromone multicomponent?, *J. Chem. Ecol.*, 21, 1065–1071, 1995.
56. Light, D.M., Flath, R.A., Buttery, R.G., Zalom, F.G., Rice, R.E., Dickens, J.C., and Jang, E.B., Host-plant, green leaf volatiles synergize the synthetic sex pheromones of the corn earworm and codling moth (Lepidoptera), *Chemoecology*, 4, 145–152, 1993.
57. Rice, R.E. and Jones, R.A., *Mating Disruption of Oriental Fruit Moth and Other Moths in Stone Fruits*, California Tree Fruit Agreement, Sacramento, CA, 1989, 8 pp.

58. Roelofs, W.L., Kochansky, J., Anthon, E., Rice, R.E., and Cardé, R.T., Sex pheromone of the peach twig borer moth (*Anarsia lineatella*), *Environ. Entomol.*, 4, 580–582, 1975.

59. Rice, R.E., Flaherty, D.L., and Bentley, W.J., Mating disruption for control of orchard pests in California, *Acta Phytopathol. Entomol. Hung.*, 27, 1–4, 1992.

60. Roitman, J., unpublished results.

61. Buttery, R.G., Seifert, R.M., Haddon, W.F., and Lundin, R.E., 2-Hexyl-3-methylmaleic anhydride: an unusual volatile component of raisins and almond hulls, *J. Agric. Food Chem.*, 28, 1336–1338, 1980.

62. Buttery, R.G., Soderstrom, E.L., Seifert, R.M., Ling, L.C., and Haddon, W.F., Components of almond hulls: possible navel orangeworm attractants and growth inhibitors, *J. Agric. Food Chem.*, 28, 353–356, 1980.

63. Phelan, P.L., Roelofs, C.J., Youngman, R.R., and Baker, T.C., Characterization of chemicals mediating ovipositional host-plant finding by *Amyelois transitella* females, *J. Chem. Ecol.*, 17, 599–613, 1991.

64. Clark, R.G. and Nursten, H.E., Volatile flavour components of walnuts (*Juglans regia* L.), *J. Sci. Food Agric.*, 27, 902–908, 1976.

65. Clark, R.G. and Nursten, H.E., The sensory analysis and identification of volatiles from walnut (*Juglans regia* L.) head space, *J. Sci. Food Agric.*, 28, 69–77, 1977.

66. Nahrstedt, A., Vetter, U., and Hammerschmidt, F.J., Zur Kenntnis des Wasserdampfdestillates der Blätter von *Juglans regia*, *Planta Med.*, 42, 313–332, 1981.

67. Buttery, R.G., Flath, R.A., Mon, T.R., and Ling, L.C., Identification of germacrene D in walnut and fig leaf volatiles, *J. Agric. Food Chem.*, 34, 820–822, 1986.

68. Binder, R.G., Benson, M.E., and Flath, R.A., Eight 1,4-naphthoquinones from *Juglans*, *Phytochemistry*, 28 (10), 2799–801, 1989.

69. Buchbauer, G., Jirovetz, L., Wasicky, M., and Nikiforov, A., Headspace constituents of fresh *Juglans nigra* L. peels, *J. Essen. Oil Res.*, 5, 455–457, 1993.

70. Buchbauer, G. and Jirovetz, L., Volatile constituents of the essential oil of the peels of *Juglans nigra* L., *J. Essent. Oil Res.*, 4, 539–541, 1992.

71. Lieu, F.Y., Rice, R.E., and Jennings, W.G., Volatile components of navel orangeworm attractants. II. Constituents of larval frass from invested [*sic*] almonds, *Chem. Mikrobiol. Technol. Lebensm.*, 7, 154–160, 1982.

72. Wearing, C.H., Connor, P.J., and Ambler, K.D., Olfactory stimulation of oviposition and flight activity of the codling moth *Laspeyresia pomonella*, using apples in an automated olfactometer, *N. Z. J. Sci.*, 16, 697–710, 1973.

73. Yan, F. and Bengtsson, M.P.W., Behavioral response of female codling moths, *Cydia pomonella*, to apple volatiles, *J. Chem. Ecol.*, 25, 1343–1351, 1999.

74. Hern, A. and Dorn, S., Sexual dimorphism in the olfactory orientation of adult *Cydia pomonella* in response to a-farnesene, *Entomol. Exper. Appl.*, 92, 63–72, 1999.

75. Landolt, P.J., Brumley, J.A., Smithhisler, C.L., Biddick, L.L., and Hofstetter, R.W., Apple fruit infested with codling moth are more attractive to neonate codling moth larvae and possess increased amounts of (*E,E*)-a-farnesene, *J. Chem. Ecol.*, 26, 1685–1199, 2000.

76. Cavill, G.W.K. and Coggiola, I.M., Photosensitized oxygenation of a-farnesene, *Aust. J. Chem.*, 24, 135–142, 1971.

77. Campbell, B.C., Merrill, G.B., Roitman, J.N., Bourgoin, T., and McGranahan, G., GCMS and cladistic analysis of walnut leaf volatiles, in *Walnut Research Reports 1998*, Ramos, D., Ed., Walnut Marketing Board of California, Sacramento, 1999, pp. 209–213.

78. Miller, R., Bills, D.D., and Buttery, R.G., Volatile components from Bartlett and Bradford pear leaves, *J. Agric. Food Chem.*, 37, 1476–1479, 1989.

79. Scutareanu, P., Drukker, B., Bruin, J., Posthumus, M.A., and Sabelis, M.W., Volatiles from *Psylla*-infested pear trees and their possible involvement in attraction of anthocorid predators, *J. Chem. Ecol.*, 23 2241–2260, 1997.

80. Takabayashi, J., Dicke, M., and Posthumus, M., Variation in composition of predator attracting allellochemicals emitted by herbivore-infested plants: relative influence of plant and herbivore, *Chemoecology*, 2, 1–6, 1991.

81. Buttery, R.G., Light, D.M., Nam, Y., Merrill, G.B., and Roitman, J.N., Volatile components of green walnut husks, *J. Agric. Food Chem.*, 48, 2858–2861, 2000.

82. Buttery, R.G., Flath, R.A., Mon, T.R., and Light, D.M., unpublished results.

83. Carle, S.A., Averill, A.L., Rule, G.S., Reissig, W.H., and Roelofs, W.L., Variation in host fruit volatiles attractive to apple maggot fly, *Rhagoletis pomonella*, *J. Chem. Ecol.*, 13, 795–805, 1987.

84. Nijssen, L.M., Visscher, C.A., Maarse, H., Willemsens, L.C., and Boelens, M.H., *Volatile Compounds in Food*, TNO Nutrition and Food Research Institute, Zeist, The Netherlands, 1996, pp. 1.1–1.18, 13.1–13.5.

85. Barnes, M.M., Codling moth occurrence, host race formation, and damage, in *Tortricid Pests: Their Biology, Natural Enemies and Control*, van der Geest, L.P.S. and Evenhuis, H.H., Ed., Elsevier, Amsterdam, 1991, pp. 313–327.

86. Light, D.M., Knight, A.L., Henrick, C.A., Rajapaska, D., Lingren, B., Dickens, J.C., Reynolds, K.M., Buttery, R.G., Merrill, G., Roitman, J., and Campbell, B.C., A pear-derived kairomone with pheromonal potency that attracts male and female codling moth, *Cydia pomonella* (L.), *Naturwissenschaften*, 88, 333–338, 2001.

87. Dandekar, A.M., McGranahan, G.H., Vail, P.V., Uratsu, S.L., Leslie, C., and Tebbets, S.J., Low levels of expression of wild type *Bacillus thuringiensis* var. *kunstaki cryl A* sequences in transgenic walnut somatic embryos, *Plant Sci.*, 96, 151–162, 1994.

88. Light, D.M. and Henrick, C.A., Bisexual Attractants, Aggregants and Arrestants for Adults and Larvae of Codling Moth and Other Species of Lepidoptera, U.S. Patent 6,264,939, July 24, 2001.

89. Rice, R.E., Sadler, L.L., Hoffman, M.L., and Jones, R.A., Egg traps for the navel orangeworm, *Paramyelois transitella* (Walker), *Environ. Entomol.*, 5, 697–700, 1976.

90. Van Steenwyk, R.A. and Barnett, W.W., Improvement of navel orangeworm (Lepidoptera: Pyralidae) egg traps, *J. Econ. Entomol.*, 78, 282–286, 1985.

91. Picuric-Jovanovic, K. and Milovanovic, M., Analysis of volatile compounds in almond and plum kernel oils, *J. AOCS*, 70, 1101–1104, 1993.

92. Millar, J., Shorey, H., and Cardé, R., Pheromone-based monitoring and mating disruption of navel orangeworm, in *Proc. 25th Almond Industry Conference*, Almond Board of California, Modesto, 1997, pp. 51–53.

93. Shorey, H., Millar, J., and Gerber, R., Disruption of pheromone communication for control of peach twig borer and navel orangeworm in almonds, in *Proc. 26th Almond Industry Conference*, Almond Board of California, Modesto, 1998, pp. 21–22.

94. Dicenta, F., Martínez-Gómez, P., Grané, N., Martín, M.L., León, A., Cánovas, J.A., and Berenguer, V., Relationship between cyanogenic compounds in kernels, leaves, and roots of sweet and bitter kernelled almonds, *J. Agric. Food Chem.*, 50, 2149–2152, 2002.

95. Ferreira, C., Torres, B.B., and Terra, W.R., Substrate specificities of midgut β-glycosidases from insects of different orders, *Comp. Biochem. Physiol. B, Biochem. Mol. Biol.*, 119, 219–225, 1998.

96. Gradziel, T., unpublished results.

97. Hamid, A.B. and Smith, J.E., Degradation of aflatoxin by *Aspergillus flavus*, *J. Gen. Microbiol.*, 133, 2023–2029, 1987.

98. D'Souza, D.H., Brackett, R.E., The role of trace metal ions in aflatoxin B-1 degradation by *Flavobacterium auantiacum*, *J. Food Protect.*, 61, 1666–1669, 1998.

99. Munimbazi, C. and Bullerman, L.B., Inhibition of aflatoxin production of *Aspergillus parasiticus* NRRL 2999 by *Bacillus pumilus*, *Mycopathologia*, 140, 163–169, 1998.

100. Klier, B. and Schimmer, O., Microsomal metabolism of dictamnine: identification of metabolites and evaluation of their mutagenicity in *Salmonella typhimurium*, *Mutagenesis*, 14, 181–185, 1999.

101. Wang, J.S. and Groopman, J.D., DNA damage by mycotoxins, *Mutat. Res. Fund. Mol. Mech. Mutagen.*, 424, 167–181, 1999.

102. Pavlovicova, R., Fundamental aspects of secondary metabolism and its expression in fungal metabolism, *Chemicke Listy*, 92, 406–414, 1998.

103. Guengrich, F.P., Johnson, W.W., Ueng, Y.F., Yamazaki, H., and Shimada, T., Involvement of cytochrome P450, glutathione *S*-transferase, and epoxide hydrolase in the metabolism of aflatoxin B_1 and relevance to risk of human liver cancer, *Environ. Health Perspect.*, 104(Suppl. 3), 557–562, 1996.

104. Raney, K.D., Meyer, D.J., Ketter, B., Harris, T.M., and Guengerich, F.P., Glutathione conjugation of aflatoxin B_1 exo- and endo-epoxides by rat and human glutathione *S*-transferase, *Chem. Res. Toxicol.*, 5, 470–478, 1992.

105. Eaton, D.L., Monroe, D.H., Bellamy, G., and Kalman, D.A., Identification of a novel dihydroxy metabolite of aflatoxin B_1 produced *in vitro* and *in vivo* in rats and mice, *Chem. Res. Toxicol.*, 1, 108–114, 1988.

106. Lamb, M.J. and Lilly, L.J., Induction of recessive lethals in *Drosophila melanogaster* by aflatoxin B_1, *Mutat. Res.*, 11, 430–433, 1971.

107. Layor, J.H., Chinnici, J.P., and Llewellyn, G.C., Effects of a fungal metabolite, aflatoxin B_1, on larval viability and gross morphology in *Drosophila melanogaster*, *Dev. Industr. Microbiol.*, 17, 443–449, 1976.

108. Moore, T.H., Hammond, A.M., and Llewellyn, G.C., Chemosterilant and insecticidal activity of mixed aflatoxins against *Anthonomous grandus* Bohemia (Coleoptera), *J. Invert. Pathol.*, 31, 365–367, 1978.

109. Gaston, J.Q. and Llewellyn, G.C., Sex-determined differential mortality of milkweed bugs, *Oncopeltus fasciatus* (Hemiptera), to aflatoxins, *J. Invert. Pathol.*, 35, 195–199, 1980.

110. Shibahara, T., Ogawa, H.I., Ryo, H., and Fujikawa, K., DNA-damaging potency and genotoxicity of aflatoxin M_1 in somatic cells *in vivo* of *Drosophila melanogaster*, *Mutagenesis*, 10, 161–164, 1995.

111. Foester, R.E. and Wurgler, F.E., *In vitro* studies on the metabolism of aflatoxin B_1 and aldrin in testes of genetically different strains of *Drosophila melanogaster*, *Arch. Toxicol.*, 56, 12–17, 1984.

112. Labrousse, H. and Matie, L., Toxicological biotest on Diptera larvae to detect ciguatoxins and various other toxic substances, *Toxicon*, 34, 881–891, 1996.

113. Feyereisen, R., Insect P450 enzymes, *Ann. Rev. Entomol.*, 44, 507–533, 1999.

114. Sherertz, P.C., Mills, R.R., and Llewellyn, G.C., Comparative dietary patterns and body weight changes in adults male American cockroaches fed pure aflatoxin B_1, *Bull. Environ. Contam. Toxicol.*, 20, 687–695, 1978.

115. Llewellyn, G.C., Gee, C.L., and Sherertz, P.C., Toxic responses of developing fifth instar milkweed bugs, *Oncopeltus fasciatus* (Hemiptera), to aflatoxin B_1, *Bull. Environ. Contam. Toxicol.*, 40, 332–338, 1988.

116. Drummond, J. and Pinnock, D.E., Aflatoxin production by entomopathogenic isolates of *Aspergillus parasiticus* and *Aspergillus flavus*, *J. Invert. Pathol.*, 55, 332–336, 1990.

117. Doster, M.A. and Michailides, T.J., *Aspergillus* molds and aflatoxins in pistachio nuts in California, *Phytopathology*, 84, 583–590, 1994.

118. Mahoney, N., Molyneux, R.J., and Campbell, B.C., Regulation of aflatoxin production by naphthoquinones of walnut (*Juglans regia*), *J. Agric. Food Chem.*, 48(9), 4418–4421, 2000.

119. Lee, S.-E. and Campbell, B.C., *In vitro* metabolism of aflatoxin B$_1$ by larvae of navel orangeworm, *Amyelois transitella* (Walker) (Insecta, Lepidoptera, Pyralidae) and codling moth, *Cydia pomonella* (L.) (Insecta, Lepidoptera, Tortricidae), *Arch. Insect Biochem. Physiol.*, 45, 166–174, 2000.

120. Neal, G.E., Judah, D.J., Strip, F., and Patterson, D.S.P., The formation of 2,3-dihydroxy-2,3-dihydro-aflatoxin B$_1$ by the metabolism of aflatoxin B$_1$ by liver microsomes isolated from certain avian and mammalian species and the possible role of this metabolite in the acute toxicity of aflatoxin B$_1$, *Toxicol. Appl. Pharmacol.*, 58, 431–437, 1981.

121. Manning, R.O., Wyatt, R.D., and Marks, H.L., Effects of phenobarbital and beta-naphthoflavone on the *in vivo* toxicity and *in vitro* metabolism of aflatoxin in an aflatoxin-resistant and control line of chickens, *J. Toxicol. Environ. Health*, 31, 291–311, 1990.

122. Lillard, H.S., Hanlin, R.T., and Lillard, D.A., Aflatoxigenic isolates of *Aspergillus flavus* from pecans, *Appl. Microbiol.*, 19, 128–130, 1970.

123. Schade, J.E., McGreevy, K., King, A.D.J., Mackey, B., and Fuller, G., Incidence of aflatoxin in California almonds, *Appl. Microbiol.*, 29, 48–53, 1975.

124. Emami, A., Suzangar, M., and Barnett, R., Contamination of pistachio nuts with aflatoxins while on the trees and in storage, *Zesz. Probl. Postepow Nauk Roln*, 189, 135–140, 1977.

125. Mojtahedi, H., Rabie, C.J., Lubben, A.M.S., and Danesh, D., Toxic aspergilli from pistachio nuts, *Mycopahtologia*, 31, 123–127, 1979.

126. Denizel, T., Jarvis, B., and Rolfe, E., A field survey of pistachio (*Pistacia vera*) nut production and storage in Turkey with particular reference to aflatoxin contamination, *J. Sci. Food Agric.*, 27, 1021–1026, 1976.

127. Heperkan, D., Aran, N., and Ayfer, M., Mycoflora and aflatoxin contamination in shelled pistachio nuts, *J. Sci. Food Agric.*, 66, 273–278, 1994.

128. Phillips, D.J., Mackey, B., Ellis, W.R., and Hansen, T.N., Occurrence and interaction of *Aspergillus flavus* other fungi in almonds, *Phytopathology*, 69, 829–831, 1979.

129. Purcell, S.L., Phillips, D.J., and Mackey, B.E., Distribution of *Aspergillus flavus* and other fungi in several almond-growing areas of California, *Phytopathology*, 70, 926–929, 1980.

130. Bayman, P.B., Baker, J.O., Doster, M.A., Michailides, T.J., and Mahoney, N.E., Ochratoxin production by the *Aspergillus ochraceus* group and *Aspergillus alliaceus*, *Appl. Environ. Microbiol.*, 68, 2326–2329, 2002.

131. Cotty, P.J., Influence of field application of an atoxigenic strain of *Aspergillus flavus* on the populations of *A. flavus* infecting cotton bolls and on the aflatoxin content of cottonseed, *Phytopathology*, 84, 1270–1277, 1994.

132. Hua, S.S., Baker, J.L., and Flores-Espiritu, M., Interactions of saprophytic yeasts with a *nor* mutant of *Aspergillus flavus*, *Appl. Environ. Microbiol.*, 65, 2738–2740, 1999.

133. Takeoka, G., Dao, L., Teranishi, R., Wong, R., Flessa, S., Harden, L., and Edwards, R., Identification of three triterpenoids in almond hulls, *J. Agric. Food Chem.*, 48(8), 3437–3439, 2000.

134. Sang, S., Lapsley, K., Rosen, R.T., and Ho, C.-T., New prenylated benzoic acid and other constituents from almond hulls (*Prunus amygdalus* Batsch), *J. Agric. Food Chem.*, 50 (3), 607–609, 2002.

135. Molyneux, R.J., Mahoney, N., and Campbell, B.C., Anti-aflatoxigenic constituents of *Pistacia* and *Juglans* species, in *Natural and Selected Synthetic Toxins*, ACS Symposium Series, American Chemical Society, Washington, D.C., 2000, pp. 43–53.

136. Hedin, P.A., Collum, D.H., Langhans, V.E., and Graves, C.H., Distribution of juglone and related compounds in pecan and their effect on *Fusicladium effusum*, *J. Agric. Food Chem.*, 28(2), 340–342, 1980.

137. Krajci, W.M. and Lynch, D.L., The inhibition of various micro-organisms by crude walnut hull extracts and juglone, *Microbios Lett.*, 4(15), 175–181, 1977.

138. Sokolov, I.N., Chekhova, A.E., Eliseev, Y.T., Nilov, G.I., and Shcherbanovskii, L.R., Antimicrobial activity of some naphthoquinones, *Prikl. Biokhim. Mikrobiol.*, 8(2), 261–263, 1972.

139. Tripathi, R.D., Tripathi, S.C., and Dixit, S.N., Structure activity relationship amongst some fungitoxic α-naphthoquinones of angiosperm origin, *Agric. Biol. Chem.*, 44(10), 2483–2485, 1980.

140. Minto, R.E. and Townsend, C.A., Enzymology and molecular biology of aflatoxin biosynthesis, *Chem. Rev. (Wash.)*, 97(7), 2537–2555, 1997.

141. Mahoney, N., Molyneux, R.J., McKenna, J., Leslie, C.A., and McGranahan, G., Resistance of "Tulare" walnut (*Juglans regia* cv. Tulare) to aflatoxigenesis, *J. Food Sci.*, 68(2), 619–622, 2002.

142. Mahoney, N. and Molyneux, R.J., Phytochemical inhibition of aflatoxigenicity in *Aspergillus flavus* by constituents of walnut (*Juglans regia*), *J. Agric. Food Chem.*, 52, 1882–1889, 2004.

143. Yamada, H., Adachi, O., Watanabe, M., and Sato, N., Studies on fungal tannase. Part 1. Formation, purification and catalytic properties of tannase of *Aspergillus flavus*, *Agric. Biol. Chem.*, 32, 1070–1078, 1968.

144. Kim, J.H. and Campbell, B.C., Targeting stress-response genes for control of mycotoxin biosynthesis in *Aspergillus*, in *Proc. 3rd Fungal Genomics, 4th Fumonisin, and 16th Aflatoxin Elimination Workshops*, Savannah, GA, 2003, p. 21.

145. Sang, S., Kikuzaki, H., Lapsley, K., Rosen, R.T., Nakatani, N., and Ho, C.-T., Sphingolipid and other constituents from almond nuts (*Prunus amygdalus* Batsch), *J. Agric. Food Chem.*, 50(16), 4709–4712, 2002.

146. Gradziel, T., Mahoney, N., and Abdallah, A., Aflatoxin production among almond genotypes is not related to either kernel oil composition of *Aspergillus flavus* growth rate, *HortScience*, 35, 937–939, 2000.

147. Crane, J.C. and Iwakiri, B.T., Shell dehiscence in pistachio, *HortScience*, 17, 797–798, 1982.

148. Schatzki, T.F. and Pan, J.L., Distribution of aflatoxin in pistachios. 3. Distribution in pistachio process streams, *J. Agric. Food Chem.*, 44, 1076–1084, 1996.

149. Mahoney, N. and Molyneux, R.J., Contamination of tree nuts by aflatoxigenic fungi: aflatoxin content of closed-shell pistachios, *J. Agric. Food Chem.*, 46 (5), 1906–1909, 1998.

150. Whitaker, T.B., Dickens, J.W., and Wiser, E.H., Comparison of the observed distribution of aflatoxin in shelled peanuts to the negative binomial, *J. AOCS*, 49, 590–593, 1972.

151. Whitaker, T.B., Dickens, J.W., and Monroe, R.J., Variability of aflatoxin test results, *J. AOCS*, 41, 214–218, 1974.

152. Whitaker, T.B., Giesbrecht, F.G., Wu, J., Hagler, W.M.J., and Dowell, F.E., Predicting the distribution of aflatoxin test results from farmers stock peanuts, *J. AOAC Int.*, 77, 659–666, 1994.

153. Schatzki, T.F., Distribution of aflatoxin in pistachios. 1. Lot distributions, *J. Agric. Food Chem.*, 43, 1561–1565, 1995.

154. Schatzki, T.F., Distribution of aflatoxin in pistachios. 2. Distribution in freshly harvested pistachios, *J. Agric. Food Chem.*, 43, 1566–1569, 1995.

155. Schatzki, T.F. and Pan, J., Distribution of aflatoxin in pistachios. 4. Distribution in small pistachios, *J. Agric. Food Chem.*, 45, 205–207, 1997.

156. Schatzki, T.F., Distribution of aflatoxin in pistachios. 5. Sampling and testing U.S. pistachios for aflatoxin, *J. Agric. Food Chem.*, 46, 2–4, 1998.

157. Schatzki, T.F. and Ong, M.S., Distribution of aflatoxin in almonds. 2. Distribution in almonds with heavy insect damage, *J. Agric. Food Chem.*, 48, 489–492, 2000.

158. Schatzki, T.F. and Ong, M.S., unpublished results.

159. Schatzki, T.F. and De Koe, W.J., Distribution of aflatoxin in pistachios. 6. Buyer's and seller's risk, *J. Agric. Food Chem.*, 47, 3771–3775, 1999.

160. Farsaie, A., McClure, W.F., and Monroe, R.J., Development of indices for sorting Iranian pistachio nuts according to fluorescence, *J. Food Sci.*, 43, 1550–1552, 1978.

161. Farsaie, A., McClure, W.F., and Monroe, R.J., Design and development of an automatic electro-optical sorter for removing fluorescent pistachio nuts, *Trans. ASAE*, 24, 1372–1375, 1981.

162. Keagy, P.M., Parvin, B., and Schatzki, T.F., Machine recognition of naval orange worm damage in x-ray images of pistachio nuts, *Lebensm.-Wiss. U. Technol.*, 29, 140–145, 1996.

163. Keagy, P.M., Schatzki, T.F., Le., L., Casasent, D., and Weber, D., Expanded image data base of pistachio x-ray images and classification by conventional methods, *SPIE Proc.*, 2907, 196–204, 1996.

164. Sim, A., Parvin, B.A., and Keagy, P.M., Invariant representation and hierarchical network for inspection of nuts from x-ray images, *Int. J. Imag. Syst. Technol.*, 7, 231–237, 1996.

165. Casasent, D., Talukter, A., Schatzki, T.F., and Keagy, P.K., Detection and segmentation of pistachio nuts from x-ray imagery, *Trans. ASAE*, 44, 337–345, 2001.

166. Pearson, T.C., Slaughter, D.C., and Studer, H.E., Physical properties of pistachio nuts, *Trans. ASAE*, 37, 913–918, 1994.

167. Pearson, T.C. and Schatzki, T.F., Machine vision system for automated detection of aflatoxin contaminated pistachios, *J. Agric. Food Chem.*, 46, 2248–2252, 1998.

168. Schatzki, T.F., Distribution of aflatoxin in almonds, *J. Agric. Food Chem.*, 44, 3595–3597, 1996.

169. Kim, S. and Schatzki, T.F., Detection of pinholes in almonds through x-ray imaging, *Trans. ASAE*, 44, 997–1003, 2001.

170. McGranahan, G., Leslie, C.A., Uratsu, S.L., and Dandekar, A.M., Improved efficiency of the walnut somatic embryo gene transfer system, *Plant Cell Rep.*, 8, 512–516, 1990.

171. Gradziel, T.M. and Kester, D.E., Breeding for resistance to *Aspergillus flavus* in almond, *Acta Hort.*, 373, 111–117, 1994.

172. Leslie, C.A., McGranahan, G.H., Mendum, M.L., Uratsu, S.L., and Dandekar, A.M., Genetic engineering of walnut (*Juglans regia* L.), *Acta Hort.*, 442, 33–41, 1997.

173. Dandekar, A.M., Fisk, H.J., McGranahan, G.H., Uratsu, S.L., Bains, H., Leslie, C.A., Tamura, M., Escobar, M., Labavitch, J., Grieve, C., Gradizel, T., Vail, P.V., Tebbets, S.J., Sassa, H., Tao, R., Viss, W., Driver, J., James, D., Passey, A., and Teo, G., Different genes for different folks in tree crops: what works and what does not, *HortScience*, 2002, 37, 281–286.

174. Moyne, A.-L., Shelby, R., Cleveland, T.E., Tuzun, S., and Bacillomycin D., An iturin with antifungal activity against *Aspergillus flavus*, *J. Appl. Microbiol.*, 90(4), 622–629, 2001.

175. Cary, J.W., Bhatnagar, D., and Linz, J.E., Aflatoxins: biological significance and regulation of biosynthesis, in *Microbial Foodborne Diseases*, Cary, J.W., Linz, J.E., and Bhatnagar, D., Eds., Technomic, Lancaster, PA, 2000, pp. 317–361.

176. Bhatnagar, D., Cotty, P.J., and Cleveland, T.E., Genetic and biological control of aflatoxigenic fungi, in *Microbial Food Contamination*, Wilson, C.L. and Samir, D., Eds., CRC Press, Boca Raton, FL, 1998, 207–240 pp.

25 Strategies for Insect Management Targeted Toward Mycotoxin Management*

Patrick F. Dowd, Eric T. Johnson, and W. Paul Williams

CONTENTS

---

* The mention of firm names or trade products does not imply that they are endorsed or recommended by the U.S. Department of Agriculture (USDA) over other firms or similar products not mentioned.

25.1 INTRODUCTION

A variety of environmental elements can interact to ultimately influence mycotoxin levels at harvest in crops such as cottonseed, figs, maize, peanuts, and tree nuts. Insects can often be important in the fungal infection process because they can carry inoculum and cause damage that facilitates colonization by mycotoxin producing fungi. An extensive review covering the inception of studies on insects and myco-toxin interactions through the mid-1990s already exists.[1] The discussion here pri-marily covers recent insights on insect–mycotoxin interactions, primarily on maize. This chapter also covers different types of insect management, primarily concen-trating on plant resistance to insects. Damage to maize ears or cotton bolls caused by insects occurs frequently and spreads the development of mycotoxin-producing fungi, thus making insect control an attractive strategy for mycotoxin management. Maize that produces the *Bacillus thuringiensis* crystal protein (Bt maize) generally offers economically advantageous yield protection from caterpillar pests and appar-ently has prevented accumulations of mycotoxins compared to when non-Bt varieties are used.

25.2 INTERACTIONS

Sometimes it is difficult to understand the importance of insect involvement in the mycotoxin problem because of other environmental factors that can influence the host plant and the mycotoxin-producing fungus. For example, where the environment is suboptimal for plant growth, defensive metabolites that influence insect or plant resistance may be up- or downregulated. Although many defensive factors can affect both insects and fungi (see later discussion), their production may not be temporally coordinated. Under conditions where the plant is healthy, layers of defenses can effectively protect against the fungus. When suboptimal conditions exist for the plant and when conditions can also be favorable for the fungus, insect damage may be relatively less important in promoting mycotoxins. Factors that affect the fungus vs. affecting mycotoxin production itself may also be different; however, studies with Bt versions of maize under field-derived natural conditions suggest that insect presence can greatly enhance mycotoxin levels in temperate areas. This information provides further incentive for considering insect directed management as an impor-tant factor in management of the mycotoxin problem in several crops. Many different species of insects can promote increased levels of mycotoxins (Table 25.1). In some cases, a particular species can be a cosmopolitan problem in different crops, while in other cases, insect involvement is species, geography, and crop specific. For example, caterpillar borers can cause problems related to mycotoxins on several different continents. Sap beetles (primarily *Carpophilus* spp.) and maize weevils (*Sitophilus zeamais*) are also important on different continents.

25.3 NEW INSIGHTS

Recent studies have provided new insights on insect involvement in mycotoxin problems, especially for caterpillars that bore into ears. Understanding these issues can help with the design of management programs; for example, *Ostrinia nubilalis* larvae can pick up the spores of *Fusarium moniliforme* (*F. verticillioides*) from plant tissue and introduce them into ears when they invade.[4] Infection caused by *F. verticillioides* introduced by *O. nubilalis* may be asymptomatic.[4] *O. nubilalis* was not found to increase infection by *Gibberella zea*.[4] Damage by the ear-boring caterpillar *Mussidia nigrivenella*, the major ear-damaging insect in a 2-year study in Benin, was significantly correlated with aflatoxin levels in both years.[3,5] Sugarcane borer (*Eldana saccharina*) and stem borer (*Sesamia calamistis*) presence or damage was also sometimes significantly correlated with aflatoxin levels in maize in Benin.[3] Stalk infection by *F. verticillioides* appears to be an important contributor of the ability of *E. saccharina* to promote ear infection.[6] Spores of *A. flavus* can multiply in the hindgut of *Helicoverpa zea*.[7] Recent studies have also further demonstrated the role of beetles, especially sap beetles, in promoting mycotoxins in maize. Aflatoxin levels of maize grown in Mexico were highly associated with the presence of sap beetles, especially *Carpophilus freemani*.[8] Aflatoxin levels of maize in Benin were also sometimes significantly correlated with the presence or damage of *Carpophilus* sap beetles, maize weevils (*Sitophilus zeamais*), and combined Coleoptera spp.[3]

The timing of ear damage by insects in relation to ear developmental stage appears to influence the impact insect damage has on promoting increases in mycotoxin levels. Fungal growth is dependent on the relative moisture levels of crop material. Thus, for example, insect damage of maize after it has dried to a moisture level that does not support growth by fumonisin-producing *Fusarium* would not be expected to greatly increase mycotoxin problems unless rainfall in opened husks rewets the kernels. Field studies have shown that insect-damaged kernels in blister through soft-dough stages have browned pericarps. These damaged kernels can contain hundreds of ppm of fumonisin and comprise the main source of fumonisin from the ear.[9] Kernels damaged during kernel drydown that are not discolored typically have very little fumonisin.[9] Understanding this concept is important in interpreting the relationship between relative insect damage in insect-resistant material (such as Bt varieties) and mycotoxin levels. Greater differences in fumonisin levels have been seen in isogenic Bt vs. non-Bt hybrids when insect damage occurs in the milk stage than when it occurs later (Dowd, unpublished data).[10,11] This concept also influences management tactics by suggesting that early planting can avoid *Ostrinia nubilalis* damage and subsequent fumonisin contamination in developing kernels (see following discussion).

25.4 MONITORING

An important part of an insect management program where "rescue" control techniques, such as insecticides, are used, is the monitoring of insect populations. Insect population monitoring is also important in predictive modeling, whether actual plant scouting or insect trapping is used. Attractants may also be used in combination with insecticides to limit environmental exposure to insecticides (see discussion section on insecticides). Pheromones for monitoring most major moth stages of pest caterpillars that damage maize (*Ostrinia nubilalis*, *Helicoverpa zea*, *Spodoptera*

TABLE 25.1
Insects and Mites Associated with Mycotoxins in Different Commodities

Insect/Mites	Scientific Name	Distribution[a]	Refs.
Coffee (Ochratoxins)			
Coleoptera:			
Coffee berry borer	*Hypothenemus hampei*	AM, AF	Vega et al.[2]
Cotton (Aflatoxins)			
Coleoptera:			
Boll weevil	*Anthonomus grandis grandis*	AM	Dowd[1]
Flea beetle	*Systena blanda*	AM	Dowd[1]
Predatory beetle	*Collops vittatis*	AM	Dowd[1]
Sap beetles	*Carpophilus* spp.	AM	Dowd[1]
Diptera:			
Fruit fly	*Drosophila melanogaster*	AM	Dowd[1]
Hemiptera:			
Lygus bug	*Lygus hesperus*	AM	Dowd[1]
Stink bug	*Chlorochroa sayi*	AM	Dowd[1]
Tarnished plant bug	*Lygus lineolaris*	AM	Dowd[1]
Lepidoptera:			
Bollworm	*Helicoverpa zea*	AM	Dowd[1]
Pink bollworm	*Pectinophora gossypiella*	AM	Dowd[1]
Figs (Aflatoxins)			
Acarina:			
Predatory mite	*Chelytus* sp.	AM	Dowd[1]
Predatory mite	*Sejus pomi*	AM	Dowd[1]
Coleoptera:			
Dried fruit beetle	*Carpophilus hemipterus*	AM	Dowd[1]
Hymenoptera:			
Fig wasp	*Blastophaga psenes*	AM	Dowd[1]
Thysanaptera:			
Flower thrip	*Franklinielli tritici*	AM	Dowd[1]
Thrip	*Heliothrips fasciatus*	AM	Dowd[1]
Thrip	*Liothrips bremneri*	AM	Dowd[1]
Thrip	*Thrips bremneri*	AM	Dowd[1]
Maize (Aflatoxins, Fumonisins)			
Acarina:			
Mite	*Caloglyphys rodriguezi*	AM	Dowd[1]
Mold mite	*Tyrophagus putrescentiae*	AM	Dowd[1]
Coleoptera:			
Corn rootworm adults	*Diabrotica* spp.	AM	Dowd[1]
Maize/rice weevils	*Sitophilus* spp.	AM, AF	Dowd,[1] Se'tamou et al.[3]
Picnic beetles	*Glischrochilus* spp.	AM	Dowd[1]
Sap beetles	*Carpophilus* spp.	AM,AF	Dowd,[1] Se'tamou et al.[3]
Scarab beetles	Not listed	AM	Dowd[1]

TABLE 25.1 (cont.)
Insects and Mites Associated with Mycotoxins in Different Commodities

Insect/Mites	Scientific Name	Distribution[a]	Refs.
Hemiptera:			
Stink bugs	e.g., *Euchistus* spp.	AM	Dowd[1]
Lepidoptera:			
Corn earworm	*Helicoverpa zea*	AM	Dowd[1]
Ear borer	*Mussidia nigrivenella*	AF	Se'tamou et al.[3]
European corn borer	*Ostrinia nubilalis*	AM, EU	Dowd[1]
Fall armyworm	*Spodoptera frugiperda*	AM	Dowd[1]
Pink scavenger caterpillar	*Sathrobrota rileyi*	AM	Dowd[1]
Southwestern corn borer	*Diatraea grandiosella*	AM	Dowd[1]
Stem borer	*Sesamia calamistis*	AF	Se'tamou et al.[3]
Sugarcane borer	*Eldana saccharina*	AF	Se'tamou et al.[3]
Psocidae:			
Bronze psocid	*Ectopsocopsis cryptomeriae*	AM	Dowd[1]
Thysanaptera:			
Western flower thrip	*Franklinella occidentalis*	AM	Dowd[1]
Peanuts (Aflatoxins)			
Acarina:			
Mite	*Caloglyphus* sp.	AF	Dowd[1]
Mite	*Tyrophagus* sp.	AF	Dowd[1]
Isoptera:			
Termite	*Odontotermes badius*	AF	Dowd[1]
Termite	*Odontotermes latericus*	AF	Dowd[1]
Lepidoptera:			
Lesser cornstalk borer	*Elasmopalpus lignosellus*	AM	Dowd[1]
Small Grains (*Claviceps* Ergot Toxins)			
Coleoptera:			
Beetle	*Cantharus melanura*	EU	Dowd[1]
Carabid beetle	Unspecified	EU	Dowd[1]
Diptera			
Fly	*Rhagonycha fulva*	EU	Dowd[1]
Fly	*Melanostoma mellina*	EU	Dowd[1]
Fungus gnat	*Sciara thomae*	EU	Dowd[1]
Tree Nuts (Aflatoxins):			
Coleoptera:			
Pecan weevil	*Curculio caryae*	AM	Dowd[1]
Hemiptera:			
Southern green stink bug	*Nezara viridula*	AM	Dowd[1]
Stink bug	*Thyanata pallidovirens*	AM	Dowd[1]
Lepidoptera			
Codling moth	*Cydia pomonella*	AM	Dowd[1]
Naval orange worm	*Amyelois transitella*	AM	Dowd[1]

[a] AF = reported from Africa, AM = reported from the Americas, EU = reported from Europe.

frugiperda, *Diatraea grandiosella*, *Heliothis virescens*, and *Cydia pomonella*) are commercially available.

Plant or fungal volatiles may also affect attractancy to insect pests and may be useful in monitoring. Levels of caterpillars such as *Sesamia calamistis* and *Eldana saccharina* were increased when maize was inoculated with *Fusarium verticillioides* in Benin.[6,12] *E. saccharina* laid significantly higher numbers of eggs on stalks of maize that were inoculated with *F. verticillioides*, and larval survival was also significantly higher on inoculated material.[13] Egg lay by *Mussidia nigrivenella* was also significantly higher on stalks inoculated with *F. verticillioides*.[13] Ethyl (2*E*,4*Z*)-2,4-decadienoate, a pear-derived compound, is attractive to both sexes of the codling moth, *Cydia pomonella*.[14] This material has been commercialized and is being tested in different formulations, including for mating disruption in combination with the pheromone.[15]

Advances in monitoring sap beetles have also occurred over the past several years. Recent studies indicate grain inoculated with *Fusarium verticillioides* was significantly more attractive to *Carpophilus dimidiatus* than uninoculated grain.[13] Larvae of *C. dimidiatus* fed *F. verticillioides*-inoculated grain had significantly shorter developmental times, and resulting adults had significantly higher egg production than larvae fed uninoculated grain.[13] Many of the same host-derived volatiles (short-chain alcohols, aldehydes, and esters) are attractive to different *Carpophilus* spp.[16–19] Formulations of natural materials can produce adequate levels of these volatiles so monitoring can occur over the critical 2-week period that sap beetles invade maize.[20–22] The pheromones of many of the *Carpophilus* sap beetles have been identified and synthesized.[23] Pheromone complexes for several different sap beetle species were produced commercially in 2002 and have proven effective in monitoring sap beetles in the field.[24,25] Various sap beetle traps that are effective in the field have also been developed.[20,21,26,27] A commercially available trap is also effective in monitoring sap beetles in the field;[24,25] thus, the tools necessary for monitoring sap beetles all became commercially available in 2002.

25.5 INSECTICIDES

Insecticides have often been tested for their ability to indirectly reduce mycotoxin levels through insect control. In most cases, insecticide use has been impractical in reducing mycotoxins to desired levels due to the cost of the multiple applications that are needed.[1] The use of insecticides for insect control is now becoming more selective than it used to be and can still play an important role in mycotoxin management through reducing insect populations. Advances in the insecticide industry have also resulted in materials that are markedly less toxic and require much less active ingredient per hectare than was formerly the case.

Recent studies on an adherent formulation of malathion indicated advantages over conventional formulations: (1) resistance to wash-off or dislodgement by equipment or crop scouts, and (2) selectivity due to reducing the mortality of beneficial insects through the use of reduced rates of application and lowered rates of exposure (the corn-flour-based granules are less likely to be eaten by beneficial compared to pest insects).[28] When properly applied so granules occur in the maize ear zone, the control of pest insects has been shown to be as good as or better than that noted with conventional formulations.[28,29] Significant reductions in pest insect populations and incidence of mycotoxin-producing fungi were noted when the adherent formulations were used in commercial fields.[9,28,29] This formulation also can be used in the field for competitors of mycotoxigenic fungi, such as *Bacillus subtilis*.[30]

"Attract and kill" formulations of insecticides and attractants for both sexes of adult insects that promote mycotoxin problems have been described but appear most relevant for higher value crops. Effective reduction of sap beetles populations in Australia (which are damaging peaches) with combinations of pheromone, host attractants (peaches), and insecticide have been described;[21] however, positioning of the bait stations is important so as to not draw beetles into the trees instead of killing them.[21] The pear volatile that attracts *Cydia pomonella* moths is also attractive to larvae and may be useful as larva-targeted, low-volume sprays.[15] Microencapsulated formulations targeted at adult control are also being evaluated.[15]

Insecticides have been used in an aflatoxin management strategy in Mexico[31] and are also proposed components of integrated management plans in the United States.[32] The life history of the insect, such as *Mussidia nigrivenella* in Benin maize,[3] may make the insect so difficult to reach with insecticides that insecticide use is impractical from a control standpoint. In lower value crops, resistance conferred by the Bt gene is much more effective and economically practical than insecticide applications. Levels of resistance to all of the insects equivalent to that for *Ostrinia nubilalis* in Bt maize do not yet exist; thus, insecticides can still play a role in rescue treatments when monitoring indicates population levels are sufficient to cause problems with regard to damage, coupled with potential losses due to mycotoxins, that makes insecticide use economically desirable.

25.6   CULTURAL PRACTICES

As discussed previously, high levels of fumonisin often accumulate in maize kernels damaged in blister through milk or soft dough stage but are much lower in kernels damaged in later stages.[9] Thus, maize planted early enough in the midwestern United States may escape caterpillar damage at stages that promote high levels of fumonisin. Data collected from central Illinois from 2001 through 2003 in commercial fields indicate that maize planted before May 1 typically escapes damage in blister through soft dough stage by *Ostrinia nubilalis* and has significantly lower levels of fumonisin compared to later planted maize (Dowd, unpublished data).[24,25] Late planting dates in the southeastern United States can reduce potential aflatoxin levels, presumably due to escaping high temperatures during kernel fill.[33] Other cultural practices, such as crop rotation, may help in reducing the levels of some insects potentially involved in mycotoxin problems, such as rootworms in maize. However, the western corn rootworm (*Diabrotica virgifera virgifera*) has recently thwarted this management strategy because it has been laying eggs in soybeans, providing hatching larvae with suitable food when maize is rotated into that field the following year.[34] Changes in crop management strategies, such as the movement from deep plowing to low or no tillage maize for soil conservation purposes, have reduced the ability to winter kill such pests as sap beetles.[35]

25.7 BIOLOGICAL CONTROL

Biological control can potentially be used not only to control pest insects but also to deliver competitive microorganisms that exclude those that produce mycotoxins. Natural agents that can be used to manage insects include a variety of microorganisms, nematodes, and other insects as parasites or predators. Frequently, natural enemies of insects already present can be exerting a significant effect, and often the best strategy is to let nature take its course and not disrupt it through unnecessary use of nonspecific control measures such as insecticides. The scope of studies addressing the biological control of insect pests that can promote mycotoxin problems is vast, but useful reviews are available.[36–38] Some more recent relevant studies not covered by these reviews will be described here.

A new species of nematode that can exert a significant effect on *Carpophilus* sap beetles was discovered in central Illinois.[39,40] This nematode appeared fairly localized in distribution;[39] although introduction of this nematode into new areas has been attempted, establishment levels have not yet been determined (Dowd, unpublished data). Commercially produced nematodes also appeared to have some potential for sap beetle control, especially in areas where beetles congregate, such as in fruit or vegetable dumps,[41] but the commercial availability of these nematodes has been inconsistent.[42]

Autoinoculative techniques have utilized sap beetles to carry sap beetle pathogens selectively to overwintering sites and to carry competitors of mycotoxigenic fungi to maize ears. The fungus *Beauveria bassiana* is a pathogen of many insect species, including beneficial ones; thus, conventional spray-type application of this or other insect pathogens may result in pest resurgence analogous to that seen when insecticides are used and beneficial insects are also killed, as pest populations tend to recover more quickly that beneficial ones. A 4-year field study indicated that a strain of *B. bassiana* effective against sap beetles could be released through autoinoculative devices in the fall and then be isolated again from overwintering sap beetles recovered from artificial overwintering sites up to 64 m from the release source.[43] Very few nontarget insects were recovered from these overwintering sites, suggesting the selectivity of this release strategy.[43] Autoinoculative techniques were also used to contaminate sap beetles with *Bacillus subtilis* so they would specifically deliver it to damaged maize ears and thereby inhibit subsequent colonization and aflatoxin production by *Aspergillus flavus*.[44] Field studies indicated that the sap beetles could disperse the *B. subtilis* up to 400 m from the initial source. Compared to ears that excluded sap beetles, the percentage of ears that had aflatoxin levels less than 20 ppb was significantly less. The frequency of ears with high levels of aflatoxin was also inversely related to the time that the ears were accessible to sap beetles.[44]

25.8 HOST PLANT RESISTANCE TO INSECTS

25.8.1 New Sources of Resistance

Because of the potentially lower overall cost, host plant resistance to insects is an attractive method for managing not only insects but also mycotoxins indirectly in lower value crops such as maize. Although many studies prior to the late 1990s indicated that managing insect pests was a useful means of indirectly managing mycotoxins, results were either variable or economically impractical enough so the incentive for pursuing this strategy appeared limited. When studies on Bt maize demonstrated how effective insect management could be in indirectly managing mycotoxins (although limitations do occur), the incentive was greater for pursuing host plant resistance of insects for managing mycotoxins. Although disciplines involving host plant resistance to insects by necessity overlap, the following discussion will involve sections devoted to discovery of insect-resistant lines associated with mycotoxin reductions; identification of insect-resistance mechanisms, genes, and loci; and the introduction of genes through breeding and genetic engineering. Impediments and strategies for genetic engineering and gene introduction are also discussed. With regard to the area of biological control, the topic of insect resistance is much broader than the coverage here, so relevant reviews should be consulted as well.[45]

Identifying plant lines with resistance to insects that promote mycotoxins continues to be pursued. Resistance traits may be introduced by breeding or genetic engineering when genes or loci have been identified. Maize germplasm has been evaluated not only for fungal resistance but also insect resistance (which may be due to many of the same mechanisms; see below) as it relates to subsequent reduction in levels of mycotoxins. For example, the maize line Mp80:04 was resistant to both aflatoxin production and *Diatraea grandiosella*.[46] A diallel cross among eight inbred lines of maize was evaluated for southwestern corn borer damage and aflatoxin accumulation.[47] Developing ears were infested with southwestern corn borer larvae 7 days after silks emerged from 50% of the plants in a plot, and silks were inoculated with a suspension of *Aspergillus flavus* conidia on the following day. Ear damage and stalk tunneling were evaluated at harvest before grain was prepared for aflatoxin analysis. Hybrids resulting from crossing Mp496, an inbred line developed and released as a source of resistance to southwestern corn borer leaf feeding, with the other parental inbred lines sustained the lowest levels of southwestern corn borer damage and aflatoxin contamination.[47] An analysis of general combining ability effects indicate that Mp496 contributed significantly to reduced ear damage, stalk tunneling, and aflatoxin contamination.[47] Insect resistance was also noted in drought-resistant germplasm that was resistant to both *A. flavus* and aflatoxin production.[48] Studies in Mississippi and Texas have indicated that hybrids developed for *Helicoverpa zea* resistance and drought tolerance are promising for reducing aflatoxin in the southern United States.[49] Tight-husked, high-maysin maize lines had increased *H. zea* resistance compared to loose-husked, high-maysin lines.[50] The maize inbred Tex6, which has resistance to *A. flavus* ear rot and aflatoxin production, also had some leaf resistance and strong silk resistance to several insect species compared to B73.[51] Corn earworm resistant hybrids have reduced aflatoxin in field studies over 2001 and 2002 in Mississippi.[52] Common insect and fungal resistance mechanisms may also be involved in almonds.[53]

An integrated data management system, including germplasm data, field data, quantitative trait loci (QTL) analysis data, proteomics data, and weather data, has been developed to assist in determining and evaluating resistance sources.[54] In addition, a consortium of scientists from the University of Arizona, the University of

Wisconsin, and the Institute for Genomic Research are developing an oligonucleotide (each 70 bases long) array of 55,000 maize gene sequences that will be released for public use (http:www.maizearray.org). This array could be very useful in identifying genes that are differentially regulated in susceptible vs. resistant maize lines. Related to this aspect, one of the objectives of the National Plant Genome Initiative for 2003–2008 is the sequencing of all the genes of maize (http:www.ostp.gov/NSTC/html/npgi2003/index.htm). This information will be an invaluable repository to identify endogenous mechanisms of resistance. The gene sequences will be correlated to available genetic and physical maps of maize, thus resistance markers identified by traditional breeding programs may one day be defined.

Studies have also identified specific loci and mechanisms of insect resistance in plant varieties being evaluated for, or targeted for, reduced levels of mycotoxins. For example, isoorientin production in silk is controlled by a single recessive gene.[55] Concurrent selection for both *Helicoverpa zea* resistance and yield may avoid later yield reduction concerns compared to when only selecting for *H. zea* resistance.[56] Markers for genes involved in maize insect resistance due to chlorogenic acid, maysin (a luteolin derivative), or maysin analog production or regulation have been identified in insect resistant lines.[57,58] Hemicellulose[59] and a cysteine protease[60–62] appear to be important sources of insect resistance in maize. Additional resistance mechanisms of maize that appear to promote both insect and fungal resistance are peroxidase[64–68] and ribosome-inactivating protein.[69–71]

25.8.2 BT GENES

25.8.2.1 Introduction

The development of Bt maize for insect control has inadvertently, but not unexpectedly, reduced the levels of mycotoxins in different commodities, as several studies have shown; however, certain mitigating factors influence the efficacy of these indirect reductions. A number of studies have demonstrated that Bt maize has the potential to greatly reduce mycotoxin levels. Both small-plot and large-field studies have demonstrated significant reductions.

25.8.2.2 Bt Gene Effects on *Fusarium* Mycotoxins

Overall reductions in fumonisins ranged from less than twofold in some years to over tenfold in others during small-plot studies in Iowa using spore contaminated larvae of *Ostrinia nubilalis* and different Bt events.[72] Correlations between insect-damaged kernels and fumonisin levels ranged from 0.50 to 0.69 in 1996 and 1997, respectively.[72] In small-plot studies in central Illinois, reductions of fumonisins up to eightfold were noted.[10] In studies using different hybrid pairs with varying resistance to *Fusarium* and *O. nubilalis* in east-central Illinois, where insects and inoculum were added under natural conditions in small-plot studies, significant reductions in fumonisin levels were noted in three of four cases for the Bt vs. non-Bt hybrid pairs.[73] Small-plot studies in Ontario, Canada, did not yield significant differences in levels of fumonisin for Bt vs. non-Bt hybrids, but mean fumonisin values were less than 0.3 ppm in all years.[74]

For studies run under natural conditions in Europe, reductions in fumonisin levels ranged from 8- to 30-fold from 1997 to 1999.[75] In small-plot studies in Spain and France,[76,77] when fumonisin levels of non-Bt hybrids were above 2 ppm, corresponding Bt hybrids had an approximately ten times or greater reduction in fumonisin levels. Significant reductions in fumonisin levels of 3- to 6-fold for Bt vs. non-Bt hybrids in 1998 and 1999 have been reported in Italy.[78]

In 0.4-ha field-based studies in Illinois under natural conditions with *Ostrinia nubilalis* infestation rates ranging from 80 to 90%, isogenic hybrids containing Bt11 and MON810 events had fumonisin levels ranging up to 40× less that non-Bt hybrids.[10] Additional studies in commercial fields up to 16 ha demonstrated significant reductions in fumonisin levels for Bt vs. non-Bt hybrids in several cases, depending on relative distribution of different insect species.[11] Significant reductions in fumonisin levels for Bt vs. non-Bt maize have also occurred in subsequent years in commercial fields in central Illinois when *O. nubilalis* was present at levels above 30 to 40% (Dowd, unpublished data).[24,25] Thus, several examples in diverse locations indicate that fumonisin levels can often be significantly less in Bt vs. non-Bt maize, depending on other mitigating factors (see below).

Some studies have looked at the effects of Bt maize on other *Fusarium* mycotoxins. For example, Bt hybrids may also significantly reduce deoxynivalenol (DON) levels in maize, which is somewhat surprising because prior studies have indicated that insect damage does not significantly affect DON levels.[4,79] DON levels in maize grown in Europe were significantly increased in Bt vs. non-Bt maize small-plot studies in one case, were unchanged in one case, and were significantly reduced in three cases.[76,77] Significant reduction in DON levels were reported for Bt vs. non-Bt maize in small-plot studies performed in Ontario, Canada.[74] Significant reductions in nivalenol levels in Bt vs. non-Bt hybrids occurred at the same sites in Spain and France that had significant reductions in DON.[76,77] Zearalenone levels were significantly reduced for some sites of Bt vs. non-Bt maize in Spain and France, but not at the same sites where DON levels were reduced.[76,77] When overall levels of DON or zearalenone were low, no significant reductions occurred for Bt vs. non-Bt maize in Italy.[78]

25.8.2.3 Bt Gene Effects on *Aspergillus* Mycotoxins

Some studies have also investigated the potential ability of Bt hybrids to reduce levels of aflatoxin compared to non-Bt versions. These studies have been performed in areas where the European corn borer is the major pest (midwestern United States and in Europe) and where this insect plus others such as the corn earworm and fall armyworm, which are not controlled well by many of the Bt hybrids available, occur (southeastern United States and Texas). No significant reductions in aflatoxin levels occurred for Bt vs. non-Bt inbreds in small-plot studies where *Ostrinia nubilalis* and *Aspergillus flavus* were added nondestructively to ears, but aflatoxin levels were quite low in all cases.[10] In small-plot studies in Iowa where nondamaging inoculation techniques were used, one case of a significant reduction in *A. flavus* levels for a Bt compared to non-Bt hybrid pair was observed;[80] however, no significant differences in *Aspergillus* ear rot or aflatoxin occurred when 11 Bt/non-Bt hybrid pairs were inoculated using a pinboard.[81] When overall levels of aflatoxin were low, no significant differences in aflatoxin levels occurred in Bt vs. non-Bt maize in Italy.[78]

Some reductions in aflatoxin were noted for Bt vs. non-Bt maize hybrids when ears were inoculated with *Diatraea grandiosella* but not *Aspergillus flavus* in Mississippi.[82] Some significant reductions in aflatoxin levels for some MON810 and Bt11 hybrids compared to non-Bt hybrids that were infested with *D. grandiosella* occurred despite *Helicoverpa zea* damage.[83] The effectiveness of the Bt hybrids in reducing aflatoxin contamination appeared to result from reduced insect damage rather than being a direct effect of the Bt hybrids on fungal infections or aflatoxin accumulation.[83] In a cooperative investigation with Monsanto, ten pairs of Bt (MON810) and non-Bt hybrids were evaluated for southwestern corn borer damage and aflatoxin accumulation using a kernel-wounding *A. flavus* inoculation technique, a nonwounding inoculation technique, and a combination of southwestern corn borer infestation and nonwounding inoculation technique.[84] The hybrids differed significantly in degree of susceptibility to aflatoxin contamination. High levels of aflatoxin contamination of both Bt and non-Bt hybrids resulted from inoculation with a kernel-wounding technique, but aflatoxin contamination was significantly lower in Bt hybrids than non-Bt hybrids following southwestern corn borer infestation of non-wounded inoculated ears. This provided further evidence that southwestern corn borer can play a significant role in increasing aflatoxin contamination and that resistance to southwestern corn borer can reduce aflatoxin contamination.[84] Most silk-inoculated Bt vs. non-Bt hybrids had significantly less aflatoxin in another study in Mississippi.[52] The aflatoxin levels from Cry2Ab hybrids (MON840) (which has more resistance to *Helicoverpa zea* than MON810 or Bt11 hybrids) were found to be significantly lower than for CryIAb hybrids and non-Bt hybrids in 2000 and were significantly lower compared to non-Bt hybrids in 2001 when infected corn kernels were distributed along rows as a source of *A. flavus* inoculum in Texas.[85] Significant reductions in aflatoxin levels were noted for Bt vs. non-Bt MON810 and Bt11 hybrids an one site but not two others in 2001 and 2002 (different sites were significantly different in the 2 years).[86] Event 176 hybrids had no significant differences in aflatoxin levels vs. their non-Bt counterparts and had fewer instances where insect damage was significantly less.[86] A consistently significant correlation occurred between insect injury ratings and aflatoxin levels for non-Bt hybrids at all sites in all years.[86]

25.8.2.4 Factors Mitigating the Efficacy of Bt Maize Hybrids in Reducing Mycotoxin Levels

Many environmental effects can affect the degree to which Bt maize hybrids indirectly prevent higher levels of mycotoxin compared to non-Bt counterparts;[10,11] however, in order to interpret the importance of these factors, studies have to be evaluated to see if comparable techniques are used. For example, based on the previous discussion, it appears that in studies where the ears are not damaged in some way significant reductions in mycotoxins tend to occur more frequently than if ears are damaged while performing fungal inoculations. This effect has been clearly demonstrated in studies performed in Mississippi, where significant reductions in aflatoxin were noted when ears were silk inoculated but not when they were pin inoculated.[83,84] As an additional factor that potentially confounds interpretation of aflatoxin studies, Bt protein is a demonstrated inhibitor of *Aspergillus flavus* at 4 to 20 ppm,[52] although these levels are higher than those that are found in field-grown Bt maize tissues that give highly effective insect control (e.g., 1 to 2 ppm).[87]

Insect pest distribution and composition, hybrid resistance, and weather factors can also influence the degree that Bt hybrids can indirectly reduce mycotoxins. Obviously, if *Ostrinia nubilalis* ear incidence is low, differences in fumonisin levels between Bt and non-Bt hybrids are not likely to be as great as if *O. nubilalis* populations are high. The breadth of resistance of the Bt hybrids, and complex of insects that attack ears in any given year can also influence the degree to which Bt hybrids can indirectly reduce mycotoxins. Under natural conditions, when *O. nubilalis* has been the predominant insect pest occurring at levels above 25 to 50%, reductions of fumonisin levels are frequently five times or more greater;[10,72,77] however, when *Helicoverpa zea* is the predominant pest under natural[11] or artificially increased conditions,[73] significant reductions in fumonisin levels are not seen for the same hybrids that show reductions for *O. nubilalis*. The greatest reductions in aflatoxin levels have occurred in the southeast under natural conditions with non-destructive additions of *Aspergillus flavus* inoculum when the most *H. zea*-resistant hybrid event (MON840) has been used.[85] Newer hybrids with enhanced resistance to insects such as *H. zea* (MON840) and *Spodoptera frugiperda* (Herculex) may show greater reductions in mycotoxin levels than previously noted for MON810 or Bt11 events when these species of insects are common; however, the degree of control for *H. zea* still is not at the 100% level that occurs for *O. nubilalis* with the MON810 or Bt11 event hybrids.[88] Other insects that are not affected by the caterpillar-targeted Bt crystal proteins, such as sap beetles, can be important contributors to the mycotoxin problem, especially when husks are open and loose.[1]

The tissues in which and levels at which the Bt protein is expressed are also important determinants of efficacy for indirectly reducing mycotoxins. As can be determined from the preceding discussion, the event 176 hybrids, for which the Bt protein is produced at low concentrations in silks and kernels, are typically less effective in indirectly reducing fumonisin or aflatoxin under the same insect pressures compared to MON 810 and Bt11 events.[10,72,86] Inherent hybrid resistance to the mycotoxin producing fungi can also mitigate the degree of efficacy seen for Bt hybrids in indirectly reducing mycotoxin levels. Correlations between insect damage and fumonisin levels have been significantly greater for some hybrids compared to others grown at the same locale in the same year,[10,11] suggesting differences in fungal reliance on insect damage to invade and spread. The one of four pairs of Bt vs. non-Bt hybrids that did not show significant differences in fumonisin levels in a study in east-central Illinois appeared to have fungal resistance that was independent of insect damage.[73] Environmental conditions that influence the hybrid resistance stability or favor the mycotoxin-producing fungi can also influence the degree of efficacy with which the Bt hybrids can indirectly reduce mycotoxin in different years. Correlations between insect damage and fumonisin levels have been significantly greater in some years compared to others for the same hybrids at the same locales.[10,11]

Bt genes have been introduced into additional plants that have been investigated or designed for the reduction of mycotoxins. Bright greenish-yellow fluorescence incidences have been reduced significantly in Bt vs. non Bt cottonseed.[89–91] These results suggest that aflatoxin may also be reduced in Bt vs. non-Bt cottonseed, but it may be important for growers to harvest immediately after boll opening to see these differences.[89–91] The Bt gene has also been introduced into walnuts[92–94] and peanuts[95,96] with the intent of reducing aflatoxin in these commodities.

25.8.3 OTHER TRANSGENES PROMOTING INSECT RESISTANCE

A variety of other genes coding for proteins have been identified as promoting enhanced resistance to insects; however, very few of these have increased insect resistance to the degree that the Bt proteins have exerted against *Ostrinia nubilalis*. It is likely that these will be of greatest value in combination, much like the resistance that naturally occurs in plants.[97] Among the more widely investigated proteins expressed transgenically and targeted toward insect resistance are protease inhibitors and lectins.[45] Tobacco anionic peroxidase has increased insect resistance in tobacco,[65] tomato,[67] sweet gum,[66] and maize.[68] Maize ribosome inactivating protein has increased insect resistance when expressed in tobacco.[70] Additional resistance proteins that have been shown to be effective against insects in transgenic plant systems include avidin,[98] alpha-amylase inhibitor,[99] and cholesterol oxidase.[100]

While Bt and other proteins have been the most thoroughly studied method of controlling insects through transgenic means, the increasing knowledge base of the synthesis of unique chemicals throughout the plant kingdom may provide new sources of insect resistance in maize or other mycotoxin susceptible crops. Increased production of tryptamine in tobacco due to enhanced expression of tryptophane decarboxylase has resulted in significantly reduced rates of survival of whitefly larvae.[102] The biosynthetic pathway for dhurrin, a cyanogenic glycoside, was transferred from *Sorghum bicolor* to *Arabidopsis thaliana*.[101] Flea beetles (*Phyllotreta nemorum*) adapted to crucifers such as *A. thaliana* were effectively killed on leaves expressing high levels of dhurrin because they did not have effective resistance mechanisms to counter this novel plant defensive compound.[101] Alternatively, an *A. thaliana* line overexpressing a number of phenylpropanoid compounds[103] significantly reduced the growth of *Spodoptera frugiperda* compared to larvae fed wild-type plant leaves.[104] The inhibitory compounds in this *A. thaliana* line may be anthocyanins, which have been shown in separate experiments to inhibit larval growth when added to insect diet.[105] One of these inhibitory anthocyanins, peonidin, is naturally produced at low levels in some maize tissues of some lines,[106] but consumers are unlikely to accept colored corn kernels. Overexpression of peonidin in plant parts that will not cause consumer rejection but are susceptible to insect damage (e.g., silks) is worth further study.

25.8.4 BENEFITS AND CONCERNS ABOUT TRANSGENE USE

Enhancing insect resistance by utilizing nonplant- or plant-derived genes through biotechnological means may be worth pursuing for additional insects not already effectively controlled by host plant resistance, provided yield is not affected. Pursuing the use of a small number of genes that promote insect resistance to a broad spectrum of insects offers potential advantages, as opposed to the use of many fairly specific genes, such as Bt. Because pests feed on plant tissues, this limits exposure of plant-contained host resistance to beneficial insects (although secondary effects may occur, depending on the resistance type, such as lectins). General insect resistance is also valuable in cases where new species of insects invade or change behavior. The advantage of using host plant resistance for managing insect damage as a technique for indirectly reducing mycotoxins is that insect resistance can provide yield protection that is economical, which explains the quick adoption of the Bt maize hybrids.

Negative impacts caused by insect-resistant Bt hybrids such as prey-independent reduction of populations of beneficial or nontarget insects have not been demonstrated under natural field conditions.[10,11,107,108] Resistance gene frequency estimates on which resistance management strategies are based have so far proved realistic.[109–112] Environmental advantages of significantly reduced pesticide use have been documented for Bt compared to non-Bt maize fields[113] and cotton.[111] No negative effects on ethanol production,[114] cattle growth, or milk production[115] due to the presence of the Bt protein have been identified.

Some environmentalist groups do not want to accept the uncertainty involved in transgene introduction, despite knowledge that more genes are moved by conventional breeding than in transgenic work. Despite the potential health benefits that may occur from transgenic insect- or fungus-resistant plants due to mycotoxin reductions, the acceptability of biotechnologically enhanced food products remains an issue. Further concerns involve uncertain copy number and insertion site (and thus unintended effects) of introduced genes, the presence of herbicide- or antibiotic-degrading selectable marker genes, and potential problems with allergenicity (despite good predictability by *in vitro* testing). The tissue-specific expression of resistance genes is possible, but plants that express low levels in tissues that require protection typically do not significantly reduce mycotoxins (e.g., event 176 maize hybrids).[10,72] Provided husk coverage is good, expression in green tissue and silks may be sufficient to prevent kernel damage at critical times. For example, an experimental inbred that produced high levels of the Bt protein in silks but not kernels, due to a pith promoter, had no corn borer damage, compared to 53% of ears damaged in the non-Bt version.[10] A promoter directing a silk-specific gene product has also been isolated from maize in an effort to make conditional female-sterile plants.[116] This information suggests that sufficient expression of insecticidal proteins in tissues not consumed by people or animals may be sufficient to control mycotoxigenic fungi indirectly.

25.8.5 DEPLOYMENT OF RESISTANCE GENES

Secondary metabolites of plants, such as anthocyanins, flavonoids, lignins, naphthoquinones, *N*-aromatics, phenolics, phytoalexins, sesquiterpene lactones, stilbenes, and terpenes can inhibit both insects and fungi.[117] Proteins such as amylase inhibitors, chitinases, lectins, lipoxygenase, peroxidase, proteinase inhibitors, and ribosome-inactivating proteins can also inhibit both insects and fungi.[45,70,118,119] Multigenic insect and disease resistance maps to many of the same sites in maize;[97] thus, it is likely that the same factors can be incorporated for control of both insects and fungi at the same time. Selection of appropriate combinations of resistance factors may be challenging due to conflicting properties of the active compounds. For example, secondary metabolites can often inhibit hydrolytic enzymes, and proteases can digest other defensive proteins. Proteins and secondary metabolites with different modes of action[108] or different functional classes[120] may need to be combined more effectively to help increase the stability of resistance and limit the number of genes necessary to confer sufficient levels of resistance.

25.9 INTEGRATED MANAGEMENT PROGRAMS

Integrated management techniques have been utilized in maize cultivation for some time and include such strategies as crop rotation. Integrated management programs for aflatoxin in maize[31] and peanuts[121] that include insect management have been practiced for many years. More recently, management programs acceptable to farmers that include predictive computer programs have evolved. An integrated pest management (IPM) program targeted toward mycotoxins in maize for the midwestern United States involves cooperation of a number of partners, including USDA personnel, extension services, farmers, industry, and farm service companies. This program has been investigated over the past 4 years. The mycotoxin levels predicted by the computer program are compared to actual values obtained in fields which are sampled for insects, mold inoculum, and mycotoxins, and adjustments are made as necessary.[32,122] Bt hybrids can be important in this system of management, but some farmers are reluctant to plant Bt hybrids, especially "stacked" versions that contain multiple introduced genes, because grain elevators to which they sell the grain will not accept it due to potential market restrictions. Insecticides are still potentially important for a rescue management approach in non-Bt maize fields with significant *Ostrinia nubilalis* presence or in other fields that have insects not well controlled by Bt proteins in respective hybrids. Although adjustments were needed in one year, predicted levels of fumonisins have been close to actual values for most hybrids examined in commercial fields.[122] Farmers are interested in the management program, but adoption is likely to be slow until elevators require fumonisin levels that affect economic productivity. A comprehensive program targeting aflatoxin in the southeastern United States includes an economic analysis of preplant and growing season issues.[123,124]

25.10 CONCLUSIONS

Insects are important in promoting high levels of mycotoxins under commonly occurring conditions in several major crops. Insect management can greatly reduce levels of mycotoxins in these crops. Insect management is often an economically effective method for protecting crop yield and quality, leading to ready adoption of insect-resistant germplasm. Bt maize and cotton have been readily adopted worldwide and have considerably reduced the amount of insect damage to these crops. Significant reductions in fumonisins have been reported in a number of studies with

Bt maize under conditions where high levels of *Ostrinia nubilalis* occur. It is likely that as greater numbers and spectrum of insect resistance traits are added to different crops, mycotoxin levels are likely to decline as a result. Additional management strategies can be combined with host plant resistance to insects as components of integrated programs utilizing predictive forecasts for mycotoxins and economic analyses for preventative measures. Such programs are likely to further contribute to the reduction of mycotoxins and thereby increase the health of people and animals worldwide.

ACKNOWLEDGMENTS

We thank the many collaborators we have had over the years for their fine efforts, and P.J. Slininger and anonymous reviewers for comments on prior versions of this manuscript. Omission of other relevant reports was unintentional.

REFERENCES

1. Dowd, P.F., Involvement of arthropods in the establishment of mycotoxigenic fungi under field conditions, in *Mycotoxins in Agriculture and Food Safety*, Sinha, K.K. and Bhatnagar, D., Eds., Marcel Dekker, New York, 1998, pp. 307–350.
2. Vega, F.E., Mercadier, G., and Dowd, P.F., Fungi associated with the coffee berry borer *Hypothenemus hampei* (Ferrari) (Coleoptera: Scolytidae), in *Proc. 18th International Scientific Colloquium on Coffee*, Helsinki, Finland, August 2–6 1999, Association Scientifique Internationale du Cafe, 1999, pp. 229–237.
3. Se'tamou, M., Cardwell, K.F., Schulthess, F., and Hell, K., Effect of insect damage to maize ears, with special reference to *Mussidia nigrivenella* (Lepidoptera: Pyralidae) on *Aspergillus flavus* (Deuteromycetes: Moniliales) infection and aflatoxin production in maize before harvest in the Republic of Benin, *J. Econ. Entomol.*, 91, 433–438, 1998.
4. Sobek, E.A. and Munkvold, G.P., European corn borer (Lepidoptera: Pyralidae) larvae as vectors of *Fusarium moniliforme*, causing kernel rot and symptomless infection of maize kernels, *J. Econ. Entomol.*, 92, 503–509, 1999.
5. Se'tamou, M., Cardwell, K.F., Schulthess, F., and Hell, K., *Aspergillus flavus* infection and aflatoxin contamination of preharvest maize in Benin, *Plant Dis.*, 81, 1323–1327, 1997.
6. Schulthess, F., Cardwell, K.F., and Gounou, S., The effect of endophytic *Fusarium verticillioides* on infestation of two maize varieties by lepidopterous stemborers and coleopteran grain feeders, *Phytopathology*, 92, 120–128, 2002.
7. Abel, C.A., Abbas, H.K., Zablotowicz, R., Pollan, M., and Dixon, K., The association between corn earworm damage and aflatoxin production in preharvest maize grain, in *Proc. 2nd Fungal Genomics, 3rd Fumonisin Elimination, and 15th Aflatoxin Elimination Workshop*, San Antonio, TX, October 23–35, 2002, Robens, J.F. and Brown, R.L., Eds., Agricultural Research Service, U.S. Department of Agriculture, Beltsville, MD, 2002, pp. 113–114.
8. Rodriguez-del-Bosque, L.R., Leos-Martinez, J., and Dowd, P.F., Effect of ear wounding and cultural practices on abundance of *Carpophilus freemani* (Coleoptera: Nitidulidae) and other microcoleopterans in maize in northeastern Mexico, *J. Econ. Entomol.*, 91, 796–801, 1998.

9. Dowd, P.F., Bennett, G.A., McGuire, M.R., Nelsen, T.C., Shasha, B.S., and Simmons, F.W., Adherent malathion flour granules as an environmentally selective control for chewing insect pests of dent corn ears: indirect reduction in mycotoxigenic ear molds, *J. Econ. Entomol.*, 92, 68–75, 1999.

10. Dowd, P.F., Indirect reduction of ear molds and associated mycotoxins in *Bacillus thuringiensis* corn under controlled and open field conditions: utility and limitations, *J. Econ. Entomol.*, 93, 1669–1679, 2000.

11. Dowd, P.F., Biotic and abiotic factors limiting efficacy of Bt corn in indirectly reducing mycotoxin levels in commercial fields, *J. Econ. Entomol.*, 94, 1067–1074, 2001.

12. Cardwell, K.F., Kling, J.G., Maziya-Dixon, B., and Bosque-Perez, N.A., Interactions between *Fusarium verticillioides*, *Aspergillus flavus*, and insect infestation in four maize genotypes in lowland Africa, *Phytopathology*, 90, 276–284, 2000.

13. Ako, M., Schulthess, F., Gumedzoe, M.Y.D., and Cardwell, K.F., The effect of *Fusarium verticillioides* on oviposition behavior and bionomics of lepidopteran and coleopteran pests attacking the stem and cobs of maize in West Africa, *Entomol. Exper. Appl.*, 106, 201–210, 2003.

14. Light, D.M., Knight, A.L., Buttery, R.G., Henrick, C.A., Rajapaska, D., Reynolds, K.M., Merrill, G., Roitman, J., Dickens, J.C., Lingren, W., and Campbell, B.C., Ethyl (2*E*,4*Z*)-2,4-decadienoate: a pear-derived kairomone with pheromonal potency that attracts both sexes of the codling moth, *Cycia pomonella* (L), *Naturwissenschaften*, 88, 333–338, 2001.

15. Light, D.M., Reynolds, K.M., and Campbell, B.C., Advances in development of kairomone-augmented control tactics for codling moth and *Aspergillus* in walnuts, in *Proc. 3rd Fungal Genomics, 4th Fumonisin Elimination, and 16th Aflatoxin Elimination Workshop*, Savannah, GA, October 13–15, 2003, Robens, J.F. and Dorner, J.W., Eds., Agricultural Research Service, U.S. Department of Agriculture, Beltsville, MD, 2003, p. 99.

16. Dowd, P.F. and Bartelt, R.J., Host-derived volatiles as attractants and pheromone synergists for the driedfruit beetle *Carpophilus hemipterus*, *J. Chem. Ecol.*, 17, 285–308, 1991.

17. Dowd, P.F. and Bartelt, R.J., Organophosphorus Insecticides as Synergizicides for *Carpophilus* spp. Pheromones, U.S. Patent 5,149,525, September 22, 1992.

18. Lin, H., Phelan, P.L., and Bartelt, R.J. Synergism between synthetic food odors and the aggregation pheromone for attracting *Carpophilus lugubris* in the field (Coleoptera: Nitidulidae), *Environ. Entomol.*, 21, 156–159, 1992.

19. Bartelt, R.J. and Wicklow, D.T., Volatiles from *Fusarium verticillioides* (Sacc.) Nireb. and their attractiveness to nitidulid beetles, *J. Agric, Food Chem.*, 47, 2447–2454, 1999.

20. James, D.G., Bartelt, R.J., and Moore, C.J., Mass-trapping of *Carpophilus* spp. (Coleoptera: Nitidulidae) in stone fruit orchards using synthetic aggregation pheromones and a coattractant: development of a strategy for population suppression, *J. Chem. Ecol.*, 22, 1541–1556, 1996.

21. James, D.G., Vogele, B., Faulder, R.J., Bartelt, R.J., and Moore, C.J. Pheromone-mediated mass trapping and population diversion as strategies for suppressing *Carpophilus* spp. (Coleoptera: Nitidulidae) in Australia stone fruit orchards, *Agric. Forest Entomol.*, 3, 41–47, 2001.

22. Dowd, P.F., Dusky sap beetles (Coleoptera: Nitidulidae) and other kernel damaging insects in Bt and non-Bt sweet corn in Illinois, *J. Econ. Entomol.*, 93, 1714–1720, 2000.

23. Bartelt, R.J., Sap beetles, in *Pheromones of Non-Lepidopteran Insects Associated with Agricultural Plants*, Hardie, J. and Minks, A.K., Eds., CAB International, Wallingford, 1999, pp. 69–89.

24. Dowd, P.F., Barnett, J, Bartelt, R.J., Beck, J.J., Berhow, M.A., Duvick, J.P., Kendra, D.A., Molid, G., and White, D.G., Insect management for reduction of mycotoxins in midwest corn: FY 2002 report, in *Proc. 2nd Fungal Genomics, 3rd Fumonisin Elimination, and 15th Aflatoxin Elimination Workshop*, San Antonio, TX, October 23–25, 2002, Robens, J.F. and Brown, R.L., Eds., Agricultural Research Service, U.S. Department of Agriculture, Beltsville, MD, 2002, pp. 117–118.

25. Dowd, P.F., Barnett, J, Bartelt, R.J., Beck, J.J., Berhow, M.A., Boston, R.S., Duvick, J.P., Johnson, E.T., Lagrimini, L.M., Molid, G., and White, D.G., Insect management for reduction of mycotoxins in midwest corn: FY 2003 report, in *Proc. 3rd Fungal Genomics, 4th Fumonisin Elimination, and 16th Aflatoxin Elimination Workshop*, Savannah, GA, October 13–15, 2003, Robens, J.F. and Dorner, J.W., Eds., Agricultural Research Service, U.S. Department of Agriculture, Beltsville, MD, 2003, pp. 13–14.

26. Dowd, P.F., Bartelt, R.J., and Wicklow, D.T., Novel insect trap useful in capturing sap beetles (Coleoptera: Nitidulidae) and other flying insects, *J. Econ. Entomol.*, 85, 772–778, 1992.

27. Williams, R.N., Fickle, D.S., Bartelt, R.J., and Dowd, P.F., Responses by adult Nitidulidae (Coleoptera) to synthetic aggregation pheromones, a coattractant, and effects of trap design and placement, *Eur. J. Entomol.*, 90, 287–294, 1993.

28. Dowd, P.F., Behle, R.W., McGuire, M.R., Nelsen, T.C., Shasha, B.S., Simmons, F.W., and Vega, F.E., Adherent malathion flour granules as an environmentally selective control for chewing insect pests of dent corn ears: insect control, *J. Econ. Entomol.*, 91, 1058–1066, 1998.

29. Dowd, P.F., Pingel, R.L., Ruhl, D., Shasha, B.S., Behle, R.W., Penland, D.R., McGuire, M.R., and Faron, II, E.J., Multiacreage evaluation of aerially applied adherent malathion granules for selective insect control and indirect reduction of mycotoxigenic fungi in specialty corn, *J. Econ. Entomol.*, 93, 1424–1428, 2000.

30. Dowd, P.F., Bennett, G.A., Richard, J.L., Bartelt, R.J., Behle, R.W., McGuire, M.R., Vega, F.E., Scott, G.E., Brandhorst, T., Kenealy, W., Ferguson, J.S., Warren, G., Kenney, D., and Lagrimini, L.M., IPM of aflatoxin in the corn belt: FY 1995 results, in *Proc. 1995 Aflatoxin Elimination Workshop*, Atlanta, GA, October 23–24, 1995, Robens, J.F., Ed., Agricultural Research Service, U.S. Department of Agriculture, Beltsville, MD, 1995, pp. 76–78.

31. CEMCA (Comite Estatal de Modernizacion del Campo del Agua), Paquete technologico integral para la siembra del maiz in riego zona norte y centro de Tamaulipas, Secretaria Agricltura y Recursos Hidraulicos, 1993.

32. Dowd, P.F., An integrated management plan for mycotoxins in midwest corn, in *Proc. 42nd Annual Corn Dry Milling Conference*, Peoria, IL, May 31–June 1, 2002, Blair, J.A. and Wicklow, D.T., Eds., North American Millers Federation, Washington, D.C., 2001, p.16.

33. Widstrom, N.W., McMillian, W.W., Beaver, R.W., and Wilson, D.M., Weather-associated changes in aflatoxin contamination of preharvest maize, *J. Prod. Agric.*, 3, 196–199, 1990.

34. Levine, E. and Oloumi-Sadeghi, H., Western corn rootworm (Coleoptera: Chrysomelidae) larval injury to corn grown for seed production following soybeans grown for seed production, *J. Econ. Entomol.*, 89, 1010–1016, 1996.

35. Connell, W.A., *Nitidulidae of Delaware*, University of Delaware, Newark, DE, 1956, 67 pp.

36. Hokkanen, H.M.T. and Lynch, J.M., *Biological Control: Benefits and Risks*, Cambridge University Press, New York, 1995, 304 pp.

37. Van Driesche, R.G. and Bellows, Jr., T.S., *Biological Control*, Chapman & Hall, New York, 1996, 539 pp.

38. Gurr, G. and Wratten, S.D., *Biological Control: Measures of Success*, Kluwer Academic, Boston, MA, 2000, 429 pp.

39. Dowd, P.F., Moore, D.E., Vega, F.E., McGuire, M.R., Bartelt, R.J., Nelsen, T.C., and Miller, D.A., Occurrence of a mermithid nematode parasite of *Carpophilus lugubris* (Coleoptera: Nitidulidae) in central Illinois, *Environ. Entomol.*, 24, 1245–1251, 1995.

40. Poiner, G.O. and Dowd, P.F., *Psammomermis nitidulensis* n. sp. (Nematoda: Mermithidae) from sap beetles (Coleoptera: Nitidulidae) with biological observations and a key to the species of *Psammomermis*, *Fund. Appl. Nematol.*, 20, 207–211, 1997.

41. Vega, F.E., Dowd, P.F., and Nelsen, T.C., Susceptibility of driedfruit beetles (*Carpophilus hemipterus* L.) (Coleoptera: Nitidulidae) to different *Steinernema* species (Nematoda: Rhabditida: Steinernematidae), *J. Invert. Pathol.*, 64, 276–277, 1994.

42. Gaugler, R. and Han, R., Production technology, in *Entomopathogenic Nematology*, Gaugler, R., Ed., CAB International, New York, 2002, pp. 289–310.

43. Dowd, P.F. and Vega, F.E., Autodissemination of *Beauveria bassiana* by sap beetles (Coleoptera: Nitidulidae) to overwintering sites, *Biocontrol Sci. Technol.*, 13, 65–75, 2003.

44. Dowd, P.F., Vega, F.E., Nelsen, T.C., and Richard, J.L., Dusky sap beetle mediated dispersal of *Bacillus subtilis* to inhibit *Aspergillus flavus* and aflatoxin production in maize *Zea mays* L., *Biocontrol Sci. Technol.*, 8, 221–235, 1998.

45. Gatehouse, J.A. and Gatehouse, A.M.R., Genetic engineering of plants for insect resistance, in *Biological and Biotechnological Control of Insect Pests*, Rechcigl, J.E. and Rechcigl, N.A., Eds., Lewis Publishers, Boca Raton, FL, 2000, pp. 211–241.

46. Williams, W.P., Buckley, P.M., and Windham, G.L., Southwestern corn borer (Lepidoptera: Crambidae) damage and aflatoxin accumulation in maize, *J. Econ. Entomol.*, 95, 1049–1053, 2002.

47. Williams, W.P., Davis, F.M., Windham, G.L., and Buckley, P.M., Southwestern corn borer damage and aflatoxin accumulation in a diallele cross of maize, *J. Genet. Breed.*, 56, 165–169, 2002.

48. Tubijika, K.M. and Damann, K.E., Sources of resistance to aflatoxin production in maize, *J. Agric. Food Chem.*, 49, 2652–2656, 2001.

49. Xu, W., Odvody, G., and Williams, W.P., Progress toward developing stress-tolerant and low-aflatoxin corn hybrids for southern states, in *Proc. 3rd Fungal Genomics, 4th Fumonisin Elimination, and 16th Aflatoxin Elimination Workshop*, Savannah, GA, October 13–15, 2002, Robens, J.F. and Dorner, J.W., Eds., Agricultural Research Service, U.S. Department of Agriculture, Beltsville, MD, 2002, p. 74.

50. Rector, B.G., Snook, M.E., and Widstrom, N.W., Effect of husk characters on resistance to corn earworm (Lepidoptera: Noctuidae) in high-maysin maize populations, *J. Econ. Entomol.*, 95, 1303–1307, 2002.

51. Dowd, P.F. and White, D.G., Corn earworm *Helicoverpa zea* (Boddie) and other insect associated resistance in the maize inbred Tex6, *J. Econ. Entomol.*, 95, 628–634, 2002.

52. Abel, C.A., Abbas, H.K., Zablotowicz, R., Dixon, K., and Pollan, M., Interactions between *Aspergillus flavus* and corn earworm on insect resistant maize, in *Proc. 3rd Fungal Genomics, 4th Fumonisin Elimination, and 16th Aflatoxin Elimination Workshop*, Savannah, GA, October 13–15, 2003, Robens, J.F. and Dorner, J.W., Eds., Agricultural Research Service, U.S. Department of Agriculture, Beltsville, MD, 2003, pp. 113–114.

53. Gradziel, T. and Dandekar, A., Aflatoxin suppression is not associated with gallic acid metabolism in almond through large-scale field trials support effective control through integrated endocarp-kernel based resistance, in *Proc. 3rd Fungal Genomics, 4th Fumonisin Elimination, and 16th Aflatoxin Elimination Workshop*, Savannah, GA, October 13–15, 2003, Robens, J.F. and Dorner, J.W., Eds., Agricultural Research Service, U.S. Department of Agriculture, Beltsville, MD, 2003, p. 64.

54. Wang, Y., Hodges, J.E., Bridges, S.M., Williams, W.P., Brooks, T., Windham, G.L., and Luthe, D.S., An integrated data management system supporting aflatoxin studies, in *Proc. 3rd Fungal Genomics, 4th Fumonisin Elimination, and 16th Aflatoxin Elimination Workshop*, Savannah, GA, October 13–15, 2003, Robens, J.F. and Dorner, J.W., Eds., Agricultural Research Service, U.S. Department of Agriculture, Beltsville, MD, 2003, p. 76.

55. Widstrom, N.W. and Snook, M.E., A gene controlling biosynthesis of isoorientin, a compound in corn silks antibiotic to the corn earworm, *Entomol. Exper. Appl.*, 89, 119–124, 1998.

56. Butron, A., Widstrom, N.W., Snook, M.E., and Wiseman, B.R., Recurrent selection for corn earworm (Lepidoptera: Noctuidae) resistance in three closely related corn southern synthetics, *J. Econ. Entomol.*, 95, 458–462, 2002.

57. Guo, B.Z., Zhang, Z.J., Li, R.G., Widstrom, N.W., Snook, M.E., Lynch, R.E., and Plaisted, D., Restriction fragment length polymorphism markers associated with silk maysin, antibiosis to corn earworm (Lepidoptera: Noctuidae) larvae, in a dent and sweet corn cross, *J. Econ. Entomol.*, 94, 564–571, 2001.

58. Guo, B.Z., Zhang, Z.J., Butron, A., Widstrom, N.W., Snook, M.E., Lynch, R.E., and Plaisted, D., Quantitative effects of loci *p1* and *a1* on the concentrations of maysin, apimaysin, methoxymaysin and chlorogenic acid in maize silk tissue, *MGCN*, 75, 64–66, 2001.

59. Williams, W.P., Davis, F.M., Buckley, P.M., Hedin, P.A., Baker, G.T., and Luthe, D.S., Factors associated with resistance to fall armyworm (Lepidoptera: Noctuidae) and southwestern corn borer (Lepidoptera: Crambidae) in corn at different vegetative stages, *J. Econ. Entomol.*, 91, 1471–1480, 1998.

60. Pechan, T., Cohen, A., Williams, W.P., and Luthe, D.S., Insect feeding metabolizes a unique plant defense protease that disrupts the peritrophic matrix of caterpillar, *Proc. Natl. Acad. Sci. USA*, 99, 13319–13323, 2002.

61. Penchan, T., Jiang, B., Steckler, D., Ye, L., Lin, L., Luthe, D.S., and Williams, W.P., Characterization of three distinct cDNA clones encoding cysteine proteinases from maize (*Zea mays* L.) callus, *Plant Mol. Biol.*, 40, 111–119, 1999.

62. Penchan, T., Ye, L., Chang, Y.M., Mitra, A., Lin, L., Davis, F.M., Williams, W.P., and Luthe, D.S., A unique 33-kD cysteine proteinase accumulates in response to larval feeding in maize genotypes resistant to fall armyworm and other Lepidoptera, *Plant Cell*, 12, 1031–1040, 2000.

63. Dowd, P.F., Examination of an *Aspergillus flavus* resistant inbred of maize for cross-resistance to sap beetle vectors, *Entomol. Exp. Appl.*, 77, 177–180, 1994.

64. Dowd, P.F., Enhanced maize (*Zea mays* L.) pericarp browning: associations with insect resistance and involvement of oxidizing enzymes, *J. Chem. Ecol.*, 20, 2777–2803, 1994.

65. Dowd, P.F. and Lagrimini, L.M., Examination of different tobacco (*Nicotiana* sp.) types under- and overproducing tobacco anionic peroxidase for their leaf resistance to *Helicoverpa zea*, *J. Chem. Ecol.*, 23, 2357–2370, 1997.

66. Dowd, P.F., Lagrimini, L.M., and Herms, D.A., Differential leaf resistance to insects of transgenic sweetgum (*Liquidambar styraciflua*) expressing tobacco anionic peroxidase, *Cell. Mol. Life Sci.*, 54, 712–720, 1998.

67. Dowd, P.F., Lagrimini, L.M., and Nelsen, T.C., Relative resistance of transgenic tomato tissues expressing high levels of tobacco anionic peroxidase to different insect species, *Nat. Toxins*, 6, 241–249, 1998.

68. Privalle, L.S., Estruch, J.J., Wright, M., Hill, M.B., Dowd, P.F., and Lagrimini, L.M., Methods for Conferring Insect Resistance to a Monocot Using a Peroxidase Coding Sequence, U.S. Patent 6,002,068, December 14, 1999.

69. Dowd, P.F., Mehta, A.D., and Boston, R.S., Relative toxicity of the maize endosperm ribosome-inactivating protein to insects, *J. Agric. Food Chem.*, 46, 3775–3779, 1998.

70. Dowd, P.F., Zuo, W.-N., Gillikin, J.W., Johnson, E.T., and Boston, R.S., Enhanced resistance to *Helicoverpa zea* in tobacco expressing an activated form of maize ribosome-inactivating protein, *J. Agric. Food Chem.*, 51, 3568–3574, 2003.

71. Nielsen, K., Payne, G.A., and Boston, R.S., Maize ribosome-inactivating protein inhibits normal development of *Aspergillus nidulans* and *Aspergillus flavus*, *Mol. Plant Microb. Interact.*, 14, 164–172, 2002.

72. Munkvold, G.P., Hellmich, R.L., and Rice, L.G., Comparison of fumonisin concentrations in kernels of transgenic Bt maize hybrids and non-transgenic hybrids, *Plant Dis.*, 83, 130–138, 1999.

73. Clements, M.J., Campbell, K.W., Maragos, C.M., Pilcher, C., Headrick, J.M., Pataky, J.K., and White, D.G., Influence of Cry1Ab protein and hybrid genotype on fumonisin contamination and *Fusarium* ear rot of corn, *Crop Sci.*, 43, 1283–1293, 2003.

74. Schaafsma, A.W., Hooker, D.C., Baute, T.S., and Illincic-Tamburic, L., Effect of Bt-corn hybrids on deoxynivalenol content in grain at harvest, *Plant Dis.*, 86, 1123–1126, 2002.

75. Hammond, B., Campbell, K., Pilcher, C., Degooyer, T., Robinson, A., Rice, L., Pietri, A., Piva, G., Melcion, D., and Cahagnier, B., Reduction of fungal and fumonisin levels in Bt corn, *Mycopathologia*, 155, 22, 2002.

76. Cahagnier, B. and Melcion, D., Mycotoxines de *Fusarium* dans les mais-grains a la recolte: relation entre la presence d'insectes (pyrale, sesamie) et la teneur en mycotoxines, in *Food Safety: Current Situation and Perspectives in the European Community*, Piva, G. and Masoero, F., Eds., Proc. 6th International Feed Production Conference, Piacenza, Italy, November 2000, pp. 237–249.

77. Bakan, B., Melcion, D., Richard-Molard, D., and Cahagnier, B., Fungal growth and *Fusarium* mycotoxin content in isogenic traditional maize and genetically modified maize grown in France and Spain, *J. Agric. Food Chem.*, 50, 728–731, 2002.

78. Pietri, A. and Piva, G., Occurrence and control of mycotoxins in maize grown in Italy, in *Food Safety: Current Situation and Perspectives in the European Community*, Piva, G. and Masoero, F., Eds., Proc. 6th International Feed Production Conference, Trieste, Italy, November 2000, pp. 226–236.

79. Lew, H., Adler, A., and Edinger, W., Moniliformin and the European corn borer (*Ostrinia nubilalis*), *Mycotoxin Res.*, 7, 71–76, 1991.

80. Munkvold, G.P., Hellmich, R.L., and Biggerstaff, C.M., Interaction among *Fusarium verticillioides*, insect pests, and *Aspergillus flavus* in transgenic and conventional maize hybrids, in *Proc. of the 1st Fumonisin Elimination and 13th Aflatoxin Elimination Workshop*, Yosemite, CA, October 25–27, 2000, Robens, J.F., Cary, J.W., and Campbell, B.C., Eds., Agricultural Research Service, U.S. Department of Agriculture, Beltsville, MD, 2000, p. 142.

81. Maupin, L.M., Clements, M.J., Walker, S.L., and White, D.G., Effect of CryIA(b) on *Aspergillus* ear rot and aflatoxin production in commercial corn hybrids, *Mycopathologia*, 155, 106, 2002.

82. Windham, G.L., Williams, W.P., and Davis, F.M., Effects of the southwestern corn borer on *Aspergillus flavus* kernel infection and aflatoxin accumulation in maize hybrids, *Plant Dis.*, 83, 535–540, 1999.

83. Williams, W.P., Windham, G.L., Buckley, P.M., and Daves, C.A., Aflatoxin accumulation in conventional and transgenic corn hybrids infested with southwestern corn borer (Lepidoptera: Crambidae), *J. Agric. Urban Entomol.*, 19, 227–236, 2002.

84. Williams, W.P., Windham, G.L., Buckley, P.M., and Perkins, J.M., Southwestern corn borer damage and aflatoxin accumulation in conventional and transgenic corn hybrids, Field Crop Res., 92, 329–336, 2005.

85. Odvody, G.N. and Chilcutt, C.F., Aflatoxin and insect response in south Texas of near-isogenic corn hybrids with Cry1Ab and Cry2Ab events, *Mycopathologia*, 155, 107, 2002.

86. Odvody, G.N. and Chilcutt, C.F., Aflatoxin and insect response of near-isogenic non-Bt and Cry1A(b) (Mon810 and Bt11) commercial corn hybrids in south Texas in 2001–2002, in *Proc. 3rd Fungal Genomics, 4th Fumonisin Elimination, and 16th Aflatoxin Elimination Workshop*, Savannah, GA, October 13–15, 2003, Robens, J.F. and Dorner, J.W., Eds., Agricultural Research Service, U.S. Department of Agriculture, Beltsville, MD, 2003, p. 120.

87. EPA Scientific Advisory Panel on Issues Pertaining to the Bt Plant Pesticides, *Risk and Benefit Assessments*, http://www.epa.gov/scipoly/sap/2000/october/.

88. Babcock, J., Bing, J., Hyronimus, S., Edwards, J., and Storer, N., Western bean cutworm management with Herculex I hybrid corn, paper presented at the Annual Meeting of the Entomological Society of America, Cincinnati, OH, October 26–29, 2003 (http://esa.confex.com/esa/2002/techprogram/paper_12848.htm).

89. Cotty, P.J., Bock, C., Howelland, D.R., and Tellez, A., Aflatoxin contamination of commercially grown transgenic Bt cottonseed, in *Proc. Beltwide Cotton Conference*, National Cotton Council of America, Memphis, TN, 1997, pp. 108–110.

90. Cotty, P.J., Howell, D.R., Bock, C., and Tellez, A., Aflatoxin contamination of commercially grown transgenic Bt cottonseed, in *Proc. 1997 Aflatoxin Elimination Workshop*, Memphis, TN, October 26–28, 1997, Robens, J.F. and Dorner, J., Eds., Agricultural Research Service, U.S. Department of Agriculture, Beltsville, MD, 1997, p.13

91. Bock, C.H. and Cotty, P.J., The relationship of gin date of aflatoxin contamination of cottonseed in Arizona, *Plant Dis.*, 83, 279–285, 1999.

92. Dandekar, A.M., McGranahan, G.H., Vail, P.V., Uratsu, S.L., Leslie, C.A., and Tebbets, J.S., High levels of expression of full-length *cryIA(c)* gene from *Bacillus thuringiensis* in transgenic somatic walnut embryos, *Plant Sci.*, 131, 181–193, 1998.

93. Dandekar, A.M., McGranahan, G., Vail, P., Molyneux, R., Mahoney, N., Leslie, C., Uratsu, S., and Tebbets, S., Genetic engineering and breeding of walnuts for control of aflatoxin, in *Proc. Aflatoxin/Fumonisin Workshop 2000*, Yosemite, CA, October 25–27, 2000, Robens, J.F., Cary, J.W., and Campbell, B.C., Eds., Agricultural Research Service, U.S. Department of Agriculture, Beltsville, MD, 2000, pp. 108–109.

94. Muir, R., Dandekar, A.M., McGranahan, G., Vail, P., Molyneux, R., Mahoney, N., Leslie, C., Uratsu, S., and Tebbets, S., Genetic engineering and breeding of walnuts for control of aflatoxin, in *Proc. 2nd Fungal Genomics, 3rd Fumonisin Elimination, and 15th Aflatoxin Elimination Workshop*, San Antonio, TX, October 23–25, 2002, Robens, J.F. and Brown, R.L., Eds., Agricultural Research Service, U.S. Department of Agriculture, Beltsville, MD, 2002, p. 79.

95. Ozias-Akins, P., Yang, H., Roberson, E., Akasaka, Y., and Lynch R., Genetic engineering of peanut for reduction of aflatoxin contamination, in *Proc. Aflatoxin/Fumonisin Workshop 2000*, Yosemite, CA, October 25–27, 2000, Robens, J.F., Cary, J.W., and Campbell, B.C., Eds., Agricultural Research Service, U.S. Department of Agriculture Beltsville, MD, 2002, p. 106.

96. Ozias-Akins, P., Yang, H., Perry, E., Akasaka, Y., Niu, C., Holbrook, C., and Lynch, R., Transgenic peanut for preharvest aflatoxin reduction, in *Proc. 1st Fungal Genomics, 2nd Fumonisin Elimination, and 14th Aflatoxin Elimination Workshop*, Robens, J.F. and Riley, R., Eds., Agricultural Research Service, U.S. Department of Agriculture, Beltsville, MD, 2001, p. 141.

97. McMullen, M.D. and Simcox, K.E., Genomic organization of disease and insect resistance genes in maize, *Mol. Plant. Micro. Int.*, 8, 811–815, 1995.

98. Kramer, K.J., Morgan, T.D., Throne, J.E., Dowell, F.E., Bailey, M., and Howard, J.A., Transgenic avidin maize is resistant to storage insect pests, *Nat. Biotechnol.*, 18, 670–674, 2000.

99. Morton, R.L., Schroeder, H.E., Bateman, K.S., Chrispeels, M.J., Armstrong, E., and Higgins, T.J.V., Bean alpha-amylase inhibitor 1 in transgenic peas (*Pisum sativum*) provides complete protection from pea weevil (*Bruchus pisorum*) under field conditions, *Proc. Natl. Acad. Sci. USA*, 97, 3820–3825, 2000.

100. Corbin, D.R., Grebenok, R.J., Ohnmeiss, T.E., Greenplate, J.T., and Purcell, J.P., Expression and chloroplast targeting of cholesterol oxidase in transgenic tobacco plants, *Plant Physiol.*, 126, 1116–1128, 2001.

101. Tattersall, D.B., Bak, S., Jones, P.R., Olsen, C.E., Nielsen, J.K., Hansen, M.L., Hoj, P.B., and Moller, B.L., Resistance to an herbivore through engineered cyanogenic glucoside synthesis, *Science*, 293, 1826–1828, 2001.

102. Thomas, J.C., Adams, D.G., Nessler, C.L., Brown, J.K., and Bohner, H.J., Tryptophane decarboxylase, tryptamine, and reproduction of the whitefly, *Plant Physiol.*, 109, 717–720, 1995.

103. Borevitz, J.O., Xia, Y., Blount, J., Dixon, R.A., and Lamb, C., Activation tagging identifies a conserved MYB regulator of phenylpropanoid biosynthesis, *Plant Cell.*, 12, 2383–2393, 2000.

104. Johnson, E.T. and Dowd, P.F., Differentially enhanced resistance, at a cost, in *Arabidopsis thaliana* constitutively expressing a transcription factor of defensive metabolites, *J. Agric. Food Chem.*, 52, 5135–5138, 2004.

105. Johnson, E.T. and Dowd, P.F., Plant anthocyanin insect feeding deterrents, in *Proc. Meeting of the Phytochemical Society of North America*, Peoria, IL, August 11–13, 2003, Berhow, M.A., Ed., Phytochemical Society of North America, University, MS, 2003, p. 8.

106. Styles, E.D. and Ceska, O., Flavonoid pigments in genetic strains of maize, *Phytochemistry*, 11, 3019–3021, 1972.

107. Sears, M.K., Hellmich, R.L., Stanley-Horn, D.E., Oberhauser, K.S., Pleasants, J.M., Mattila, H.R., Siegfried, B.D., and Dively, G.P., Impact of Bt corn pollen on monarch butterfly populations: a risk assessment, *Proc. Natl. Acad. Sci. USA*, 98, 11937–11942, 2001.

108. Gatehouse, A.M.R., Ferry, N., and Raemaekers, R.J.M., The case of the monarch butterfly: a verdict is returned, *Trends Genet.*, 18, 249–251, 2002.

109. Andow, D.A., Olson, D.M., Hellmich, R.L., Alstad, D.N., and Hutchinson, W.D., Frequency of resistance to *Bacillus thuringiensis* toxin CryIAb in an Iowa population of European corn borer (Lepidoptera: Crambidae), *J. Econ. Entomol.*, 93, 26–30, 2000.

110. Bourguet, D., Chaufaux, J., Seguin, M., Buisson, C., Hinton, J.L., Stodola, T.J., Porter, P., Cronholm, G., Buschman, L.L., and Andow, D.A., Frequency of alleles conferring resistance to Bt maize in French and U.S. corn belt populations of the European corn borer, *Ostrinia nubilalis*, *Theor. Appl. Genet.*, 106, 1225–1233, 2003.

111. Tabashnik, B.E., Patin, A.L., Dennehy, T.J., Liu, Y.B., Carriere, Y., Sims, M.A., and Antilla, L., Frequency of resistance to *Bacillus thuringiensis* in field populations of pink bollworm, *Proc. Natl. Acad. Sci. USA*, 97, 12980–12984, 2001.

112. Tabashnik, B.E., Carriere, Y., Dennehy, T.J., Morin, S., Sisterson, M.S., Roush, R.T., Shelton, A.M., and Zhao, J.-Z., Insects resistance to transgenic Bt crops: lessons from laboratory and field, *J. Econ. Entomol.*, 96, 1031–1038, 2003.

113. Carpenter, J.E. and Gianessi, L.P., *Agricultural Biotechnology: Updated Benefit Estimates*, National Center for Food and Agricultural Policy, Washington, D.C., November 6, 2002 (www.ncfap.org/pub/biotech/updatedbenefits.pdf).
114. Dien, B.S., Bothast, R.J., Iten, L.B., Barrios, L.B., and Eckhoff, S.R., Fate of Bt protein and influence of corn hybrid on ethanol production, *Cereal Chem.*, 79, 582–585, 2002.
115. Folmer, J.D., Grant, R.J., Milton, C.T., and Beck, J., Utilization of Bt corn residues by grazing beef steers and Bt corn silage and grain by growing beef cattle and lactating dairy cows, *J. Animal Sci.*, 80, 1352–1361, 2002.
116. Harper, S.M., Crossland, L.D., and Pascal, E., Female-Preferential Promoters Isolated from Maize and Wheat, U.S. Patent 6,392,123, May 21, 2002.
117. Dowd, P.F., Insect interactions with mycotoxin-producing fungi and their hosts, in *Handbook of Applied Mycology*, Vol. 5, *Mycotoxins in Ecological Systems*, Bhatnagar, D., Lillehoj, E.B., and Arora, D.K., Eds., Marcel Dekker, New York, 1992, pp. 137–155.
118. Bell, E.A., Biochemical mechanisms of disease resistance, *Annu. Rev. Plant Physiol.*, 32, 21–81, 1981.
119. Selitrennikoff, C.P., Antifungal proteins, *Appl. Environ. Microbiol.*, 67, 2883–2894, 2001.
120. Dowd, P.F., A functional approach to more effective multigenic host plant pest resistance, *Mycopathologia*, 155, 46, 2002.
121. Wilson, D.M., Management of mycotoxins in peanut, in *Peanut Health Management*, Melouk, H.A. and Shokes, F.M., Eds., American Phytopathological Society, St. Paul, MN, 1995, pp. 87–92.
122. Dowd, P.F., Reliability of a computer program for predicting mycotoxin levels in midwestern USA corn, in *Proceedings of the XI International IUPAC Symposium on Mycotoxins and Phycotoxins*, Bethesda, MD, May 17–21, 2004, Park, D.L., Ed., National Institute of Health, Bethesda, MD, 2004, p. 102.
123. Widstrom, N.W., Lamb, M.C., and Williams, R.G., Economic input for an "expert management system" to minimize risk of aflatoxin contamination of maize, in *Proc. Aflatoxin/Fumonisin Workshop 2000*, Yosemite, CA, October 25–27, 2000, Robens, J.F., Cary, J.W., and Campbell, B.C., Eds., Agricultural Research Service, U.S. Department of Agriculture, Beltsville, MD, 2000, p. 64.
124. Widstrom, N.W., Lamb, M., and Johnson, J., Corn aflatoxin management system (CAMS): assessing risks and a timeline for completion, *Mycopathologia*, 155, 47, 2002.

26 Chemical Detoxification of Aflatoxins in Food and Feeds

Joan M. King and Alfredo D. Prudente, Jr.

CONTENTS

26.1 INTRODUCTION

Aflatoxins are a group of mycotoxins that are produced primarily by *Aspergillus flavus* Link ex Fries and *Aspergillus parasiticus* Speare. Fungi producing aflatoxin can affect crops such as corn, cottonseed, and groundnuts and can infect or spread while the crops are in the field or while the products are stored. Aflatoxins, particularly aflatoxin B_1, have been a focus of much attention because of their acute toxicity and carcinogenicity. Aside from their carcinogenic potential, aflatoxins cause significant economic losses to agriculture. Direct economic losses due to aflatoxins include reduced crop yields and lower quality, reduced animal performance and reproduction capabilities, and increased incidence of diseases.[1] It has been estimated that the annual costs related to mycotoxins for crop loss, research, and monitoring range from $0.5 million to over $1.5 billion a year in the United States alone.[2] Further, it is estimated that the annual losses associated with mycotoxins in the feed and livestock industries are of the order of $5 billion in the United States and Canada.[3] The best way to control aflatoxin contamination would be prevention, if economically feasible;[4] however, prevention is not always possible for certain agronomic and storage practices.[5] When contamination has occurred, alternative measures must be implemented to reduce exposure risks to these toxins. Some current practices of detoxifying aflatoxin-contaminated products involve physical, biological, and chemical methods.[6] This chapter focuses on an overview of the chemical methods used to decontaminate products after harvest.

26.2 CHEMICAL DETOXIFICATION

Chemical detoxification of aflatoxins in food is currently one of the practical post-harvest approaches. Some chemicals that have been investigated as potential agents for the degradation of aflatoxins include acids and bases, bisulfites, chlorinating compounds, and oxidizing agents.

26.2.1 ACID TREATMENT

Strong acids convert aflatoxin to its hemiacetal form through hydration.[7] Pons et al.[8] studied acid conversion of AFB_1 and AFG_1 to AFB_{2a} and AFG_{2a}, respectively, forms that are much less toxic. They found that the rate of conversion increased as the pH decreased or the temperature increased. It was also observed that AFB_2 and AFG_2 were less susceptible to acid degradation than AFB_1 and AFG_1. The effectiveness of acids to degrade aflatoxins was demonstrated in naturally contaminated peanut meal. The addition of 3-M hydrochloric acid during the manufacture of hydrolyzed vegetable proteins in a reactor with steam at 129°C and 160 kPa totally degraded aflatoxins without the production of toxic or mutagenic compounds.[9] In another study, 5-N hydrochloric acid completely destroyed aflatoxin B_1 in peanut flour at 100°C in sealed culture tubes placed in an oil bath.[10] Both studies show that an aflatoxin-free hydrolyzed vegetable protein could be made from aflatoxin-contaminated peanuts under certain conditions. Not all acids are as effective in destroying aflatoxin-contaminated commodities. Addition of citric acid to milk, prior to ultra-filtration or diafiltration, did not enhance the removal of aflatoxin M_1.[11] At a concentration of 3 N, salicylic, sulfamic, and sulfosalicylic acids reduced 1-ppm AFB_1 by 90% in 25% moisture sorghum stored for 72 hours at 25°C in cotton-stoppered Erlenmeyer flasks.[12] In the same study, a concentration of 5-N anthranilic, benzoic, boric, oxalic, and propionic acids also reduced 1-ppm AFB_1 by 90% or more in sorghum. Although treatment with strong acids has been shown to effectively degrade AFB_1, acid treatment has little or no effect on AFB_2 or AFG_2, and AFB_{2a} is still toxic.

26.2.2 ALKALINE TREATMENT WITH HYDROXIDE

Several studies have shown that alkali treatment, using inorganic or organic bases, is an effective and economically feasible method of degrading aflatoxins. Alkalis cause the hydrolysis of the lactone ring in AFB_1; however, evidence suggests that the hydrolyzed lactone ring can close again under acidic conditions and regenerate back to AFB_1. Alkaline treatments have been studied for the destruction of aflatoxins because of the conditions used during the making of tortillas from corn. Treatment of corn with less than 0.5% calcium hydroxide decreased aflatoxin levels by 43%. Reversion tests with acid treatment resulted in conversion back to the original concentration.[13] Higher levels of calcium hydroxide did not improve aflatoxin degradation and resulted in a less sensory acceptable product that broke easily and had too strong of an alkaline flavor.[14] Typical conditions of nixtamalization only raise pH levels in corn products to about 7.0. At these pH levels, the aflatoxin detoxification process can be reversed by acid treatment, resulting in the original AFB_1 structure being reformed.[15] Boiling 1600-ppb naturally contaminated corn with 3% NaOH at 100°C for 4 minutes decreased total AFB_1 and AFB_2 levels by 93%.[16] A reversion level of 18% back to the original AFB_1 structure was observed after treatment with acid. Further heat processing by autoclaving and deep frying at 196°C for 15 minutes to make a corn snack resulted in a product with acceptable levels of less than 20 ppb of aflatoxin for human food and nondetectable mutagenicity.[4] An earlier study used a combination of 2% calcium hydroxide based on sample weight followed by 0.5% methylamine to decontaminate peanut meal with aflatoxin levels of 400 ppb and found that the level was reduced to acceptable standards with no reversion.[17] A study was conducted to determine the effects of nixtamalization on decontamination of corn co-contaminated with aflatoxin and fumonisin. Nixtamalization alone resulted in aflatoxin levels being decreased from 300 ppb to 5 ppb, and complete decontamination was achieved when combined with ammonium hydroxide.[18] Fumonisin levels were reduced by 100% using this procedure, but it was not known whether the reduction was due to loss in the water soaking step or if chemical modification occurred. Extracts of tortillas made with the nixtamalized corn from the same study did not show teratogenic effects by the avian embryo assay,[18] but mixed results were found in the mutagenicity assay by the Ames test.[19]

26.2.3 BISULFITE TREATMENT

Bisulfite is a highly reactive chemical that is commonly used in some foods and beverages because of its ability to inhibit both enzymatic and nonenzymatic browning, to inhibit growth of many microorganisms, and to act as an antioxidant and a reducing agent. Bisulfite has also been tested for its ability to degrade aflatoxin. Sodium bisulfite was hypothesized to react with the double bond on position 8,9 of the terminal furan ring to make it more water soluble. Aflatoxin B_2 does not have this double bond; hence, degradation by bisulfite is not possible. The formation of sodium sulfonate (B_1S) was confirmed to be the major reaction product of aflatoxin with sulfonic acid.[20,21] Aflatoxin B_1 was completely destroyed after soaking corn with aflatoxin levels in excess of 1900 ppb in 10% sodium bisulfite for 72 hours followed by filtering, drying, and incubation at 50°C for 21 days.[22] Moisture, sodium bisulfite level, time, and temperature have significant effects on AFB_1 degradation whereas AFB_2 is not affected. Doyle and Marth[23] observed that the presence of citric acid or methanol decreased the rate at which sodium bisulfite destroyed aflatoxins in a pH 5.5 buffered system. For aflatoxin levels of about 235 ppb in corn, lower concentrations of 0.5% and 1% sodium bisulfite were more effective at destroying AFB_1 than NaOH or aqueous ammonia at the same level, while at 2% NaOH or aqueous ammonia were more effective than bisulfite.[24] When figs contaminated with

250 ppb AFB_1 were treated with 0.2% hydrogen peroxide minutes before a 1% bisulfite treatment, 57% more AFB_1 was destroyed in 72 hours at 25°C than with bisulfite alone.[25] Treatment of naturally contaminated groundnut cake with sodium bisulfite and sodium hydroxide separately decreased aflatoxin levels for up to 24 hours of storage, but samples showed an increase in total aflatoxin content after 10 and 20 days of storage at ambient temperature, most likely due to regrowth of fungus seen at longer time periods.[26] Treatment of *Aspergillus flavus* inoculated groundnut cake with 1% sodium bisulfite at 10% moisture completely inhibited mold growth and aflatoxin production at room temperature.[27]

26.2.4 HYPOCHLORITE TREATMENT

Aqueous chlorine is used in the food industry in disinfecting food processing equipment and to wash a variety of raw materials including fruits, nut meats, and meat prior to processing.[5] Chlorine is also used in the flour industry as a bleaching and an oxidizing agent.[28] Sodium hypochlorite was more effective in reducing fluorescence detection of AFB_1 at concentrations much lower (4.6 to 22% aqueous solution) than those required for sodium hydroxide or ammonium hydroxide.[29] It was not possible to measure toxicity by the Ames or brine shrimp assays due to the toxicity of the sodium hypochlorite to the organisms. Sodium hydroxide and ammonium hydroxide reduced mutagenicity of pure AFB_1 and decreased the toxicity to brine shrimp.[29] Soaking of parboiled rice in water was observed to increase AFB_1 levels, but the addition of 10 ppm calcium hypochlorite significantly reduced AFB_1 levels.[30] Hypochlorous acid was shown to be more effective than sodium hypochlorite in degrading AFB_1 and reducing mutagenicity due to oxidation through the OH radical.[31]

26.2.5 AMMONIATION TREATMENT

Chemical inactivation by ammoniation has achieved widespread use and acceptance by the corn production industry.[32–35] Lee et al.[36] showed that 4% ammonia treatment of AFB_1 on silica gel in a pressurized chamber at 40 psi and 100°C for 30 minutes could degrade 99% of pure AFB_1, but two new compounds with molecular weights of 286 and 206 were formed. Solvent fractions showed 2000 to 20,000 times less toxicity than that with the untreated AFB_1.[37] Solvent fractionation of a nonammoniated cottonseed meal found 90% of radiolabeled product in the methylene chloride fraction, whereas in the ammoniated meal only 25% was found in the methylene chloride fraction.[38] About 19% of the radiolabeled product was found in the pronase digestion fraction of the ammoniated meal, indicating that protein bound the radiolabeled product. Analysis of these fractions showed that products formed by ammoniation treatment of aflatoxin-contaminated cottonseed had little to no Ames test mutagenic potential.[39] The enzymatic digestion was the only fraction showing mutagenicity at higher concentrations. For the enzymatic digestion fraction to show a mutagenic response, 36,000 times the concentration of untreated AFB_1 was required.

Similar studies were completed with corn meal treated with 2% ammonia at 45°C for 60 minutes at a pressure of 55 psi. The methylene chloride, sodium hydroxide, and proteolytic enzyme digestion fractions contained about 19% each of ammoniation products, whereas the methanol fraction contained about 13% of the products.[33] The differences in the concentrations of products found in the various fractions between ammoniated cottonseed and corn was hypothesized to be due to the different matrices or the different bases used for extraction or the ammoniation conditions. Copra contaminated with 500-ppb AFB_1 could be detoxified by 1.5% ammonium hydroxide at a moisture content of 20% in 5 days to levels below 20 ppb with no reversion back to the parent compound.[40] Another study indicated that the moisture content of the aflatoxin-contaminated corn and the holding temperature during ammoniation were the most important factors for decontamination.[41] Higher temperature and moistures (121°C and 16%) were more efficient, as corn could be 99% decontaminated under these conditions. The products were also shown to be quite stable to stomach acidity, as less than 0.05% of the product reverted back to aflatoxin under those conditions.

A commercial-scale study showed that aflatoxin-contaminated cottonseed meal could be 97% detoxified with a treatment of 1% ammonia at 99°C and 0.7 bar steam pressure without affecting the quality of the meal.[42] One study showed that 2% ammonium persulfate could degrade AFB_1 in corn without affecting production of ethanol during fermentation.[43] Addition of benzoyl peroxide could enhance the decontamination and ethanol production. More detailed information on reducing aflatoxin hazards through ammoniation has been reviewed by Park and Price.[44]

26.2.6 OZONATION

Ozone is becoming a widely used replacement for chlorine-based chemicals for sanitation purposes in food processing, especially in the meat industry and for water quality purposes, such as bacterial, odor, pesticide, and hazardous compound degradation. Ozonation may now be a useful process in the decontamination of grains containing aflatoxin. Compared to ammoniation treatment at $20/ton, decontamination with ozonation is estimated to cost only about $4 per ton (Lynntech, Inc., pers. comm.).

Early studies showed that aflatoxin-contaminated cottonseed and peanut meal ozonated at high moisture (30%) and temperature (100°C) for 2 hours could completely degrade AFB_1 levels, but 9% of the original AFB_2 remained.[45] The treated peanut meal was fed to ducklings at 60% of their diet and was found to result in ducklings with lower body weights than those fed aflatoxin-contaminated meal.[46] Lower protein efficiency ratios were also found with the ozone-treated meal, when compared with aflatoxin-contaminated corn. These results indicated that, although most of the aflatoxin was no longer detected in the meal, either a destruction of essential nutrients or production of new toxins occurred.

Maeba et al.[47] studied the ozonation of individual 5% solutions of pure AFB_1, AFB_2, AFG_1, and AFG_2. Aflatoxin B_2 and G_2 were more resistant than AFB_1 and AFG_1 to oxidation by ozone and required higher concentrations and longer times for oxidation. Ozone-treated aflatoxins were not toxic, as shown by the chick embryo assay. Ozonated AFB_1 and AFG_1 were not mutagenic, as determined by the Ames test.[47] Ozonation was also shown to destroy the immunity-impairing activity of AFB_1.[48] Each of the above-mentioned studies utilized ozone produced by electric (corona) discharge.

A new ozonation process was developed as a potential procedure for the decontamination of aflatoxin in grains, which could then be utilized in animal feeds. This method differs from conventional methods, which utilize oxygen and corona discharge for ozone production, because it produces ozone through the use of water and an electrolysis cell.[49] Recent experiments with 30-kg batches of corn kernels have shown that aflatoxin could be reduced by 95% in corn samples treated with this ozonation process for 92 hours at a flow rate of 200 mL/min of 12 wt% ozone gas.[49] Turkey poults fed ozone-treated corn, ground and mixed with soybean meal, did not differ from controls in weight gain, liver weight, and blood chemistry, whereas those fed aflatoxin-contaminated grain did differ negatively.[49] The results were the same whether the treated corn was previously contaminated or uncontaminated. This indicates that no harmful compounds are formed by the ozonation process, but this finding has not been proven, and the long-term effects, such as mutagenicity of ozonated corn, have not been tested. Ozonation has, therefore, not yet been fully proven to be a safe and effective method for decontamination of aflatoxin-contaminated grains.

Aflatoxin-free (clean corn) and naturally contaminated corn, with and without ozone treatment, were analyzed for their concentration of AFB_1. Results of the analysis showed that untreated and ozone-treated clean corn contained less than 2 parts per billion (ppb) AFB_1, while 48 ppb and 587 ppb were detected in ozone-treated and untreated contaminated corn, respectively.[50] This reduction in AFB_1 concentration in contaminated corn represents about a 92% reduction. This result indicates that the application of ozone (10 to 12 wt%) could effectively reduce aflatoxin levels in contaminated corn. Results of the study showed no reversion of inactivated aflatoxin to the parent compound. The initial level of 47 ppb AFB_1 in the ozone-treated contaminated sample was further reduced to about 29 ppb after exposure to an acidic environment. The acid treatment leads to hydration of AFB_1 at the 8,9-olefinic bond of the terminal furan ring to form AFB_{2a}, which has a toxicity of less than 1/200 that of AFB_1.[5] Hexane extracts consistently lowered the mutagenic potential of pure AFB_1.[50] This result confirmed the presence of materials in crude corn extracts that interfered with the mutagenic activity of aflatoxin. In addition, it was observed that the extract from ozone-treated contaminated corn had less inhibitory effect compared to other extracts. This result might be an indication that the ozonation process has produced reaction products that have mutagenic potentials. It is also possible that the ozonation process might have destroyed the natural mutagen inhibitors in contaminated corn. For naturally contaminated corn, treatment with ozone resulted in an increase in palmitic acid from 15.8 to 18.2% and a decrease in linoleic acid from 58.7 to 56.2%.[50] After ozonation, the percentage of unsaturated fatty acid in contaminated sample was significantly reduced from 82.0 to 79.1%.

Aikawa and Komatsu,[51] Aikawa,[52] and Ho et al.[53] reported the antimutagenic effects of linoleic acid in the *Salmonella* mutagenicity assay. Aikawa and Komatsu[51] reported the mutagenic activity of autoxidized linoleic (peroxide value [POV] = 1482 mEq/kg) and oleic (POV = 690 mEq/kg) acids. Malonaldehyde has been found to react with DNA to cause mutation.[51,54,55] Studies conducted by Smith et al.[56] and Benamira et al.[57] showed that acrolein is mutagenic in the V79 and Ames assays, respectively. Medina et al.[58] identified acrolein from the ozone oxidation of unsaturated fatty acids.

26.3 NATURAL INHIBITION

An antimutagenic factor was found in corn. Extracts of ammoniated and nonammo-niated corn, which had been naturally contaminated with aflatoxin or which was aflatoxin free, did not show mutagenicity by the Ames test.[32] Methylene chloride extracts from ammoniated aflatoxin-free corn that was then spiked with aflatoxin also showed no mutagenic potential. Only pure aflatoxin B_1 showed mutagenicity; therefore, the results indicated no differences between pure aflatoxins and naturally contaminated corn in mutagenic potential. It was hypothesized that antimutagenic compounds in the corn may have been bound to the aflatoxin after ammoniation or were extracted together with aflatoxin by methylene chloride.[32]

Burgos-Hernandez[59] also found an antimutagenic factor in contaminated corn that was not seen in the pure aflatoxin B_1 control. An attempt was made to isolate and identify the antimutagenic compounds. These compounds were separated from the aflatoxin B_1 by thin-layer chromatography. The antimutagenic compounds were shown to have a dose–response relationship, were intrinsic to the corn not the fungi, and were linoleic acid like, as determined by mass spectroscopy.[59]

Further research was done on aflatoxin and fumonisin co-contaminated corn. Treatments of corn with 3% hydrogen peroxide and 2% sodium bicarbonate were effective in reducing toxin levels without producing mutagenic products as measured by the Ames test using tester strain TA-100.[60] *Fusarium moniliforme* was shown to either inhibit aflatoxin formation by *Aspergillus flavus* or enhance its degradation in mixed cultures of these fungi. A dose–response relationship between fumonisin and aflatoxin was also observed. Fumonisin, up to 1×10^2 ng/plate, acted as an anti-mutagen to 1×10^3 ng/plate of aflatoxin in the Ames assay, whereas higher levels of fumonisin resulted in increased or original levels of mutagenicity.[60] The interaction between these compounds may be chemical or fumonisin could be interfering with an enzyme system in the xenobiotic activation/deactivation pathways.

Many phytochemicals in vegetables and fruits have been isolated and identified as agents that can block different stages in the carcinogenic process in several animal models.[61] In addition to minimizing the formation of aflatoxin, these compounds mitigate the toxic or mutagenic effects of aflatoxin.[62–64] Norton[65] reported that pure, β-carotene and lutein reduced the mutagenic effect of aflatoxin to 2%. In addition, Mejia et al.[66] reported that pure lutein and xanthophylls from Aztec Marigold inhib-ited the mutagenic potential of AFB_1 in the Ames assay using tester strains TA-98 and TA-100. Furthermore, Rauscher et al.[67] found that carotenoids extracted from fruits and vegetables inhibited (<20%) the mutagenicity induced by AFB_1 in the Ames assay using both TA-98 and TA-100 tester strains.

26.4 SUMMARY

Chemical detoxification of aflatoxins in foods and feeds is important as a short-term postharvest solution to the problem. Although there are many chemicals methods, ammoniation is still the most utilized approved method for decontamination. New methods such as ozonation treatment do show promise, but require further testing for safety and scalability. With any chemical method, studies must be done to determine if new toxins are formed as a result of the treatment. It is also important to determine whether the treatment will alter the functional and nutritional characteristics of the products.

REFERENCES

1. Smith, J.E., Aflatoxins, in *Handbook of Plant and Fungal Toxicants*, Felix, J.P., Ed., CRC Press, Boca Raton, FL, 1997, pp. 269–285.

2. Rubens, J. and Cardwell, K., The cost of mycotoxins management to the USA: management of aflatoxins in the United States, *J. Toxicol. Toxin Rev.*, 22(2–3), 139–152, 2003.

3. Coker, R.D., The chemical detoxification of aflatoxin-contaminated animal feed, in *Natural Toxicants in Food*, Watson, D., Ed., Sheffielf Academic Press, Kent, 1998, pp. 284–298.

4. Park, D.L., Perspectives on mycotoxin decontamination procedures, *Food Addit. Contam.*, 10, 49–60, 1993.

5. Samarajeewa, U., Sen, A.C., Cohen, M.D., and Wei, C.I., Detoxification of aflatoxins in foods and feeds by physical and chemical methods, *J. Food Protect.*, 53(6), 489–501, 1990.

6. Park, D.L., Controlling aflatoxin in food and feed, *Food Technol.*, 10, 92–96, 1993.

7. Ellis, W.O., Smith, J.P., Simpson, B.K., and Oldham, J.H., Aflatoxins in food: occurrence, biosynthesis, effects on organisms, detection, and method of control, *CRC Crit. Rev. Food Sci. Nutr.*, 30(3), 403–439, 1991.

8. Pons, Jr., W.A., Cucullu, A.F., Lee, L.S., and Janssen, H.J., Kinetic study of acid-catalyzed conversion of aflatoxins B_1 and G_1 to B_{2a} and G_{2a}, *J. AOCS*, 49, 124–128, 1972.

9. Williams, K.R. and Dutton, M.F., Destruction of aflatoxin during the production of hydrolysed vegetable protein, *J. Food Prot.*, 51, 887–891, 1988.

10. Wattanapat, R. Nakayama, T., and Beuchat, L.R., Characteristics of acid hydrolysate from defatted peanut flour, *J. Food Sci.*, 60, 443–445, 1995.

11. Higuera-Ciapara, I. Esqueda-Valle, M., and Nieblas, J., Reduction of aflatoxin M_1 from artificially contaminated milk using ultrafiltration and diafiltration, *J. Food Sci.*, 60, 645–647, 1995.

12. Hasan, H.A.H., Destruction of aflatoxin B_1 on sorghum grain with acids, salts and ammonia derivatives, *Crypogamie Mycol.*, 17, 129–134, 1996.

13. Price, R.L. and Jorgensen, K.V., Effects of processing on aflatoxin levels and on mutagenic potential of tortillas made from naturally contaminated corn, *J. Food Sci.*, 50, 347–357, 1985.

14. Carmen de Arriola, M., Porres, E., Cabrera, S., Zepeda, M., and Rolz, C., Aflatoxin fate during alkaline cooking of corn for tortilla preparation, *J. Agric. Food Chem.*, 36, 530–533, 1988.

15. Torres, P. Gomez-Ortiz, M., and Ramirez-Weng, B., Revising the role of pH and thermal treatments in aflatoxin content reduction during the tortilla and deep frying processes, *J. Agric. Food Chem.*, 49, 2825–2829, 2001.

16. Camou-Arriola, J.P. and Price, R.L., Destruction of aflatoxin and reduction of mutagenicity of naturally contaminated corn during production of a corn snack, *J. Food Prot.*, 52, 814–817, 1989.

17. Park, D.L. et al., Decontamination of aflatoxin contaminated peanut meal using monoethylamine:Ca(OH)$_2$, *J. AOCS*, 12, 995A–1002A, 1981.

18. Trujillo, S., Reduction and Management of Risks Associated with Aflatoxin and Fumonisin Contamination in Corn, Ph.D. dissertation, Louisiana State University, Baton Rouge, LA, 1997.

19. Ames, B.N., McCann, J., and Yamasaki, E., Methods for detecting carcinogens and mutagens with the *Salmonella*/mammalian-microsome mutagenicity test, *Mutation Res.*, 31, 347–356, 1975.

20. Hagler, W.M., Hutchins, J.E., and Hamilton, P.B., Destruction of aflatoxin B_1 with sodium bisulfite: isolation of the major product aflatoxin B_1S, *J. Food Prot.*, 46, 295–300, 1983.

21. Yagen, B., Hutchins, J.E., Cox, R.H., Hagler, W.M., and Hamilton, P.B., Aflatoxin B_1S: revised structure for the sodium bisulfonate formed by destruction of aflatoxin B_1 with sodium bisulfite, *J. Food Prot.*, 52, 574–577, 1989.

22. Hagler, Jr., W.M.. Hutchins, J.E., and Hamilton, P.B.. Destruction of aflatoxin in corn with sodium bisulfite, *J. Food Protect.*, 45, 1287–1291, 1982.

23. Doyle, M.P. and Harth, E.H., Bisulfite degrades aflatoxin: effect of citric acid and methanol and possible mechanism of degradation, *J. Food Prot.*, 41, 891–896, 1978.

24. Moerck, K.E. McElfresh, P. Wohlman, A., and Hilton, B.W., Aflatoxin destruction in corn using sodium bisulfate, sodium hydroxide and aqueous ammonia, *J. Food Prot.*, 43, 571–574, 1980.

25. Altug, T., Yousef, A.E., and Martin, E.H., Degradation of aflatoxin B_1 in dried figs by sodium bisulfite with or without heat, ultraviolet energy or hydrogen peroxide, *J. Food Prot.*, 53, 581–582, 628, 1990.

26. Ghosh, M.K. and Chhabra, A., Aflatoxin detoxification in naturally contaminated groundnut cake, *Indian J. Animal Nutr.*, 1995, 12, 105–107.

27. Ghosh, M.K., Chhabra, A., Atreja, P.P., and Chopra, R.C., Effect of treating with propionic acid, sodium bisulfite and sodium hydroxide on the biosynthesis of aflatoxin on groundnut cake, *Animal Feed Sci. Technol.*, 60, 43–49, 1996.

28. Wei, C.I., Cook, D.L., and Kirk, J.R., Use of chlorine compounds in the food industry, *Food Technol.*, 39, 107–115, 1985.

29. Draughon, F.A. and Childs, E.A., Chemical and biological evaluation of aflatoxin after treatment with sodium hypochlorite, sodium hydroxide and ammonium hydroxide, *J. Food Prot.*, 45, 703–706, 1982.

30. Bandara, J.M.R.S., Vithanege, A.K., and Bean, G.A., Effect of parboiling and bran removal on aflatoxin levels in Sri Lankan rice, *Mycopathologia*, 115, 31–35, 1991.

31. Suzuki, T., Noro, T., Kawamura, Y., Fukunaga, K., Watanabe, M., Ohta, M., Sugiue, H., Sato, Y., Kohno, M., and Hotta, K., Decontamination of aflatoxin forming fungus and elimination of aflatoxin mutagenicity with electrolyzed NaCl anode solution, *J. Agric. Food Chem.*, 50, 633–641, 2002.

32. Weng, C.Y., Martinez, A.J., and Park, D.L., Anti-aflatoxin mutagenic factors in corn, *Food Addit. Contamin.*, 14, 269–279, 1997.

33. Martinez, A.J., Weng, C.Y., and Park, D.L., Distribution of ammonia/aflatoxin reaction products in corn following exposure to ammonia decontamination procedure, *Food Addit. Contamin.*, 11(6), 649–658, 1994.

34. Park, D.L., Lee, L.S., Price, R.L., and Pohland, A.E., Review of the decontamination of aflatoxins by ammoniation: current status and regulation, *J. AOCS*, 71(4), 685–703, 1988.

35. Park, D.L. and Njapau, H., Aflatoxin contamination issues, technology, *J. AOCS*, 66, 1402–1407, 1989.

36. Lee, L.S. Koltun, S.P., and Stanley, J.B., Ammoniation of aflatoxin B_1 in a pressure chamber used to decontaminate toxin containing cottonseed meal, *J. AOCS*, 61, 1607–1608, 1984.

37. Haworth, S.R., Lawlor, T.E., Zeiget, E., Lee, L.S., and Park, D.L., Mutagenic potential of ammonia related aflatoxin reaction products in a model system, *J. AOCS*, 66, 102–104, 1989.

38. Park, D.L., Lee, L., and Koltun, S.A., Distribution of ammonia-related aflatoxin reaction products in cottonseed meal, *J. AOCS*, 61, 1071–1074, 1984.

39. Lawlor, T.E., Hayworth, S.R., Zeigler, E., Park, D.L., and Lee, L., Mutagenic potential of ammoniation-related aflatoxin reaction-products isolated from cottonseed meal, *J. AOCS*, 62, 1136–1138, 1985.

40. Mercado, C.J., Real, M.P.N., and Del Rosario, R.R., Chemical detoxification of aflatoxin containing copra, *J. Food Sci.*, 56, 733–735, 1991.

41. Weng, C.Y., Martinez, A.J., and Park, D.L., Efficacy and permanency of ammonia treatment in reducing aflatoxin levels in corn, *Food Addit. Contamin.*, 11, 649–658, 1994.

42. Ahmed, M.A. Shamsudding, Z.A., and Khan, B.A., Elimination of naturally occurring aflatoxins in cottonseed meal, *Pak, J. Sci. Ind. Res.*, 39, 183–185, 1996.

43. Burgos-Hernandez, A., Price, R.L. Jorgensen-Kornman, K., Lopez-Garcia, R., Njapau, H., and Park, D.L., Decontamination of aflatoxin B_1 contaminated corn by ammoniation persulphate during fermentation, *J. Sci. Food Agric.*, 82, 546–552, 2002.

44. Park, D.L. and Price, R.L., Reduction of aflatoxin hazards using ammoniation, *Rev. Environ. Contamin. Toxicol.*, 136, 4816, 2001.

45. Dwarakanath, C.T., Rayner, E.T., Mann, G.E., and Dollear, F.G., Reduction of aflatoxin levels in cottonseed and peanut meals by ozonation, *J. AOCS*, 45, 93–95, 1968.

46. Dollear, F.G., Mann, G.E., Codifer, L.P., Gardner, H.K., Koltun, S.P., and Vix, H.L.E., Elimination of aflatoxins from peanut meal, *J. AOCS*, 45, 862–865, 1968.

47. Maeba, H., Takamoto, Y., Kamimura, M., and Miura, T., Destruction and detoxification of aflatoxins with ozone, *J. Food Sci.*, 53, 667–668, 1988.

48. Chatterjee, D. and Mukherjee, S.K., Destruction of phagocytosis-suppressing activity of aflatoxin B_1 by ozone, *Lett. Appl. Microbiol.*, 17, 52–54, 1993.

49. McKenzie, K.S., Kubena, L.F., Denvir, A.J., Rogers, T.D., Hitchens, G.D., Bailey, R.H., Harvey, R.B., Buckley, S.A., and Phillips, T.D., Aflatoxicosis in turkey poults is prevented by treatment of naturally contaminated corn with ozone generated by electrolysis, *Poultry Sci.*, 77, 1094–1102, 1998.

50. Prudente, A.D. and King, J.M., Efficacy and safety evaluation of ozonation to degrade aflatoxin in corn, *J. Food Sci.*, 67(8), 2866–2872, 2002.

51. Aikawa K. and Komatsu Y., Antimutagenic effects of autoxidized linoleic and oleic acids on UV-induced mutagenesis in *Escherichia coli*, *Agric. Biol. Chem.*, 51(10), 2717–2720, 1987.

52. Aikawa K., Effect of s-9 mix on antimutagenic activity of autoxidized linoleic acid, *Agric. Biol. Chem.*, 52(8), 2115–2116, 1988.

53. Ho, K.I., Sook, C.H., and Wha, M.T., Constituents of antimutagenic factor from brown rice, *Agric. Chem. Biotechnol.*, 38(5), 478–483, 1995.

54. Dennis K.J. and Shibamoto T., Gas chromatographic analysis of reactive carbonyl compounds formed from lipids upon UV-irradiation, *Lipids*, 25(8), 460–464, 1990.

55. Plastaras, J.P., Riggins, J.N., Otteneder, M., and Marnett, L.J., Reactivity and mutagenicity of endogenous DNA oxopropenylating agents: base propenals, malondialdehyde, and nepsilon-oxopropenyllysine, *Chem. Res. Toxicol.*, 13(12), 1235–1242, 2000.

56. Smith, R.A., Cohen, S.M., and Lawson, T.A., Acrolein mutagenicity in the V79 assay, *Carcinogenesis (Lond.)*, 11(3), 497–498, 1990.

57. Benamira, M. and Marnett, L.J., The lipid peroxidation product 4-hydroxynonenal is a potent inducer of the SOS response, *Mutat. Res.*, 293(1), 1–10, 1992.

58. Medina, N.R., Mercado, P.E., Hernandez, P.O., and Hicks, J.J., Identification of acrolein from the ozone oxidation of unsaturated fatty acids, *Hum. Exp. Toxic.*, 18(11),677–682, 1999.

59. Burgos-Hernandez, A., Evaluation of Chemical Treatments and Intrinsic Factors that Affect the Mutagenic Potential of Aflatoxin B_1-Contaminated Corn, Ph.D. dissertation, Louisiana State University, Baton Rouge, LA, 1998, 201 pp.

60. Lopez-Garcia, R., Aflatoxin B_1 and Fumonisin B_1 Co-Contamination: Interactive Effects, Possible Mechanisms of Toxicity, and Decontamination Procedures, Ph.D. dissertation, Louisiana State University, Baton Rouge, LA, 1998.

61. Huang, M.T., Ferraro, T., and Ho, C.T., Cancer chemoprevention by phytochemicals in fruits and vegetables: an overview, in *Food Phytochemicals for Cancer Prevention I. Fruits and Vegetables*, Huang, M.T., Osawa, T., Ho, C.T., and Rosen, R.T., Eds., ACS Symposium Series 546, American Chemical Society, Washington, D.C., 1994.

62. Gasiorowski, K., Szyba, K., Brokos, B., and Kozubek, A., Antimutagenic activity of alkylresorcinols from cereal grains, *Cancer Lett.*, 106, 109–115, 1996.

63. Kriskova, L., Nagy, M., Polonyi, J., and Ebringer, L., The effect of flavanoids on ofloxacin induced mutagenicity in *Euglena gracilis*, *Mutation Res.*, 414, 85–92, 1998.

64. Masuda, T., Hidaka, K., Shinohara, A., Maekawa, T., Takeda, Y., and Yamaguchi, H., Chemical studies on antioxidant mechanism of curcuminoid analysis of radical reaction products from curcumin, *J. Agric. Food Chem.*, 47, 71–77, 1999.

65. Norton, R.A., Effects of carotenoids on aflatoxin B_1 synthesis by *Aspergillus flavus*, *Phytopathology*, 87(8), 815–821, 1997.

66. Mejia, E.G., Piña, G.L., and Gomez, M.R., Antimutagenic activity of natural xanthophylls against aflatoxin B_1 in *Salmonella typhimurium*, *Environ. Mol. Mutagen.*, 30, 346–353, 1997.

67. Rauscher, R., Edenharder, R., and Platt, K.L., *In vitro* antimutagenic and *in vivo* anticlastogenic effects of carotenoids and solvent extracts from fruits and vegetables rich in carotenoids, *Mutat. Res.*, 413, 129–142, 1998.

27 Feedborne Mycotoxins in Aquaculture Feeds: Impact and Management of Aflatoxin, Fumonisin, and Moniliformin

Bruce B. Manning, Menghe H. Li, and Edwin H. Robinson

CONTENTS

27.1 INTRODUCTION

Feeds for aquaculture have evolved over the past decade to include reduced levels of animal protein products such as fish meal, meat and bone meal, and poultry byproduct meal. Levels of animal protein products have declined to less than 5% in commercial channel catfish feeds.[1] The factors promoting this trend in feed formulation include higher costs of animal protein products, conservation of depleted marine fisheries, and concerns about transmission of animal-derived diseases such as bovine spongiform encepthalopathy (BSE) to humans. Feeds for warmwater aquaculture fish can easily include higher levels of cereal grains and plant protein products without incurring deleterious effects on growth or health of the fish. Development of feeds with higher levels of plant-derived ingredients designated for use in coldwater aquaculture systems has proved to be more challenging, because coldwater fish such as salmonids do not grow as well on these feeds as those that contain higher proportions of animal products. Still, current research efforts are aimed toward genetically improving the feeding value of cereal grains and plant protein products for salmonids.[2] As the levels of plant-derived ingredients increase in aquaculture diets, so will the opportunity for mycotoxin contamination of these feeds. This chapter reviews the effects of feedborne mycotoxins on aquatic animals and the prevention and reduction of mycotoxins in aquaculture feeds.

27.2 AFLATOXIN

Early interest in the effects of mycotoxin contamination of animal diets occurred in 1960 with reports of high mortality in flocks of domesticated turkeys in the United Kingdom. The condition was initially referred to as turkey X disease and was later found to be caused by feeds that were prepared with peanut meal contaminated with aflatoxin.[3] About the same time, rainbow trout (*Onchorhyncus mykiss*) cultured in commercial and governmental facilities in the United States were experiencing high incidences of liver tumors. These lesions were determined to be hepatocellular carcinomas (HCCs) and were found to be caused by the inclusion of aflatoxin-contaminated cottonseed meal in pelletized dry trout diets.[4] Because rainbow trout appeared to be very sensitive to dietary aflatoxin, considerable research was conducted to evaluate the effects of aflatoxin exposure on trout. In some cases, mere exposure of developing trout eggs by immersion in solutions of aflatoxin B_1 (AFB_1) resulted in significant numbers of trout developing HCC many months later. Sinnhuber et al.[5] reported that immersion of rainbow trout embryos or fry in 0.5 ppm AFB_1 for 0.5 hour resulted in 30 to 40% incidence of HCC in fingerlings after 9 months. Feeding rainbow trout diets contaminated with only 0.4 ppb AFB_1 for 15 months produced HCC at a 14% rate.[6] Salmonid fish appear to exhibit species differences in their susceptibility to aflatoxin. Rainbow trout are generally the most susceptible, with coho salmon (*Onchorhyncus kisutch*) and brown trout (*Salmo trutta*) demonstrating the least susceptibility.[6] The differences in aflatoxin susceptibility appear to be attributed to the increased ability of rainbow trout to form the −8,9 epoxide of the furan ring of aflatoxin molecule compared to other fish species. The epoxide compound of AFB_1 is the proposed carcinogenic form that acts as a mitogen by forming adducts with the guanine base of DNA.[7]

Warmwater species of fish demonstrate reduced sensitivity to feedborne aflatoxin. Jantrarotai and Lovell[8] found that feeding a semipurified diet containing purified AFB_1 at 2154 ppb for 10 weeks to channel catfish (*Ictalurus punctatus*) had no effect on growth and feed conversion ratio (FCR), and no internal lesions were found. Feeding AFB_1 at 10,000 ppb in this study did result in significant reduction of catfish growth, hematocrit value, hemoglobin concentration, erythrocyte count, and leukocyte count. Also, histopathological examination revealed moderate lesions of the liver, hematopoietic areas of the anterior kidney, and the gastric glands. These lesions included evidence of necrosis of hepatocytes and the gastric glands with infiltrating macrophages. No neoplasms of the liver were observed.

Another laboratory study was conducted with channel catfish fed practical diets formulated with moldy corn naturally infected with *Aspergillus flavus* and containing a known high level of aflatoxin (550 ppb).[9] Four nutritionally complete diets containing 20 or 40% clean, nonmoldy corn and 20 or 40% moldy corn were fed twice daily to catfish maintained in flowing-water aquaria. Aflatoxin concentrations were 9 and 18 ppb for the two diets with clean corn and 110 and 220 ppb for the two diets containing moldy corn. Results after 12 weeks showed that normal, expected growth was attained with no significant differences among treatment groups for growth, FCR, survival, liver weight, or hematocrit. Gross examination indicated there were no liver lesions among the 50 fish examined from each treatment. A pond study was conducted with channel catfish fingerlings fed practical diets formulated with the same moldy corn used for the aquarium study. The study was conducted in 0.04-hectare earthen ponds, each stocked with approximately 600 fingerlings that were fed the experimental diets once daily for 130 days. The three diets contained 50% clean corn and 50% moldy corn, or 25% each of clean corn and moldy corn with mean aflatoxin contents of 1, 88, or 47 ppb, respectively. Fish growth was normal with no significant differences among treatments for growth, FCR, survival, hematocrit, or liver weights. Again, no liver lesions were found. These results indicate that channel catfish are not adversely affected by the consumption of naturally occurring aflatoxin either under controlled laboratory conditions or in a practical pond study during a normal production cycle.

The effect of aflatoxin-containing diets on another species of warmwater aquaculture fish has been examined. Nile tilapia (*Oreochromis nilotica*), initial weight 0.5 g/fish, were fed diets containing 0, 0.94, 1.88, 3.75, 7.52, 15.0, or 30.0 mg AFB_1/kg diet for 25 days followed by a 50-day feeding period of the control diet.[10] Reductions in growth and feed consumption were observed from the onset of the experiment for all treatment groups containing AFB_1, but significant reductions for these variables were observed only for treatments fed diets with 1.88 mg AFB_1/kg or greater. Survival was not affected by aflatoxin concentration. Cellular changes were observed in liver and posterior (excretory) kidney upon histological examination of fish fed diets with 1.88 mg AFB_1 or above. Lesions included fatty degeneration and focal necrosis of liver and shrunken glomeruli. Development of precancerous liver lesions was observed in tilapia fed with 7.52 mg AFB_1 per kg diet or above, but these did not advance to carcinomas. More recently, the effect of AFB_1 on growth and development of hepatic lesions in Nile tilapia was also evaluated by Nguyen et al.[11] In this study, juvenile tilapia with body weights of 2.7 g/fish were fed a semipurified diet with 0, 0.25, 2.5, 10, or 100 mg AFB_1 per kg of diet for 8 weeks. The mycotoxin was supplied from a culture material (CM) of *Aspergillus parasiticus* containing a known concentration of AFB_1. Results showed that levels of AFB_1 of 2.5 mg/kg of diet or above had deleterious effects on the growth, FCR, and hematocrit. Survival was significantly lower only for the highest level of AFB_1 inclusion; 60% of the fish died in this treatment. Histological examination of liver, spleen, heart, anterior kidney, stomach, and pyloric intestine revealed that tilapia fed diets with 0, 0.25, or 2.5 mg AFB_1 per kg had no lesions. Fish fed the diet of 10 or 100 mg AFB_1 per kg had lesions of the liver only. The lesions were characterized as cells with pleomorphic nuclei, accumulations of lipofuscin as a result of cellular breakdown, and evidence of necrotic hepatocytes. Results of the two experiments with tilapia are essentially in agreement in that they show that levels above the range of 0.25 to 0.94 mg AFB_1

per kg of diet resulted in lower weight gain. Cellular changes were observed in liver tissue for both experiments, but only at the higher levels of dietary aflatoxin. Based on the previously described results, tilapia appear to be more sensitive to dietary aflatoxin than channel catfish. Generally, the results of these experiments indicate that tilapia feeds should be monitored for aflatoxin content and that feeds should be maintained in adequate storage facilities to prevent proliferation of *Aspergillus* spp. and subsequent production of aflatoxin.

The sensitivity of cultured shrimp to aflatoxin has been evaluated. The sensitivity of Pacific white shrimp (*Penaeus vannamei*) to AFB_1 was tested by Ostrowski-Meissner[12] under controlled environmental conditions. Shrimp were fed diets containing purified AFB_1 at seven dietary levels: 0, 15, 20, 60, 300, 400, or 900 ppb for 8 weeks. Results show that growth and FCR of white shrimp fed diets containing 400 or 900 ppb were significantly poorer than shrimp fed diets with lower concentrations of AFB_1. Survival was not significantly different among the treatment groups. Histological examination showed that lesions were present in shrimp fed diets with all levels AFB_1, but severity was dose related. These lesions consisted of necrosis of the hepatopancreas and antennal gland. Another more recent experiment conducted by Boonyaratpalin et al.[13] confirmed the results of the previously described study. Black tiger shrimp (*Penaeus monodon*) were fed diets containing 0, 50, 100, 500, 1000, or 2500 ppb AFB_1 for 8 weeks. Weight gain and survival were significantly reduced for shrimp fed 2500 ppb AFB_1 when compared to control-fed shrimp or shrimp fed the lower dietary levels of AFB_1. Histological evaluation showed that shrimp fed diets containing 500, 1000, or 2500 ppb AFB_1 for 8 weeks had incidence of hepatopancreatic lesions of 40, 100, and 100%, respectively. The lesions consisted of inflammation, necrosis, and degeneration of the tubules with infiltration of intertubular tissue by hemocytes and fibroblastic cells.

The results of these studies with aflatoxin-contaminated feeds suggest that warm-water aquatic animals are less sensitive to aflatoxin than coldwater fish. Halver[4] ranked the susceptibility of fish to deleterious effects of exposure to aflatoxin, in descending order, as rainbow trout, coho salmon, and channel catfish. Based on the results of the studies presented above, one could insert Pacific white shrimp, Nile tilapia, and black tiger shrimp between coho salmon and channel catfish.

27.3 *FUSARIUM* MYCOTOXINS: FUMONISIN AND MONILIFORMIN

Fumonisin, the recently discovered mycotoxin of great interest,[14] has been studied extensively in animal systems because of its association with many animal diseases of previously unknown etiology. After its isolation and chemical characterization, its identification as the causative agent of equine leukoencephalomalacia (ELEM)[15] and porcine pulmonary edema (PPE)[16] was confirmed. Research continued with these species and others including poultry such as chickens[17] and turkeys.[18] Research to evaluate the effect of fumonisin on warmwater fish began at Auburn University, AL, by Lovell and associates in the early 1990s using channel catfish.

Interest in studying the toxic effects of fumonisin on channel catfish and other warmwater fish arises from the extensive use of corn, which may be contaminated with fumonisin, in the commercial feeds for these aquaculturally important fish.[1]

Initially, a method for laboratory production of culture material (CM) was developed using sterilized corn as the substrate and inoculation with conidia from a toxigenic isolate of *Fusarium verticillioides* (formerly *F. moniliforme*). The CM was incubated at ambient temperature for 5 weeks.[19] After drying and grinding the CM, its fumonisin B_1 (FB_1) and fumonisin B_2 (FB_2) contents were determined by a high-performance liquid chromatography (HPLC) method.[20] Fumonisin B_1 concentration was determined to be 1600 mg/kg, and FB_2 was present at 365 mg/kg. Practical-type, nutritionally complete diets were formulated to contain appropriate amounts of CM in place of control corn (FB_1 content of control corn was 0.7 mg/kg) to provide dietary levels of FB_1 of 0.3 (control), 20, 80, 320, and 720 mg/kg of diet.[19] These diets were tested on two sizes of channel catfish nominally referred to as year-1 fish (fry weight, 1.2 g/fish) and year-2 fish (fingerling weight, 31 g/fish). Results after feeding the diets to year-1 catfish for 10 weeks showed that fish fed diets containing 20 mg FB_1 per kg of diet or greater had significantly lower weight gains than the control fish. Year-1 catfish fed 80 mg FB_1 per kg of diet had significantly lower hematocrit and blood cell counts (red and white) than fish fed the control diet or the diet containing 20 mg FB_1 kg. Year-2 catfish fed FB_1 at 80 mg/kg of diet had significantly lower weight gains than fish fed the control diet or the diets with lower concentrations of FB_1. Hematocrit values and blood cell counts (red and white) of the fish fed diets containing 320 or 720 mg FB_1 per kg were lower than those of the control fish. These results clearly indicate a dose-related response to the consumption of diets containing FB_1 and that smaller catfish are more sensitive to this feedborne mycotoxin than larger catfish. Histological examination of tissues from various organs including liver, brain, kidney, and spleen revealed that fish fed diets with FB_1 concentrations of 20 mg/kg or greater had foci of swollen hepatocytes and hepatocytes with lipid-containing vacuoles. No histological lesions were detected in the other tissues.[19]

In another experiment conducted in the same laboratory, the effects of moniliformin supplied from *Fusarium proliferatum* CM was studied with channel catfish. Yildirim et al.[21] found that juvenile channel catfish (initial weight, 1.5 g/fish) fed diets containing 0, 20, 40, 60, or 120 mg moniliformin per kg of diet had significantly decreased growth for levels of 20 mg/kg or above. Additional treatments in the 10-week study demonstrated that feeding diets with 20 or 40 mg FB_1 per kg of diet resulted in significantly reduced weight gains. Likewise, feeding combinations of moniliformin:FB_1 of 40:20 mg/kg or 40:40 mg/kg produced weight gains that were significantly lower than fish fed the control, 20, or 40 mg moniliformin per kg diets. Significantly reduced weight gain was observed for fish fed the combination diet with 40:40 mg moniliformin:FB_1 per kg when compared to the response of fish fed diets with either 40 mg moniliformin per kg or 40 mg FB_1 per kg individually. The reduced weight gain of fish fed the 40:40 combination diet was equivalent to that of fish fed the diet containing 60 mg moniliformin per kg. Feed conversion ratios for all treatment groups fed the mycotoxins singly or in combination were significantly poorer than the FCR of the control-fed fish or the fish fed diets with 20 or

40 mg moniliformin per kg. Hematocrit values were significantly lower than control values for catfish fed diets containing 60 or 120 mg moniliformin per kg, 40 mg FB_1 per kg, or the 40:40 combination of moniliformin and FB_1.

In a separate study conducted in the same laboratory, similar responses were observed after feeding diets containing FB_1 or moniliformin to Nile tilapia for 8 weeks.[22] Tilapia with an initial weight of 2.7 g/fish had significantly lower weight gains when fed diets containing 70 mg moniliformin per kg of diet or 40 mg FB_1 per kg of diet. Tilapia fed the same dietary concentrations of these mycotoxins had significantly poorer feed conversion values than control fish or fish fed diets with lower concentrations of FB_1 or moniliformin.

Consumption of diets containing either FB_1 or moniliformin produces biochemical changes in animals. In the case of FB_1, it was found that feeding ponies diets contaminated with fumonisins altered the sphinganine to sphingosine ratio (SA:SO) of serum.[23] The mechanism of the alteration is competitive inhibition of the enzyme sphinganine N-acyltransferase by FB_1, thus blocking the conversion of sphinganine to dihydroceramide, the precursor to ceramide. Ceramide is an important component of the axon nerve cell covering sphingomyelin. The result is greatly increased levels of tissue sphinganine in comparison to sphingosine which elevates SA:SO. This response was demonstrated for catfish in the feeding study described by Lumlertdacha et al.[19] and reported by Goel et al.,[24] in the catfish study of Yildirim et al.,[21] and in the tilapia study of Nguyen et al.[22] Disruption of sphingolipid metabolism after exposure to FB_1 reduces biosynthesis of ceramide. Apart from their function as components of sphingomyelin, sphingolipids have important functions as second messengers in cell-to-cell signaling. Moniliformin, on the other hand, affects a major biochemical pathway by blocking conversion of pyruvate to acetyl-CoA, the starting intermediate of the tricarboxylic acid cycle. Moniliformin competitively inhibits the enzyme complex pyruvate dehydrogenase; thus, moniliformin reduces metabolic energy that would be derived, under normal circumstances, from glycolysis. Increased serum pyruvate levels were observed in the feeding studies with moniliformin that have been described for channel catfish[21] and for Nile tilapia.[22]

27.4 IMPACT OF FEEDBORNE MYCOTOXINS ON DISEASE RESISTANCE OF FISH

Disease resistance of fish can be impaired following consumption of feeds contaminated with mycotoxins. Lumlertdacha and Lovell[25] found that feeding 2-year-old channel catfish diets containing FB_1 from *Fusarium verticillioides* CM reduced survival after challenge with the catfish pathogenic bacteria *Edwardsiella ictaluri*. Catfish fed a diet containing 80 mg FB_1 per kg of diet, as described in Lumlertdacha et al.,[19] had significantly lower survival than catfish fed the control diet or a diet containing 20 mg FB_1 per kg. Fifteen days after initiation of the challenge, catfish fed the diet with 80 mg FB_1 per kg had a survival of 11% compared to 72% for the control fish and 57% for catfish fed 20 mg FB_1 per kg of diet. Antibody titer at 14 days after bacterial challenge was significantly higher for the control fish than catfish fed diets containing 20 or 80 mg FB_1 per kg, and antibody titer of catfish fed 20 mg FB_1 per kg was higher than the titer of catfish fed the 80 mg FB_1 per kg of diet.[25] Channel catfish fed diets containing the purified *Fusarium* mycotoxin, T-2 toxin, or ochratoxin A from *Aspergillus ochraceus* CM experienced significantly greater mortality after challenge with *Edwardsiella ictaluri* compared to catfish fed a diet with no mycotoxin.[26] Catfish fed diets with 1 or 2 mg T-2 toxin per kg had mortality rates of 84.1% and 99.3%, respectively, and 80.3% and 80.5% for diets fed with 2 or 4 mg ochratoxin A per kg. These mortality rates compare with 68.3% for catfish fed the control diet.

Other studies have shown that Black tiger shrimp (*Panaeus monodon*) had reduced numbers of hemocytes in response to consumption of a diet containing 2500 ppb of AFB_1.[13] Hemocytes in combination with fixed phagocytes form important elements of the shrimp immune system. Reduction in their numbers can impair disease resistance of shrimp. Indian major carp *Labeo rohita* had decreased disease resistance to challenges from *Edwardsiella tarda* or *Aeromonas hydrophila* after an intraperitoneal injection of AFB_1.[27]

A number of important mycotoxins appear to impair immune response by inhibiting protein synthesis by mechanisms that are somewhat different for each mycotoxin. Of the mycotoxins reviewed in this section, AFB_1 inhibits protein synthesis by forming mutagenic adducts between the $-8,9$ epoxide of AFB_1 and guanine of DNA or RNA.[28] Fumonisin B_1 inhibits the synthesis of proteins that function in immune response by preventing incorporation of valine in rat primary hepatocytes.[29] Ochratoxin A inhibits protein synthesis at a translational step by competitive inhibition of the enzyme phenylalanine–tRNA synthetase resulting in decreased levels of circulating antibodies.[30] Mycotoxins also adversely affect immune response by suppressing the activity of the cellular components of the immune system. Aflatoxin suppresses phagocytosis by macrophages, resulting in decreased uptake and presentation of antigen to B lymphocytes which decreases antibody production.[28] As previously stated, feeding diets containing 2500 ppb of AFB_1 to black tiger shrimp caused reductions in hemocytes.[13] T-2 toxin impairs immune system response, in part, by inhibiting protein synthesis. T-2 toxin also reduces the numbers of macrophages, which decreases antigen uptake and presentation to B lymphocytes with consequential reductions in antibody production.[28] Obviously, consumption of aquaculture feeds containing toxic concentrations of mycotoxins could seriously weaken the ability of fish to fight off naturally occurring pathogens.

27.5 REDUCTION OF MYCOTOXIN CONTAMINATION IN AQUACULTURE FEEDS

Various methods have been used to reduce mycotoxin contamination in animal feeds and feed ingredients. Among these are ammoniation of corn and cottonseed meal and roasting of corn. Reduction of aflatoxin content of these commodities can be achieved by ammoniation with gaseous ammonia (NH_3) or use of solutions of ammonium hydroxide under various conditions of pressure, temperature, and reaction time. Successful reduction of aflatoxin has been achieved with cottonseed meal contaminated with high concentrations of aflatoxin after ammoniation treatment.

Meal that initially contained 500 ppb aflatoxin was reduced to less than 5 ppb after ammoniation for 30 minutes at 48 psi and 118°C.[31] Ammoniated corn and cottonseed products have been used for ruminant, swine, and poultry feeds. Roasting aflatoxin-contaminated corn is an effective means to reduce aflatoxin levels. The aflatoxin content of corn was reduced 40 to 48% after heating at 145°C in a continuous roaster and 58 to 66% after heating to 165°C.[32] The appearance of products from these processes was dark colored. It is important to ensure that any detoxification process that is applied to aflatoxin-contaminated feed ingredients does not degrade the nutritional value of the ingredient.

Buser and Abbas[33] found that extrusion of cottonseed contaminated with aflatoxin reduced the concentration of aflatoxin by 50% without diminishing the nutritional value of the cottonseed for ruminants. Extrusion is commonly used to manufacture commercial aquaculture feeds, because careful adjustment of the extrusion processing equipment can produce pellets that float when applied to the surface of pond water. The floating characteristic allows for adjustment of the amount of feed applied to any pond based on feeding activity of the fish. Other adjustments of the same equipment allow for production of sinking pellets that are preferred for other aquaculture species such as trout and shrimp. Production of experimental catfish feeds containing moldy corn contaminated with aflatoxin for the feeding study previously described[9] showed that the aflatoxin levels could be reduced by over 60% after completing the cooker-extrusion and heated drying processes.[9] Catfish fed these feeds during the course of the study grew at normal rates, indicating that the feed caused no adverse nutritional degradation. Application of the cooker–extrusion process to reduce the levels of mycotoxins other than aflatoxin may be ineffective. Fumonisin and trichothecene mycotoxins appear to tolerate high-temperature processing to remain intact and thus toxic.

Hydrated sodium calcium aluminosilicate (HSCAS) adsorbent clays have been demonstrated to bind aflatoxin in contaminated feeds thereby reducing its bioavailability. It has been suggested that these clay products and other binding agents may also sequester other mycotoxins, but this is apparently not the case. Ledoux and Rottinghaus[34] found that binding agents tested with poultry did not provide protection against FB_1, moniliformin, ochratoxin A, or deoxynivalenol. It is generally agreed that laboratory *in vitro* testing does not always predict the ability of the binding agent to sequester mycotoxins under practical conditions. While the U.S. Food and Drug Administration permits use of HSCAS at up to 2% in animal feeds under the generally regarded as safe (GRAS) category, it is recommended that this binding agent and others be tested on the intended animal species for safety and efficacy.[35]

27.6 PREVENTION OF MYCOTOXIN CONTAMINATION IN AQUACULTURE FEEDS

Prevention of mycotoxin contamination in aquaculture feeds is important to maintaining the health and productivity of cultured fish. The first step in prevention is to control mycotoxin contamination of feed ingredients. Examination of feed ingredients before they are unloaded from rail cars or grain-hauling trucks is essential. Grains can be examined for appearance such as evidence of water damage or the presence of mold. Grains that are suspect based on appearance can be subjected to rapid assays for mycotoxins using commercially available enzyme-linked immunosorbent assay (ELISA) kits. Shipments of ingredients that fail to meet specifications should be rejected before unloading. During manufacture of aquaculture feeds, it is critical that processed feed pellets are properly cooled and dried to a moisture content of 11 to 12% or less to prevent significant mold growth. In some cases, mold inhibitors such as propionic acid are sprayed-on cooled pellets to retard the growth of fungal organisms. Because aquaculture is conducted in wet and in many cases hot, humid environments, caution must be taken to provide storage conditions for feeds that exclude moisture and water. Use of moldy feed should be considered very risky, especially in light of the potential damage that can be incurred to a valuable crop of fish.

27.7 CONCLUSIONS

Information regarding the effects of feedborne mycotoxins on the performance and health of cultured fish is important because of the increasing use of plant-derived ingredients in commercial aquaculture feeds. Researchers are currently attempting to develop new strains of cereal grains and plant protein sources from oil seeds that are nutritionally better suited for use in aquaculture feeds. Use of these new feed ingredients in addition to the plant-derived ingredients already in use will increase the risk of mycotoxin contamination of aquaculture feeds. Species differences in response to the consumption of mycotoxin contaminated feeds can be interpreted based on the results of the studies presented in this section. Generally, it appears that coldwater fish are more sensitive to the toxic effects of mycotoxins than warmwater fish. Fish produced in aquaculture systems have become an increasingly important source of food for people over the past three decades. This trend should continue as new, stronger economies emerge in developing counties and there is continued growth in established economies with increasing demand for high quality protein.

REFERENCES

1. Robinson, E.H., Li, M.H., and Manning, B.B., Evolving catfish diets, *Feed Manage.*, 54(1), 18–23, 2003.
2. Overturf, K., Cereal grains for use in aquaculture feeds, in *Proc. Fish Feed and Nutrition Workshop*, University of California, Davis, June 22–25, 2003.
3. Blount, W.P., Turkey "X" disease, *J. Br. Turkey Fed.*, 9(2), 52, 55–58, 1961.
4. Halver, J.E., Aflatoxicosis and trout hepatoma, in *Aflatoxin: Scientific Background, Control, and Implications*, Goldblatt, L.A., Ed., Academic Press, New York, 1969, pp. 265–306.
5. Sinnhuber, R.O., Hendricks, J.D., Wales, J.H., and Putman, G.B., Neoplasms in rainbow trout, a sensitive animal model for environmental carcinogenesis, *Ann. N.Y. Acad. Sci.*, 298, 389–408, 1977.

6. Lee, D.J., Wales J.H., Ayres, J.L., and Sinnhuber, R.O., Synergism between cyclopropenoid fatty acids and chemical carcinogens in rainbow trout (*Salmo gairdneri*), *Cancer Res.*, 28, 2312–2318, 1968.

7. Coulombe, R.A., Biological action of mycotoxins, *J. Dairy Sci.*, 76, 880–891, 1993.

8. Jantrarotai, W. and Lovell, R.T., Subchronic toxicity of dietary aflatoxin B$_1$ to channel catfish, *J. Aquat. Animal Health*, 2, 248–254, 1990.

9. Manning, B.B., Li, M.H., and Robinson, E.H., Aflatoxins from moldy corn cause no reductions in channel catfish *Ictalurus punctatus* performance, *J. World Aquaculture Soc.*, 36, 59–67, 2005..

10. Chavez-Sanchez, M.C., Martinez, C.A., and Osorio Moreno, I., Pathological effects of feeding young *Oreochromis niloticus* diets supplemented with different levels of aflatoxin B$_1$, *Aquaculture*, 127, 49–60, 1994.

11. Nguyen, A.T., Grizzle, J.M., Lovell, R.T., Manning, B.B., and Rottinghaus, G.E., Growth and hepatic lesions of Nile tilapia (*Oreochromis niloticus*) fed diets containing aflatoxin B$_1$, *Aquaculture*, 212, 311–319, 2002.

12. Ostrowski-Meissner, H.T., B.R. Leamaster, B.R., Duerr, E.O., and Walsh, W.A., Sensitivity of the Pacific white shrimp, *Panaeus vannamei,* to aflatoxin B$_1$, *Aquaculture*, 131, 155–164, 1995.

13. Boonyaratpalin, M., Supamattaya, K., Verakunpiriya, V., and Suprasert, D., Effects of aflatoxin B$_1$ on growth performance, blood components, immune function and histopathological changes in black tiger shrimp (*Panaeus monodon* Fabricius), *Aquaculture Res.*, 32(Suppl. 1), 388–398, 2001.

14. Gelderblom, W.C.A., Jaskiewicz, K., Marasas, W.F.O., Thiel, P.G., Horak, R.M., Vleggar, R., and Kriek, N.P.J., Fumonisins: novel mycotoxins with cancer promoting activity produced by *Fusarium moniliforme*, *Appl. Environ. Microbiol.*, 54, 1806–1811, 1988.

15. Wilson, T.M., Ross, P.F., Owens, D.L., Rice, L.G., Green, S.A., Jenkins, S.J., and Nelson, H.A., Experimental reproduction of ELEM, *Mycopathologia*, 117, 115–120, 1992.

16. Harrison, L.R., Colvin, B.M., Greene, J.T., Newman, L.E., and Cole, Jr., R.J., Pulmonary edema and hydrothorax in swine produced by fumonisin B$_1$, a toxic metabolite of *Fusarium moniliforme*, *J. Vet. Diagn. Invest.*, 2, 217–221, 1990.

17. Weibking, T.S., Ledoux, D.R., Bermudez, A.J., Turk, J.R. Rottinghaus, G.E., Wang, E. and Merrill, Jr., A.H., Effects of feeding *Fusarium moniliforme* culture material, containing known levels of fumonisin B$_1$, on the young broiler chick, *Poultry Sci.*, 72, 456–466, 1993.

18. Weibking, T.S., Ledoux, D.R., Brown, T.P., and Rottinghaus, G.E., Fumonisin toxicity in turkey poults, *J. Vet. Diagn. Invest.*, 5, 75–83, 1993.

19. Lumlertdacha, S., Lovell, R.T., Shelby, R.A., Lenz, S.D., and Kemppainen, B.W., Growth, hematology, and histopathology of channel catfish, *Ictalurus punctatus*, fed toxins from *Fusarium moniliforme*, *Aquaculture*, 130, 201–218, 1995.

20. Shephard, G.S., Sydenham, E.W., Thiel, P.G., and Gelderblom, W.C.A., Quantitative determination of fumonisin B$_1$ and B$_2$ by high performance liquid chromatography with fluorescence detection, *J. Liquid Chromatogr.*, 13, 2077–2087, 1992.

21. Yildirim, M., Manning, B., Lovell, R.T., Grizzle, J.M., and Rottinghaus, G.E., Toxicity of moniliformin and fumonisin B$_1$ fed singly and in combination in diets for channel catfish, *J. World Aquaculture Soc.*, 31, 599–608, 2000.

22. Nguyen, A.T., Manning, B.B., Lovell, R.T., and Rottinghaus, G.E., Responses of Nile tilapia (*Oreochromis niloticus*) fed diets containing different concentrations of moniliformin or fumonisin B$_1$, *Aquaculture*, 217, 515–528, 2003.

23. Wang, E., Ross, P.F., Wilson, T.M., Riley, R.T. and Merrill, Jr., A.H. Increases in serum sphingosine and sphinganine and decreases in complex sphingolipids in ponies given feed containing fumonisins, mycotoxins produced by *Fusarium moniliforme*, *J. Nutr.*, 122, 1706–1716, 1992.

24. Goel, S., Lenz, S.D., Lumlertdacha, S., Lovell, R.T., Shelby, R.A., Li, M., Riley, R.T., and Kemppainen, B.W., Sphingolipid levels in catfish consuming *Fusarium moniliforme* corn culture material containing fumonisin, *Aquat. Toxicol.*, 30, 285–294, 1994.

25. Lumlertdacha, S. and Lovell, R.T., Fumonisin-contaminated dietary corn reduced survival and antibody production by channel catfish challenged with *Edwardsiella ictaluri*, *J. Aquat. Animal Health*, 7, 1–8, 1995.

26. Manning, B.B., Terhune, J.S., Li, M.H., Robinson, E.H., Wise, D.J., and Rottinghaus, G.E., Exposure to feedborne mycrotoxins T-2 toxin or ochratoxin A causes increased mortality of channel catfish *Ictalurus punctatus* challenged with *Edwardsiella ictaluri*, *J. Aquat. Animal Health*, 17, 147–152, 2005.

27. Sahoo, P.K. and Mukherjee, S.C., Influence of high dietary α-tocopherol intakes on specific immune response, nonspecific resistance factors and disease resistance of healthy and aflatoxin B$_1$-induced immunocompromised Indian major carp, *Labeo rohita* (Hamilton), *Aquaculture Nutr.*, 8, 159–167, 2002.

28. Pier, A.C., The influence of mycotoxins on the immune system., in *Mycotoxins in Animal Foods*, Smith, J.E., and Henderson, R.S., Eds., CRC Press, Boca Raton, FL, 1991, pp. 489–497.

29. Norred, W.P., Wang, E., Yoo, H., Riley, R.T. and Merrill, Jr., A.H., *In vitro* toxicology of fumonisins and the mechanistic implications, *Mycopathologia*, 177, 73–78, 1992.

30. Kuiper-Goodman, T. and Scott, P.M., Risk assessment of the mycotoxin ochratoxin A, *Biomed. Environ. Sci.*, 2, 179–248, 1989.

31. Gardner, Jr., H.K., Koltun, S.P., Dollear, F.G., and Rayner, E.T., Inactivation of aflatoxins in peanut and cottonseed meals by ammoniation, *J. AOCS*, 48, 70–73, 1971.

32. Conway, H.F., Anderson, R.A., and Bagley, E.B., Detoxification of aflatoxin-contaminated corn by roasting, *Cereal Chem.*, 55, 115–117, 1978.

33. Buser, M.D. and Abbas, H.K., Mechanically processing cottonseed to reduce gossypol and aflatoxin levels, *J. Toxicol. Toxin Rev.*, 20(3,4), 179–208, 2001.

34. Ledoux, D.R. and Rottinghaus, G.E., *In vitro* and *in vivo* testing of adsorbents for detoxifying mycotoxins in contaminated feedstuffs, in *Biotechnology in the Feed Industry*, Proc. Alltech's Fifteenth Annual Symposium, Lyons, T.P. and Jacques, K.A., Eds., Nottingham University Press, Nottingham, 1999, pp. 369–379.

35. CAST, *Mycotoxins: Risks in Plant, Animal, and Human Systems*, Report No. 139, Council for Agricultural Science and Technology, Ames, IA, 2003.

Index